RABIES IN BATS

Natural History and Public Health Implications

Danny A. Brass, D.V.M.

Livia Press
Ridgefield, Connecticut

Rabies in Bats
Natural History and Public Health Implications

Livia Press
Ridgefield, Connecticut

ISBN 0-9637045-1-6
Library of Congress Catalogue Card Number 93-78291

First Edition, First Printing 1994
Manufactured in the United States of America

For my parents, who have enthusiastically encouraged my many interests and, in teaching me to regard all living creatures with respect, instilled in me a sense of value in all creation; truly, a gift beyond price.

FOREWORD

Rabies in bats fascinates the reader and the viewer, bringing up images of Dracula, vampires, and the whole aura of rabies infection in man and beast. One can just imagine the surprise of the Spanish troops when they rode out into the Mexican and South American countryside in the early 1500's and were bitten by beasts that latched onto their horses and even themselves, and caused deaths from what must have been rabies. Outbreaks of rabies in cattle were also reported. Vampire rabies continues to cause the death of hundreds of thousands of cattle in the Americas every year, from northern Mexico to northern Argentina. In one recent and massive outbreak in southern Bolivia, for instance (in 1954 and 1955), 260,000 cattle died.

Bat rabies in the United States is totally different. Only insectivorous bats, not vampire bats, are found in the United States. From the first few cases reported in 1953, the number has now risen to 500 to 600 every year, reported from the majority of the states. Since that first year, there have also been 18 human deaths from exposure to rabid bats. There is also evidence that rabid insectivorous bats sporadically infect terrestrial animals, mostly foxes and cats, but also occasional horses and cows. Obviously, the rabies researcher delves into this movement of the disease, attempting to establish infection rates in bats and the animals they bite, in order to better understand the disease and its control. The mammalogist, on the other hand, seeks to understand the movement of this intriguing, nocturnal flying mammal, its classification, hibernation, migration, and behavior in and out of caves. Then there is the caver, who sometimes climbs and clambers around caves with bats.

Dr. Danny Brass has gathered together a massive amount of information on rabies in bats and has put it into a tome with all the relevant bits and pieces, but it is nevertheless a work that is very well written and exciting to read. Bats are wonderful creatures and enrich our animal world; those of us who have worked with them admire their versatility, habits, and prowess. We need to do as much as possible to preserve this rich order of mammals, the Chiroptera, but also should realize that they are occasionally infected with rabies, a disease to be respected. Those who may come into contact with bats, including cavers, should be vaccinated against rabies.

This book should be read by all those people who work with bats and those who work with rabies. It is an exhaustive and admirable account of the disease in those flying mammals.

George M. Baer, D.V.M., M.P.H.
Chief, Rabies Laboratory (1966-1991)
Centers for Disease Control
Atlanta, Georgia

PREFACE

The pioneering age of rabies research was followed by one of tremendous expansion. With the advent of ever more sophisticated technologies, impressive progress has been made in our ability to probe the intricacies of the rabies virus. In the search for a broader understanding of the relationship between urban and sylvatic rabies cycles, a variety of immunological differences among the many variants of rabies and rabies-related viruses have become targets of modern investigation. Use of monoclonal antibodies has become an important yardstick for characterizing variants of rabies virus. What began in a few prestigious research centers, has gradually became a more widely available tool at many institutions and laboratories. The unique achievements made possible by the application of monoclonal antibody technology have revolutionized our understanding of rabies epidemiology.

The yield from monoclonal analyses has been substantial, but even more impressive genetic technologies are being developed to study the relationships between different viral variants, providing new insight into their evolutionary history and global distribution. Ongoing analysis continues to further our understanding of the dynamic nature of rabies epidemiology.

Our perceptions of the role played by bats in rabies epidemiology have changed vastly during the course of the last half century. From the initial discovery of rabies in North American bats in 1953 through the latest serologic and genetic analyses of bat-rabies isolates, scientific thought on the subject has evolved in dramatic fashion. As such, this book has been written from an historical perspective, tracing the evolution of thought and knowledge on bat rabies through many decades. Aspects of bat physiology and natural history have been included where appropriate to the discussion of rabies epidemiology. This is particularly true for several discussions on vampire bats, since their characteristic hunting behavior and dependence on nightly meals of blood is so intimately related to their role as disease vectors.

In tracing our understanding of the role of bats in rabies epidemiology, this text represents a complete and up-to-date reference, containing the very latest information available on the subject. However, it is, by no means, meant to be the final word on rabies in bats. Rabies epidemiology remains a dynamic field, steadily changing with the expanding fabric of our technology. Rather, the book is meant to provide the interested reader with a comprehensive review of this disease in bats, encompassing discussions of rabies in the hematophagous vampire bats of Latin America, the frugivorous bats of Africa, and the insectivorous bats of North America, Africa, Europe, and Asia. Discussion focuses on the prevalence and distribution of rabies in bats, mechanisms whereby disease is maintained within bat populations, the relationship of bat rabies to rabies in other animals (both wild and domestic), and the public-health significance of this disease in bat populations.

Regrettably, many of these issues have been grossly magnified and carried far out of proper perspective by sensation-seeking reporting, designed to prey on deep-rooted cultural phobias. The irresponsible reporting that characterizes tabloid journalism has continued to fuel public fear of bats, helping to forge an image of these animals not at all consistent with scientific fact. It is, therefore, important to acknowledge the ecological importance of bats worldwide and to recognize the significance that ongoing conservation efforts have played in helping to safeguard their populations. In many countries, bats remain endangered species. Not only are they a fascinating group of animals, but bats do indeed play integral roles in the complex web of ecology worldwide.

In attempting to distill the available literature on rabies in bats, development of this manuscript has been both challenging and informative, as well as laborious. Compared to other fields of scientific endeavor, the published studies on bat rabies are somewhat limited. Thus, while the writing of this book certainly constituted a Herculean effort, it was not an impossible one. It is hoped that it will be of value to physicians, veterinarians, and public-health authorities, as well as virologists, zoologists, and naturalists. However, it is not intended to be beyond the grasp of lay persons who might have an interest in bats. In this regard, the biomedical background needed to understand the text is minimal and relatively few demands are placed on prerequisite knowledge. Furthermore, I have tried as much as possible to avoid a significant language barrier to those readers without a medical or biological background, while not sacrificing scientific accuracy.

Bridging the gap between those with and without such backgrounds has proven to be a formidable task. Several explanatory notes have been included to help readers unfamiliar with certain biological concepts required for appreciation of a particular discussion. Introductory chapters on general aspects of rabies as well as clinical manifestations in humans and selected animals serve to highlight the nature of this disease and provide a framework, if needed, for appreciation of the full spectrum of clinical rabies.

With all due respect for basic research into the epidemiologic aspects of urban and sylvatic rabies cycles, these investigations would be shallow and barren without application of the knowledge gained to methods of disease control. In this regard, rabies researchers have not confined themselves to epidemiological studies alone. New and improved treatment protocols for persons exposed to rabies are continually being evaluated. Tremendous gains are also being made in attempts to eradicate the disease on a global level. Significant advances made in both laboratory studies and field trials have paved the way for use of revolutionary new recombinant oral rabies vaccines. Their widespread application, in attempts to immunize wildlife, will reflect the next major step in the study of rabies and pursuit of a goal of worldwide control or eradication of the disease.

Danny A. Brass

ACKNOWLEDGMENTS

I would like to express my deepest appreciation to the several scientists who critically reviewed the manuscript, in whole or in part at various stages in its development, offering valuable suggestions and giving generously of their time:

I am particularly indebted to Dr. George Beran, Professor of Veterinary Epidemiology and Public Health, Department of Veterinary Microbiology and Preventive Medicine, College of Veterinary Medicine, Iowa State University. Dr. Beran is also a consultant to the World Health Organization Expert Committee on Rabies. Dr. Beran's preeminence in teaching/research and dedication to excellence provided the initial inspiration to undertake this project. His expertise in rabies epidemiology and willingness to communicate his excitement in this field to others is gratefully acknowledged.

Dr. Denny Constantine, Public Health Veterinarian, California Department of Health Services, widely recognized as one of the world's foremost authorities on the relationship between bats and public health.

Dr. George Baer, former Chief of the Rabies Laboratory, Centers for Disease Control, advisor to the World Health Organization Expert Committee on Rabies, and Director of the World Health Organization's Collaborating Center for Reference and Research on Rabies. Dr. Baer is world renowned for his research in the field of rabies epidemiology. I am also very grateful to Dr. Baer for writing a foreword to the book.

Dr. Charles Rupprecht, Associate Professor, Department of Microbiology and Immunology, Center for Neurovirology, Thomas Jefferson University, Jefferson Medical College. Dr. Rupprecht's extensive research has helped pave the way for development of programs to control wildlife rabies in the United States. He is currently Chief of the Rabies Laboratory, Centers for Disease Control.

Mr. Charles Trimarchi, Director of the Rabies Laboratory, New York State Department of Health, and Dr. Stephen Frantz, Vertebrate Vector Specialist, Virology Laboratory, New York State Department of Health, whose efforts to institute comprehensive and ecologically sound public-health programs to help manage bat-related problems should serve as an example for public-health departments nationwide.

Ms. Jean Smith, Research Microbiologist, Rabies Laboratory, Centers for Disease Control, whose substantial research efforts have helped to define the relationship between terrestrial and nonterrestrial rabies. I am also grateful to Jean for many valuable discussions regarding her work with monoclonal antibody and genetic analyses of viral isolates.

Dr. Arthur King, Rabies Research Leader, Central Veterinary Laboratory, United Kingdom. Dr. King's extensive studies of viral isolates have helped to define the nature of rabies epidemiology in much of Africa and Europe. Dr. Monique Lafon, Rabies Unit, Pasteur Institute, Paris, France, whose work has been instrumental in clarifying the nature and extent of bat rabies in Europe and in helping to develop improved post-exposure treatment protocols for persons exposed to bat rabies of European origin.

Dr. Carlos Arellano-Sota, Regional Officer on Animal Production and Health, Food and Agriculture Organization of the United Nations, Santiago, Chile, and Dr. G. Clay Mitchell, Denver Wildlife Research Center, U. S. Department of Agriculture, who have both played leading roles in development of our understanding of rabies in vampire bats and methods of control. Mr. Timothy J. McCarthy, Section of Mammals, Carnegie Museum of Natural History. Mr. McCarthy was in charge of the Vampire Bat Education and Control Programme in Belize from 1975 to 1978 and is currently an advisor to the Belize Ministry of Agriculture and Fisheries on matters of vampire-bat control. Dr. Bert Prins, Animal Diseases Research Institute, Alberta, who has played a considerable role in defining the epidemiology of rabies in Canada.

The staff of the computer facility of the Iowa State University College of Veterinary Medicine has been of enormous help in the preparation of this manuscript. Grateful appreciation is extended to Mr. Craig McClanahan, Mr. Steve Pendry, Dr. Roger Hogle, Mr. Bruce Eveland, and Mr. Art Anderson. Thanks also to Dr. Nathan M. Appel, Center for Drug Evaluation and Research, Food and Drug Administration; Dr. Etsuro Uemura, Department of Anatomy, College of Veterinary Medicine, Iowa State University; Dr. David Hopper, Diagnostic Laboratory, College of Veterinary Medicine, Iowa State University; Dr. Scott B. Plummer, Veterinary Neurological Center, Phoenix, Arizona; and the New York State College of Veterinary Medicine, Cornell University for generous use of their computer facilities. I am also grateful for computer facilities provided by MaxGraphics Printing, Venice, Florida, courtesy of Mr. Steven R. Moore.

Grateful acknowledgment is extended to Mr. Joseph Senulis, Department of Psychology, University of Wisconsin for reading an earlier draft of the manuscript in its entirety and providing valuable editorial comment; to Mr. David McClurg, Chairman, Special Publications Committee, National Speleological Society for very helpful discussion and advice; and to Mr. Scott E. Tensen, a graduate of the College of Design, Iowa State University, for many of the fine pen-and-ink illustrations that appear in the text.

My most sincere gratitude is extended to Dr. Robert Carithers, teacher and friend, Department of Veterinary Clinical Sciences, College of Veterinary Medicine, Iowa State University, and to H. V. Grey, former publications editor, Cave Diving Section of the National Speleological Society, who have both been a source of constant encouragement.

I am especially indebted to my close friends at the Iowa State University College of Veterinary Medicine, who have added immeasurably to the quality of my life in Iowa, and to the students, interns, residents, faculty, and staff of both the College of Veterinary Medicine, Iowa State University, and the New York State College of Veterinary Medicine, Cornell University, who have been extraordinarily understanding of my idiosyncracies during the completion of this manuscript.

Finally, it is my pleasure to extend heartfelt thanks to the many persons who have helped foster my interest in caves, caving, and life underground. Special thanks to members of the caving section of the Rutgers University Outdoors Club. Kevin Psarianos, Rich Joswick, Joe Senulis, Chuck Chapman, and Drs. Margaret Kruse and Fred Miller made up the nuclear group of my early (dry) caving experiences. In introducing me to the intricacies of technical caving, they opened my eyes to a fascinating new horizon deep below ground. To glimpse the pristine beauty of these darkened corridors is to be mesmerized and captivated by worlds frozen in time. I am particularly indebted to Kevin, Rich, and Peggy—companions and guides on my first adventure underground.

This work was supported, in part, by a grant from the National Speleological Society.

Danny A. Brass

TABLE OF CONTENTS

SECTION I
Rabies: Disease and Nature of the Infective Process

1. General Nature of the Disease . . . 3
- Global Distribution . . . 3
- The Causative Agent . . . 4
- Routes of Transmission . . . 6
- Centripetal Migration of Virus . . . 8
- Centrifugal Migration of Virus . . . 8
- Continuity of Viral Transmission . . . 10

2. Rabies in Terrestrial Animals . . . 13
- Animal Reservoirs of Virus . . . 13
- Skunks . . . 13
- Raccoons . . . 14
- Foxes . . . 17
- Dogs . . . 19
- Cats . . . 21

3. Rabies in Humans . . . 25
- Prevalence of Human Rabies in the United States . . . 25
- Major Sources of Human Exposure to Virus . . . 26
- Pre-Exposure Rabies Prophylaxis . . . 26
- Post-Exposure Rabies Prophylaxis . . . 28
- Clinical Manifestations . . . 34
- Documented Cases of Humans Surviving Rabies . . . 35

SECTION II
Vampire Bats and Rabies in Latin America

4. Vampire Bats and Bovine Paralytic Rabies . . . 41
- Vampire Bats and Livestock Production . . . 41
- Brazil . . . 43
- Trinidad . . . 44
- Mexico . . . 47

5. Rabies and the Bats of Latin America . . . 51
- Alleged Correlations Between Behavior and Disease . . . 51
- Early Studies . . . 51

6. Vampire Bats of the American Tropics . . . 57
- Myth, Superstition, and Medical Oddities . . . 57
- General Description . . . 58
- Vampire Roosts . . . 59
- Distribution and Energetics of the Vampire Bat . . . 60
- Fossil Remains of Vampire Bats in the Americas . . . 62
- Hunting and Feeding Characteristics . . . 62
- Host Selection . . . 62
- Detection and Tracking of Hosts . . . 65
- Distribution of Bites on Animal Hosts . . . 67
- The Vampire-Bat Bite . . . 69
- The Feeding Process . . . 72
- Anticoagulation and Fibrinolysis . . . 73
- Flight after Feeding . . . 75
- Roosts and Digestion . . . 76
- Metabolic Waste and Water Consumption . . . 76

7. Clinical Manifestations of Rabies in the Vampire Bat . . . 83
- Early Descriptions of Clinical Disease . . . 83
- Asymptomatic Salivary Carrier State . . . 83

8. Epizootiology of Vampire-Bat Rabies . . . 85
- Economic Impact of Bovine Paralytic Rabies . . . 85
- Social Grooming . . . 88
- Reciprocal Food Sharing . . . 90
- Intraspecific Aggression Among Vampire Bats . . . 93
- Interactions Among Vampires at Feeding Sites . . . 93
- Propagation of the Vampire Rabies Epizootic . . . 94
- Seasonal Influences on the Incidence of Bovine Paralytic Rabies . . . 97

9. Human Exposure to Rabies of Vampire-Bat Origin . . . 101
- Reports of Vampire-Inflicted Human Rabies in Latin America . . . 101
- Availability of Animal Food Sources and Human Depredation by Vampire Bats . . . 105
- Risks Associated with Handling and Ingestion of Infected Cattle . . . 107
- Risk Assessment and the Implementation of Public-Health Programs . . . 108

10. Methods in the Control of Vampire-Bat Rabies . . . 111
- Prevention of Bat Bites . . . 111
- Prophylactic Vaccination of Livestock . . . 112
- Vampire Population Control . . . 113
- Economic Significance of Vampire Population Control . . . 120
- Efficacy of Available Control Methods . . . 121
- Future Trends in Vampire Control . . . 123
- Impact of Random Bat Destruction . . . 123

SECTION III
Insectivorous Bats and Rabies in North America

11. Prevalence and Distribution of Rabies in Insectivorous Bats . . . 131
Compartmentalization of Rabies Virus . . . 131
Relationship Between Terrestrial and Nonterrestrial Rabies . . . 132
Early Reports of Rabies in Bats . . . 133
Distribution of Bat Rabies in the United States . . . 137
Inherent Difficulties in Studying Wildlife Disease . . . 139
Prevalence of Rabies in Colonial versus Solitary Species . . . 142
Biased Perspectives . . . 147
Species-Associated Geographic Distribution of Bat Rabies . . . 147

12. Clinical Manifestations of Rabies in Insectivorous Bats . . . 151
Incubation Period . . . 151
Lethal versus Nonlethal Cycles of Infection . . . 151
Disorientation and Abnormalities of Flight . . . 151
Furious versus Paralytic Disease and Provoked versus Unprovoked Attacks . . . 152
Salivary Carrier State and the Rio Bravo Virus . . . 154
The Role of Hibernation in Rabies Pathogenesis . . . 155
Significance of Naturally Occurring Rabies-Neutralizing Antibodies . . . 157

13. Maintenance of Enzootic Rabies in Insectivorous Bats . . . 163
Potential Sources of Virus . . . 163
Horizontal Transmission of Virus Among Insectivorous Bats . . . 166
Vertical Transmission of Virus Among Insectivorous Bats . . . 167

14. Airborne Transmission of Rabies Virus . . . 169
Human Case Studies . . . 169
Bat Populations of Frio Cave . . . 169
Experimental Studies Within Frio Cave . . . 170
Evidence in Support of Inhalation Exposure . . . 171
Inhalation Exposure in Frio Cave? . . . 173

15. Viral Transmission Studies and Retrospective Analyses . . . 177
Are Insectivorous Bats a Special Link in the Spread of Disease? . . . 177
Limitations of Inoculation and Forced-Bite Studies . . . 179
Experimental Parenteral Transmission of Rabies Virus . . . 179
Experimental Transmission of Rabies Virus by Forced Biting . . . 180
Experimental Transmission of Rabies Virus by Ingestion . . . 180
Retrospective Analyses: Associations on a Local Level . . . 181
Retrospective Analyses: Associations on a National Level . . . 183
Insectivorous Bats and Sylvatic Rabies Cycles . . . 184

16. Monoclonal Antibody Characterization of Bat-Rabies Isolates . . . 189
Value in Epidemiologic Investigation . . . 189
Compartmentalization of Rabies Variants . . . 189
Antigenic Characterization of Bat-Rabies Isolates . . . 190
Transmission of Nonterrestrial Virus to Terrestrial Species . . . 193
Insectivorous Bats and Sylvatic Rabies Cycles . . . 200
Genetic Analysis of Rabies Isolates . . . 203

17. Insectivorous Bats and Rabies in Canada . . . 207
Reservoirs of Disease . . . 207
Epidemiology and Epizootiology . . . 207
Antigenic Characterization of Rabies Isolates from Canadian Bats . . . 209
British Columbia . . . 212
Alberta . . . 212
Early Reports of Human Exposure . . . 213
Human Rabies of Bat Origin in Canada . . . 214

18. Human Exposure to Rabies Virus of Insectivorous-Bat Origin . . . 217
Limitations in the Collection of Human Exposure Data . . . 217
Limited Survey Information . . . 218
Common Circumstances of Human Exposure . . . 219
Bat/Human Exposure Histories . . . 219

19. Human Rabies of Insectivorous-Bat Origin . . . 229
Recognizing the Source of Exposure . . . 229
Clinical Case Histories: The United States . . . 229
Clinical Case Histories: Canada . . . 237
Clinical Case Histories: Africa, Europe, and Asia . . . 238
Public-Health Implications of Rabies in Insectivorous Bats . . . 240

20. Management of Unwanted Bats in the Home . . . 243
General Considerations . . . 243
Possible Health Hazards Associated with Bats in the Home . . . 244
Health Concerns Related to the Chemical Extermination of Bats . . . 245
Batproofing Homes as an Effective Means of Controlling House Bats . . . 247

21. Control of Rabies in Wild Bat Populations . . . 251
Programs for Oral Vaccination of Wildlife . . . 251
Vaccinia Virus as a Recombinant Vaccine . . . 252
Field Trials of Recombinant Vaccine Products . . . 254
Possibility of Immunizing Bats Against Rabies . . . 255

SECTION IV
Rabies Infection in Old World Bats

22. Rabies and the Rabies-Related Viruses of Africa 263
The Lyssavirus Genus 263
Serotype 1 265
Serotype 2 265
Serotype 3 266
Serotype 4 270
Serotype 5 270

23. Rabies-Related Viruses From Bats in Europe and Asia 275
Reports of Bat Rabies in Europe 275
Antigenic Characterization of Rabies Isolates from European Bats 280
Genetic Analysis of Rabies-Related Lyssaviruses 284
Migratory Behavior of Bats and the European Bat Lyssaviruses 285
Pathogenicity of European Bat Lyssaviruses 287
Transmission of Nonterrestrial Virus to Terrestrial Species in Europe 288
Human Exposure to European Bat Lyssavirus 288
Bat Rabies in the Former Soviet Union 290
Bat Rabies in Asia 290
Public-Health Recommendations 291
Vaccination Against European Bat Lyssaviruses 291

SECTION V
Public Health Concerns

24. Bat Rabies and the General Public 303
Routes of Human Exposure 303
Handling of Bats 304
Potential Exposure of Pets 305
Hazard to Human Health 306
First Aid for Bat Bite 308
Role of Pre-Exposure Rabies Prophylaxis 308

25. Concerns in Cave Exploration 311
Encounters with Bats in Restricted Passageway 311
Risk to Cave Explorers 311
Can Probabilities of Exposure Be Defined? 314
Exposure to Viral Aerosols 315
Maximizing Safety Underground 316
Should Cavers Seek Pre-Exposure Rabies Prophylaxis? 316
Specific Recommendations for the Caving Community 318
Cavers, Caves, and Caving — A Perspective 320

Index 323

SECTION I

Rabies: Disease and Nature of the Infective Process

Chapter 1:
GENERAL NATURE OF THE DISEASE

Global Distribution

Rabies is a viral infection of the central nervous system, causing a fatal encephalitis (inflammation of the brain) or encephalomyelitis (inflammation of the brain and spinal cord). An ancient disease, its recorded history is shrouded in ambiguity. Some believe that the first recognizable written description of rabies is contained in the writings of Aristotle, circa 300 B.C. (Wilkinson, 1977). In his *Natural History of Animals*, Aristotle wrote,

> *Rabies drives the animal mad, and any animal whatever, excepting man, will take the disease if bitten by a mad dog so afflicted; the disease is fatal to the dog itself and to any animal it may bite, man excepted.*

Others believe that references to rabies may be found in the writings of Democritus, circa 500 B.C., or even in the Laws of Eshnunna, circa 2000 B.C. (Sureau, 1988).[1] The earliest collection of laws known, the Laws of Eshnuna predate the Code of Hammurabi by almost two centuries and state,

> *If a dog is mad and the authorities have brought the fact to the knowledge of its owner; if he does not keep it in, and it bites a man and causes his death, then the owner shall pay two-thirds of a mine (40 shekels of silver). If it bites a slave and causes his death he shall pay 15 shekels of silver.*

Although primarily a disease of animals, humans may be exposed by bites from infected animals. In the United States, approximately two million people sustain animal bites each year, mostly from nonrabid domestic species. However, bites inflicted by wildlife may cause victims considerable anxiety due to threat of possible rabies transmission.

Although all mammals may become infected with rabies, their public-health significance is highly variable. Moreover, even among the common reservoir hosts, species-associated epidemiologic importance differs markedly from country to country and even geographically within a particular country. It is, therefore, important that physicians, veterinarians, and public-health officials have a broad understanding of rabies epidemiology and a working knowledge of the major reservoir species in their practice locale.

Except in those countries that have managed to eradicate it or those that have been historically free, rabies is a worldwide disease. Although not present in all countries, the disease is of global concern. Even though the likelihood of imported rabies becoming established in a rabies-free country is extremely small, these countries require constant vigilance to maintain their rabies-free status. Detailed guidelines for the importation of animals from rabies-free and rabies-infected countries are contained in the International Animal Health Code (Office International des Épizooties, 1993).

Worldwide, more than 30,000 human deaths from rabies are believed to occur annually, principally following bites from rabid dogs. Each year, approximately four million people require post-exposure rabies prophylaxis in more than 80 countries (World Health Organization, 1992). Three principal world areas of rabies have been defined, differing in both the magnitude and nature of the disease (Baer, 1985) and include the

[1]The Laws of Eshnunna were contained on two clay tablets discovered in 1947 in the village of Tell Harmal, on the outskirts of Baghdad. Tell Harmal represents ancient Shaduppum, part of the kingdom whose capital was centered at Eshnunna (Saggs, 1983).

EPIDEMIOLOGY AND EPIZOOTIOLOGY

Epidemiology is the study of diseases in human populations. The study of epidemiology entails observation of naturally occurring disease, study of disease in populations versus individuals, and the elucidation of associations via inference. If a disease occurs rarely and without regularity in a human population, its occurrence is called sporadic in nature. Diseases that occur with predictable regularity and with only minor variations in frequency are known as endemic.

Disease may be endemic at various levels within a population, including: 1) holoendemic disease, when most individuals are affected; 2) hyperendemic disease, when a high proportion of individuals is affected; 3) mesoendemic disease, when a moderate proportion of individuals is affected; and 4) hypoendemic disease, when a relatively small proportion of individuals is affected.

A disease is said to be epidemic within a human population if it occurs in excess of its expected frequency. The term epidemic does not imply large numbers of diseased individuals. Even a small number of cases, when the expected frequency is zero, constitutes an epidemic. A mass epidemic, encompassing several countries (or even global in nature) is called a pandemic.

The terms epizootiology, enzootic, and epizootic have similar meanings to epidemiology, endemic, and epidemic respectively, but refer to disease in animal, rather than human, populations. In many instances, epidemiology is used in a generic fashion, referring to disease in both human and animal populations.

following:

1) Countries with enzootic dog rabies (including almost all of Asia, Latin America, and Africa).

2) Countries in which wildlife rabies predominates, dog rabies having been brought under control (including western Europe, Canada, and the United States).

3) Rabies-free countries (mostly islands, including England, Australia, Japan, and others).

Countries are accorded a rabies-free status if, in the face of appropriate surveillance and an effective import policy, no cases of indigenously acquired rabies have been confirmed in humans or any animal species during the previous two years (World Health Organization, 1992; Office International des Épizooties, 1993). Rabies is a notifiable disease in such countries. Rabies-free countries (Table 1-1) maintain rigorous quarantine programs to prevent introduction of virus. The Expert Committee on Rabies (World Health Organization, 1984, 1992) recommends that the importation of certain species of mammals (including bats) into rabies-free countries be prohibited, or permitted only under license and quarantine conditions approved by the government veterinary service. Horst and Langworthy (1972) reported an incident of rabies in a colony of captive vampire bats, pointing out the importance of maintaining newly captured specimens in quarantine.

The Causative Agent

The causative agent of rabies is a bullet-shaped virus (Figure 1-1) belonging to the genus *Lyssavirus* (from the Greek *lyssa*, meaning frenzy) of the family known as Rhabdoviridae. The family Rhabdoviridae belongs to the order Mononegavirales (*mono* = single; *nega* = negative-stranded; *virales* = viruses), a classification which it shares with two other groups of viruses, Filoviridae and Paramyxoviridae (Pringle, 1991). In addition to the rabies virus itself, the rabies subgroup of the Rhabdoviridae contains a number of related viruses (Lagos bat, Mokola, Duvenhage, and European bat lyssavirus) that may produce neurological disease in humans or animals and which have no specific vaccines available against them. These agents are discussed more fully in Chapters 22 and 23.

Individual rabies viral particles (virions) are round at one end and blunt at the other. Average

Table 1-1

Countries Where No Rabies Cases Were Reported in the Year 1991

Continent	Country
Africa	Equatorial Guinea Libyan Arab Jamahiriya Mauritius
Americas	Antigua/Barbados Bahamas British Virgin Islands Saint Lucia Uruguay Vanuatu
Asia	Bahrain Brunei Darussalam Japan Malaysia (Island) Malaysia (Peninsula) Maldives Qatar Singapore Tonga
Europe	Cyprus Denmark Finland Gibraltar Greece Iceland Ireland Malta Norway (except Svalbard Islands) Portugal Sweden United Kingdom
Oceania	Australia French Polynesia Hong Kong New Caledonia New Zealand Niue Island (New Zealand) Papua New Guinea Republic of Seychelles

From the World Health Organization. *World Survey of Rabies 27 (for the year 1991).* © World Health Organization, Veterinary Public Health Unit, Division of Communicable Diseases. Geneva, Switzerland. WHO/Rabies/93.209, 1993. Reproduced with permission.

dimensions are 180 x 75 nanometers. They are covered by glycoprotein surface projections, called spikes. The virus is not very resistant to environmental factors and is quickly inactivated outside of the body. It is readily inactivated by heat, drying, sunlight, ultraviolet light, ethanol, formalin, aqueous quaternary ammonium compounds, soap and water, and a 1:10 dilution of household bleach in water. Disinfection of an area is a relatively simple procedure (Anderson et al, 1981).

Naturally occurring variants of rabies virus, isolated from animals in the wild, are referred to as "street virus" (*virus rué* of Pasteur). Street viruses are characterized by a long and variable incubation period and the production of Negri bodies (see page 8) in the brains of infected animals. If virus is experimentally passaged (transferred) from one individual to another for enough generations, the resulting viral isolate is referred to as a fixed virus (*virus fixé* of Pasteur). Fixed viruses tend to have a shortened and more uniform (i.e., "fixed") incubation period in those species in which they were fixed.

Until relatively recently, it was believed that the rabies viruses isolated from various species were identical. Today, it is known that such isolates are similar, but not identical (Wiktor and Clark, 1973; Wiktor and Koprowski, 1978, 1980). They can now be differentiated according to their reactions with various panels of monoclonal antibodies and by genetic analysis. Recognition of both antigenic and genetic differences among rabies viruses provides at least one explanation for earlier findings that suggested species differences in both susceptibility and reaction to infection.

Antigenic characterization of rabies and rabies-related viruses has revealed a variety of viral strains. A distinct species-associated variant characterizes each of the major terrestrial hosts. Multiple bat variants are known. With the development of monoclonal antibody analysis as a means of differentiating viruses, a powerful tool for studying the epidemiology and epizootiology of assorted variants of rabies and rabies-related viruses became available. The yield from newly applied techniques of genetic analysis will provide even greater understanding of rabies epidemiology worldwide.

Our ability to distinguish among the many isolates of virus with which animals or humans may become infected has been of inestimable value in shaping our understanding of rabies epidemiology worldwide. In particular, the finding that bat variants of rabies virus can be distinguished from those of terrestrial species has led to significant alterations in epidemiologic perspectives voiced in preceding decades.

Routes of Transmission

Rabies virus does not penetrate intact skin. Infection is dependent upon the virus coming into contact with deeper tissues or with mucous membranes, such as those of the nose, eyes, or mouth. Bite wounds from rabid animals represent the major source of exposure for both humans and animals. In those nations in which canine rabies has been largely controlled by vaccination, wild animal bites are the predominant source of exposure for the human population. By contrast, in many developing nations, where widespread canine immunization programs do not exist, most human rabies is spread by dogs. Worldwide, dogs are responsible for the overwhelming majority of human deaths from rabies.

Nonbite routes of exposure to rabies virus are extremely rare. Potential sources include contact of viral-laden saliva with open wounds, abrasions, or mucous membranes. Four cases of human rabies following inhalation of aerosolized virus have been reported. Two of these cases were

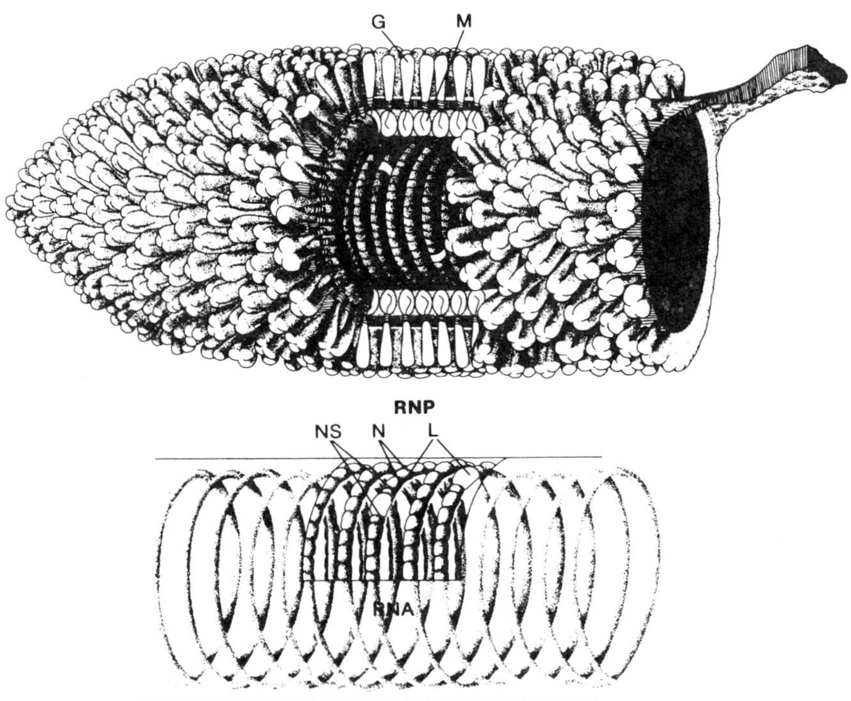

Figure 1-1. Drawing of rabies virus (*top*) showing surface glycoprotein (*G*) projections (peplomers) extending from the lipid envelope that surrounds the internal nucleocapsid. Matrix (*M*) protein is shown lining the viral envelope and interacting with the cytoplasmic domain of the surface glycoprotein. The helical nucleocapsid core (*bottom*) comprises the ribonucleoprotein RNP (i.e., the single-stranded RNA genome plus nucleoprotein [*N*]), phosphoprotein (*NS*), and virion transcriptase (*L*) molecules. The membrane "tail" of the virus represents the frequently observed irregular shape of particles budding from the plasma membrane of the infected cell. (From Wunner, W. H., Larson, J. K., Dietzschold, B., and C. L. Smith. The molecular biology of rabies viruses. *Rev. Infect. Dis.* 10(Suppl. 4): S771, 1988. © by The University of Chicago. All rights reserved. Reproduced with permission.)

BRITISH QUARANTINE REGULATIONS

British dog and cat breeders import and export large numbers of animals annually. In the years between 1911 and 1982, 152,917 dogs were imported. Between 1931 and 1982, 36,218 cats were imported. Quarantine regulations, and legislation governing the muzzling of dogs and the elimination of stray animals have been in effect since 1897. By 1922, rabies had been eradicated from Great Britain. A rigid quarantine is still imposed on all imported mammals in order to safeguard its rabies-free status.

The duration of this quarantine is meant to cover the average incubation period of the disease in dogs and cats, which is 2 to 3 months. Thus, a quarantine period of six months is in effect. On occasion, rabies may incubate for longer than six months. It is believed, however, that increasing the length of the quarantine period beyond six months would be counter-productive, leading to wide-scale animal smuggling. In fact, some investigators have recommended a quarantine time of less than six months as being adequate. Imported vampire bats and their offspring are required to remain in quarantine for life.

The *Rabies Importation of Dogs and Cats or Other Mammals Order* specifies that all mammals, other than man, be landed at specified ports or airports and transported to a quarantine facility by an authorized agent. An import license must accompany each animal. Between 1979 and 1982, 221 dogs and 125 cats are known to have been landed illegally in England. A provision exists for destruction of animals landed illegally.

Between 1922 and 1970, 26 dogs and two cats (one a leopard) have died of rabies in quarantine facilities. No other cases were reported until 1990, when one dog was confirmed as rabid within a quarantine facility (Editorial, 1990). Since 1971, none of close to 200,000 animals immunized in quarantine have developed rabies following release (King and Turner, 1993).

Increasing numbers of families are pleasure boating on the English Channel. In spite of widespread publicity, many of these boat outings include the family pet. Even if the boat has not landed on mainland Europe, the animals are subject to quarantine upon return. Drive-on, drive-off ferry boats have increased the risk of potentially infected animal "stowaways." There is also increasing concern that completion of the Channel Tunnel may provide a possible route of entry of rabid animals into England (Tyrrell and Nicholson, 1990).

Artificial insemination of dogs in many European countries is a common practice. Importation of canine semen into Great Britain is strictly regulated. The donor animal is required to be certified rabies-free and kept in a certified rabies-free area for 12 months prior to collection (Turner, 1984).

Currently, significant political and economic pressures are being placed on the United Kingdom by the European Community to eliminate its quarantine programs (Editorial, 1992; Hewett, 1992; Holt, 1992). Other nations with a rabies-free status that are members of the EC include Ireland and Portugal. Rabies-free countries that reduce quarantine requirements may increase their possibility of importing the disease (World Health Organization, 1992; Gorman, 1993).

Other nations that have adopted similar quarantine programs include Australia, New Zealand, the Netherlands, Ireland, and some Caribbean nations (Held et al, 1991; Forman, 1993). Hawaii also maintains a strict rabies quarantine (Frankel, 1978; Fishbein et al, 1990; Sasaki et al, 1992). Shorter quarantine programs or predominant dependence on prior immunization of imported animals may be in use elsewhere.

laboratory accidents and two were naturally occurring (see page 169). Six human cases are known in which rabies developed in recipients of corneal transplants from undiagnosed rabid human donors (see page 234). Rarely, cases of transplacental or transmammary transmission have been claimed.

As with all infectious diseases, distinction must be made between exposure, infection, and clinical disease (Bernard, 1985). Contact with rabies virus constitutes an exposure. This is not synonymous with infection, which refers to the presence of virus in deep body tissues. For example, exposure to the infectious saliva of a rabid animal will not lead to infection when applied to intact skin, because the virus cannot penetrate unbroken skin. If applied to abraded skin, to mucous membranes, or if introduced directly into a bite wound, the virus may gain access to deeper tissue, resulting in infection. Viral infection may or may not lead to clinical disease, depending on a variety of factors.

Centripetal Migration of Virus

Following deposition of virus in body tissues by the bite of a rabid animal, the virus may replicate at the site of injury, primarily in muscle, but also in nerves. Virus may also invade nerve endings directly, without prior replication in muscle (Shankar et al, 1991). Rabies virus may persist at the wound site in an "eclipse" phase for an extended period of time. The key to progression of the infection is the presence of nerve endings at the site of viral replication. Virus will enter exposed nerve endings and be carried passively along the many nerve processes to the central nervous system.

Retrograde transport along nerves from the periphery to the central nervous system occurs at a rate of about 8 to 20 mm per day. En route to the brain, multiplication of virus occurs in neurons of the dorsal root ganglia and spinal gray matter. An amplified viral population, therefore, reaches the brain (Kaplan, 1985). In the case of bites sustained about the head, or exposure of membranes of the eyes, mouth, or nose, virus may migrate directly to the brain (Murphy, 1985).

During the course of its centripetal migration, movement of the rabies virus occurs almost exclusively along nerve-tissue pathways. Virus is generally not present in the blood. Within various neuronal processes, virus is effectively isolated from both the body's immune system and from antiviral medications. Although not considered a method of preventing clinical disease following the bite of a rabid animal, it has been shown experimentally that if ascent of virus through nerves to the brain is prevented by amputation of the bitten limb, progression of the infection will be stopped (Baer and Cleary, 1972).

Virus may remain at its peripheral site of deposition for much of the incubation period (Baer and Cleary, 1972). Viral entry into nerve cells during this time is not immediate. Rather, intramuscular harborage prior to intraneural infection, in contrast to viral sequestration within peripheral nerves, might account for longer incubation times (Murphy et al, 1973a, 1973b).

By nature, the rabies virus is highly neurotropic. It has a predilection for infecting nervous tissue. Virtually all portions of the brain become rapidly infected with virus and, as neuronal infection progresses, a variety of neurologic abnormalities become evident. Histopathologically, infection is typically described as a nonsuppurative encephalomyelitis with ganglioneuritis and diffuse or focal gliosis. Lymphoplasmacytic infiltration with perivascular cuffing is common. Inclusion bodies are characteristic of viral-infected cells. These represent areas of the cell which can be perceived microscopically as regions of altered stain uptake. Inclusion bodies develop during the course of viral replication and may represent sites at which viral nucleic acid or protein synthesis is occurring. Negri bodies are the intracytoplasmic inclusion bodies found in nerve cells infected with rabies virus (Negri, 1903).

Clinical signs of rabies do not appear until several cycles of viral replication have occurred in the brain (Kaplan, 1985). Varying distribution of virus within the brain may be responsible for the different manifestations (i.e., furious versus paralytic) of clinical rabies (Jackson and Reimer, 1989). The precise lesions in the brain ultimately responsible for the diverse neurologic manifestations of rabies are, as yet, poorly understood. Infection of nerve cells in the limbic system (a portion of the brain related to the expression of emotion) may be an integral component of the bizarre behavior that often characterizes rabies infection. However, recent studies have shown that viral infection of other regions of the brain may also be involved in development of the behavioral changes characteristic of rabies infection in animals and humans (Smart and Charlton, 1992).

Centrifugal Migration of Virus

After a variable period of time, virus will undergo a movement away from the brain, outward through the body along nerve axons. In this fashion, rabies virus will become widely distributed throughout the body (Duenas et al, 1973; Balachandran and Charlton, 1994). Structures shown to become secondarily invaded by virus during this centrifugal migration include the heart, lungs, skin, pancreas, thymus, kidneys, ovaries, uterus, adrenal glands, liver, spleen, intestines, smooth and skeletal muscles, salivary glands, and the nerve bundles of hair roots, eyes, and taste buds. The amount of virus distributed to various organs correlates well with the density of each organ's nerve supply, but may also be related to the variant and dose of virus, species infected, and route of exposure.

Further replication of virus occurs in the salivary glands (Wunner and Dietzschold, 1987). Relatively enormous amounts of virus may be present in saliva of infected animals. For example, enough virus may be contained in a 1 ml suspension of rabid fox salivary gland to infect 34 million other foxes (Blancou et al, 1979 [cited by Macdonald and Voigt, 1985]).

The passage of virus from brain to salivary glands is a critical element in completion of the rabies transmission cycle. Rabies virus may be present in saliva at the time aggressive behavior appears and a bite capable of transmitting disease. Viral-induced behavioral alterations are important for the transmission of virus from animal to animal and for maintenance of the viral life cycle in many reservoir species. However, paralytic rabies (without development of furious signs) may also be important to the maintenance of virus in a reservoir species, preventing rapid and wide-

Table 1-2

Alternative Strategies of Rabies Viruses and of Carnivore Hosts: Consequences and Constraints

Strategy	Consequences + Constraints
Rabies Virus	
change of receptor (cell) specificity	loss of easy access to central nervous system (as in some attenuated virus strains)
change of host specificity	loss of epidemiological correlation with parameters of host population
change in pathogenicity	loss of behavioral mechanisms of virus transmission
Carnivore Rabies Host	
improvement of peripheral immune surveillance for an early virus recognition and immune response	increase in number of allergic responses (?)
increase in number of molecular sites functioning as virus receptors on peripheral cells (increased peripheral virus replication, earlier immune response)	loss of physiological function of receptors
structural change in molecular sites functioning as virus receptors (reduction in susceptibility)	loss of physiological function of receptors
avoidance of all contacts with potentially infectious conspecifics	abstinence from competition (resource defense), cooperation, mating, etc.
recognition of infective animals (avoidance of contacts with infective animals)	no constraints (?)

From Wandeler, A. Carnivore rabies: Ecological and evolutionary aspects. *Hystrix.* 3: 121, 1991. Reproduced with permission.

spread death among the infected host population.

Continuity of Viral Transmission

Establishment of enzootic rabies in a susceptible wild population is a very unlikely event, requiring an uncommon combination of features related to both the virus and its potential host. Once established, however, optimal conditions for maintenance of virus in an infected population generally include a highly susceptible target species, a high titer of salivary viral excretion, and an absence of postinfection immunity (Blancou, 1988). Under these circumstances, there will be no break between the exposure of one individual and that of another and an immune population will not survive to impair progressive infection.

Continuity of viral transmission is related to both the infective and pathogenic nature of the virus. Both may change in time, evolving as required to best accommodate the biology of a particular reservoir host. This dynamic development is a manifestation of reciprocal evolution, with "mutual adjustments between the host and the parasite" (Abdussalam, 1959). Hall (1978 [cited by Carey, 1985]) referred to such adaptable obligate viral parasites as "dynamic disease entities."

Animal populations and their respective environments are dynamic in nature. Persistence of a disease in such a system requires that one or more of several criteria be met (Tinline, 1988), including:

1) A pathogen's ability to develop new strains to suit new conditions.
2) Variability in a pathogen's characteristics that permit it to take advantage of a broad range of conditions.
3) Alterations in the host or its environment that create a new set of opportunities for the pathogen to exploit, without itself changing.

Each major reservoir host has its own species-adapted strain of virus. Although coadaptation and coevolution are terms commonly employed in discussions of host/virus interactions, the relationship is more closely akin to an "arms race" between the two, with the host building up its defenses and the virus attempting to counter them (Wandeler, 1991). There are limitations placed on the respective strategies employed by each (Table 1-2).

A variety of properties associated with either the host or the virus influence the incidence and prevalence of disease, as well as morbidity and mortality in specific animal populations at risk (Wandeler, 1991). Features related to the virus include pathogenicity, cell and species specificity, incubation period, nature of viral excretion, and clinical manifestations. Those related to the host include rate of population growth, habitat use, social organization and behavior, and mortality from causes other than rabies.

References

Abdussalam, M. (1959). Significance of ecological studies of wild animal reservoirs of zoonoses. *Bull. Wld. Hlth. Org.* 21: 179

Anderson, L. J., Hattwick, M. A., and M. B. Gregg (1981). Rabies. In J. P. Sanford and J. P. Luby (eds.) *Infectious Diseases—The Science and Practice of Clinical Medicine.* Volume 8. Grune and Stratton. New York.

Baer, G. M. (1985). Rabies Virus. In H. N. Fields et al (eds.) *Virology.* Raven Press. New York.

Baer, G. M. and W. F. Cleary (1972). A model in mice for the pathogenesis and treatment of rabies. *J. Infect. Dis.* 125(5): 520

Balachandran, A. and K. Charlton (1994). Experimental rabies infection of nonnervous tissues in skunks (*Mephitis mephitis*) and foxes (*Vulpes vulpes*). *Vet. Pathol.* 31(1): 93

Bernard, K. W. (1985). Clinical Rabies in Humans. In W. G. Winkler (ed.) *Rabies Concepts for Medical Professionals.* Merieux Institute, Inc. Miami, Florida.

Blancou, J. (1988). Ecology and epidemiology of fox rabies. *Rev. Infect. Dis.* 10(Suppl. 4): S607

Blancou, J., Aubert, M. F. A., Andral, L., and M. Artois (1979). Rage experimental du renard roux (*Vulpes vulpes*). *Rev. Med. Vet.* (Toulouse). 130: 1001.

Carey, A. B. (1985). Multispecies Rabies in the Eastern United States. In P. J. Bacon (ed.) *Population Dynamics of Rabies in Wildlife.* Academic Press. New York.

Duenas, A., Belsey, M. A., Escobar, J., Medina, P., and C. Sanmartin (1973). Isolation of rabies virus outside the human central nervous system. *J. Infect. Dis.* 127(6): 702

Editorial (1990). Rabies case found in quarantine kennels. *Vet. Rec.* 127(12): 294

Editorial (1992). Comment: Keeping rabies at bay. *Vet. Rec.* 130(7): 129

Fishbein, D. B., Corboy, J. M., and D. M. Sasaki (1990). Rabies prevention in Hawaii. *Hawaii Med. J.* 49(3): 98

Forman, A. J. (1993). The threat of rabies introduction and establishment in Australia. *Aust. Vet. J.* 70(3): 81

Frankel, R. I. (1978). Hawaii's quarantine regulations and the epidemiology of rabies. *Hawaii Med. J.* 37(1): 16

Gorman, N. (1993). Of medicines, rabies control, and the continuing development of practice. *Vet. Rec.* 132(14): 336

Held, J. R., Escalante, J. A., and W. G. Winkler (1991). The International Management of Rabies. In G. M. Baer (ed.) *The Natural History of Rabies*. 2nd Edition. CRC Press, Inc. Boca Raton, Florida.

Hewett, G. R. (1992). Rabies requirements—Letter to the editor. *Vet. Rec.* 130(9): 191

Holt, E. A. (1992). Rabies requirements—Letter to the editor. *Vet. Rec.* 130(9): 192

Horst, R. and M. Langworthy (1972). Rabies in a colony of vampire bats. *J. Mammal.* 53(4): 903

Jackson, A. C. and D. L. Reimer (1989). Pathogenesis of experimental rabies in mice: An immunohistochemical study. *Acta Neuropath.* 78: 159

Kaplan, C. (1985). Rabies: A Worldwide Disease. In P. J. Bacon (ed.) *Population Dynamics of Rabies in Wildlife*. Academic Press. New York.

King, A. A. and G. S. Turner (1993). Rabies: A review. *J. Comp. Path.* 108(1): 1

Macdonald, D. W. and D. R. Voigt (1985). The Biological Basis of Rabies Models. In P. J. Bacon (ed.) *Population Dynamics of Rabies in Wildlife*. Academic Press. New York.

Murphy, F. A. (1985). The Rabies Virus and Pathogenesis of the Disease. In W. G. Winkler (ed.) *Rabies Concepts for Medical Professionals*. Merieux Institute, Inc. Miami, Florida.

Murphy, F. A., Bauer, S. P., Harrison, A. K., and W. C. Winn (1973a). Comparative pathogenesis of rabies and rabies-like viruses. Infection and transit from inoculation site to the central nervous system. *Lab. Invest.* 28(3): 361

Murphy, F. A., Harrison, A. K., Winn, W. C., and S. P. Bauer (1973b). Comparative pathogenesis of rabies and rabies-like viruses. Infection of the central nervous system and centrifugal spread of virus to peripheral tissues. *Lab. Invest.* 29(1): 1

Negri, A. (1903). Beitrag zum studium der aetiologie der tollwut. *Zeitschrift fur Hygiene und Infektionskrankheiten.* 43: 507

Office International des Épizooties (1993). Chapter 3.1.5. Rabies. *International Animal Health Code.* Office International des Épizooties. Paris, France.

Pringle, C. R. (1991). The order *Mononegavirales*. *Arch. Virol.* 117: 137

Saggs, H. W. F. (1983). *The Greatness that was Babylon.* Sidgwick and Jackson. London.

Sasaki, D. M., Middleton, C. R., Sawa, T. R., Christensen, C. C., and G. Y. Kobayashi (1992). Rabid bat diagnosed in Hawaii. *Hawaii Med. J.* 51(7): 181

Shankar, V., Dietzschold, B., and H. Koprowski (1991). Direct entry of rabies virus into the central nervous system without prior local replication. *J. Virol.* 65: 2736

Smart, N. L. and K. M. Charlton (1992). The distribution of challenge virus standard rabies virus versus skunk street rabies virus in the brains of experimentally infected rabid skunks. *Acta Neuropath.* 84: 501

Sureau, P. (1988). History of rabies: Advances in research towards rabies prevention during the last 30 years. *Rev. Infect. Dis.* 10(Suppl. 4): S581

Tinline, R. R. (1988). Persistence of Rabies in Wildlife. In J. B. Campbell and K. M. Charlton (eds.) *Rabies.* Kluwer Academic Publications. Boston.

Turner, T. (1984). The risks and problems associated with the importation of dogs, cats and other mammals. I. Rabies. *Br. Vet. J.* 140: 96

Tyrrell, D. A. and K. G. Nicholson (1990). Rabies in Britain: Britain remains vigilant and safe. *Br. Med. J.* 300: 137

Wandeler, A. I. (1991). Carnivore rabies: Ecological and evolutionary aspects. *Hystrix.* 3: 121

Wiktor, T. J. and H. F. Clark (1973). Comparison of rabies virus strains by means of the plaque reduction test (abstract). *Ann. Microbiol.* (Paris). 124: 283

Wiktor, T. J. and H. Koprowski (1978). Monoclonal antibodies against rabies virus produced by somatic cell hybridization: Detection of antigenic variants. *Proc. Natl. Acad. Sci.* USA. 75: 3938

Wiktor, T. J. and H. Koprowski (1980). Antigenic variants of rabies virus. *J. Exp. Med.* 152: 99

Wilkinson, L. (1977). The development of the virus concept as reflected in corpora of studies on individual pathogens. Rabies—Two millennia of ideas and conjecture on the aetiology of a virus disease. *Med. Hist.* 21: 15

World Health Organization (1984). *Expert Committee on Rabies. Seventh Report.* WHO Tech. Rpt. No. 709. Geneva.

World Health Organization (1992). *Expert Committee on Rabies. Eighth Report.* WHO Tech. Rpt. No. 824. Geneva.

World Health Organization (1993). *World Survey of Rabies 27 (for the year 1991).* WHO/Rabies/93.209, 1993. Unpublished document (reviewed with permission).

Wunner, W. H. and B. Dietzschold (1987). Rabies virus infection: Genetic mutations and the impact on viral pathogenicity and immunity. *Contr. Microbiol. Immunol.* 8: 103

Wunner, W. H., Larson, J. K., Dietzschold, B., and C. L. Smith (1988). The molecular biology of rabies viruses. *Rev. Infect. Dis.* 10(Suppl. 4): S771

Chapter 2:
RABIES IN TERRESTRIAL ANIMALS

Animal Reservoirs of Virus

Although all mammals are susceptible to rabies infection, their significance to rabies epidemiology may be highly variable. Species susceptibility to clinical rabies may vary, depending, in part, on both the dose of virus and route of exposure, as well as the individual variant of infecting virus. In the United States, several wildlife species, notably raccoons, skunks, bats, and foxes, are important reservoirs of virus. Since the 1950's, the relative importance of wildlife in rabies epidemiology has increased, while that of domestic animals has declined (Figures 2-1 and 2-2). Reported cases of rabies in wild animals first exceeded those in domestic species in the late 1950's and have continued to do so each year since. In 1992, wildlife accounted for 91.5% (7,912 of 8,645) of rabies cases reported to the Centers for Disease Control (Figures 2-3 and 2-4).

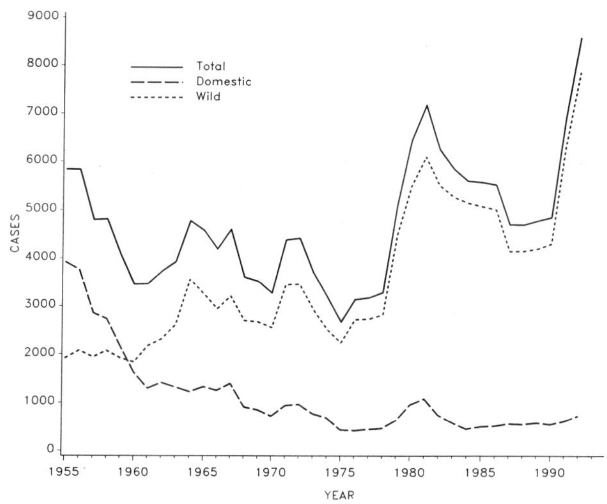

Figure 2-1. Cases of animal rabies in the United States, by year, 1955-1992. (From Krebs, J. W., Strine, T. W., and J. E. Childs. Rabies surveillance in the United States during 1992. *J. Am. Vet. Med. Assoc.* 203(12): 1718, 1993. Reproduced with permission.)

Rabies is enzootic and sometimes epizootic in certain wildlife species.

The progression of clinical signs in rabid animals is comparable to that in humans, but there is a degree of species variability. Following the incubation period, three stages of illness are generally recognized. The prodromal stage is a period of altered behavior and is followed by a stage of aggression (fury). Finally, animals enter into a stage of paralysis and death. The duration of fury and paralysis are highly variable (see page 21). Common elements of rabies infection in animals include a loss of their natural wariness of humans, exhibition of markedly abnormal behavior, and, in the case of nocturnal animals, an increased measure of activity during daylight hours. Although all wildlife should be left strictly alone, those noted to be behaving in an abnormal fashion (especially a member of a reservoir species) should be considered potentially rabid, unless proven otherwise.

Skunks

Skunks are important reservoirs of rabies virus in the midwestern United States and California (Figure 2-5). The midwest band of skunk rabies may have begun as two separate foci: an older focus in Minnesota/Iowa and a newer one in Texas. These foci expanded during the 1970's, ultimately encompassing Missouri and Arkansas. Viral isolates from rabid skunks in Minnesota and Iowa are antigenically different from those in Texas. A mixture of both isolates is present in infected skunks of Missouri and Arkansas (Smith et al, 1986; Smith and Baer, 1988).

The striped skunk has been most studied because of its wide distribution and close association with human populations. Incubation period (duration of time from initial exposure to onset of clinical signs or symptoms) generally varies between 3 weeks and 6 months. The prodromal phase is usually 1 to 3 days in duration and characterized by alterations in normal behavior. Normally nocturnal in habit, rabid skunks become active during daylight hours and lose their natural fear of humans. They are often killed as they wander about during their daytime excursions. Virus may be present in saliva at this time and a bite may be infectious. Rabid skunks generally have higher levels of virus in their saliva than either foxes or raccoons.

The aggressive stage is brief, usually lasting 1 to 2 days. Rabid skunks may be very aggressive, often biting farm machinery and farm animals, and commonly attacking dogs (frequently biting them on the muzzle). They are known to react in a violent manner to a variety of environmental stimuli. When attacking, the rabid skunk may cling tenaciously to its victim. Virus is not present in scent glands and so spraying is not a route of viral transmission. The paralytic stage is generally 2 to 4 days in duration. Paralysis usually begins in the hind limbs and animals are commonly seen dragging themselves along the ground. The paralysis gradually spreads cranially, with death following soon after.

In 1992, 27% (2,334 of 8,645) of all animals reported rabid in the United States were skunks, a 12.6% increase over the number reported in 1991. California, Iowa, Kansas, Minnesota, New York, North Dakota, Oklahoma, and Texas each reported more than 100 cases, accounting for 49% of all skunk rabies in the country. Most cases of skunk rabies in the Northeast and mid-Atlantic states are the result of spillover from rabies in the local raccoon population (Krebs et al, 1992, 1993).

Raccoons

Rabies in raccoons was first identified in California in 1936. Sporadic reports of infection were subsequently noted across the country. In the mid 1950's, the disease became a major problem in Florida and has since spread throughout the state, as well as into Georgia and parts of South Carolina and Alabama. In the late 1970's, an outbreak of raccoon rabies occurred in the mid-Atlantic states and the disease continued spreading north towards New England (Israel et al, 1982; Pacer et al, 1985). Presently, the northernmost extent of the epizootic stretches across Ohio, Pennsylvania, New York, and New Hampshire (Trimarchi, 1990, 1991, 1992; Cartter et al, 1992; Smith, 1992; Uhaa et al, 1992a) and threatens to extend into southern Ontario (Rosatte et al, 1993). Raccoons are major reservoirs of rabies from Florida to Connecticut (Figure 2-6) and the epizootic will likely continue to expand further north and west (Centers for Disease Control, 1992). This growing urban threat will likely have a significant impact on public health.

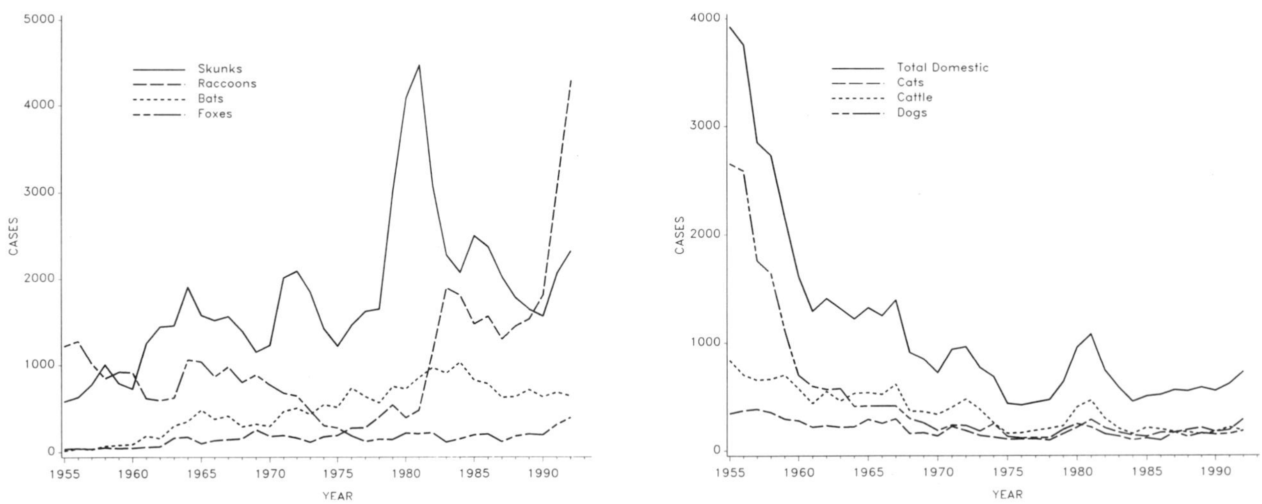

Figure 2-2. Cases of rabies in wild animals (left) and domestic animals (right) in the United States, by year and species, 1955-1992. (From Krebs, J. W., Strine, T. W., and J. E. Childs. Rabies surveillance in the United States during 1992. *J. Am. Vet. Med. Assoc.* 203(12): 1718, 1993. Reproduced with permission.)

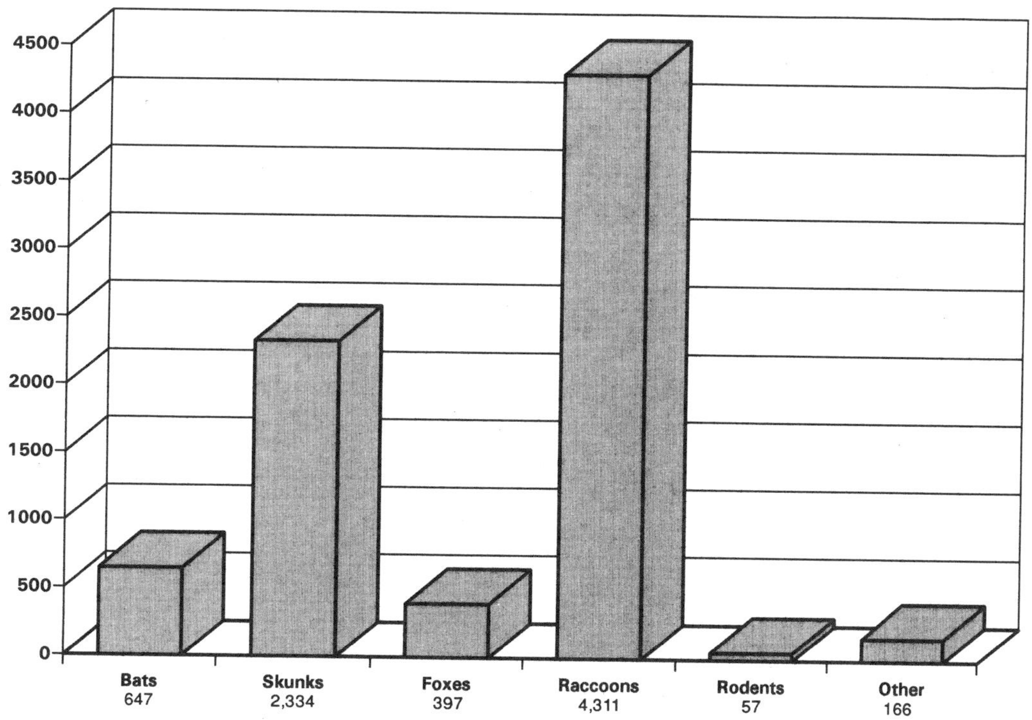

Figure 2-3. Cases of rabies in wildlife in the United States, by year and species, 1992. Other "wild" includes 1 badger, 2 ringtails, 4 opossums, 6 deer, 6 otters, 20 bobcats, 51 mongooses (Puerto Rico), and 75 coyotes. (Data from Krebs, J. W., Strine, T. W., and J. E. Childs. Rabies surveillance in the United States during 1992. *J. Am. Vet. Med. Assoc.* 203(12): 1718, 1993.)

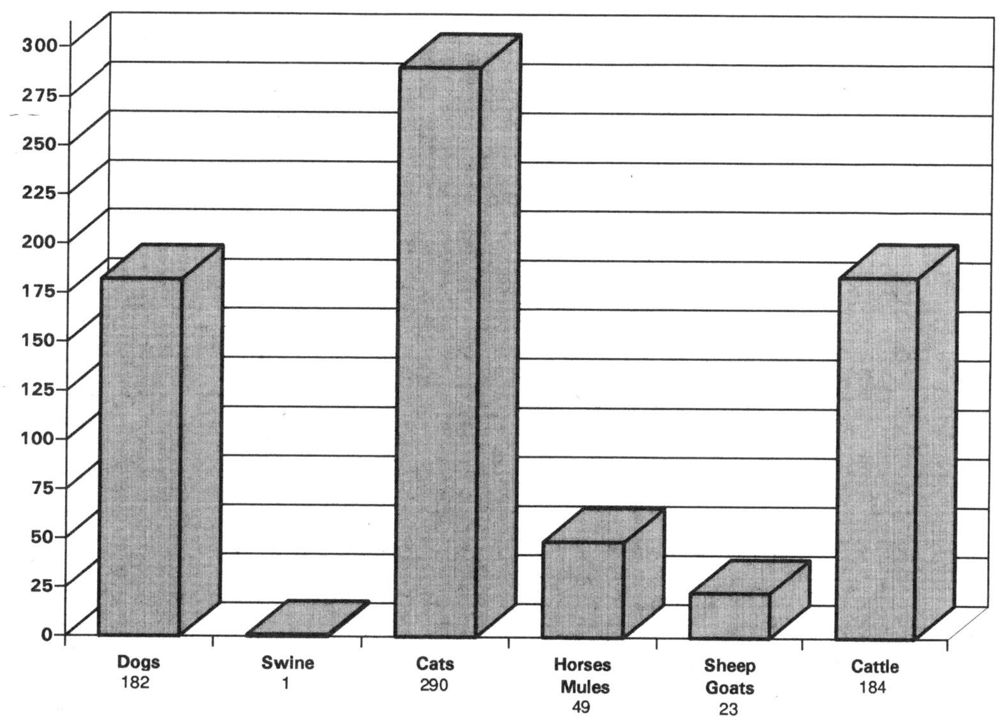

Figure 2-4. Cases of rabies in domestic animals in the United States, by species, 1992. Other "domestic" includes 1 llama and 2 ferrets. (Data from Krebs, J. W., Strine, T. W., and J. E. Childs. Rabies surveillance in the United States during 1992. *J. Am. Vet. Med. Assoc.* 203(12): 1718, 1993.)

With respect to the origin of the mid-Atlantic outbreak, several theories have been advanced, including exposure to rabid bats and transportation of rabid raccoons from the southeastern focus of disease. There has been no evidence to implicate bats as agents in the spread of raccoon rabies northward (see page 199). However, many thousands of raccoons have been illegally transported into mid-Atlantic states by private hunting clubs seeking to bolster the animal's population. Between 1977 and 1981, for example, more than 3,500 raccoons were translocated from Florida to southwest Virginia (Jenkins et al, 1988). Nettles et al (1979) reported finding two rabid animals out of 165 translocated raccoons examined between 1976 and 1978. Many of these imported raccoons were released for pursuit and capture by dogs, thereby adding to the potential public-health burden. Additionally, persons handling these animals risked exposure to infectious material.

Results of monoclonal antibody analyses are consistent with a traffic of rabid raccoons from the Southeast to mid-Atlantic states. The variant of rabies virus isolated from raccoons in the mid-Atlantic states is identical to that of infected animals in Florida, but dissimilar to variants of virus found in bats (Smith et al, 1984, 1990; Rupprecht et al, 1987; Jenkins et al, 1988). The mid-Atlantic epizootic of raccoon rabies has had no detectable effect on reported cases of bat rabies, consistent with the existence of separate and unrelated cycles of infection (Winkler, 1985).

Continued development of wilderness areas has resulted in a diminished range of the raccoon and a concentration of its population in urban environments, to which it readily adapts (Burridge et al, 1986). Forty-nine rabid raccoons were found in metropolitan New York between January of 1992 and April of 1993 (Trimarchi, 1993a, 1993b). They coexist well in association with hu-

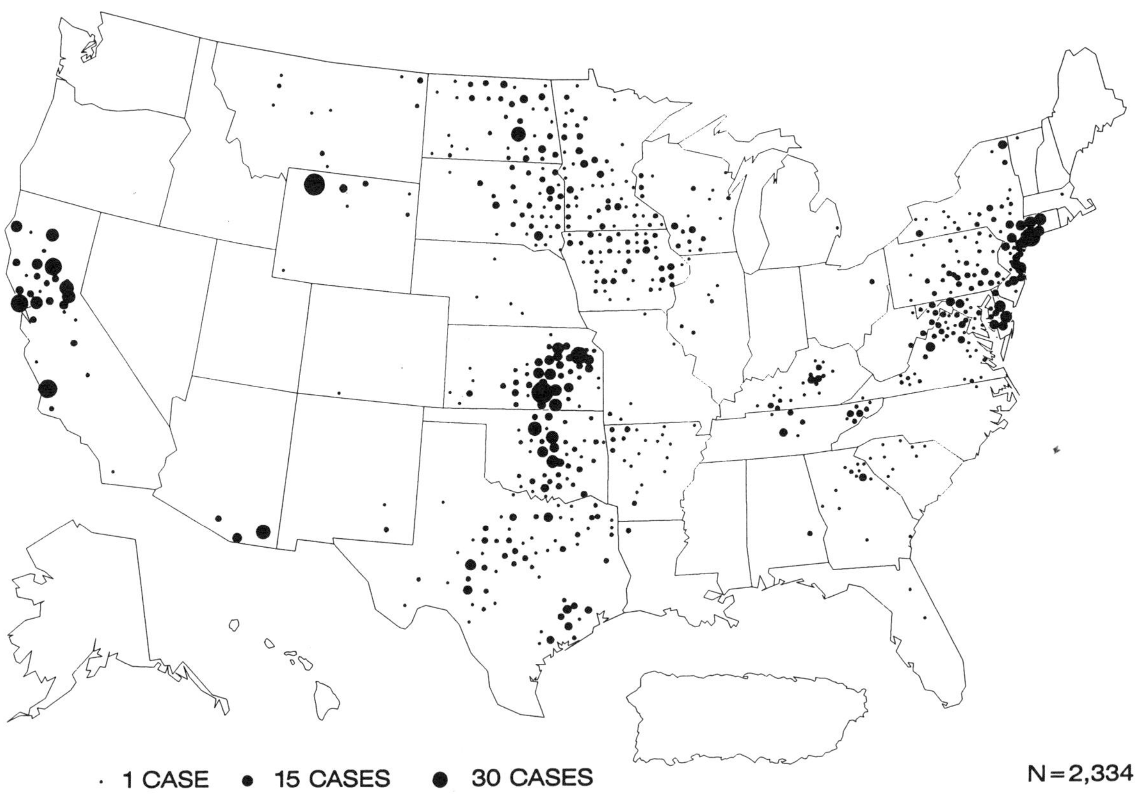

Figure 2-5. Reported cases of rabies in skunks, by county, 1992. Dot size is proportional to the number of cases in the county. (From Krebs, J. W., Strine, T. W., and J. E. Childs. Rabies surveillance in the United States during 1992. *J. Am. Vet. Med. Assoc.* 203(12): 1718, 1993. Reproduced with permission.)

mans, increasing their potential threat to public health (Uhaa et al, 1992b). Rabid raccoons commonly walk into the backyards of homes during daylight hours and are often involved in attacks on dogs. This behavior increases the likelihood of human exposure as well. A higher incidence of raccoon rabies is related to adult male aggression during breeding seasons.

In one study of captured raccoons in Virginia and mid-Atlantic states, 12% to 16% of randomly selected, normal-appearing individuals, and 38% to 71% of abnormal-appearing raccoons were positive for rabies (Jenkins et al, 1988). In 1990, raccoons accounted for 37.3% (1,821 of 4,881) of all animals reported rabid in the United States, making them the most commonly reported rabid animal in the country during that year. The number of reported rabid raccoons exceeded that of skunks for the first time since wildlife surveillance began in the 1950's (Uhaa et al, 1992a). In 1992, raccoons accounted for 49.9% (4,311 of 8,645) of all animals reported rabid, a 40% increase over the number reported in 1991 and the largest number ever reported (Krebs et al, 1993). The greatest number were reported from New York (1,392), followed by Connecticut (720), and New Jersey (579). New York reported the largest number of rabid raccoons ever recorded from a single state (Trimarchi, 1993a). In 1993, 2,369 confirmed cases of rabies in raccoons were reported in New York State, a 70% increase over 1992 (Trimarchi, 1994). In some states, limited field trials using an orally effective, genetically engineered rabies vaccine are being carried out in attempts to control rabies in free-ranging raccoons (see page 254).

Foxes

Once an important reservoir of virus from the Ohio River Valley through New England, foxes

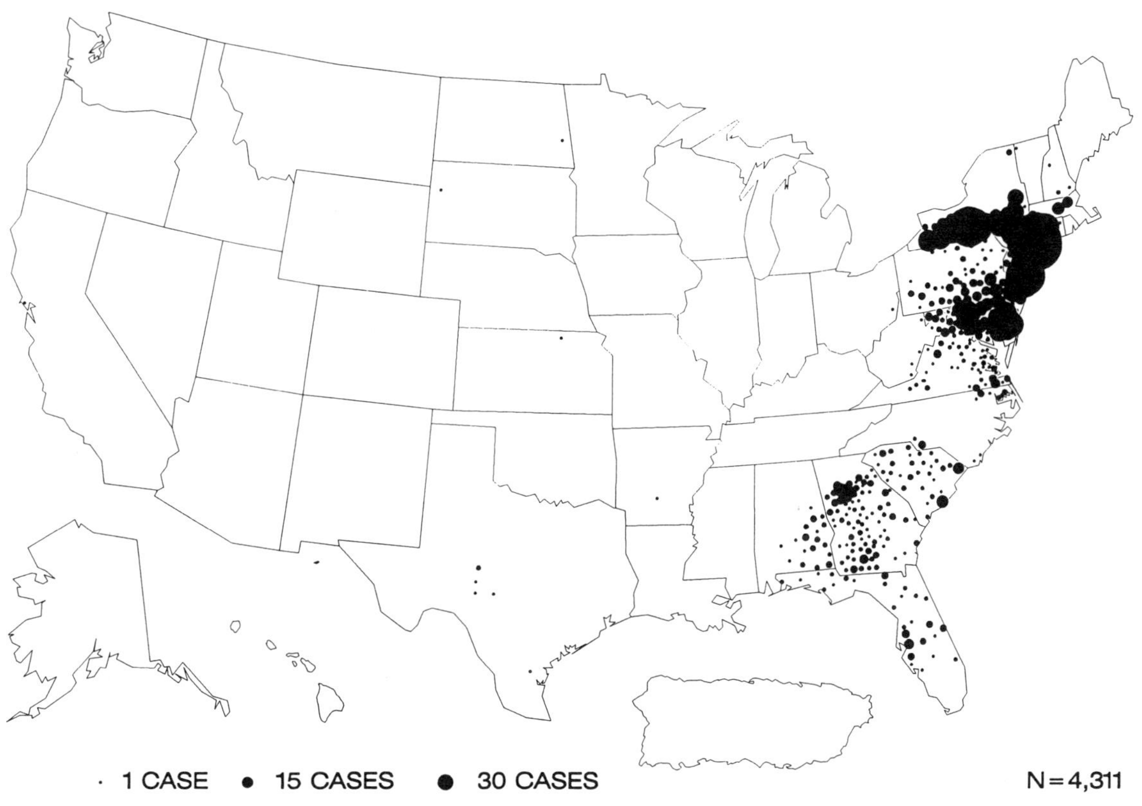

Figure 2-6. Reported cases of rabies in raccoons, by county, 1992. Dot size is proportional to the number of cases in the county. (From Krebs, J. W., Strine, T. W., and J. E. Childs. Rabies surveillance in the United States during 1992. *J. Am. Vet. Med. Assoc.* 203(12): 1718, 1993. Reproduced with permission.)

are no longer major reservoirs of rabies in the United States (Figure 2-7). A region of enzootic red fox rabies exists in northern New York, along the border with southern Ontario. Central Texas and Arizona consistently report rabies at low frequencies (generally less than 20 cases per year) in gray foxes. Isolates from foxes in both states are readily distinguished from those of skunks in surrounding enzootic skunk rabies areas, suggesting two independent cycles (Smith and Baer, 1988). In other areas of enzootic skunk rabies, rabid foxes are typically infected with a skunk variant of virus following spillover from the local skunk reservoir. Currently, about 200 to 300 cases of fox rabies are reported annually in the United States.

The incubation period has been observed to vary from 9 to 109 days. During the prodromal stage, rabid foxes tend to dart out, bite people, and then quickly disappear. The most notable sign in the prodrome is an increase in daytime activity (Andral et al, 1982). Their violent prodromal period blends imperceptibly into an aggressive phase and the two are difficult to differentiate. Aggression or confusion are common manifestations in the rabid fox.

Rabid foxes frequently attack porcupines, often resulting in severe facial mutilation. The finding of porcupine quills embedded in the skin of a fox is highly suggestive of a rabid individual (Macdonald, 1980). Animals lose their fear of humans, but may only bite people or animals that approach them. They may appear docile and friendly, often approaching children. The aggressive stage is followed by paralysis and death (usually within four days of onset of clinical signs).

Illegal transportation of enormous numbers of foxes to supply fox-chasing enclosures for recreational pursuit by hunting clubs is becoming an increasingly common practice (Davidson et al,

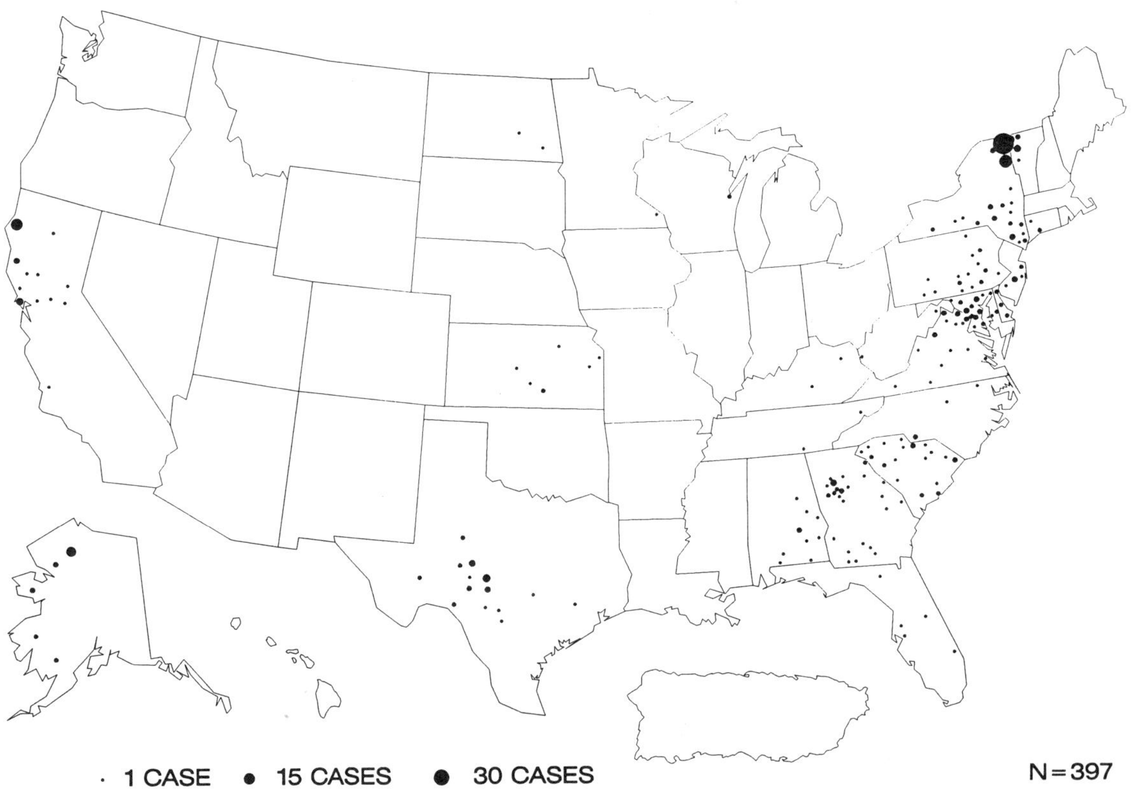

Figure 2-7. Reported cases of rabies in foxes, by county, 1992. Dot size is proportional to the number of cases in the county. (From Krebs, J. W., Strine, T. W., and J. E. Childs. Rabies surveillance in the United States during 1992. *J. Am. Vet. Med. Assoc.* 203(12): 1718, 1993. Reproduced with permission.)

1992). The public-health hazards associated with these practices should be considered. In 1992, foxes accounted for 4.6% (397 of 8,645) of all animals reported rabid in the United States, a 24.8% increase over the number reported in 1991 (Krebs et al, 1992, 1993).

Dogs

Worldwide, dogs are the most important vectors of human rabies. Rabid dogs are responsible for 99% of human rabies cases worldwide. In most developing countries of Asia, Africa, and Latin America, control of canine rabies has not been effective and these countries remain plagued by rabid dogs. The public-health significance of rabies in any country is best correlated with the prevalence of rabies in its canine population.

In industrialized nations of Europe and North America, vaccination and stray-dog removal programs have significantly reduced the threat of canine rabies. In the United States, dogs are now infected by local wildlife, but the disease is no longer maintained within the canine population. The maintenance of an immunized population of dogs is the single most important element in the prevention of human rabies. All dogs should be vaccinated against rabies at three months of age, revaccinated one year later, and then vaccinated regularly by a veterinarian using an approved vaccine (AVMA Council on Biologic and Therapeutic Agents, 1989; National Association of State Public Health Veterinarians, 1992, 1993, 1994).

The incubation period in dogs varies between 10 days and 6 months, averaging 3 to 8 weeks. It is followed by a prodromal phase which usually lasts 2 to 3 days. Behavioral alterations in the prodrome are generally recognized by the owner. House dogs may show a tendency to wander and previously affectionate animals may become excitable and ill-tempered. The normally free-

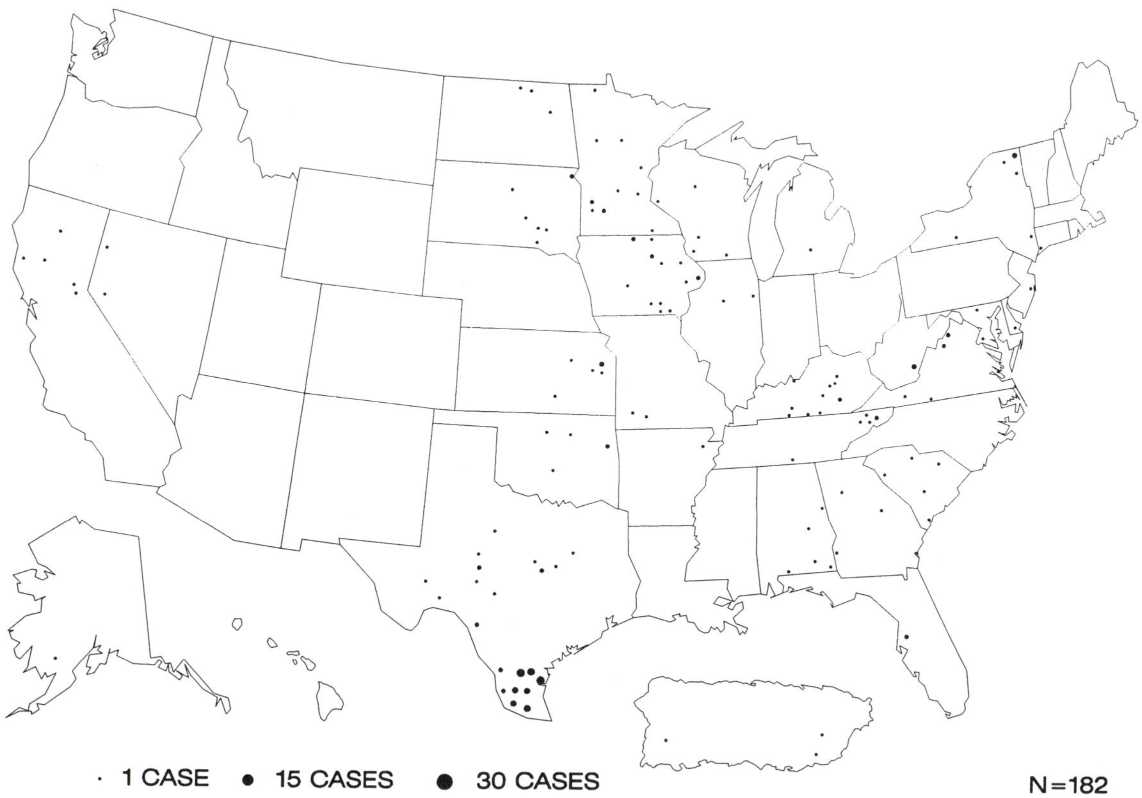

Figure 2-8. Reported cases of rabies in dogs, by county and municipio (Puerto Rico), 1992. Dot size is proportional to the number of cases in the county. (From Krebs, J. W., Strine, T. W., and J. E. Childs. Rabies surveillance in the United States during 1992. *J. Am. Vet. Med. Assoc.* 203(12): 1718, 1993. Reproduced with permission.)

roaming dog may become affectionate and home bound. Owners may be pleased by such a change in disposition, hardly suspecting its frightening cause. Rabid dogs generally recognize and respond to their owners and can still find their way home (Beran, 1981).

The aggressive stage is very pronounced. It usually lasts from 1 to 7 days, but may be as brief as a few hours. Rabid dogs are extremely irritable and tend to bite at anything, including people, other animals, cars, fence posts, houses, etc. Noise may invite attack. They may even snap at insects and imaginary objects. Their face conveys a look of alertness and anxiety. Periods of calm may alternate with those when the dog is "clearly mad." Rabid dogs frequently eat unusual objects (a condition known as pica), such as sticks, stones, straw, and earth, and then vomit. Prior to the 19th century, the presence of pica was a common means of diagnosing rabies in dogs (Tierkel, 1975).

Rabid dogs shun light, preferring to hide in dark places (photophobia) and may experience hyperesthesia (excessive sensitivity to sensory stimuli such as bright light, loud noises, gentle breezes, or touch). Irritability and aggressive tendencies increase and animals tend to wander aimlessly. If caged, they will viciously bite at cage bars and chains, often breaking teeth and damaging oral tissue in the process (Tierkel, 1975). The aggressive stage is followed by one of paralysis.

Signs of imminent paralysis include a change in the animal's bark ("rabies howl") due to paralysis of the laryngeal muscles. This is a choking-like sound and owners, thinking that the animal has a foreign object lodged in its throat, may reach into the animal's mouth and accidentally scratch themselves on the dog's teeth, unwittingly exposing themselves to infectious saliva.

Paralysis in affected dogs may begin at the

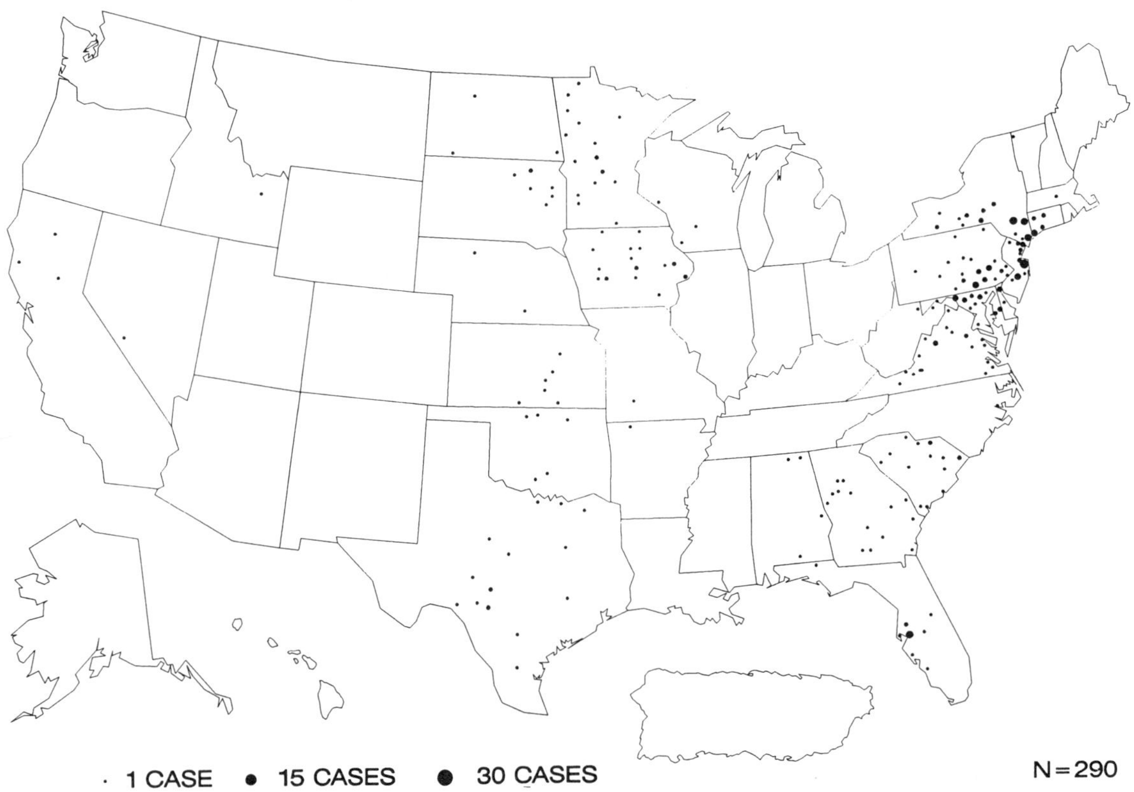

Figure 2-9. Reported cases of rabies in cats, by county, 1992. Dot size is proportional to the number of cases in the county. (From Krebs, J. W., Strine, T. W., and J. E. Childs. Rabies surveillance in the United States during 1992. *J. Am. Vet. Med. Assoc.* 203(12): 1718, 1993. Reproduced with permission.)

site of exposure, the hind limbs, or the jaw. It subsequently progresses throughout the body. Paralysis of the jaw is marked by a hanging jaw and protruding tongue. It is caused by paralysis of the muscles of mastication. At this stage, animals can neither eat nor drink and have saliva constantly drooling from their mouth. This is the most characteristic sign of the paralytic stage in dogs.

The paralytic stage, like the aggressive stage, may last from a few hours to a few days. In general, if the aggressive stage is long, the paralytic stage is short and vice versa. Thus, in a given rabid dog, aggression or paralysis may dominate. When the aggressive stage is preeminent, the condition is referred to as the furious form of rabies. In the dumb form of rabies, the paralytic stage is predominant and "the dog's appearance is such as to inspire pity rather than fear" (West, 1973). Furious or dumb rabies develops with about equal frequency. The entire clinical course of disease in dogs rarely exceeds ten days.

Unlike humans, rabid dogs do not develop an aversion to water (hydrophobia). They do try to drink but, because of a progressive paralysis, they are unable to swallow water. Saliva drools from the mouth and, as the animal breathes through the saliva, it foams with air. This leads to the classic image of the rabid dog, foaming at the mouth.

According to Parrish et al (1959), 39% of humans bitten by dogs are bitten on the lower extremities; 37% on the upper extremities; 16% on the head, face, and neck; and 8% on the trunk, back, and buttocks. Comparable figures were reported by Hanna and Selby (1981) and Szpakowski et al (1990). Age-related data are shown in Table 2-1. Human mortality following untreated bites by rabid dogs is approximately 15% when bitten on the hands or fingers, 60% when bitten on the face, and 50% when bitten elsewhere about the head. Comparable figures for cat bites are 20%, 70%, and 50%, respectively.

Unvaccinated dogs or cats that have been bitten by a suspected rabid animal should be destroyed immediately. If owners do not wish to comply with this recommendation, animals should be maintained in strict isolation for a period of six months and, pending no overt manifestations of neurologic disease, be vaccinated one month prior to release. In one experimental study, limited success was reported in protecting dogs against rabies using a post-exposure prophylaxis schedule and biologicals similar to those recommended for human patients (Cho and Lawson, 1989). Vaccinated dogs or cats that are bitten by a suspected rabid animal should be revaccinated immediately and carefully observed by the owner for a period of 45-90 days (National Association of State Public Health Veterinarians, 1992, 1993, 1994). In 1992, dogs accounted for 2.1% (182 of 8,645) of all animals reported rabid in the United States (Figure 2-8), a 17.4% increase over the number reported in 1991 (Krebs et al, 1992, 1993).

Table 2-1

Distribution of the Sites of Animal Bite Injuries for Children as well as Teenagers and Adults Evaluated at the Hermosillo Centro de Salud, 1 January to 31 December 1987

	Number of		
Site of Injury	Children	Teenagers & Adults	Total
Head, face or neck	47 (30)[a]	2 (2)	49; *19*[b]
Upper extremities	52 (33)	39 (38)	91; *35*
Trunk	16 (10)	4 (4)	20; *8*
Lower extremities	59 (38)	67 (65)	126; *48*

[a] Figures in parentheses indicate the percent of all persons in the age group concerned (157 children and 103 teenagers and adults). Column totals may be greater than the number of persons in an age group because some patients were bitten at more than one site.

[b] Figures in italics are the percent of the total number of individuals (260).

From Eng, T. R. et al. Urban epizootic of rabies in Mexico: Epidemiology and impact of animal bite injuries. *Bull. Wld. Hlth. Org.* 71(5): 615, 1993. Reproduced with permission.

Cats

Rabies in cats is similar, in most respects, to that in dogs. Cats are not primary reservoirs of rabies, however, and there is no feline-specific variant of virus. They are exposed by wild animal bites and become infected with the variant of virus present in local wildlife (Blancou and Pastoret, 1992a, 1992b; Rodl, 1992; Fogelman et al, 1993). In those countries in which effective vaccination programs have brought canine rabies under control, but in which sylvatic (wildlife) rabies remains prevalent, the incidence of rabies in cats may be greater than that in dogs (Bunn, 1991). Cats are highly susceptible to infection, but transmission from cat to cat is rare (Ott, 1983; Fogelman et al, 1993). The disease is not known to be self-perpetuating in cats.

The incubation period in cats has been observed to vary from 9 to 84 days. The prodromal period lasts a day at most and is marked by behavioral alterations which may include either an eagerness for human affection or a tendency towards solitude (Abelseth, 1987). Some cats may simply seek out a hiding place to die. The aggressive phase usually lasts 2 to 4 days, sometimes less than one or as long as seven. A furious phase in cats is almost always present and is very pronounced (Bunn, 1991; Blancou and Pastoret, 1992a, 1992b). If caged, they will bite and lash out with claws at all objects around them. The furious cat is an extremely dangerous animal, often lashing out at the head. According to Cushman (1960 [cited by Abelseth, 1987]),

> *...some become frankly maniacal, hurtling from an open cage, attacking attendants, and battering themselves against wall and furniture until they collapse from sheer exhaustion.*

Human exposure to cat bites forces many to seek post-exposure rabies prophylaxis (Diesch et al, 1982; Kihm et al, 1982; Sureau, 1990; Eng and Fishbein, 1990; Fogelman et al, 1993).

Increased sensitivity (hyperesthesia) may lead to violent spasms when touched. Rabid farm cats may attack cows. Unlike the rabid dog, which may often respond to and can be quieted by its owner (although owners may be bitten), the rabid cat is generally not responsive to family members. In the paralytic stage, the hanging jaw so typical of dogs is rarely observed (Vaughn, 1975). Muscles of deglutition, however, are paralyzed and eating or drinking is difficult. Death usually occurs within 3 to 5 days.

In 1988, 192 cases of cat rabies were reported in the United States (Centers for Disease Control, 1989). For the first time since the Centers for Disease Control began reporting in 1960, cats were the most commonly reported rabid domestic animal in the country. This trend continued in 1989, 1990, and 1992, with annual increases in the number of reported cases (Reid-Sanden et al, 1990; Krebs et al, 1992; Uhaa et al, 1992a). In 1992, 290 cases of rabid cats were reported (Figure 2-9), a 53.4% increase over the number reported in 1991. States reporting more than ten cases of cat rabies in 1992 were Connecticut, Florida, Georgia, Iowa, Maryland, Minnesota, New Jersey, New York, Pennsylvania, South Carolina, Texas, and Virginia (Krebs et al, 1993).

There is no general requirement for compulsory vaccination of cats in this country, although local ordinances in various states may require cat vaccination. Public and veterinary compliance with such ordinances, however, is variable. Legislating control measures for cat rabies is often met with considerable resistance (Diesch et al, 1982). One reason for this is the difficulty in establishing ownership of some outdoor cats. Farm cats, for example, while often appreciated because of their efficacy in rodent control, are generally not considered pets by farmers. In fact, farm cats may actually travel widely from one farm to another (Bunn, 1991). While the rural farm cat is most likely to come into contact with a rabid wild animal, all cats may be exposed to potentially rabid animals. Many reports exist of indoor cats interacting with commensal bats in homes and apartments (Frantz and Trimarchi, 1984; Frantz, 1988). All pet cats should be vaccinated against rabies (Diesch et al, 1982; Eng and Fishbein, 1990; Varughese, 1987; Blancou and Pastoret, 1992a, 1992b; Brass, 1993; Fogelman et al, 1993; Hoff et al, 1993; Spencer, 1994).

References

Abelseth, R. H. (1987). Rabies. In J. Holzworth (ed.) *Diseases of the Cat—Medicine and Surgery.* W. B. Saunders Co. Philadelphia.

Andral, L., Artois, M., Aubert, M. F. A., and J. Blancou (1982). Radio-tracking of rabid foxes. *Comp. Immunol. Microbiol. Infect. Dis.* 5(1-3): 113

AVMA Council on Biologic and Therapeutic Agents (1989). Canine and feline immunization guidelines. Council Report. *J. Am. Vet. Med. Assoc.* 195(3): 314

Beran, G. W. (1981). Rabies and Infections by Rabies-Related Viruses. In G. W. Beran (ed.) *CRC Handbook Series in Zoonosis. Section B: Viral Zoonoses.* Volume II. CRC Press, Inc. Boca Raton, Florida.

Blancou, J. and P.-P. Pastoret (1992a). Rabies and its prevention in cats (English abstract). *Recueil de Med. Vet. de L'Ecole D'Alfort.* 168(2): 117

Blancou, J. and P.-P. Pastoret (1992b). Rabies in cats and its prophylaxis (English abstract). *Magyar Allatorvosok Lapja.* 47(5): 217

Brass, D. A. (1993). Insectivorous bats as reservoirs of rabies. *Compen. Cont. Educ. Pract. Vet.* 15(12): 33

Bunn, T. O. (1991). Cat Rabies. In G. M. Baer (ed.) *The Natural History of Rabies.* 2nd Edition. CRC Press, Inc. Boca Raton, Florida.

Burridge, M. J., Sawyer, L. A., and W. J. Bigler (1986). *Rabies in Florida.* Health Program Office, Department of Health and Rehabilitative Services. Tallahassee, Florida.

Carey, A. B. (1985). Multispecies Rabies in the Eastern United States. In P. J. Bacon (ed.) *Population Dynamics of Rabies in Wildlife.* Academic Press. New York.

Cartter, M. L., Hadler, J. L., Smith, M. G., Sorhage, F. E., Spitalny, K. C., Debbie, J. G., Morse, D. L., Hunter, J. L., MacCormack, J. N., Smith, K. A., Halpin, T. J., Jenkins, S. R., and L. E. Haddy (1992). Extension of the raccoon rabies epizootic—United States, 1992. *MMWR.* 41(36): 661

Centers for Disease Control (1988). *Rabies Surveillance Report. Annual Summary for the Year 1987.* U. S. Department of Health and Human Services, Public Health Service. Atlanta, Georgia.

Centers for Disease Control (1989). *Rabies Surveillance Report. Annual Summary for the Year 1988.* U. S. Department of Health and Human Services, Public Health Service. Atlanta, Georgia.

Centers for Disease Control (1992). Editorial note. *J. Am. Med. Assoc.* 268(13): 1646

Cho, H. C. and K. F. Lawson (1989). Protection of dogs against death from experimental rabies by postexposure administration of rabies vaccine and hyperimmune globulin (human). *Can. J. Vet. Res.* 53: 434

Davidson, W. R., Appel, M. J., Doster, G. L., Baker, O. E., and J. F. Brown (1992). Diseases and parasites of red foxes, gray foxes, and coyotes from commercial sources selling to fox-chasing enclosures. *J. Wildl. Dis.* 28(4): 581

Diesch, S. L., Hendricks, S. L., and R. W. Currier (1982). The role of cats in human rabies exposures. *J. Am. Vet. Med. Assoc.* 181(12): 1510

Eng, T. R. and D. B. Fishbein (1990). Epidemiologic factors, clinical findings, and vaccination status of rabies in cats and dogs in the United States in 1988. *J. Am. Vet. Med. Assoc.* 197(2): 201

Eng, T. R., Fishbein, D. B., Talamante, H. E., Hall, D. B., Chavez, G. F., Dobbins, J. G., Muro, F. J., Bustos, J. L., de los Angeles Ricardy, M., Munguia, A., Carrasco, J., Robles, A. R., and G. M. Baer (1993). Urban epizootic of rabies in Mexico: Epidemiology and impact of animal bite injuries. *Bull. Wld. Hlth. Org.* 71(5): 615

Fogelman, V., Fischman, H. R., Horman, J. T., and J. K. Grigor (1993). Epidemiologic and clinical characteristics of rabies in cats. *J. Am. Vet. Med. Assoc.* 202(11): 1829

Frantz, S. C. (1988). Architecture and Commensal Vertebrate Pest Management. In R. B. Kundsin (ed.) *Architectural Design and Indoor Microbial Pollution.* Oxford University Press. New York.

Frantz, S. C. and C. V. Trimarchi (1984). Bats in human dwellings: Health concerns and management. In D. J. Decker (ed.) *Proceedings of the First Eastern Wildlife Damage Control Conference.* Cornell University. Ithaca, New York. September 27-30, 1984

Hanna, T. L. and L. A. Selby (1981). Characteristics of the human and pet populations in animal bite incidents recorded at two air force bases. *Pub. Hlth. Repts.* 96(6): 580

Hoff, G. L., Mellon, G. F., Thomas, M. C., and D. H. Giedinghagen (1993). Bats, cats, and rabies in an urban community. *South. Med. J.* 88(10): 1115

Israel, E., Hays, C. W., Miller, G. B., Haddy, L. E., and M. E. Levy (1982). Rabies: Mid-Atlantic States. *MMWR.* 31(44): 592

Jenkins, S. R., Perry, B. D., and W. G. Winkler (1988). Ecology and epidemiology of raccoon rabies. *Rev. Infect. Dis.* 10(Suppl. 4): S621

Kihm, U., Lazarowicz, M., Bommeli, W., and R. Zutter (1982). Potency of two rabies vaccines in cats as determined by antibody assay and virulent virus challenge. *Comp. Immunol. Microbiol. Infect. Dis.* 5(1-3): 227

Krebs, J. W., Holman, R. C., Hines, U., Strine, T. W., Mandel, E. J., and J. E. Childs (1992). Rabies surveillance in the United States during 1991. *J. Am. Vet. Med. Assoc.* 201(12): 1836

Krebs, J. W., Strine, T. W., and J. E. Childs (1993). Rabies surveillance in the United States during 1992. *J. Am. Vet. Med. Assoc.* 203(12): 1718

Macdonald, D. W. (1980). *Rabies in Wildlife—A Biologist's Perspective.* Oxford University Press. Earth Resources Research Limited. New York.

National Association of State Public Health Veterinarians (1992). Compendium of Animal Rabies Control. *J. Am. Vet. Med. Assoc.* 200(2): 145

National Association of State Public Health Veterinarians (1993). Compendium of Animal Rabies

Control. *J. Am. Vet. Med. Assoc.* 202(2): 199

National Association of State Public Health Veterinarians (1994). Compendium of Animal Rabies Control. *J. Am. Vet. Med. Assoc.* 204(2): 173

Nettles, V. F., Shaddock, J. H., Sikes, R. K., and C. R. Reyes (1979). Rabies in translocated raccoons. *Am. J. Pub. Hlth.* 69: 601

Ott, R. L. (1983). Neurologic Viral Infections. In P. W. Pratt (ed.) *Feline Medicine*. American Veterinary Publishing, Inc. Goleta, California.

Pacer, R. E., Fishbein, D. B., Baer, G. M., Jenkins, S. R., and J. S. Smith (1985). Rabies in the United States and Canada, 1983. *MMWR.* 34(1SS): 11SS

Parrish, H., Clack, F. B., Brobst, D., and J. F. Mock (1959). Epidemiology of dog bites. *Pub. Hlth. Repts.* 74: 891

Reid-Sanden, F. L., Dobbins, J. G., Smith, J. S., and D. B. Fishbein (1990). Rabies surveillance in the United States during 1989. *J. Am. Vet. Med. Assoc.* 197(12): 1571

Rodl, P. (1992). Health impact of stray and wild cats on the environment of man (English abstract). *Ceskoslovenska Epidemiologie Mikrobiologie Immunologie.* 41(3): 169

Rossate, R. C., MacInnes, C. D., Power, M. J., Johnston, D. H., Bachmann, P., Nunan, C. P., Wannop, C., Pedde, M., and L. Calder (1993). Tactics for the control of wildlife rabies in Ontario (Canada). *Rev. Sci. Tech. Off. Int. Epiz.* 12(1): 95

Rupprecht, C. E., Glickman, L. T., Spencer, P. A., and T. J. Wiktor (1987). Epidemiology of rabies virus variants: Discrimination using monoclonal antibodies and discriminant analysis. *Am. J. Epidemiol.* 126(2): 298

Smith, W. G. (1992). Rabies in New York and New England States, 1990-1991. *Anim. Hlth. Insights.* 1992: 19

Smith, J. S. and G. M. Baer (1988). Epizootiology of Rabies in North and South America. In *Developments in Veterinary Virology*. Martinus Nijhoff. Boston.

Smith, J. S., Sumner, J. W., Roumillat, L. F., Baer, G. M., and W. G. Winkler (1984). Antigenic characteristics of isolates associated with a new epizootic of raccoon rabies in the United States. *J. Infect. Dis.* 149(5): 769

Smith, J. S., Reid-Sanden, F. L., Roumillat, L. F., Trimarchi, C., Clark, K., Baer, G. M., and W. G. Winkler (1986). Demonstration of antigenic variation among rabies virus isolates by using monoclonal antibodies to nucleocapsid proteins. *J. Clin. Microbiol.* 24(4): 573

Smith, J. S., Yager, P. A., Bigler, W. J., and E. D. Hartwig, Jr. (1990). Surveillance and epidemiologic mapping of monoclonal antibody-defined rabies variants in Florida. *J. Wildl. Dis.* 26(4): 473

Spencer, L. M. (1994). Taking a bite out of rabies. *J. Am. Vet. Med. Assoc.* 204(4): 479

Sureau, P. (1990). Recent data on the epidemiology and prophylaxis of human rabies in France. *Comp. Immunol. Microbiol. Infect. Dis.* 13(2): 107

Szpakowski, N. M., Bonnett, D. M., and S. W. Martin (1990). An epidemiological investigation into the reported incidents of dog biting in the city of Guelph (Ontario, Canada). *Can. Vet. J.* 30(12): 937

Tierkel, E. S. (1975). Canine Rabies. In G. M. Baer (ed.) *The Natural History of Rabies*. Vol. II. Academic Press. New York.

Trimarchi, C. V. (1990). *New York State Rabies Annual Summary, 1989.* Wadsworth Center for Laboratories and Research, New York State Department of Health. Albany, New York.

Trimarchi, C. V. (1991). *New York State Rabies Annual Summary, 1990.* Wadsworth Center for Laboratories and Research, New York State Department of Health. Albany, New York.

Trimarchi, C. V. (1992). *New York State Rabies Annual Summary, 1991.* Wadsworth Center for Laboratories and Research, New York State Department of Health. Albany, New York.

Trimarchi, C. V. (1993a). *New York State Rabies Annual Summary, 1992.* Wadsworth Center for Laboratories and Research, New York State Department of Health. Albany, New York.

Trimarchi, C. V. (1993b). *Laboratory confirmed rabies in New York State, 1/1/93-5/30/93.* Wadsworth Center for Laboratories and Research, New York State Department of Health. Albany, New York.

Trimarchi, C. V. (1994). *New York State Rabies Annual Summary, 1993.* Wadsworth Center for Laboratories and Research, New York State Department of Health. Albany, New York.

Uhaa, I. J., Mandel, E. J., Whiteway, R., and D. B. Fishbein (1992a). Rabies surveillance in the United States during 1990. *J. Am. Vet. Med. Assoc.* 200(7): 920

Uhaa, I. J., Dato, V. M., Sorhage, F. E., Beckley, J. W., Roscoe, D. E., Gorsky, R. D., and D. B. Fishbein (1992b). Benefits and costs of using an orally absorbed vaccine to control rabies in raccoons. *J. Am. Vet. Med. Assoc.* 201(12): 1873

Varughese, P. V. (1987). Rabies and post-exposure treatment in Canada—1985. *Can. Dis. Wkly. Rept.* 13(5): 17

Vaughn, J. B. (1975). Cat Rabies. In G. M. Baer (ed.) *The Natural History of Rabies*. Vol. II. Academic Press. New York.

West, G. P. (1973). *Rabies in Animals and Man.* Arco Publishing Co., Inc. New York.

Winkler, W. G. (1985). Current Status of Rabies in the United States. In W. G. Winkler (ed.) *Rabies Concepts for Medical Professionals*. Merieux Institute, Inc. Miami, Florida.

World Health Organization (1992). *Expert Committee on Rabies. Eighth Report*. WHO Tech. Rpt. No. 824. Geneva.

Chapter 3:
RABIES IN HUMANS

Prevalence of Human Rabies in the United States

Human rabies is presently an uncommon condition in the United States. In the years following the mid-1950's, the number of reported cases declined markedly (Figure 3-1). This drastic fall in human disease was directly related to the introduction of canine immunization programs in the late 1940's (Burridge et al, 1986). The scarcity of human deaths, however, does not mean that rabies is no longer a threat to human health. It has been estimated that between 215 and 809 people per 100,000 are bitten by animals each year in the United States (Currier, II et al, 1975). Approximately 20,000 to 30,000 receive post-exposure rabies prophylaxis annually (Helmick, 1986), at an average cost of about $500 to $1,000 per exposure.

Administration of post-exposure rabies prophylaxis is seasonal, peaking in spring, summer, and fall (Figure 3-2). This coincides with the times of greatest human contact with wild and domesticated animals (Helmick, 1983, 1986). The incidence of post-exposure rabies prophylaxis is higher in rural areas (Figure 3-3), where human/animal contacts are statistically more probable, and in younger persons (Figure 3-4),

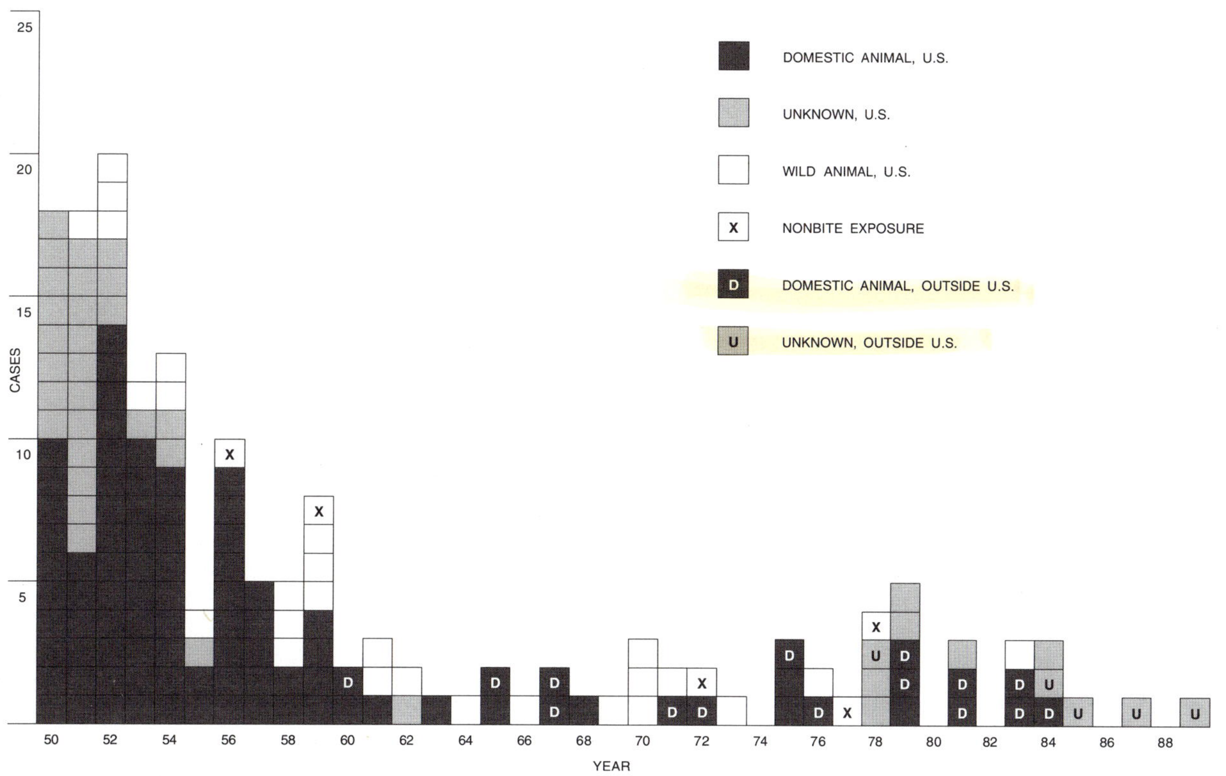

Figure 3-1. Human Rabies in the United States, 1950-1989, including two Americans who died outside of the United States. (From Fishbein, D. Rabies in Humans. In G. M. Baer (ed.) *The Natural History of Rabies*. 2nd Edition. © CRC Press, Inc. Boca Raton, Florida, 1991. Redrawn with permission.)

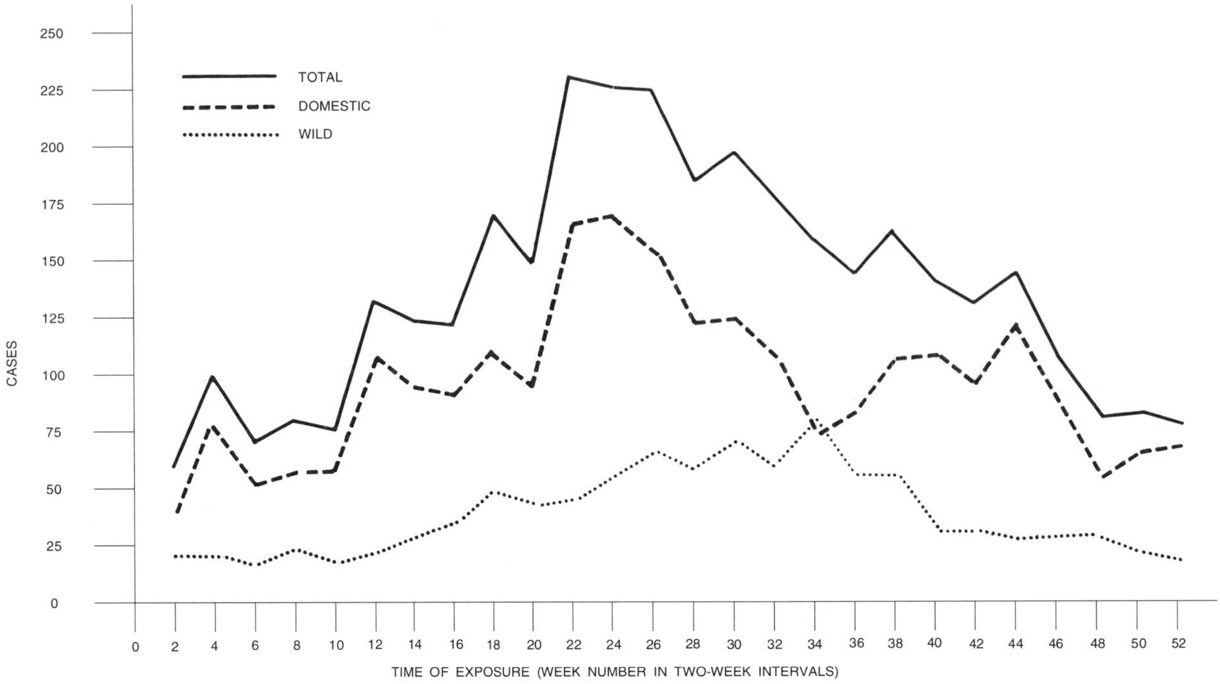

Figure 3-2. Post-exposure rabies prophylaxis, by week and type of animal exposure, 20 states, 1981. (From Helmick, C. G. The Epidemiology of Human Rabies Postexposure Prophylaxis, 1980-1981. *J. Am. Med. Assoc.* 250(15): 1990, 1983. Redrawn with permission.)

who are believed to have more frequent animal contacts (Helmick, 1983, 1986; Eng et al, 1993).[1] Although a large percentage of these exposures do not warrant post-exposure rabies prophylaxis, the fact that treatments are administered is an expression of the concern that medical authorities have for this disease.

Major Sources of Human Exposure to Virus

Although domestic animals account for the majority of animal bites, they do not cause the majority of human exposures to rabies virus in the United States (Martin et al, 1969; Currier, II et al, 1975). Results of epidemiologic studies in the United States during 1981 indicated that domestic animals accounted for approximately 66% of post-exposure rabies prophylaxis, despite the fact that they accounted for only about 13% of proven rabid animals (Helmick, 1986). Thus, as Helmick observed, "...domestic animals, especially dogs and cats, play a significant role in post exposure [rabies] prophylaxis—far out of proportion to their small role as animal rabies vectors." Wildlife, on the other hand, only accounted for about 28% of post-exposure rabies prophylaxis, even though they constituted as much as 87% of proven rabid animals. "Thus, wild animals play a relatively smaller role in human post exposure [rabies] prophylaxis—far out of proportion to their large role in animal rabies" (Helmick, 1986). These findings are consistent with the relative extent of human contact with wild and domestic species (Table 3-1).

Pre-Exposure Rabies Prophylaxis

Once the nervous system has become infected with the rabies virus, the disease is almost universally fatal. No effective medical therapy yet exists. As such, the major efforts of the biomedical community have focused on the development

[1]Human fatality from rabies throughout the Americas is also more common among younger persons (Figure 3-5).

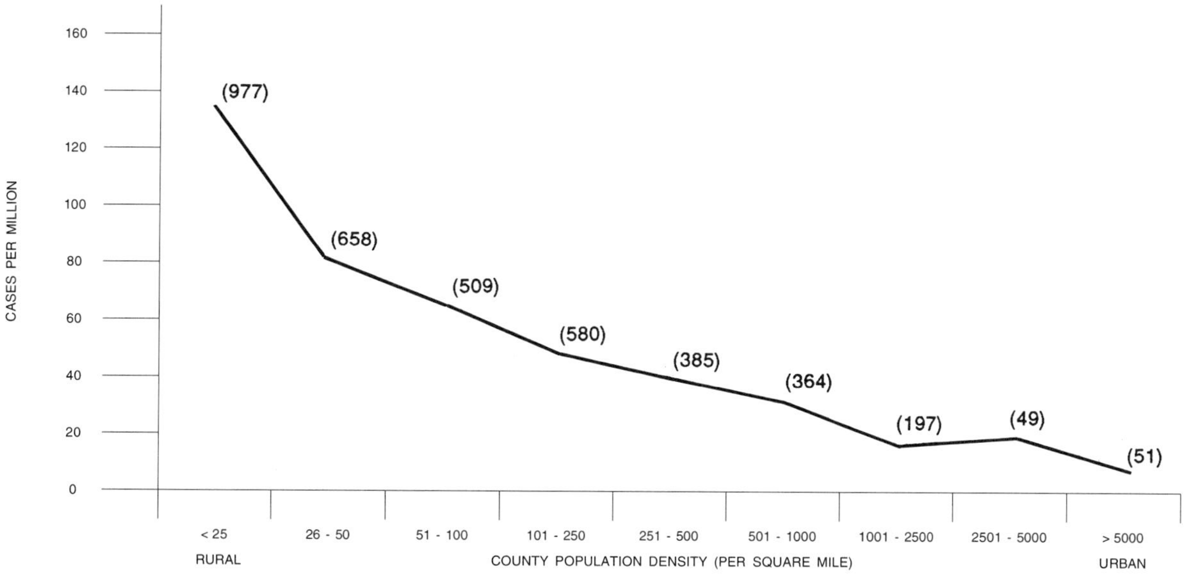

Figure 3-3. Incidence of post-exposure rabies prophylaxis, by population density of county of exposure, 21 states, 1981. Numbers in parentheses represent the actual number of cases. (From Helmick, C. G. The Epidemiology of Human Rabies Postexposure Prophylaxis, 1980-1981. *J. Am. Med. Assoc.* 250(15): 1990, 1983. Redrawn with permission.)

of effective prophylaxis, of both a pre- and post-exposure nature.

The value of pre-exposure rabies immunization lies in its capacity to afford a margin of protection for those individuals who have been unknowingly exposed to rabies virus and for those in whom an exposure is known, but there is a delay in initiation of proper post-exposure therapy. Pre-exposure immunization simplifies, but does not eliminate, the need for post-exposure rabies prophylaxis following exposure to a potentially rabid animal.

Persons generally considered to be at high risk of exposure, and who often undergo routine pre-exposure immunization, include veterinarians, veterinary students, veterinary hospital employees, animal control officers, animal handlers in zoos, and wildlife workers. Pre-exposure immunization is also very important for professional staff working in rabies research and diagnostic laboratories. People living in or visiting developing countries in which rabies is endemic or where post-exposure rabies prophylaxis with potent vaccines is not readily available, may also be candidates for pre-exposure immunization (Centers for Disease Control, 1984a, 1984b, 1985; Nicholson, 1987; Kagawa et al, 1992; World Health Organization, 1992; Wilde et al, 1994). The Immunization Practices Advisory Committee recommends that anyone whose vocational or avocational pursuits bring him into contact with potentially rabid animals consider pre-exposure immunization (Centers for Disease Control, 1991). Rabies also presents an unpredictable threat to field soldiers operating in theaters in which the disease is prevalent (Jorgenson, 1990; Flores-Crespo, 1991).

Approximately 18,000 people are pre-exposure immunized against rabies in the United States annually (Centers for Disease Control, 1991). Criteria for pre-exposure rabies prophylaxis recommended by the Immunization Practices Advisory Committee (Centers for Disease Control, 1991) are shown in Table 3-2. Despite the fact that this table places spelunkers in a category of frequent-risk exposure, there is no substantive evidence to justify this classification. This does not mean that pre-exposure rabies immunization is not justified. But the chances of a spelunker being exposed to a rabid animal (i.e., a bat) pall by comparison with other individuals in the same risk category.

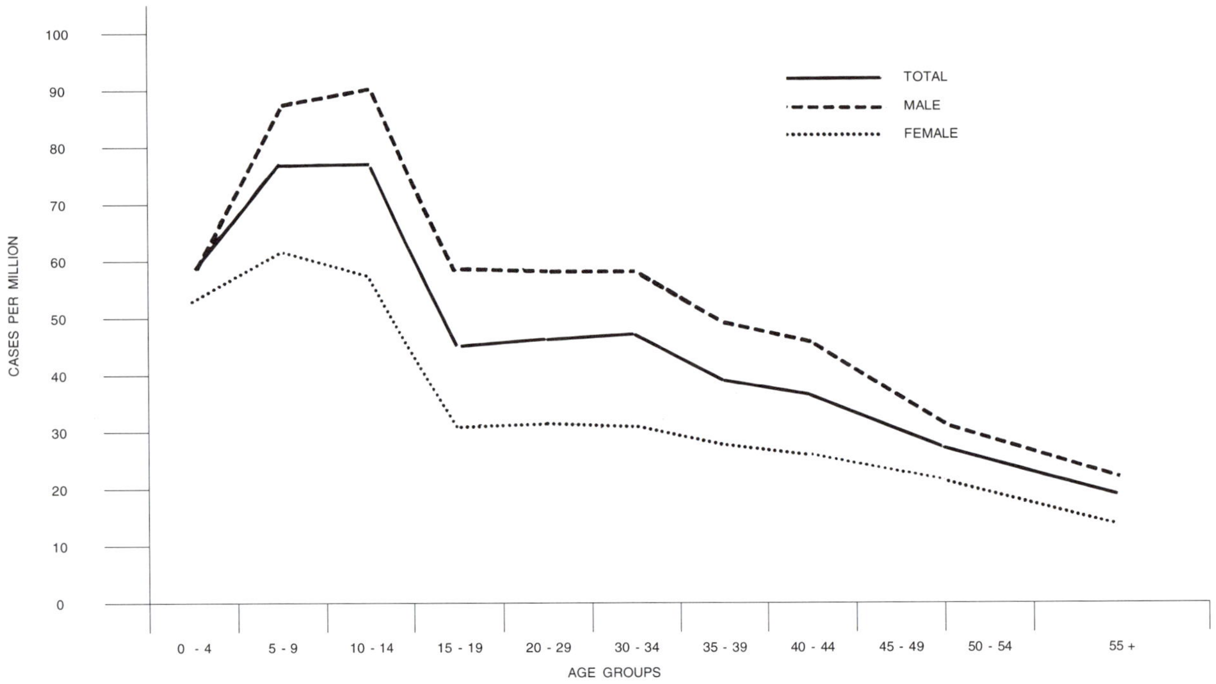

Figure 3-4. Incidence of post-exposure rabies prophylaxis, by age group and sex, 21 states, 1981. (From Helmick, C. G. The Epidemiology of Human Rabies Postexposure Prophylaxis, 1980-1981. *J. Am. Med. Assoc.* 250(15): 1990, 1983. Redrawn with permission.)

Three doses of vaccine (days 0, 7, and 21 or 28) are used for pre-exposure rabies prophylaxis. These are administered either intramuscularly (deltoid region of adults or the anterolateral thigh in small children) or intradermally. If traveling to malaria-endemic countries, physicians should be advised prior to initiation of either rabies or malarial prophylaxis. Requirements for serum testing (to determine level of neutralizing antibody in the blood) vary with the risk status of the individual (World Health Organization, 1992). However, the assumption of an adequate immune response (in the absence of serologic testing) in those immunized intradermally has recently been questioned (Trimarchi and Safford, Jr., 1992).

Post-Exposure Rabies Prophylaxis

The need for post-exposure rabies prophylaxis requires a careful consideration of the circumstances surrounding an encounter with a potentially rabid animal. Prior to making a decision, the attending physician may find it necessary to consult with public-health authorities. Numerous factors must be taken into account when making decisions regarding the need for post-exposure rabies prophylaxis (Fishbein, 1991a; Hemachudha et al, 1991; World Health Organization, 1992; Fishbein and Robinson, 1993; Dutta and Dutta, 1994) and include:

1) The nature of the contact.
2) The presence of rabies in the area where the exposure occurred or from which the animal involved came.
3) The species of animal involved.
4) The vaccination and clinical status of the exposing animal, the type of vaccine used, and the availability of the animal for observation or testing.
5) The results of laboratory testing of the animal for rabies, if available.

Categories of injury that have been adopted by the World Health Organization and which also need to be taken into consideration are outlined in Table 3-3. Recommendations for post-expo-

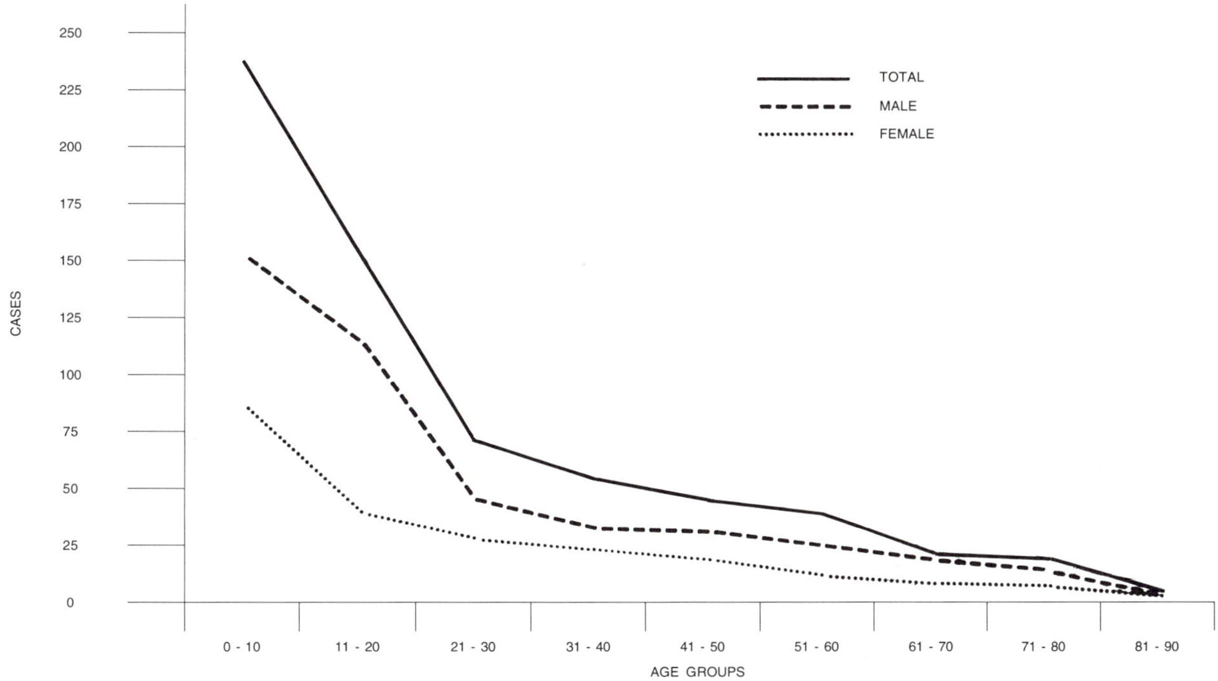

Figure 3-5. Distribution of 635 cases of human rabies in the Americas, by age group and sex, 1986-1990. (Data from *Epidemiological Surveillance of Rabies for the Americas*. Pan American Zoonoses Center, Pan American Health Organization.

sure rabies prophylaxis may vary in areas of enzootic dog rabies (Hemachudha et al, 1991).

Post-exposure rabies prophylaxis, following exposure to a potentially rabid animal, includes both proper wound management and the administration of appropriate biologicals. Wound management must entail immediate and thorough cleansing with soap and water, followed by application of either alcohol, tincture or aqueous solution of iodine, or quaternary ammonium compounds. A physician should then be contacted immediately. In view of the recently reported possibility of lengthy incubation times (as long as 6 to 7 years) for human rabies (Smith et al, 1991; Bek et al, 1992; Grattan-Smith et al, 1992; McColl et al, 1993), post-exposure rabies prophylaxis should still be obtained, even if a long period of time has elapsed since the original exposure (World Health Organization, 1992). Pregnancy is not a contraindication to treatment (see page 223).

For persons not previously immunized against rabies, both rabies human diploid cell vaccine (HDCV) and human or equine rabies immunoglobulin (HRIG or ERIG) are administered.[2] A skin test must be performed prior to the admini-

[2]Because of the high costs of HRIG, the potential for adverse reactions when using immune sera from animals (ERIG), the potential danger of transmitting human pathogens as a result of inappropriate inactivating procedures or inadequate choice of donors, and the possibility of developing more specific protection regimens, several investigators have suggested the potential for use of selective monoclonal antibodies in post-exposure rabies prophylaxis (Dietzschold et al, 1990; Lafon et al, 1990; Dietzschold and Ertl, 1991; Enssle et al, 1991; World Health Organization, 1990, 1992; Montano-Hirose et al, 1993). A "cocktail" of monoclonal antibodies of differing specificities may be helpful in obviating possible development of escape variants. These have been successful in experimental trials, although in some experimental studies, monoclonal antibodies interfered with the ability of test animals to mount an antibody response to rabies vaccine (Schumacher et al, 1992). Use of interferon and interferon-inducers are also being evaluated (World Health Organization, 1992).

Table 3-1

Source Characteristics of Human Rabies Exposure[a]

Source of Exposure	Percentage of Persons Receiving PEP	Percentage of Rabid Animals	Frequency of Rabies in Animals Examined	Percentage of Sources Exposing Two or More Persons
		All Sources		
Domestic Animals	66%	13%	1.8%	14%
Wild Animals	28%	87%	16.4%	8%
"Pet" Wild Animals	5%	<1%		33%
Lab Accidents	1%			8%
Human Cases	1%			100%
Unknown	1%			1%
Total	100%	100%		
		Animal Sources		
Dogs (D)[b]	32%	2%	0.7%	10%
Cats (D)	23%	4%	1.1%	12%
Bats (W)	10%	11%	9.6%	4%
Raccoons (W)	8%	10%	11.0%	10%
Cattle (D)	8%	5%	13.8%	44%
Skunks (W)	6%	63%	49.9%	13%
Other Domestic[c]	3%	1%	7.6%	52%
Other Wild[c]	2%	<1%	1.9%	6%
Foxes (W)	1%	3%	12.3%	19%
Rodents or Lagomorphs	2%	<<1%	0.05%	2%
"Pet" Raccoons	3%			75%
"Pet" Fox				100%
"Pet" Skunks				60%
Other "Pet" Wild[c]				15%
Total	100%	100%		

[a] Based on data from 20 states reporting exposures and animal rabies surveillance for the 12 months of 1981 only. Wild animals are not classified as pets, so they are all considered to be truly wild animals for calculating these figures.

[b] Letter in parentheses describes source as domestic (D) or wild (W) animal.

[c] Other domestic animals (persons exposed)—49 horses (131 persons), 7 sheep (24), 6 pigs (7), 1 mule (6), and 3 goats (5). Other wild animals—32 opossums (32), 12 coyotes (13), 9 wild felines (11), 3 badgers (9), 3 wolves (7), 4 minks (5), 4 weasels (4), 3 ring tails (3), 2 coatimundi (2), 2 wild pigs (2), 1 mongoose (1), 1 woodchuck (1), and 1 otter (1). Other "pet" wild—9 ferrets (13), 7 monkeys (7), 1 lion (1), 1 tiger (1), 1 bear (1), and 1 coyote (1).

From Helmick, C. G. The Epidemiology of Human Rabies Postexposure Prophylaxis in the United States. In D. B. Fishbein, L. A. Sawyer, and W. G. Winkler (eds.) *Rabies Concepts for Medical Professionals*. 2nd Edition. Merieux Institute. Miami, Florida, 1986. Reproduced by permission of Connaught Laboratories.

Table 3-2

Criteria for Pre-Exposure Rabies Prophylaxis

Risk Category: Rare (population-at-large)	
Nature of Risk	Exposure always episodic, with source recognized; mucous membrane or bite exposure.
Typical Populations	U.S. population-at-large, including hunters, trappers, and most individuals in rabies-epizootic areas.
Pre-Exposure Regimen	No pre-exposure immunization.
Risk Category: Infrequent (greater than population-at-large)	
Nature of Risk	Exposure nearly always episodic, with source recognized; mucous membrane, bite, or nonbite exposure.
Typical Populations	Veterinarians and animal control and wildlife workers in areas of low rabies endemnicity.
Pre-Exposure Regimen	Primary pre-exposure immunization course; no routine booster immunization or serology.
Risk Category: Frequent	
Nature of Risk	Exposure usually episodic, with source recognized, but exposure may also be unrecognized; aerosol, mucous membrane, bite, or nonbite exposure.
Typical Populations	Rabies diagnostic laboratory workers, spelunkers, veterinarians, and animal control and wildlife workers in rabies epizootic areas.
Pre-Exposure Regimen	Primary pre-exposure immunization course; booster immunization or serology every two years.
Risk Category: Continuous	
Nature of Risk	Virus present continuously in high concentrations; specific exposures may go unrecognized; aerosol, mucous membrane, bite, or nonbite exposure possible.
Typical Populations	Rabies research laboratory workers; rabies biologics production workers.
Pre-Exposure Regimen	Primary pre-exposure immunization course; serology every six months; booster immunization when antibody titer falls below an acceptable level.

From the Centers for Disease Control. Recommendations of the Immunization Practices Advisory Committee (ACIP). Rabies Prevention—United States, 1991. *MMWR.* 40(No. RR-3): 1, 1991. Reproduced with permission.

stration of ERIG. Rabies vaccine will stimulate an immune response in the victim, resulting in the production of neutralizing antibodies against the rabies virus. This requires about 7 to 10 days to occur. In the interim, the HRIG, which consists of pre-formed rabies-neutralizing antibodies derived from the plasma of hyperimmunized donors, will provide passive protection for category III exposures (Table 3-3).

Up to 50% of the HRIG is administered at the site of the wound, if possible. The remainder is given intramuscularly in the gluteal region. Rabies vaccine is administered intramuscularly in the deltoid region, although the anterolateral as-

Table 3-3

Guide for Post-Exposure Rabies Treatment

Category	Type of contact with a suspect or confirmed rabid domestic or wild[a] animal, or animal unavailable for observation	Recommended post-exposure treatment
I	Touching or feeding of animals. Licks on intact skin.	None, if reliable case history is available.
II	Nibbling of uncovered skin. Minor scratches or abrasions without bleeding. Licks on broken skin.	Administer rabies vaccine immediately.[b] Stop treatment if animal remains healthy throughout an observation period[c] of 10 days, or if animal is humanely killed and found to be negative for rabies by appropriate laboratory techniques.
III	Single or multiple transdermal bites or scratches. Contamination of mucous membrane with saliva (i.e., licks).	Administer rabies immunoglobulin and rabies vaccine immediately.[b] Stop treatment if animal remains healthy throughout an observation period[c] of 10 days, or if animal is humanely killed and found to be negative for rabies by appropriate laboratory techniques.

[a] Exposure to rodents, rabbits, and hares seldom, if ever, requires specific anti-rabies treatment.
[b] If an apparently healthy dog or cat in or from a low-risk area is placed under observation, the situation may warrant delaying initiation of treatment.
[c] This observation period applies only to dogs and cats. Except in the case of threatened or endangered species, other domestic and wild animals suspected as rabid should be humanely killed and their tissues examined using appropriate laboratory techniques.

From the World Health Organization. *Expert Committee on Rabies. Eighth Report.* Annex 2. WHO Tech. Rpt. No. 824. Geneva, 1992. Reproduced with permission.

pect of the thigh may be used for vaccine administration in children. It should never be administered in the gluteal region. Vaccine is administered as soon as possible (day 0) following exposure. Additional doses are given on days 3, 7, 14, and 30. Intradermal administration of vaccine is also possible, but should be done only by staff specifically trained in this technique (World Health Organization, 1992). Recommendations for abbreviated schedules are being evaluated (World Health Organization, 1992).

Post-exposure rabies prophylaxis in nonimmunized persons who have sustained a category III exposure requires administration of both HRIG and vaccine. For those who have been pre-exposure immunized against rabies with a modern cell-culture vaccine, have previously received a full course of post-exposure rabies prophylaxis with a potent cell-culture vaccine, or have been immunized with other vaccines and have a documented titer of rabies-neutralizing antibodies, post-exposure rabies prophylaxis consists of administration of vaccine only. HRIG should not be administered.

Two intramuscular or intradermal doses of vaccine are required, one immediately and a second one three days later. Individuals who may have previously received pre- or post-exposure treatments with vaccines of unproven potency, or without a documented antibody titer, should receive a complete course of post-exposure rabies prophylaxis, including immunoglobulin if needed (World Health Organization, 1992). Regardless of the immune status of the patient and the sub-

MAIN CLINICAL ABNORMALITIES	None	Fever Anorexia, nausea, vomiting Headache Malaise, lethargy Pain or paresthesias at site of bite	Anxiety, agitation, depression Hyperventilation, hypoxia Aphasia, incoordination or other CNS signs Paresis, paralysis Hydrophobia, pharyngeal spasms Confusion, delirium, hallucinations Marked hyperactivity	Pituitary dysfunction Hypoventilation, apnea Hypotension Cardiac arrhythmia, cardiac arrest	Pneumothorax Intravascular thrombosis Secondary infection
	Exposure	First symptom	First neurological sign	Onset of coma	Death occurs or recovery begins
Clinical Stage	Incubation Period	Prodrome	Acute Neurological Phase	Coma	Recovery
Usual Duration	18 to 60 days	2 to 10 days	2 to 7 days	0 to 14 days	Several Months

Figure 3-6. The natural history of clinical rabies in man, hypothetical composite case. All clinical abnormalities need not be present in each case. (From Bernard, K. W. Clinical Rabies in Humans. In D. B. Fishbein, L. A. Sawyer, and W. G. Winkler (eds.) *Rabies Concepts for Medical Professionals.* 2nd Edition. Merieux Institute, Inc. Miami, Florida, 1986. Reproduced by permission of Connaught Laboratories.)

sequent post-exposure rabies prophylaxis regimen used, immediate wound cleansing is always essential.

If exposure to a potentially rabid animal occurs while abroad, careful consideration must be given to the adequacy of medical attention available locally (Campbell, 1993). It is imperative that human diploid vaccine (and rabies immunoglobulin, if required) be administered. In general, American victims are well advised to seek attention at a U. S. Embassy or Consulate. If these are not readily accessible, American Mission Hospitals or hospitals in large urban centers often have proper (and efficacious) vaccines available (Beran, 1988).

According to Recommendations of the Immunization Practices Advisory Committee (Centers for Disease Control, 1991),

> *U.S. citizens and residents who are exposed to rabies while traveling outside the United States in countries where rabies is endemic may sometimes receive post-exposure therapy with regimens or biologics that are not used in the United States... If post-exposure treatment is begun outside the United States using one of these regimens or biologics of nerve tissue origin, it may be necessary to provide additional treatment when the patient reaches the United States. State or lo-*

cal health departments should be contacted for specific advice in such cases.

Clinical Manifestations

The clinical signs of rabies in humans are similar, in many respects, to those observed in animals. Even though the virus is widely disseminated throughout the body, the predominant clinical features are manifestations of a viral encephalomyelitis and are, therefore, neurological in nature (Figure 3-6). Clinical manifestations in any one individual may, to some extent, be a reflection of the variant of virus involved, as well as of several host-related factors (Lanska, 1992). The disease in humans is generally divided into five phases: incubation period, prodromal phase, acute neurologic phase, coma, and death (Koprowski, 1979; Corey, 1983; Bernard, 1985; Muhsin, 1986).

The incubation period is highly variable. Some of the factors involved include location and severity of the bite (or bites), density of peripheral nerves at the site of injury, dose of virus inoculated into the wound, variant of infecting virus, and the age and immunologic status of the victim.

Clinical signs might appear in as short a time as 9 to 10 days or as long as one year or more following exposure. On average, disease becomes evident within 1 to 3 months of exposure, with a tendency for the incubation period to be shorter if the site of bite is on the head, compared to an extremity. Of 1,555 cases of human rabies for which the incubation period was known, 0% had an incubation period less than 10 days, 29.8% (464) had an incubation period of 10 to 30 days, 54.4% (846) had an incubation period of 31 to 90 days, 14.5% (226) had an incubation period of 91 to 365 days, and 1.2% (19) had an incubation period greater than 365 days (Fishbein, 1991b). Incubation times may be shorter in children. Recent evidence is consistent with incubation times in humans extending for as long as 6 to 7 years on rare occasions (Smith et al, 1991, 1992; Bek et al, 1992; Grattan-Smith et al, 1992; Smith and Seidel, 1993). With the exception of the bite trauma itself, there is no evidence of illness during the incubation period of the disease.

Clinical symptoms are first noted during the prodromal phase. Initially, they are nonspecific and begin with vague feelings of malaise. Early symptoms include pruritus (itching) at the site of exposure, headache, fatigue, sore throat, nonproductive (dry) cough, chills, nausea and vomiting, diarrhea, abdominal pain, anorexia, hyperesthesia, and a fever (as high as 105° F). There may be pain and paresthesia (abnormal sensations). Paresthesia may manifest as burning, pricking, and tingling at the site of exposure or as a feeling of ants crawling over the body (formication). A prodromal feeling of fear may manifest as a sense of impending doom (Beran, 1992).

The prodromal period (2 to 10 days in duration) is followed by a period of acute neurologic signs that may include depression, disorientation, incoordination, dilated and irregular pupils, double vision, optic neuritis, facial palsies, stiff neck, increased lacrimation, salivation and perspiration, postural hypotension, paralysis of vocal cords, difficulty swallowing, seizures, paresis (partial loss of motor function due to neurologic impairment in one or more limbs), and paralysis (complete loss of motor function in one or more limbs) that may be either upper motor neuron (UMN) or lower motor neuron (LMN) in nature. Involvement of the amygdaloid nucleus in the brain may result in priapism (persistent penile erection unrelated to sexual stimulation) and spontaneous ejaculation. These are common features of the human disease and often a source of embarrassment for the patient.

Neurologic abnormalities are of a furious nature in about 80% of cases (Fishbein, 1991b). These are characterized by hyperactivity, anxiety, agitation, and hallucinations. Periods of bizarre behavior, including thrashing, running, biting, or tearing clothing may occur for several minutes at a time, followed by periods of calm or anxiety. An exaggerated reflex protecting the respiratory tract is common, leading to choking and gagging. Episodes may be brought on by eating, drinking, seeing water, or by air gently blowing on the face. Fear of these painful occurrences may lead patients to stop eating and drinking (hydrophobia). By not swallowing, copious amounts of saliva drool from the mouth and may be a source of infection for hospital personnel, although, in the cycle of rabies transmission, humans are considered to be dead-end hosts in the sense that human patients are not known to infect others (see page 234). Nevertheless, medical staff attending human rabies patients in endemic areas should be pre-exposure immunized and avoid contamination with infectious secretions.

In about 20% of patients, neurologic signs are primarily paralytic in nature. This condition is characterized by numbness, pain, weakness, and flaccid paralysis of the bitten area. This will progress to paraplegia, triplegia, or tetraplegia. Manifestations usually typifying furious disease (including hydrophobia) may develop terminally or not at all. Paralytic rabies may be more common in patients that have been bitten by a bat (especially a vampire) or have been infected with a fixed strain of virus (Fishbein, 1991b).

The period of acute neurologic signs usually lasts for 2 to 7 days, the latter portion being marked by paralysis and deterioration of mental acuity. Periods of confusion alternate with periods in which the patient is fully lucid. There is a gradual mental deterioration, progressing from confusion to disorientation and stupor.

Patients may die at this time or lapse into a coma of variable duration. Coma, in turn, is followed by death due to multiple organ dysfunction, including, but not limited to, cardiac arrhythmias, congestive heart failure, acute respiratory distress (ARDS), autonomic nervous system dysfunction, and pulmonary or circulatory collapse (Baevsky and Bartfield, 1993).

Death commonly occurs within one week in untreated patients and within about three weeks in hospitalized patients. In the United States, most victims of rabies are hospitalized within four days after the onset of clinical signs. Rabies is not usually diagnosed during initial medical evaluation because of the nonspecific nature of initial clinical presentation (Centers for Disease Control, 1993).

Intensive care may offer some shred of hope, however small, for affected individuals and tertiary care centers continue to investigate new treatment protocols (World Health Organization, 1984, 1992). If patients are supported by intensive care, a variety of late-appearing medical complications may become apparent. Despite the vast amount of information that has been accumulated about this disease, there is still much to be learned. Even the mechan leading to the death of an infecteu main unknown.

Documented Cases of Huma. Surviving Rabies

Although generally considered to be a fatal disease once clinical signs appear, three documented cases of persons surviving rabies are known. The first case was that of a 45-year-old woman from Argentina who developed rabies three weeks after being bitten by an aggressive dog. Post-exposure rabies prophylaxis included 12 doses of suckling-mouse brain vaccine. Clinical signs included depression, headache, paresthesia at the location of the bite, and a cerebellar striatal syndrome. Over the course of the next 13 months, she slowly recovered (Porras et al, 1971).

The second case involved a six-year-old boy from Lima, Ohio who was bitten on his thumb by a rabid bat while asleep in his bed. The wound was washed with soap and water and a 14-day course of duck-embryo vaccine started. He was admitted to the hospital with signs of progressive neurologic disease (see page 235 for additional medical details). After about one week, he began to improve and exhibited minimal neurological signs. Although rabies virus was not isolated from the boy, the clinical, laboratory, and epidemiologic findings strongly supported a diagnosis of rabies (Centers for Disease Control, 1971; Hattwick et al, 1972; Carlson and Beran, 1986).

The third case involved a 32-year-old laboratory technician working at the New York State Department of Health, who was accidentally exposed to a heavy dose of aerosolized virus. Although he suffered from a confirmed case of paralytic rabies, he survived (see page 172 for additional medical details). With time, he has recovered use of his arms and legs, and partial recovery of speech (Tillotson et al, 1977a, 1977b), although considerable neurologic impairment remains to date.

References

Baevsky, R. H. and J. M. Bartfield (1993). Human rabies: A review. *Am. J. Emerg. Med.* 11(3): 279

Bek, M. D., Smith, W. T., Levy, M. H., Sullivan, E., and G. L. Rubin (1992). Rabies case in New South Wales, 1990: Public health aspects. *Med. J. Aust.* 156(9): 596

Beran, G. W. (1988/92). Professor of Veterinary Epidemiology and Public Health. Department of Veterinary Microbiology and Preventive Medicine. College of Veterinary Medicine, Iowa State University. Ames, Iowa. Personal communication.

Bernard, K. W. (1985). Clinical Rabies in Humans. In W. G. Winkler (ed.) *Rabies Concepts for Medical Professionals*. Merieux Institute, Inc. Miami, Florida.

Burridge, M. J., Sawyer, L. A., and W. J. Bigler (1986). *Rabies in Florida*. Health Program Office, Department of Health and Rehabilitative Services. Tallahassee, Florida.

Campbell, A. G. M. (1993). Is a change in rabies vaccine schedule necessary for travellers? *The Lancet*. 341(8843): 500

Carlson, T. A. and G. W. Beran (1986). The first well documented case of recovery from clinical rabies in a human being. *ISU Vet.* 48(2): 107

Centers for Disease Control—Miscellaneous Pathogens Unit (1971). Followup on probable human rabies—Lima, Ohio. *MMWR.* 20(7): 54

Centers for Disease Control (1984a). Adult Immunization. Recommendations of the Immunization Practices Advisory Committee. *MMWR.*, Supplement. 33(1S): 26S

Centers for Disease Control (1984b). Rabies Prevention—United States, 1984. Recommendation of the Immunization Practices Advisory Committee. *MMWR.* 33(28): 393

Centers for Disease Control (1985). Human rabies acquired outside the United States. *MMWR.* 34(17): 235

Centers for Disease Control (1991). Recommendations of the Immunization Practices Advisory Committee (ACIP). Rabies Prevention—United States, 1991. *MMWR.* 40(No. RR-3): 1

Centers for Disease Control (1993). Editorial note. *MMWR.* 42(41): 799

Corey, L. (1983). Rabies and Other Rhabdoviruses. In R. G. Petersdorf, R. D. Adams, E. Braunwald, K. J. Isselbacher, J. B. Martin, and J. D. Wilson (eds.) *Harrison's Principles of Internal Medicine*. McGraw-Hill Book Co. New York.

Currier, II, R. W., McCroan, J. E., Dreesen, D. W., Winkler, W. G., and R. L. Parker (1975). Epidemiology of antirabies treatment in Georgia, 1967-71. *Pub. Hlth. Repts.* 90(5): 435

Dietzschold, B. and H. C. J. Ertl (1991). New developments in the pre- and post-exposure treatment of rabies. *Crit. Rev. Immunol.* 10(5): 427

Dietzschold, B., Gore, M., Casali, P., Ueki, Y., Rupprecht, C. E., Notkins, A. L., and H. Koprowski (1990). Biological characterization of human monoclonal antibodies to rabies virus. *J. Virol.* 64(6): 3087

Dutta, J. K. and T. K. Dutta (1994). Rabies in endemic countries. *Br. Med. J.* 308(6927): 488

Eng, T. R., Fishbein, D. B., Talamante, H. E., Hall, D. B., Chavez, G. F., Dobbins, J. G., Muro, F. J., Bustos, J. L., de los Angeles Ricardy, M., Munguia, A., Carrasco, J., Robles, A. R., and G. M. Baer (1993). Urban epizootic of rabies in Mexico: Epidemiology and impact of animal bite injuries. *Bull. Wld. Hlth. Org.* 71(5): 615

Enssle, K., Kohler, K. R., Muller, H., Kanzy, E. J., Hilfenhaus, J., and F. R. Seiler (1991). A rabies-specific human monoclonal antibody that protects mice against lethal rabies. *Hybridoma.* 10(5): 547

Fishbein, D. B. (1991a). Latent rabies—Letter to the editor. *New Engl. J. Med.* 324(26): 1891

Fishbein, D. (1991b). Rabies in Humans. In G. M. Baer (ed.) *The Natural History of Rabies*. 2nd Edition. CRC Press, Inc. Boca Raton, Florida.

Fishbein, D. B. and L. E. Robinson (1993). Rabies—Current concepts. *New Engl. J. Med.* 329(22): 1632

Flores-Crespo, R. (1991). Techniques to Control Vampire Bats. In *Expert Consultation on the Care of Persons Exposed to Rabies Transmitted by Vampire Bats*. PAHO/WHO. Programs for Veterinary Public Health. Washington, D.C. April 1-5, 1991

Gardner, A. M. N. (1970). An unusual case of rabies. *The Lancet*. 2: 523

Grattan-Smith, P. J., O'Regan, W. J., Ellis, P. S. J., O'Flaherty, S. J., McIntyre, P. B., and C. L. Barnes (1992). Rabies—A second Australian case, with a long incubation period. *Med. J. Aust.* 156: 651

Hattwick, M. A., Weiss, T. T., Stechschulte, C. J., Baer, G. M., and M. B. Gregg (1972). Recovery from rabies. A case report. *Ann. Int. Med.* 76: 931

Helmick, C. G. (1983). The Epidemiology of Human Rabies Postexposure Prophylaxis, 1980-1981. *J. Am. Med. Assoc.* 250(15): 1990

Helmick, C. G. (1986). The Epidemiology of Human Rabies Post-Exposure Prophylaxis in the United States. In D. B. Fishbein, L. A. Sawyer, and W. G. Winkler (eds.) *Rabies Concepts for Medical Professionals*. 2nd Edition. Merieux Institute, Inc. Miami, Florida.

Hemachudha, T., Chutivongse, S., Wilde, H., and P. Phanuphak (1991). Latent rabies. *New Engl. J. Med.* 324(26): 1890

Jorgenson, R. R. (1990). Rabies in wildlife: A consideration of its epidemiology in the countries of the European continent and the USA. *Revue Internationale des Services de Sante des Forces Armees.* 82(10-12): 310

Kagawa, K. J., Chomel, B. B., and L. Lery (1992). Rabies and brucellosis immunization status and adverse reactions to rabies vaccines in veterinary students. *Comp. Immunol. Microbiol. Infect. Dis.* 15(2): 79

Koprowski, H. (1979). Rabies. In P. B. Beeson, W. McDermott, and J. B. Wyngaarden (eds.) *Cecil's Textbook of Medicine*. W. B. Saunders Co. Philadelphia.

Lafon, M., Edelman, L., Bouvet, J. P., and M. Lafage (1990). Human monoclonal antibodies specific for the rabies virus glycoprotein and N protein. *J. Gen. Virol.* 71: 1689

Lanska, D. J. (1992). Rabies virus, paralytic and classical. *The Lancet.* 339: 809

Martin, R. J., Schnurrenberger, R. R., and N. J. Rose (1969). Epidemiology of rabies vaccinations of persons in Illinois, 1967-68. *Pub. Hlth. Repts.* 84: 1069

McColl, K. A., Gould, P. W., Hooper, P. T., Westbury, H. A., and J. S. Smith (1993). Polymerase chain reaction and other laboratory techniques in the diagnosis of long incubation rabies in Australia. *Aust. Vet. J.* 70(3): 84

Montano-Hirose, J. A., Lafage, M., Weber, P., Badrane, H., Tordo, N., and M. Lafon (1993). Protective activity of a murine monoclonal antibody against European bat lyssavirus 1 (EBL1) infection in mice. *Vaccine.* 11(12): 1259

Muhsin, M. A. (1986). *Studies on the Epidemiology and Control of Rabies*. PhD Dissertation. Iowa State University. Ames, Iowa.

Nicholson, K. G. (1987). Rabies. In A. J. Zuckerman, J. E. Banatuala, and J. R. Pattison (eds.) *Principles and Practice of Clinical Virology*. John Wiley and Sons, Ltd. New York.

Porras, C., Barboza, J. J., Fuenzalida, E., Adaros, H. L., de Diaz, A. M. O., and J. Furst (1971). Recovery from rabies in man. *Ann. Intern. Med.* 85: 44

Schumacher, C. L., Ertl, H. C., Koprowski, H., and B. Dietzschold (1992). Inhibition of immune response against rabies virus by monoclonal antibodies directed against rabies virus antigens. *Vaccine.* 10(11): 754

Smith, J. S. and H. D. Seidel (1993). Rabies: A new look at an old disease. *Prog. Med. Virol.* 40: 82

Smith, J. S., Fishbein, D. B., Rupprecht, C. E., and K. Clark (1991). Unexplained rabies in three immigrants in the United States. *New Engl. J. Med.* 324(4): 205

Smith, J. S., Orciari, L. A., Yager, P. A., Seidel, H. D., and C. K. Warner (1992). Epidemiologic and historical relationships among 87 rabies virus isolates as determined by limited sequence analysis. *J. Infect. Dis.* 166: 296

Tillotson, J. R., Axelrod, D., and D. O. Lyman (1977a). Rabies in a laboratory worker—New York. *MMWR.* 26(22): 183

Tillotson, J. R., Axelrod, D., and D. O. Lyman (1977b). Follow-up on rabies—New York. *MMWR.* 26(31): 249

Trimarchi, C. V. and M. Safford, Jr. (1992). Poor response to rabies vaccination by the intradermal route—Letter to the editor. *J. Am. Med. Assoc.* 268(7): 874

Wilde, H., Chutivongse, S., and T. Hemachudha (1994). Tropical health. 26. Rabies and its prevention. *Med. J. Austral.* 160(2): 83

World Health Organization (1984). *Expert Committee on Rabies. Seventh Report*. WHO Tech. Rpt. No. 709. Geneva.

World Health Organization/Veterinary Public Health (1990). *Report of the Sixth WHO Consultation on Monoclonal Antibodies in Rabies Diagnosis and Research*. The Wistar Institute. Philadelphia, Pennsylvania, USA. April 2-3, 1990. WHO/Rab. Res./ 90.34. Unpublished document (reviewed with permission).

World Health Organization (1992). *Expert Committee on Rabies. Eighth Report*. WHO Tech. Rpt. No. 824. Geneva.

SECTION II

Vampire Bats and Rabies in Latin America

Chapter 4:
VAMPIRE BATS AND BOVINE PARALYTIC RABIES

Vampire Bats and Livestock Production

Like the rodents and roaches who have thrived in company with man, populations of vampire bats in Latin America have increased sharply in areas where European-type livestock have been introduced. Presumably, livestock production practices have created a more favorable, or more readily obtainable, food supply for the vampire bat than that afforded by wildlife alone. Creation of more favorable roosting habitats, such as mines, wells, and aqueducts, has also led to an expansion in the population and distribution of vampire bats. Results of population studies of vampire bats in northeast Argentina have shown that vampire populations are almost twice as large in cattle-raising ecosystems as in natural ecosystems (Delpietro et al, 1993).

Parasitizing domestic animals may also improve the vampire's overall feeding efficiency. In their study in northeast Argentina, Delpietro et al (1993) found that none of the vampire bats captured from natural ecosystems between sunset and midnight had fed prior to capture, whereas 33% of those captured from cattle-raising ecosystems had fed prior to capture. The energetic stress of foraging is greatly reduced for vampires feeding on livestock compared to that of vampires foraging in natural ecosystems (McCarthy, 1976).

Turner (1975) observed that the average cow sustained visits from 10.5 bats per evening. Since each bat may drink between 15 and 25 ml of blood, a cow can lose as much as 0.25 liters of blood in a night (not counting the loss from continued post-feeding hemorrhage). According to Goodwin and Greenhall (1961), a vampire may be responsible for as much as 5.75 gallons of blood loss annually. This includes both ingested blood and that which continues to bleed from open wounds. If an animal were bled continuously, as may be the case when bats revisit animals each night, the blood loss could be significant and such animals could become severely debilitated. Such debilitated cattle have been observed in some areas where vampires return to feed on the same individual each night.

In the course of their nightly blood meals, vampire bats have the potential to spread a variety of diseases. The wounds they leave can provide a portal of entry for secondary bacterial or viral infection, as well as attract a host of blood- and tissue-feeding parasites. Many species of parasitic flies, particularly primary screw-worms, whose larvae feed in fresh or healing wounds (myiasis), are attracted to stricken livestock (Gilyard, 1945; Prieto and Baer, 1972; Rawlins, 1985). Between the parasite burden, secondary infection, and blood loss incurred, cattle may succumb, or they may weaken sufficiently to cause a significant drop in milk production, weight gain, or reproductive capacity (Thompson et al, 1977).

Compounding this is the periodic threat of rabies, transmitted while the bats drink blood. Bovine paralytic rabies has been variously referred to as *derriengue* (limping illness), *mal de caderas* (hip illness), *tumbi baba* (dripping saliva), *rabia paresiante* (rabies with paresis), and *rabia paralitica* (paralytic rabies).[1] In his comprehensive review of rabies worldwide, Beran (1981) referred to vampire bats as "the best adapted of all mammalian hosts to rabies." In regard to their parasitic mode of existence, however, Beran

[1]Bovine rabies of vampire origin is typically paralytic in nature. Hence the name, bovine paralytic rabies.

MYIASIS

Both adult and immature forms of flies may be parasitic. Adult flies are often blood-sucking ectoparasites (external parasites) and may be important vectors of disease. Parasitic larvae, however, may be devastating to a parasitized animal. The infection or damage caused by the invasion of either superficial or deep body tissues by larval flies is called myiasis. Another commonly applied name is "strike." The common flies that may invade wounds such as those made by vampire bats are flesh flies and blow flies, including *Cochliomyia hominivorax*, the primary screw-worm.

Most blow flies are scavengers; the larvae feed on the decaying flesh of carrion, thereby serving an important housekeeping role in nature. However, some species (called secondary screw-worms) are attracted by the foul-smelling exudates of putrefying tissues, depositing their eggs in old and infected wounds. They are not attracted to freshly made wounds. The feeding of the larvae serves to further contaminate and extend the wound. Flesh flies are similar to blow flies in their habits, but eggs are not deposited in putrid flesh. Rather, the flesh fly deposits larvae (immature flies) directly. Thus, larvae appear "spontaneously" in wounds.

The primary screw-worm is one of the most dangerous of the parasitic flies. It is called primary because the female deposits its eggs in living tissues, laying masses of eggs next to open wounds. The larvae crawl into the wounds and devour living flesh, penetrating deeper and deeper into the host's body and causing extensive damage. Victimized animals often die from severe hemorrhage. The dead tissue left in the wake of these parasites is attractive to secondary screw-worms, which compound the damage.

Fortunately, the primary screw-worm has been eradicated from the United States. Eradication of the primary screw-worm from the southern part of the country took advantage of the fact that the female fly mates only once in its lifetime. Widespread programs were implemented to irradiate and release millions of male flies. The irradiated males would compete with wild males for females, but the irradiated ones were sterile. Females that mated with an irradiated male would produce no young and the population of flies began to decline. The numbers of irradiated males eventually outweighed the fertile wild males and the balance was tipped in favor of extinction of the fly from the country. The United States was finally declared free of the primary screw-worm in 1977 (Mertins, 1993). It was not until the primary screw-worm had been eradicated from the southern half of the country that cattle raising could be successfully undertaken there.

Similar control programs, in various phases, are currently underway in Mexico and throughout Central America (Editorial, 1994). Guatemala and Belize are reportedly screw-worm free. Mexico had been declared free in 1991, but a reinfestation began in 1992. Infected cattle have been observed in Aldamas, within 200 miles of Brownsville, Texas, posing a serious threat to the United States. Although highly speculative, it has been suggested that Mexico's reinfestation was secondary to an illegal trafficking of less expensive cattle from infected countries in Central and South America. Mexico continues its eradication efforts, but most of Latin America is still plagued by the presence of the primary screw-worm.

noted that because they are so efficient in transmitting the rabies virus to cattle, they wreak great havoc on the population of their preferred hosts. According to reports of the Expert Committee on Rabies (World Health Organization, 1957, 1966, 1973, 1984), as well as the First International Conference on Rabies in the Americas (1967 [cited by Greenhall, 1970]), rabies of vampire-bat origin has been a major obstacle to expansion of the livestock industry in Latin America. In 1973, Steele wrote, "...control of vampire bat rabies is probably the biggest challenge facing animal authorities today."

Vampire bats are commonly found throughout the more tropical regions of Latin America. The number of acceptable habitats for vampire bats is increased wherever livestock are raised, and a variety of man-made structures prove suitable as roosting places (Malaga-Alba, 1954, 1966; Greenhall, 1974, 1988; Kverno and

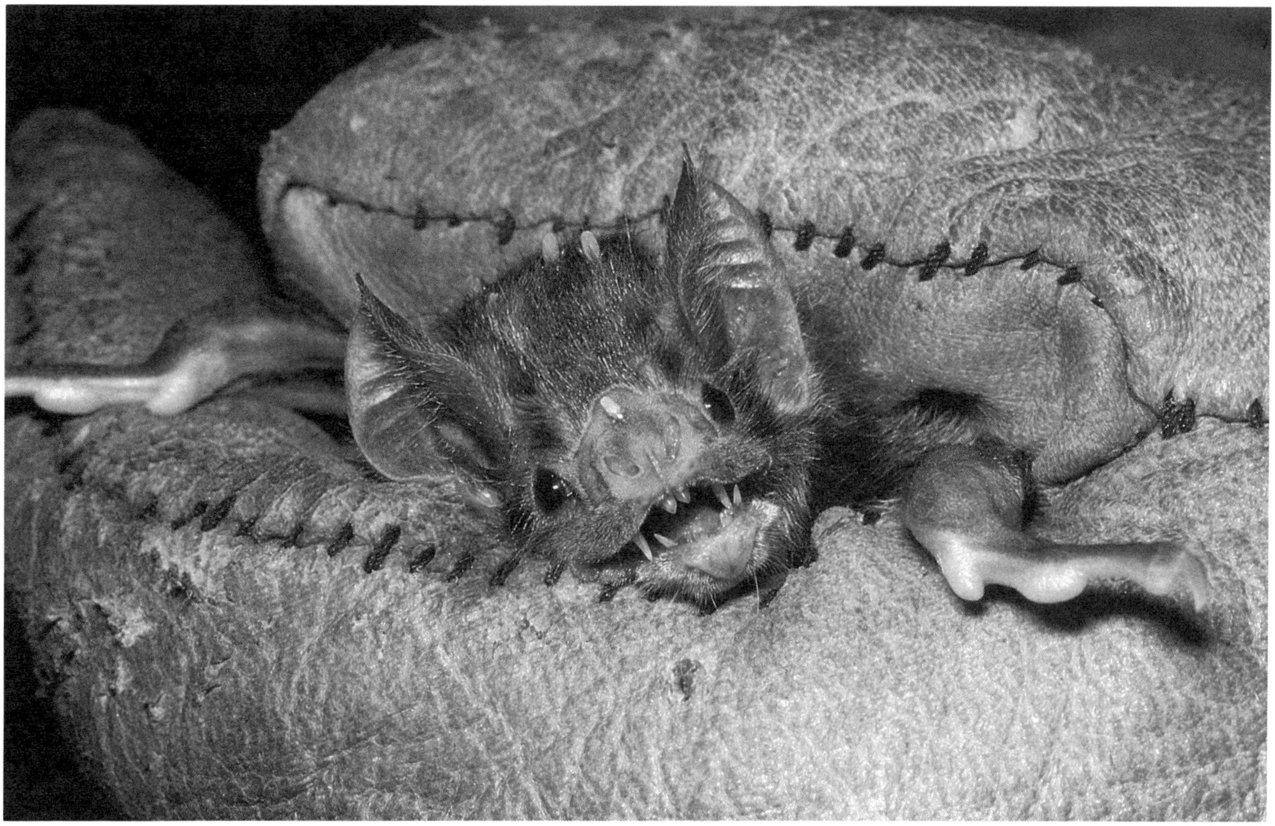

Figure 4-1. Closeup of *Desmodus rotundus*, the common vampire bat. Bats should never be handled without good reason, and then, only with gloves. Photo © Randall D. Babb.

Mitchell, 1976; Acha, 1981; Beran, 1981; Acha and Arambulo, III, 1985). The existence of rabies in vampire populations has had devastating effects on cattle-production operations in the past century. With confirmation of bat-inflicted paralytic rabies in Latin America and the ensuing struggle with repeated outbreaks, it has been a constant battle for livestock producers to survive. Since the turn of the century, ranchers have been embroiled in an ongoing war with a small flying mammal, no larger that a child's fist (Figure 4-1).

Brazil

A link between bat bites and death of both humans and animals was observed by Spanish colonists in Panama, Colombia, Venezuela, and the Mexican Peninsula of Yucatan as early as the 16th century (de Oviedo, 1526).[2] Despite historical testimony of the presence of bat rabies in the Americas (Villa-Ramirez, 1969; Acha and Arambulo, III, 1985), the first modern evidence of the existence of rabies in bats is generally considered to date from 1906. At that time, an outbreak of disease known locally as *mal de caderas de bovinos* (hip disease of cattle) occurred among the livestock in the state of Santa Catarina, Brazil.

Animals principally affected were cattle, horses, and mules, with those raised in the close vicinity of forests more commonly afflicted. Animals developed a paralytic condition, the clinical course of which was uniformly fatal. Early in the history of the disease, it had been mistakenly diagnosed as rinderpest, trypanosomiasis, Aujeszky's disease, hemorrhagic septicemia, and poisoning by the plant *Ipomohea digitata* (Metivier, 1935; Enright, 1956). By 1908, over 4,000 cows and 1,000 horses and mules had died (Haupt and

[2]An interesting summary of early naturalists' initial encounters with vampire bats can be found in the work by Brown (1994).

Rehaag, 1921).

The eventual diagnosis of paralytic rabies in Santa Catarina and various neighboring districts in South Brazil was a surprising one since, as Carini reported in 1911 (cited by Pawan, 1936a), rabies was extremely rare among the indigenous canine population. Indeed, the knowledge was made even more remarkable by observation that the rabies epizootic spread across rivers that were clearly an impassable barrier to dogs. But, Carini believed the disease to have been a form of rabies and that an animal other than the dog must have been the vector.

By 1913, thc disease had spread to the German settlement of Blumenau, causing heavy losses among cattle and horses. Two German veterinary researchers (H. Haupt in 1914 and H. Rehaag in 1916-1918) were sent from Europe to help with the investigations. They confirmed the findings of Carini that the condition was rabies (Haupt and Rehaag, 1921). The diagnosis of rabies was regarded with distrust and resistance and, in many instances, rejected outright (Carneiro, 1954).

Despite the lack of enzootic canine rabies in the region, a massive depopulation of dogs was initiated in an attempt to contain the disease in livestock. Close to 7,000 dogs were destroyed in 1912. The outbreaks, nevertheless, were not curtailed, spreading throughout Brazil until 1920. Curiously, it seemed that dogs and humans had been unaffected by the early outbreaks (Pawan, 1936a).

Trinidad

Trinidad and Tobago are continental islands of northern South America. Trinidad, the larger island, is just seven miles east of Venezuela. Tobago is 20 miles northeast of Trinidad. In July of 1925, an outbreak of a mysterious new disease led to the death of numerous cattle grazing on the St. Ann's and Queen's Park Savannahs, two government pastures used for grazing by dairy herders from Trinidad's capital city, Port-of-Spain (Director of Agriculture, 1925).

Although animals had been removed from the savannahs at the urging of the government, livestock continued to die for varying periods of time. Only those animals that had been outside on one of the government pastures died. Those stabled indoors remained unaffected, even if housed in a stall adjacent to one that subsequently died. By the end of 1925, similar outbreaks had occurred in cattle grazing on several other government and private pastures in and around the district of Port-of-Spain.

Initial signs in livestock included straying from the herd, dilated pupils, drowsiness, depression, loss of appetite and thirst, grinding of teeth, constipation, dribbling of urine, increased salivation, involuntary tremors, and a stiff, incoordinated gait. With progression of illness, additional abnormalitics included dehydration, sunken flanks, continuous bellowing, flapping of the ears, nervousness and excitability, straining to defecate, and production of a thick, malodorous feces. Violence was very rare, but the zebu (brahma or Indian-humped) cattle reportedly charged people frequently.

Progressive incoordination and weakness, particularly of the hind limbs, led to frequent stumbling. Animals often remained on their sides for a prolonged period, making incoordinated running movements with their front legs on attempting to rise. Many animals would dig a circular hole about themselves. Progressive paralysis developed, culminating in respiratory failure and death about a week after the onset of clinical signs. Clinical signs in affected animals, as well as gross and histologic descriptions of lesions, have been recounted in detail by Hurst and Pawan (1931, 1932), Metivier (1935), Gilyard (1945), Bush (1961), and Baer (1975).

It is interesting to note that other puzzling cattle deaths had been recorded earlier in Trinidad. Several deaths in March of 1923 at Debé Village, Maraval had been attributed to consumption of Oleander leaves. Additional deaths in Maraval in 1924 were also diagnosed as Oleander poisoning. In April of 1923, the sudden deaths of seven head of cattle had been reported from the Queen's Park Savannah in the district of Port-of-Spain (Director of Agriculture, 1923). Oleander poisoning had been suggested as the cause of these deaths also; however, the plant could not be found on the pasture (Waterman, 1959a). Two suspicious-looking plants failed to produce clinical signs in cattle when ingested. Although other suggested causes included herbicide/insecticide poisoning or an illness borne by blood-sucking insects, the general consensus was that the deaths had been due to sodium chloride intoxication (Freeman, 1923). When Dr. J. L. Pawan, the Government Bacteriologist, reported isolating *Bacillus botulinus* from clinical material and from soil and water samples from "infected" pastures, botulism seemed to have been confirmed as cause of the most recent cattle deaths (Hurst and Pawan, 1931).

The Governor had closed the Queen's Park Savannah to livestock for all of 1926 and no outbreaks of what was believed to have been botulism were reported that year. However, since livestock producers came to recognize the characteristic signs in affected animals as being invariably fatal, veterinarians were less frequently consulted. Lack of official notification, therefore, did not necessarily prove that disease was no longer present on the island (Waterman, 1959a).

In 1927, two cases were reported at River Estate (a government cocoa plantation with a public savannah maintained for the "peasantry"), and the condition was reported to be prevalent in the Diego Martin Valley (Director of Agriculture, 1927; Metivier, 1935). For the first time, reports were also received of cattle deaths in animals housed in stalls, although peasant farmers generally housed their cattle in open sheds with only a roof overhead (Metivier, 1935).

In 1928, a few more cases were reported from the Diego Martin and Maraval districts. The Department of Agriculture ordered a supply of Botulinus antitoxin. However, the outbreaks appeared to cease and the antitoxin was not tested at that time (Director of Agriculture, 1928; Waterman, 1959a).

Between August and December of 1929, disease was quite prevalent. It was first reported from the southern districts of Siparia (55 miles from Port-of-Spain), Penal, La Brea, Parry Lands, and Oropouche, but cases later occurred in the central part of the island as well (Director of Agriculture, 1929). Although cattle were the most commonly affected species, disease also occurred in horses, mules, and donkeys. Occasional cases were reported in goats, sheep, and pigs (Metivier, 1935). The incidence of disease was highest among animals on pasture, particularly those left out overnight.

In subsequent years, outbreaks were noted throughout the island, occurring at intervals of approximately five years. Greenhall (1965) reported that on two occasions, he had been able to predict the development of an epizootic based on numerous factors. Within ten years of the initial outbreak, many thousands of animals had died, at an average rate of 1,000 per year (Metivier, 1935; de Verteuil and Urich, 1936; Pawan, 1936a, 1936b, 1955). Epizootics were not reported from Tobago (Greenhall, 1959; Goodwin and Greenhall, 1961).

In contrast to the Brazilian outbreak, a paralytic disease of humans was first observed in Trinidad in 1929. On July 15, a 15-year-old boy living in de Gannes Village, Siparia was diagnosed with an acute ascending myelitis (Waterman, 1959a). Between 1929 and 1931, 16 similar cases were identified and diagnosed as acute anterior poliomyelitis, a diagnosis supported by the Office of the Surgeon General. Typical of human cases was the initial development of localized symptoms of paresthesia, progressing to paresis and paralysis of the foot, toe, and occasionally the arm. Human cases were uniformly fatal (Hurst and Pawan, 1931, 1932). Clinical signs in affected humans, as well as gross and histologic descriptions of lesions, have been recounted in detail by Hurst and Pawan (1931, 1932), Metivier (1935), Gilyard (1945), and Baer (1975).

Disease among the island's inhabitants occurred in small, local epidemics lasting from 1 to 10 weeks, after which isolated cases would persist in endemic form. The majority of cases (64%) occurred between May and August (de Verteuil and Urich, 1936). By 1937, 89 human deaths had been reported. Despite the widespread continuance of disease in cattle, no further human deaths in Trinidad have been recorded (Butcher, 1959; Goodwin and Greenhall, 1961; Baer, 1991; Lopez et al, 1992).

Suggestions of a relationship between the human condition and the disease ravaging the island's livestock were received with skepticism (Waterman, 1959a, 1959b). The Public Health Department expressed the view that the diseases were not the same for two principal reasons:

1) On the basis of clinical signs and bacteriological findings, veterinarians had already diagnosed the disease in livestock as botulism. There was no reason for this diagnosis to be challenged by physicians.
2) Disease in livestock was first observed in 1925 and had remained epizootic for some time after. Disease in humans, however, had not been described until four years later, suggesting that they were not the same.

Convinced that the diseases in cattle and humans were related, Waterman (1959b) in 1930 attempted to transmit disease to calves by inoculation (intrathecal, intramuscular, and subcutaneous) of cerebrospinal fluid obtained from one of the human patients. These attempts were unsuccessful. Samples of brain and spinal cord parenchyma obtained from two human cases had been sent by Pawan to Dr. W. Hurst of the Lister Institute in London (Hurst and Pawan, 1931). Four rhesus monkeys were inoculated intracerebrally with an emulsion of spinal cord from one of the human patients. After incubation periods ranging from 15 to 42 days, the animals developed unusual clinical signs, including clinging to cage bars, repeatedly uttering peculiar piercing shrieks, apparent states of extreme terror, reluctance to move, marked weakness of the legs progressing to flaccid paralysis, lack of response to painful stimuli, and a state of increasing stupor.

Virus isolated from these monkeys was used to infect five generations of others. The clinical signs and histological lesions observed in secondarily infected monkeys were very similar to those of monkeys inoculated with a known strain of fixed rabies virus (Hurst and Pawan, 1931, 1932). Clinical signs included periods of active aggression, dazed expressions, occasional self-mutilation, and violent muscular spasms, which gradually progressed to generalized weakness and death.

Viral isolates from monkeys, as well as from material obtained from one of the human cases, were passaged through multiple generations of rabbits. Clinical signs in experimentally infected rabbits were typical of paralytic rabies and could not be distinguished from those produced by a fixed strain of rabies virus. In all experimentally infected animals, lesions in the central nervous system were similar to those characteristically produced by rabies virus. Negri bodies were found in the brains of all infected monkeys and in some of the rabbits (Hurst and Pawan, 1931), confirming earlier findings of Pawan.

Clinical material from Trinidad had also been sent to Dr. S. Flexner of the Rockefeller Institute in New York, Dr. Andrews of the Ministry of Agriculture and Fisheries in London, Dr. Krause of Vienna, Drs. Remlinger and Bailly of the Pasteur Institute in Algiers, and Professor Finzi of Milan (Metivier, 1935). Similar conclusions had been reached by these investigators, based on serological findings and studies of central nervous system pathology in experimentally infected animals.

Hurst and Pawan (1931, 1932) reported finding Negri bodies in the brains of cows allegedly suffering from botulism. Intracerebral or intramuscular inoculation of monkeys and rabbits with brain emulsions obtained from affected cows resulted in development of a rabies-like disease with demonstrable Negri bodies in some of the experimental animals. Hurst and Pawan (1931) concluded that these findings left "little doubt that the virus responsible for both the human and the cattle disease is that of rabies." In July of 1931, Dr. Wise, Trinidad's Surgeon General, declared that both the human and animal diseases were due to the virus of rabies (Waterman, 1959a).

Hurst pointed out that the existence of a similar illness among livestock in South America had been known of for several years and described as paralytic rabies. The vector was believed to be the vampire bat. Moreover, Dr. Roux of the Pasteur Institute and Professor Finzi of Milan both reported that the virus obtained from patients in Trinidad was identical to that received from investigators in South America (Metivier, 1935). Vampire bats were common in Trinidad.

In September of 1931, Dr. Pawan demonstrated the presence of Negri bodies in the brain of a bat with unusual habits and in March of 1932 identified Negri bodies in the brain of a vampire bat (Pawan, 1936a). In his report to the Director of Agriculture in 1931, Dr. H. V. Metivier, Trinidad's Government Veterinary Surgeon, related the results of experiments with three bats captured early one morning in the poultry compound at the Government Stock Farm. The bats had been fighting and biting each other and had subsequently been diagnosed as rabid. Metivier inoculated a calf, a guinea pig, and a rabbit subcutaneously with an emulsion made from the brains and salivary glands of these bats. All three experimentally infected animals developed clinical signs typical of paralytic rabies (Metivier, 1931).

Despite initial misdiagnosis, the true nature of the disease was uncovered and, in time, both the animal and human conditions in Trinidad were identified as paralytic rabies, confirming the suspicions of earlier investigators, as well as those of livestock owners. As was the case in Brazil, recognition of the condition as rabies led to consideration of dogs as vectors. However, a rigidly enforced quarantine law existed in Trinidad at the time. With the exception of animals from the United Kingdom (which was known to be free of rabies), all dogs were required to spend six months in a quarantine facility and be issued a certificate of inspection by the Government Veterinary Surgeon before they could be brought onto the island. Rabies in the island's canine population had not been observed since 1914 (Hurst and Pawan, 1931).

Over the course of several years following the outbreaks in Brazil and Trinidad, the epidemiology of the diseases was elucidated. In a series of rather classic studies in medical detection, involving many investigators, the reservoir of virus was ultimately identified. Medical case histories, clinical studies, and experimental findings conclusively documented the fact that vampire bats were responsible for both human and animal disease. Dr. Pawan has generally been credited with the first identification of Negri bodies in the brains of animals, humans, and vampire bats in Trinidad and Dr. Metivier with establishing a plausible relationship between bites of bats and the development of paralytic rabies.

With confirmation of the vampire bat as an important vector of rabies in Latin America, bats emerged as agents of significant concern in areas of human and animal health. Bats had never before been incriminated as vectors of human disease (Waterman 1959a).

Mexico

In 1943, scientists from New York's Rockefeller Foundation were asked to help devise an agricultural development program in Mexico. At the time, *derriengue* (referring to a break or injury of the spine, limping illness) was considered to be one of the major diseases affecting livestock.

Derriengue was characterized by restlessness or excitement, followed by rear-limb paralysis. Early in the clinical course of the disease, animals would salivate excessively due to difficulty in swallowing. Affected animals would rapidly lose weight and die in a few days (Johnson, 1948; Enright, 1956; Ornelas and Aranalde, 1964).

The condition had been known in Mexico since 1910, at which time there had been an epizootic in the state of Colima. Epizootics have subsequently been reported in Michoacan, Nayarit, Guerrero, Jalisco, Oaxaca, Chiapas, Sinaloa, and Chihuahua. *Derriengue* gradually spread from the coast to inland sites. It was most commonly found in Mexico's valleys and arroyos.

The disease was cyclic in a given area, usually lasting 1 to 2 months and then disappearing for 1 to 2 years. Outbreaks were most numerous between October and April, generally clustering in January and February. Typically, 20% to 50% of the cattle in affected areas died during an outbreak. It has been reported that *derriengue* claimed the lives of about 50,000 head of cattle in the years between 1939 and 1943. Arellano-Sota (1986) reported that as many as 120,000 head of cattle died annually in Mexico prior to control methods. Currently, Mexican cattle losses reportedly average 30,000 head annually.

Epizootics occurred in areas in which canine rabies was not present. Despite the characteristic signs and the isolation of a viral agent believed to be the cause of the illness, local veterinarians did not believe the problem to have been rabies. A concurrent paralytic disease of horses, believed to be some form of equine encephalitis, led investigators to search for a relationship between the disease in horses and that in cattle. Sheep and swine were rarely affected.

In 1944, members of the Rockefeller delegation found vampire bats in caves around Michoacan and Jalisco, two regions which had recently suffered through an outbreak of *derriengue*. Virus, serologically related to rabies virus, was isolated from these bats, as well as from a paralyzed cow of the region. Salivary gland and brain tissue obtained from both this cow and from captured bats, produced a paralytic condition in mice following intracerebral inoculation. Various isolates of virus obtained from cattle afflicted in previous years were found to be serologically related to rabies virus. Outbreaks of *derriengue* did not appear to be fundamentally different, either clinically or epidemiologically, from episodes of paralytic rabies described elsewhere in Latin America. Tellez-Giron (1937, 1944) had suggested involvement of vampire bats in rabies epidemiology in Mexico several years earlier.

Through 1990, 137 human deaths due to vampire-inflicted rabies have been reported in Mexico (Ornelas and Aranalde, 1964; Ruiz and Diaz, 1990; Flores-Crespo, 1991; PAHO/WHO, 1991). Between 1970 and 1986, human deaths due to vampire-induced rabies accounted for 7.1% of all reported human deaths due to rabies in the country. As a vector species, only dogs (82.3% of cases) surpassed vampire bats in transmitting rabies to humans (Vargas Pino, 1987 [cited by Flores-Crespo, 1991]). Between January and mid-November of 1990, 262 people were reportedly attacked by vampire bats in different municipalities of Jalisco, Mexico (Flores-Crespo, 1991).

The presence of vampire bats in Mexico is a matter of concern to U. S. public-health authorities in states bordering Mexico. Vampire bats may range to within about 150 miles of the international border (Irons et al, 1954; Dalquest, 1955). Circumstantial evidence has been presented suggesting the presence of vampire bats in San Diego, California in the 1940's and 1950's (Enright, 1956; Maddy et al, 1958). In 1967, a hairy-legged vampire bat was found in an unused railroad tunnel on the Brotherton-Calk Ranch, 12 miles west of Comstock, Val Verde Co., Texas. This was the first documented instance in modern history of a vampire bat being found in the United States (Reddell, 1968; West, 1973). It is unlikely that vampire bats will become established in the United States (see pages 60-61). Isolated occurrences, however, may be reported from time to time. These stray bats may or may not be rabid, but must be considered of potential public-health significance (Dalquest, 1955).

References

Acha, P. N. (1981). *A Review of Rabies Prevention and Control in the Americas 1970 to 1980—Overall Status of Rabies*. Presented at the Joint C.N.E.R.-WHO Scientific Meeting on Animal Rabies, Nancy and Malzeville, France. June 3-5, 1981

Acha, P. N. and P. V. Arambulo, III (1985). Rabies in the Tropics—History and Current Status. In E. Kuwert, C. Merieux, H. Koprowski, and K. Bogel (eds.) *Rabies in the Tropics*. Springer-Verlag. New York.

Arellano-Sota, C. (1986). Vampire Bat Rabies. *Rabies Control Symposium*. Washington, D. C. November 3-5, 1986

Baer, G. M. (1975). Bovine Paralytic Rabies and Rabies in the Vampire Bat. In G. M. Baer (ed.) *The Natural History of Rabies*. Vol. II. Academic Press. New York.

Baer, G. M. (1991). Vampire Bat and Bovine Paralytic Rabies. In G. M. Baer (ed.) *The Natural History of Rabies*. 2nd Edition. CRC Press, Inc. Boca Raton, Florida.

Beran, G. W. (1981). Rabies and Infections by Rabies-Related Viruses. In G. W. Beran (section ed.) *CRC Handbook Series in Zoonoses. Section B: Viral Zoonoses*. Volume II. CRC Press, Inc. Boca Raton, Florida.

Brown, D. E. (1994). *Vampiro: The Vampire Bat in Fact and Fantasy*. High-Lonesome Press. Silver City, New Mexico.

Busch, C. (1988). Consumption of blood, renal function and utilization of free water by the vampire bat, *Desmodus rotundus*. *Comp. Biochem. Physiol.* 90A(1): 141

Bush, D. L. (1961). Epizootic bat rabies in Surinam—Effectiveness of a mass field immunization program. *J. Am. Vet. Med. Assoc.* 138(7): 36

Butcher, L. V. (1959). The present status of paralytic rabies (bat-transmitted) in Trinidad. *Carib. Med. J.* XXI (1-4): 166

Carini, A. (1911). Sur une grande epizootie de rage. *Ann. Inst. Pasteur*. 25: 843

Carneiro, V. (1954). Transmission of rabies by bats in Latin America. *Bull. Wld. Hlth. Org.* 10: 775

Constantine, D. G. (1971). Bat Rabies: Current Knowledge and Future Research. In Y. Nagano and F. M. Davenport (eds.) *Rabies*. Sponsored by the Japan-United States Cooperative Medical Science Program. University Park Press. Baltimore.

Dalquest, W. W. (1955). Natural history of the vampire

bats of eastern Mexico. *Am. Midl. Nat.* 53(1): 79

de Diego, A. and J. R. Valotta (1973). Rabia transmitida por murcielagos. Situacion en la Republica Argentina. (Bat-transmitted rabies. Situation in Argentina.) *Revista de Medicina Veterinaria, Argentina.* 54(4): 275 (English abstract) in *Vet. Bull.* (1974). 44(4): 217

Delpietro, H. A., Marchevsky, N., and E. Simonetti (1993). Relative population densities and predation of the common vampire bat (*Desmodus rotundus*) in natural and cattle-raising areas in north-east Argentina. *Prev. Vet. Med.* 14: 13

de Oviedo, G. F. (1526). *Natural History of the West Indies.* Translated and edited by S. A. Stoudemire. University of North Carolina Studies in the Romance Languages and Literature. Number 32, 1959. The University of North Carolina Press. Chapel Hill, North Carolina.

de Verteuil, E. and F. W. Urich (1936). The study and control of paralytic rabies transmitted by bats in Trinidad, British West Indies. *Trans. Roy. Soc. Trop. Med. Hyg.* XXIX(4): 317

Director of Agriculture (1923-1929). *Administration Reports of the Director of Agriculture (Trinidad) for the Years 1923-1929.* Reported in *Carib. Med. J.* (1959). XXI (1-4): 172

Editorial (1994). Screwworm laboratory to be built in Panama. *J. Am. Vet. Med. Assoc.* 204(8): 1127

Enright, J. B. (1956). Bats and their relation to rabies. *Ann. Rev. Microbiol.* 10: 369

Flores-Crespo, R. (1991). Techniques to Control Vampire Bats. In *Expert Consultation on the Care of Persons Exposed to Rabies Transmitted by Vampire Bats.* PAHO/WHO. Programs for Veterinary Public Health. Washington, D.C. April 1-5, 1991

Freeman, W. G. (1923). Deaths of Cattle in the Queen's Park Savannah—Report by the Director of Agriculture. *Proceedings of the Agricultural Society of Trinidad and Tobago.* 23: 284. Reported in *Carib. Med. J.* (1959). XXI (1-4): 185

Gilyard, R. T. (1945). Bat transmitted paralytic rabies. *Cornell Vet.* XXXV(3): 195

Goodwin, G. C. and A. M. Greenhall (1961). A review of the bats of Trinidad and Tobago. *Bull. Am. Mus. Nat. Hist.* 122: 187

Greenhall, A. M. (1959). The ecological role of Trinidad bats, especially the vampire, and bat rabies. *Vet. Rec.* 71(10): 188

Greenhall, A. M. (1965). Notes on behavior of captive vampire bats. *Mammalia.* 29(4): 441

Greenhall, A. M. (1970). Vampire Bat Control: A Review and Proposed Programme for Latin America. In R. H. Dana (ed.) *Proceedings of the Fourth Vertebrate Pest Conference.* California Vertebrate Pest Committee. West Sacramento, California. March 3-5, 1970

Greenhall, A. M. (1971). Trinidad and bat research. *Nat. Hist.* 74: 14

Greenhall, A. M. (1974). Vampire bat control in the Americas: A review and proposed program for action. *Bull. Pan Am. Hlth. Org.* 8(1): 30

Greenhall, A. M. (1988). Feeding Behavior. In A. M. Greenhall and U. Schmidt (eds.) *The Natural History of Vampire Bats.* CRC Press, Inc. Boca Raton, Florida.

Haupt, H. and H. Rehaag (1921). Durch fledermause verbreitete seuchenhafte Tollwut unter Viehbestanden in Santa Catharina (Sud-Brasilien). *Ztschr. f. Infecktionskr. Haustiere.* 22: 76. English translation courtesy of Dr. Volker Moenig.

Hurst, E. W. and J. L. Pawan (1931). An outbreak of rabies in Trinidad without history of bites, and with the symptoms of acute ascending myelitis. *The Lancet.* 221: 622

Hurst, E. W. and J. L. Pawan (1932). A further account of the Trinidad outbreak of acute rabic myelitis: Histology of the experimental disease. *J. Path. Bact.* XXXV(3): 301

Irons, J. V., Eads, R. B., Sullivan, T., and J. E. Grimes (1954). The current status of rabies in Texas. *Texas Repts. Biol. Med.* 12: 489

Johnson, H. N. (1948). Derriengue: Vampire bat rabies in Mexico. *Am. J. Hyg.* 47: 189

Kverno, N. B. and G. C. Mitchell (1976). Vampire bats and their effect on cattle production in Latin America. *Wld. Anim. Rev.* (FAO). 17: 1

Lopez-R., A., Miranda-P., P., Tejada-V., E., and D. B. Fishbein (1992). Outbreak of human rabies in the Peruvian jungle. *The Lancet.* 339: 408

Maddy, K. T., Cockrum, E. L., and H. G. Crecelius (1958). Bat rabies in Arizona. *Arizona Med.* 15(5): 344

Malaga-Alba, A. (1954). Vampire bat as a carrier of rabies. *Am. J. Pub. Hlth.* 44: 909

Malaga-Alba, A. (1966). Ecological Relationship of Rabies in Wildlife. *International Symposium on Rabies.* Symp. Series Immunobiol. Standard. Vol. I. Karger, Basel. New York. Talloires, 1965

McCarthy, T. J. (1976). Vampire bat control in Belize. Comments on ecology and a program of education, research and control. *First International Symposium on Vampire Bat Control.* Managua, Nicaragua. June 29-30, 1976

Mertins, J. W. (1993). Medical Entomologist. National Veterinary Services Laboratory. Ames, Iowa. Personal communication.

Metivier, H. V. (1931). *The Administration Reports of the Director of Agriculture for 1931.* Reported in *Carib. Med. J.* (1959). XXI (1-4): 174

Metivier, H. V. (1935). Paralytic rabies in livestock. *J. Comp. Path. Ther.* 48: 245

Migone, L. E. and R. Pena (1932). Le Mal de Caderas

de bovides du Paraguay. *Bull. Soc. Path. Exot.* XXV.

Ornelas, O. and G. Aranalde (1964). Bat rabies in Mexico. *Southern Vet.* 1: 13

PAHO/WHO (1991). Consideration on the prevention, control and epidemiologic surveillance of vampire bat-transmitted rabies in man in the Americas. In *Expert Consultation on the Care of Persons Exposed to Rabies Transmitted by Vampire Bats.* PAHO/WHO Programs for Veterinary Public Health. Washington, D.C. April 1-5, 1991

Pawan, J. L. (1936a). The transmission of paralytic rabies in Trinidad by the vampire bat (*Desmodus rotundus murinus* Wagner, 1840). *Ann. Trop. Med. Parasit.* 30: 101

Pawan, J. L. (1936b). Rabies in the vampire bat of Trinidad, with special reference to the clinical course and latency of infection. *Ann. Trop. Med. Parasit.* 30: 401

Pawan, J. L. (1955). Rabies in bats. *Vet. Bull.* 14(4): 52

Prieto, J. F. and G. M. Baer (1972). An outbreak of bovine paralytic rabies in Tuxtepec, Oaxaca, Mexico. *Am. J. Trop. Med. Hyg.* 21(2): 219

Quiroga, S. S., Rottdart, A., and J. Acosta (1932). Mal de Caderas bovino (rabia paresiante). *Laboratorio de Bacteriologia del Ministeria de Agriculture (Buenos Aires).*

Rawlins, S. C. (1985). Current trends in screwworm myiasis in the Caribbean region. *Vet. Parasitol.* 18(3): 241

Reddell, J. R. (1968). The hairy-legged vampire, *Diphylla ecaudata*, in Texas. *J. Mammal.* 49(4): 769

Ricciardi, I. D., Nunes, M. P., Andrade, C. M., and A. G. da Silva (1976). Anti-Brucella agglutinins in bats and "Callithrix" monkeys. *J. Wildl. Dis.* 12: 52

Ruiz, A. and A. M. Diaz (1990). Epidemiology of Rabies Transmitted by Vampire Bats. Subject 3.8. Pan American Health Organization, Pan American Sanitary Bureau, Regional Office of the World Health Organization. *WHO Seminar on Wildlife Rabies Control.* Geneva. July 2-5, 1990

Steele, J. H. (1973). The epidemiology and control of rabies. *Scand. J. Infect. Dis.* 5: 312

Tellez-Giron, A. (1937). Los murcielagos portadores de virus del derriengue. (Encefalomielitis Bovina). *Revista Medica. Mexico.* 5: 6

Tellez-Giron, A. (1944). El vampiro portador del virus del derriengue. *Rev. Soc. Mex. Hist. Nat.* 5: 32

Thompson, R. D., Elias, D. J., and G. C. Mitchell (1977). Effects of vampire bat control on bovine milk production. *J. Wildl. Manage.* 41(4): 736

Turner, D. C. (1975). *The Vampire Bat—A Field Study in Behavior and Ecology.* The Johns Hopkins University Press. Baltimore.

Vargas Pino, F. (1987). Situacion actual de la rabia en Mexico. Memoria Simposio. *La atencion medida de las personas involucradas en un incidente de rabia.* Mexico, D. F., SSA,OPS. IMSS, p. 17

Villa-Ramirez, B. (1969). *The Ecology and Biology of Vampire Bats and Their Relationship to Paralytic Rabies.* Report to the Government of Brazil. United Nations Development Programme/Food and Agriculture Organization. FAO No. TA2656. Rome, 1969

Waterman, J. A. (1959a). The history of the outbreak of paralytic rabies in Trinidad transmitted by bats to human beings and the lower animals from 1925. *Carib. Med. J.* XXI (1-4): 1

Waterman, J. A. (1959b). Acute ascending rabic myelitis: Rabies—Transmitted by bats to human beings and animals. *Carib. Med. J.* XXI (1-4): 46

West, G. P. (1973). *Rabies in Animals and Man.* Arco Publishing Co., Inc. New York.

Wimsatt, W. A. and A. Guerriere (1962). Observations on the feeding capacities and excretory functions of captive vampire bats. *J. Mammal.* 43(1): 17

World Health Organization (1957). *Expert Committee on Rabies. Third Report.* WHO Tech. Rpt. No. 121. Geneva.

World Health Organization (1966). *Expert Committee on Rabies. Fifth Report.* WHO Tech. Rpt. No. 321. Geneva.

World Health Organization (1973). *Expert Committee on Rabies. Sixth Report.* WHO Tech. Rpt. No. 523. Geneva.

World Health Organization (1984). *Expert Committee on Rabies. Seventh Report.* WHO Tech. Rpt. No. 709. Geneva.

Chapter 5:
RABIES AND THE BATS OF LATIN AMERICA

Alleged Correlations Between Behavior and Disease

Of striking interest to the inhabitants of both Trinidad and southern Brazil during the early epizootics of paralytic rabies was the unusual occurrence of bats flying in apparent frenzy during daylight hours (Haupt and Rehaag, 1921; Pawan, 1936a). These bats would reportedly screech wildly and fight with each other in flight, often just over the heads of stunned observers. Such bats were frequently knocked to the ground by observers and sent to laboratories for study.

Seemingly reliable accounts accumulated that told of "crazed" vampire bats repeatedly crashing into obstacles. The bats allegedly behaved as "mad dogs," baring their teeth and snapping at animals and men alike. Livestock were viciously attacked and violent, unprovoked attacks on humans were not unknown. Such observations, Pawan (1936b) noted, were unusual within the collective memory of the existing generation of islanders. Haupt and Rehaag (1921) had considered this aberrant behavior to be a reflection of some disease within the local bat populace.

To the inhabitants of Trinidad and southern Brazil, there seemed to be a close correlation between the frequency with which such odd incidents of bat behavior were reported and the prevalence of paralytic disease in area livestock. It was frequently observed that cattle bitten by bats during daylight hours subsequently developed paralytic disease and died (Carini, 1911; Haupt and Rehaag, 1921). Indeed, an unusually large number of abnormally behaving bats was generally regarded by local ranchers as heralding the development of disease in cattle (Pawan, 1936a).

In southern Brazil, many ranchers were convinced that *mal de caderas*, the disease that was ravaging their livestock, was being spread by maddened vampire bats, wildly biting their cattle during daylight hours. Such attention-getting reports should not be completely accepted at face value. Numerous cases of "bat attacks" in the United States are grossly exaggerated and misperceived. There have been no recent confirmed reports of similar behavior in vampire bats (Schroeder et al, 1952; Constantine, 1987).

The suggestion that vampire bats (Figure 5-1) may have been the agents responsible for the epizootics would explain both the prevalence of the disease, in the absence of demonstrable enzootic rabies in the canine population, as well as its progression across natural barriers, seemingly insurmountable except by flight. Some time after the recognition by Carini (1911 [cited by Gilyard, 1945]) that cattle deaths were caused by paralytic rabies, investigators began testing the possibility that bats were the principal reservoir of virus.

Early Studies

In Brazil, Haupt and Rehaag (1921) described the case of a leaf-nosed bat, *Artibeus lituratus* (formerly known as *Phyllostoma superciliatum*), captured on the back of an eight-day-old calf. The calf subsequently died of paralytic rabies and the bat was diagnosed rabid by demonstration that its brain and salivary glands could induce a rabies-like disease when injected into test subjects. Baer (1975a) suggested that this may have been a misidentified vampire bat.

In 1931, a specimen of *Artibeus planirostris trinitatis* was captured one morning in a chemist's shop in Trinidad and Metivier captured three specimens of *Artibeus sp.* fighting and biting each other early one morning on one of the government farms. All four specimens were diagnosed positive for rabies (Metivier, 1931; de Verteuil and Urich, 1936).

These were the first cases of bat rabies to be reported in Brazil and Trinidad, respectively, and were of interest because *Artibeus* are not vampire bats. They are, in fact, fruit-eating bats, known to bite no animal and drink no blood. Even so, Haupt and Rehaag (1921) did report finding partially digested blood in the stomachs of fruit-eating bats and, during the years between 1929 and 1931, incidents were reported of bats, believed to have been fruit-eating species, allegedly swooping down from fruit trees in Trinidad and biting both humans and animals. Whether justified or not, fruit-eating bats were considered as possible components in this newly recognized sylvatic rabies cycle. Addressing this concern, Pawan (1948) reported that species of *Artibeus* would develop rabies following the bite of a rabid vampire bat. The saliva of such infected fruit bats could, in turn, produce paralysis in rabbits.

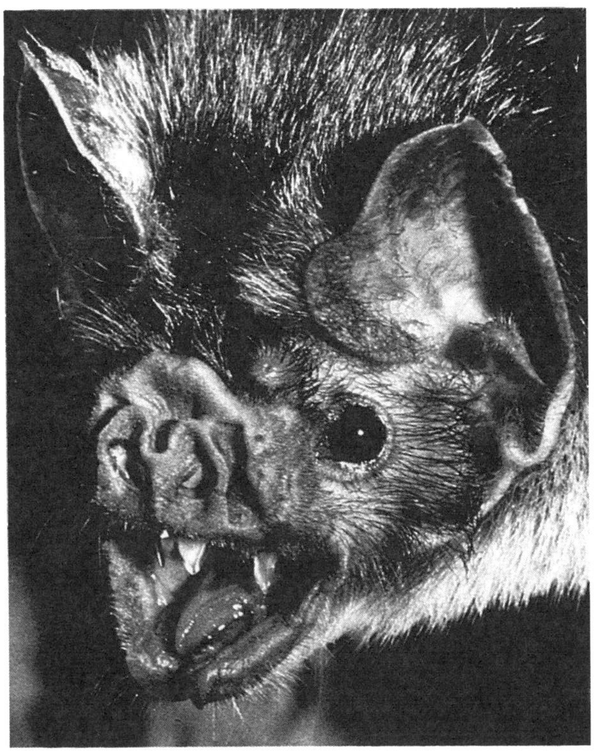

Figure 5-1. Facial features of the common vampire bat. (From Schmidt, U. Orientation and Sensory Function in *Desmodus rotundus*. In A. M. Greenhall and U. Schmidt (eds.) *Natural History of Vampire Bats*. © CRC Press, Inc. Boca Raton, Florida, 1988. Reproduced with permission.)

Pawan (1936a, 1936b) described early studies of the brains and salivary glands of day-flying vampire bats caught while attacking livestock or humans. He found that extracts of salivary glands or brain emulsions from these bats produced disease when inoculated into rabbits and calves. These animals subsequently became severely emaciated and paralyzed. Negri bodies could often be demonstrated in their brains. Furthermore, bites by naturally infected vampire bats were shown to cause paralytic rabies in calves.

Prior to the development of modern methods of rabies identification, the demonstration of Negri bodies, in the face of appropriate clinical signs, was the principle means of diagnosing the disease. Today, the accuracy of this test, when used alone, is considered questionable. At present, it is known that Negri bodies cannot be universally demonstrated in cases of rabies confirmed by fluorescent antibody test (a highly accurate test that is currently the gold standard for rabies diagnosis). They are demonstrable in only about 85% of animal rabies cases (Kaplan, 1985). Bat variants of rabies virus may have a reduced negrigenesis, perhaps as low as 50% to 60% (Tjalma and Wentworth, 1957; Burns et al, 1958). It is entirely possible that bats with no demonstrable Negri bodies in their brains, but extracts of whose brains produced a paralytic condition in challenged test animals, were rabid. This is possible regardless of whether or not Negri bodies could be demonstrated in the brains of challenged test subjects. It is also possible that false positives were diagnosed due to the mistaken identification of Negri bodies. Diagnosis by experimental salivary transmission of rabies-like disease to laboratory animals might also have been complicated by the presence of other bat salivary gland viruses, which may have led to false-positive results (see page 154).

Pawan's work confirmed and extended earlier studies of Queiroz Lima (1934a, 1934b) and Torres and Queiroz Lima (1936) in Brazil. These workers had also shown that extracts of the brain of a dead vampire bat would produce paralytic rabies (with demonstrable Negri bodies) when inoculated into an eight-day-old calf and into several rabbits.

Pawan (1936a) discussed the possibility that

THE FLUORESCENT ANTIBODY TEST

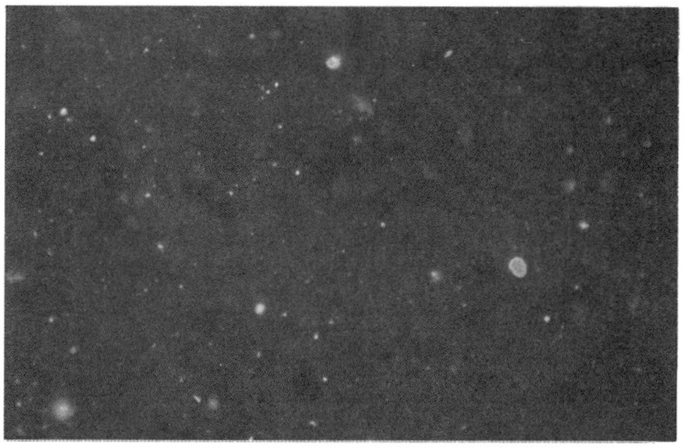

Green fluorescence characteristic of a positive FAT test for rabies on a brain specimen. Photo courtesy of Dr. D. Kinker. Diagnostic Laboratory, College of Veterinary Medicine, Iowa State University.

The fluorescent antibody test, or FAT, remains the most reliable microscopic method currently available for the diagnosis of rabies. Diagnosis can be made within a matter of hours, at most, of receiving appropriate specimens.

The test utilizes fluorescence microscopy to help identify rabies antigen within the tissues of a suspect specimen. The technique entails use of a combined reagent, consisting of an antibody against the rabies virus and an attached fluorochrome. When exposed to ultraviolet light, the fluorochrome will fluoresce (emit light of a different wavelength). This can be detected by a trained technician. Fluorescein isothiocyanate is the fluorochrome most frequently used.

Generally, an impression smear of the brain is made on a glass slide. Once done, the rabies antibody/fluorochrome conjugate is applied. If rabies antigen is present, the conjugate will bind to it and remain fixed as the unbound conjugate is washed off. If no rabies antigen is present, all of the conjugate will be washed off. When adequately stimulated by light of the correct wavelength, the fluorochrome component of the bound conjugate will fluoresce, showing the green fluorescence characteristic of a positive fluorescent antibody test. If the brain was negative for rabies, no fluorescence will be seen because all of the conjugate was washed off. Positive and negative controls are run with each test.

virus isolated from alleged cases of rabies was, in fact, the virus of pseudorabies (Aujeszky's disease). He considered that the pseudorabies and rabies viruses coexisted in the bat population and that the severe emaciation and paralysis produced in rabbits following challenge with viral isolates from brains of afflicted bats may have been due to pseudorabies infection. Reagan et al (1953) demonstrated that the big brown bat, *Eptesicus fuscus*, could be experimentally infected with pseudorabies virus.

On the basis of initial serological tests, Remlinger and Bailly (1931a, 1931b) believed that the cattle disease in Latin America was due to *Maladie d'Aujeszky*. In a second report of the same year, however, Remlinger and Bailly indicated that the epizootics of bovine paralysis were not due to pseudorabies, but were caused by paralytic rabies (Metivier, 1935). Limited serological testing (serum-neutralization and cross-immunity tests) at the time indicated an antigenic relatedness of virus isolated from outbreaks in Latin America to a fixed strain of rabies virus (Pawan, 1936a).

During 1934 and 1935, Pawan had examined 2,292 bats in Trinidad for rabies. Of these, 88 (3.8%) were confirmed positive. Fifty-nine rabies-positive bats were identified as vampires, four were species of *Artibeus*, and one was *Hemiderma/Carollia sp.* (another fruit-eating species that shares caves with the vampire bat, with *Artibeus*, and with various insectivorous bats). Twenty-four were not clearly identified. To what extent the sampling was representative of the local bat population was not known. Rabies has since been reported in over 50 species of nonhematophagous bats from Latin America (see Baer, 1975b). However, findings in some of the early studies (prior to the advent of fluorescent antibody testing) may have been inaccurate.

Sugay and Nilsson (1966 [cited by Constantine, 1970]), reported that 1.6% (9 of 554) of vampire bats examined in Brazil were confirmed positive for rabies, and Williams (1960) reported that 0.46% (26 of 5,709) of vampires in Trinidad were positive for rabies. The observed prevalence of rabies in a population of vampire bats is now known to be cyclic in nature (see page 94) and will be biased by the time of sampling with respect to the appearance of epizootic disease in local livestock (Delpietro et al, 1972; Fornes et al, 1974; Lord et al, 1975; Delpietro and Konolsaisen, 1991).

References

Amasino, C. F., Avolio, J., Fava, F., Fernandez, R., and D. Pereira (1986). Rabies en murcielagos insectivoros: Nuevos diagnosticos efectuados en el laboratorio central de salud publica de la Pcia. de Buenos Aires (Rabies in insectivorous bats: New diagnoses at the Central Public Health Laboratory of Buenos Aires province). *Veterinaria Argentina.* 3(28): 735 (English abstract) in *Vet. Bull.* (1987). 57(2): 104

Baer, G. M. (1975a). Bovine Paralytic Rabies and Rabies in the Vampire Bat. In G. M. Baer (ed.) *The Natural History of Rabies.* Vol. II. Academic Press. New York.

Baer, G. M. (1975b). Rabies in Nonhematophagous Bats. In G. M. Baer (ed.) *The Natural History of Rabies.* Vol. I. Academic Press. New York.

Burns, K. F., Shelton, D. F., and E. W. Grogan (1958). Bat rabies: Experimental host transmission studies. *Ann. N. Y. Acad. Sci.* 70: 452

Carini, A. (1911). Sur une grande epizootie de rage. *Ann. Inst. Pasteur.* 25: 843

Constantine, D. G. (1970). Bats in Relation to the Health, Welfare, and Economy of Man. In W. Wimsatt (ed.) *Biology of Bats.* Vol. II. Academic Press. New York.

Constantine, D. G. (1987). Public Health Veterinarian. Department of Health Services, State of California—Health and Welfare Agency, Veterinary Public Health Unit. Berkeley, California. Personal communication.

de Amorim, A. F., da Silva, R. A., and N. M. da Silva (1970). Isolamento do virus rabico de morcego insectivoro, *Histiotus velatus*, capturado no estado de Santa Catarina (Isolation of rabies virus from an insectivorous bat, *Histiotus velatus*, captured in Santa Catarina State, Brazil). *Pesquisa Agropecuaria Brasileira.* 5: 433 (English abstract) in *Vet. Bull.* (1972). 42(2): 73

Delpietro, H. A. and J. F. Konolsaisen (1991). Dinamica da raiva em uma populacao de morcegos hematofagos (*Desmodus rotundus*) no nordeste Argentino, e sua relacao com a raiva paralitica dos herbivoros. *Arq. Biol. Tecnol.* 34(3/4): 381

Delpietro, H., de Diaz, A. M. C., Fuenzalida, E., and J. F. Bell (1972). Determinacion de la tasa de ataque de rabia en murcielagos (Determination of the frequency of rabies in vampire bats). *Bol. Of. Sanit. Panam.* 73(3): 222 (English abstract) in *Vet. Bull.* (1973). 43(8): 415

de Verteuil, E. and F. W. Urich (1936). The study and control of paralytic rabies transmitted by bats in Trinidad, British West Indies. *Trans. Roy. Soc. Trop. Med. Hyg.* XXIX(4): 317

Fornes, A., Lord, R. D., Kuns, M. L., Larghi, O. P., Fuenzalida, E., and L. Lazara (1974). Control of bovine rabies through vampire bat control. *J. Wildl. Dis.* 10: 310

Gilyard, R. T. (1945). Bat transmitted paralytic rabies. *Cornell Vet.* XXXV(3): 195

Haupt, H. and H. Rehaag (1921). Durch fledermause verbreitete seuchenhafte Tollwut unter Viehbestanden in Santa Catharina (Sud-Brasilien). *Ztschr. f. Infecktionskr. Haustiere.* 22: 76 English translation courtesy of Dr. Volker Moenig.

Kaplan, C. (1985). Rabies: A Worldwide Disease. In P. J. Bacon (ed.) *Population Dynamics of Rabies in Wildlife.* Academic Press. New York.

Lord, R. D., Fuenzalida, E., Delpietro, H., Larghi, O. P., de Diaz, A. M. O., and L. Lazaro (1975). Observations on the epizootiology of vampire bat rabies. *Bull. Pan Am. Hlth. Org.* IX(3): 189

Metivier, H. V. (1931). *The Administration Reports of the Director of Agriculture for 1931.* Reported in *Carib. Med. J.* (1959). XXI (1-4): 174

Metivier, H. V. M. (1935). Paralytic rabies in livestock. *J. Comp. Path. Ther.* 48: 245

Nilsson, M. R. and C. A. Nagata (1975). Isolamento do virus rabico do cerebro, glandulas salivares e interescapular, coracao, pulmoes e testiculos de morcego *Desmodus rotundus* (Geoffry, 1810), no Estado de Sao Paulo (Isolation of rabies virus from brain, salivary and interscapular glands, heart, lungs and testis of the bat *Desmodus rotundus*, (Geoffrey, 1810) in the State of Sao Paulo, Brazil). *Arquivos do Instituto Biologico, Sao Paulo, Brazil* (English abstract) in *Vet. Bull.* (1978). 48(4): 309.

Pawan, J. L. (1936a). The transmission of paralytic rabies in Trinidad by the vampire bat (*Desmodus rotundus murinus* Wagner, 1840). *Ann. Trop. Med. Parasit.* 30: 101

Pawan, J. L. (1936b). Rabies in the vampire bat of Trinidad, with special reference to the clinical course and latency of infection. *Ann. Trop. Med. Parasit.* 30: 401

Pawan, J. L. (1948). Fruit-eating bats and paralytic rabies in Trinidad. *Ann. Trop. Med. Parasit.* 42: 173

Queiroz Lima, E. (1934a). A transmissao da raiva bovina pelo morcego hematophago *Desmodus rotundus. Brazil Med.* 48: 38

Queiroz Lima, E. (1934b). A transmissao da raiva dos herbivoros pelos morcegos hematophagos da familia Desmodontidae. *Rev. Dep. Nac. Prod. Anim.* 1: 165

Reagan, R. L., Day, W. C., Marley, R. T., and A. T. Bruekner (1953). Effect of pseudorabies virus (Aujeszky strain) in the large brown bat (*Eptesicus fuscus*). *Am. J. Vet. Res.* 14: 331

Remlinger, P. and J. Bailly (1931a). Les confusions entre le virus neurotropes et le virus rabique; moyens de les eviter. *Bull. Inst. Pasteur.* XXIX

Remlinger, P. and J. Bailly (1931b). Etudes sur la rage. *Ann. Inst. Pasteur.* XLVII

Schmidt, U. (1988). Orientation and Sensory Function in *Desmodus rotundus.* In A. M. Greenhall and U. Schmidt (eds.) *Natural History of Vampire Bats.* CRC Press, Inc. Boca Raton, Florida.

Schroeder, C. R., Black, J., Burkhart, R. L., and H. Koprowski (1952). Rabies in cattle. I. Prevention of vampire bat paralytic rabies, derriengue, by vaccination with chick-embryo-adapted rabies virus. *Vet. Med.* 47: 502

Stouraitis, P. and J. Salvatierra (1978). Isolation of rabies virus from bats in Bolivia. *Trop. Anim. Hlth. Prod.* 10(2): 101 (English abstract) in *Vet. Bull.* (1978). 48(11): 934

Sugay, W. and M. R. Nilsson (1966). Isolamentode virus da raiva de morcegos hematofogos do estado de Sao Paulo, Brasil. *Bol. Of. Sanit. Panam.* 60: 310

Tjalma, R. A. and B. B. Wentworth (1957). Bat rabies—Report of an isolation of rabies virus from native Ohio bats. *J. Am. Vet. Med. Assoc.* XXX: 68

Torres, S. and E. Queiroz Lima (1936). A raiva e os morcegos hematophagos. Morcegos que resistem a infeccao tornam-se portadores e eliminadores de virus. *Rev. Dep. Nac. Prod. Anim.* 3: 165

Williams, H. E. (1960). Bat transmitted rabies in Trinidad. *Can. Vet. J.* 1(1): 20

Yepez, A. R., La Mata, M., and A. Fornes (1972). Aislamiento de virus rabico en cerebro y glandulas de un murcielago insectivoro, *Lasiurus cinereus villosissimus* (Isolation of rabies from the brain and salivary glands of an insectivorous bat, *Lasiurus cinerueu villosissimus*). *Revista de Medicina Veterinaria, Buenos Aires.* 53(4): 281 (English abstract) in *Vet. Bull.* (1973). 43(4): 190.

Chapter 6:
VAMPIRE BATS OF THE AMERICAN TROPICS

Myth, Superstition, and Medical Oddities

The term vampire comes from the Magyar (Hungarian) word *vampir*, meaning a person who comes back from the dead to feed on the blood of the living (Fenton, 1983). In discussing vampire-bat lore and the blood-feeding undead, Gilyard (1945) wrote,

> *When the sanguinivorous behavior of the Desmodus "family" was first observed by early South American conquerors the common name "vampire" was appropriately applied. Its origin is found in an ancient slavonic superstition in which it was believed that deceased people of questionable character became reanimated and prowled about at night sucking the blood from sleeping brethren. When individuals suspected of such behavior were disinterred, their cadavers were found to be fresh, as if decomposition were being averted by their nocturnal blood foraging expeditions. To prevent "vampire" ghosts the practice of driving a huge stake through the body at the time of interment came into being. This procedure was believed to prevent the escape of an evil soul. It was at one time regularly practiced if the character of the late personality suggested that he might become addicted to vampirism in after life.*

Dalquest (1955) related an interesting account of vampire bites in eastern Mexico. In this region, local inhabitants denied any possibility that they could be bitten by bats and were actually repulsed by the thought that such a circumstance might occur. They did admit, however, that brujas, or witches, frequently bit their children at night. A similar belief existed in southern Belize (McCarthy, 1993). In northeastern Mexico, many local ranchers believe that wounds on apparently healthy cattle are made by blood-feeding bats other than vampires. Only when concurrent rabies-related cattle deaths occur are wounds attributed to attacks by vampire bats (Babb, 1993; Brown, 1993). Regarding human attacks by vampire bats in Trinidad, Goodwin and Greenhall (1961) wrote,

> *Many country people or peasants in Trinidad, when questioned about wounds that had obviously been inflicted on them by vampire bats, frequently and resolutely state that they had been bitten by a soucouyant, a blood-sucking supernatural jumbie, or evil spirit, well known in Trinidad folklore. The soucouyant is usually an old woman, who at night sheds her skin, generally hiding it under a mortar, and flies off through the air as a ball of fire. She can only pass through a keyhole or crack in the house and, as does the vampire bat, attacks some person for her nightly meal of blood. There are several methods of trapping this jumbie. One is to locate the shed skin and sprinkle hot pepper on it which may burn the soucouyant to death when she returns and replaces her skin. A less drastic method is to scatter several pounds of rice outside her house which she must count, grain by grain, before she can re-enter. If the jumbie is caught without her skin, the villagers may decide to dispose of the soucouyant by placing her in a nail-spiked barrel full of tar and then roll the barrel into the ocean. Complete household protection may be afforded by the elimination of keyholes and the filling in of all cracks in the house.*

In considering the reality of vampirism, Heick (1992) compared the behavior of the mythical human vampire to a psychotic rabid state. He speculated that a genuine human vampire may simply have been "a poor, rabid peasant who ended up buried with a stake driven through his heart." Hemphill and Zabow (1983), on the other hand, suggested that the actions of human vampirists may have been the source of the original vampire myths. Clinical vampirism is a rare and frightening human condition. A human displaying the three essential characteristics of vampirism is called a vampirist. The triad of signs typifying the psychopathology of human vampirism includes:

1) A lack of absolute self-identity (patients often being unable to identify their own face in a mirror).
2) A periodic craving to drink fresh blood, either one's own (auto-vampirism associated with self-mutilation), that of another person (often associated with violence), or that of an animal. The craving is often associated with intense recurrent blood dreams.
3) A nonsexual fascination with the dead, or a desire to experience death and dying. This fixation with death and dying is not of a suicidal nature. Human vampirists do not seek to find, in death, peace and release from their aberrant existence in life. Rather, they are searching to experience the existence of a "living death."

Drinking blood temporarily relieves the vampirist's cravings and characteristically induces a period of calm and relaxation. Auto-vampirists are primarily non-criminal females, whereas taking blood from others appears to be an exclusively male purview, possibly because of the requisite force involved. Clinical vampirism may be associated with serial murder in attempts to obtain blood from others. According to Hemphill and Zabow (1983), the vampirist's sole desire is to procure blood and not to indulge in acts of cruelty and violence. They do not consider the condition to be a form of sadomasochism. The vampirist may show no outward signs of a mental disorder and may, in fact, be an otherwise pleasant person. Additional information concerning vampires in myth and superstition can be found in the works by Villa-C. and Canela-R. (1988) and Brown (1994).

General Description

Among the many and diverse species of bats inhabiting Latin America are insectivorous, frugivorous, piscivorous, and carnivorous species, plus one group of hematophagous bats, the vampire bats. Because of their specialized feeding habits, some taxonomists have considered that the vampire bats should hold status as a distinct family, the Desmodontidae, of the order Chiroptera. Immunologic, morphologic, and chromosomal studies, however, are most consistent with the evolutionary perspective that vampire bats be considered as a subfamily (Desmodontinae) of the New World leaf-nosed bats, the Phyllostomidae (Greenhall, 1974; Handley, Jr., 1980; Baker et al, 1988; Koopman, 1988; Anderson, 1990; Morgan, 1991).

The vampire bats comprise three genera and three species: the common vampire bat (*Desmodus rotundus rotundus*, Geoffrey, 1810), the hairy-legged vampire bat (*Diphylla ecaudata*, Spix, 1823), and the white-winged vampire bat (*Diaemus youngi*, Jentinck, 1893).[1]

Although they may become infected with the rabies virus, *Diaemus* and *Diphylla* are generally not considered to be significant in the cycle of rabies transmission to livestock or humans. Few investigations have been made of these bats and

[1]The hairy-legged vampire bat has also gone by the name of *Diphylla centralis* (Thomas, 1903). The white-winged vampire bat has also gone by the name of *Diaemus youngi cypselinus* (Thomas, 1928). The common vampire bat has gone by the various names of *Phyllostoma rotundum* (Geoffrey, 1810), *Rhinolophus ecaudatus* (Schinz, 1821), *Desmodus rufus* (Wied, 1826), *Edostoma cinerea* (D'Orbigny, 1835), *Desmodus d'orbignyi* (Waterhouse, 1839), *Desmodus murinus* (Wagner, 1840), *Desmodus fuscus* (Burmeister, 1854), and *Desmodus mordax* (Burmeister, 1879). Although once considered a subspecies of *Desmodus rotundus*, *Desmodus murinus* may simply reflect individual species variation (Koopman, 1988).

little is known of their habits or biology (Greenhall, 1972a). *Desmodus* is the most common of the vampires, has the widest distribution, and is the most well known of the three. *Diaemus* is the rarest and least studied. The relative abundance of *Desmodus* may be related to its more liberal tastes in animal blood and the wider range of its host animal populations (Villa-Ramirez, 1969). Of the three species of vampire bats, the common vampire bat, *Desmodus rotundus*, is implicated almost exclusively in the transmission of paralytic rabies to livestock (Greenhall, 1974) and will be referred to by the common name, vampire bat, throughout this text.

Among the vertebrates, the vampire bat is unique in its adaptations to a diet consisting solely of blood. In regard to blood meals, it is believed that a component of plasma, rather than red blood cells, attracts the bats (Busch, 1988). Turner (1975) advanced an evolutionary hypothesis to explain the hematophagous habits of the vampire bat. Accordingly, he believed it to be plausible that vampire bats acquired their initial taste for blood by feeding on parasitic moths, such as the Noctuid (*Calyptra eustrigata*). Moths which pierce the skin of cattle to suck their blood and those which drink blood from previously inflicted wounds or from blood droplets shed by mosquitos have been described (Banziger, 1968). Others have suggested that their taste for blood was acquired from feeding on engorged ticks parasitizing large mammals, or on adult and larval insects (especially screw-worms) feeding in flesh wounds (Gillette, 1975; Fenton, 1992a, 1992b). Mills (1980) observed a captive vampire bat regurgitating blood into the mouth of her offspring when it was only one week of age and suggested that young vampires may receive their first taste of blood in this manner.

The vampire bat has a wingspan averaging 350 to 400 mm and a combined head and body length of about 70 to 90 mm. The female is somewhat larger than the male. They have a modified (small) nose-leaf (a leaf-like appendage found in association with the nasal region in other species of phyllostomid bats) and a highly reduced interfemoral membrane. They lack external tails. Adult bats weigh between 15 and 60 grams (Greenhall, 1972b; Bhatnagar, 1988).

Although occasionally hopping like toads, vampire bats are adept at scurrying along the ground and are, in fact, unique among bats in their agility at walking on all fours (Figure 6-1). With wings compactly folded and using their thumbs as forefeet, they can shuffle about with their body raised fully two inches off the ground (Ditmars, 1934; Ditmars and Greenhall, 1935, 1960). In searching for vampires in the caves of Panama, Ditmars and Greenhall (1935) wrote of the bats scurrying along cave walls like rodents, this habit being sufficiently distinct among bats as to allow identification of vampires at a glance (Figure 6-2). Altenbach (1979) has discussed the unique locomotor ability of the vampire bat in detail.

Vampires may live a long time, both in captivity and in the wild. Trapido (1946) reported keeping one individual alive for as long as 12 years. Delpietro et al (1993) captured three specimens in Argentina that had been banded as adults 12, 13, and 15 years earlier and Wimsatt (cited by Schmidt et al, 1980) reportedly kept one alive in captivity for as long as 19.5 years.

Vampire Roosts

During the day, vampire bats have been found to occupy caves, culverts, hollow trees, underground drains, dilapidated houses, empty garrets, cellars, bridges, wells (both active and in disuse), tunnels, buildings, steeples, archaeological ruins, and crevices in stone walls. They have been found deep in the forest, as well as in and about Trinidad's capital city. Roost requirements of *Desmodus* include an average ambient temperature between 21° C (70° F) and 23° C (73° F) and a minimum humidity of 45% (Flores-Crespo and Arellano-Sota, 1991). Like other bats, the vampire rests hanging head down, both when roosting and when digesting its blood meal.

Vampires do not always utilize a solitary roost, to which all individuals in the colony return on a daily basis. Multiple roosts may be used and the factors which govern the movement between them is poorly understood (Greenhall, 1985). A vampire roost is readily recognized. Beneath the clusters of bats is a "deep pool of (dark) stinking liquid or semi-liquid feces" (Dalquest, 1955). This is the remains of many blood meals. Dalquest referred to it as the "vampire pool." As

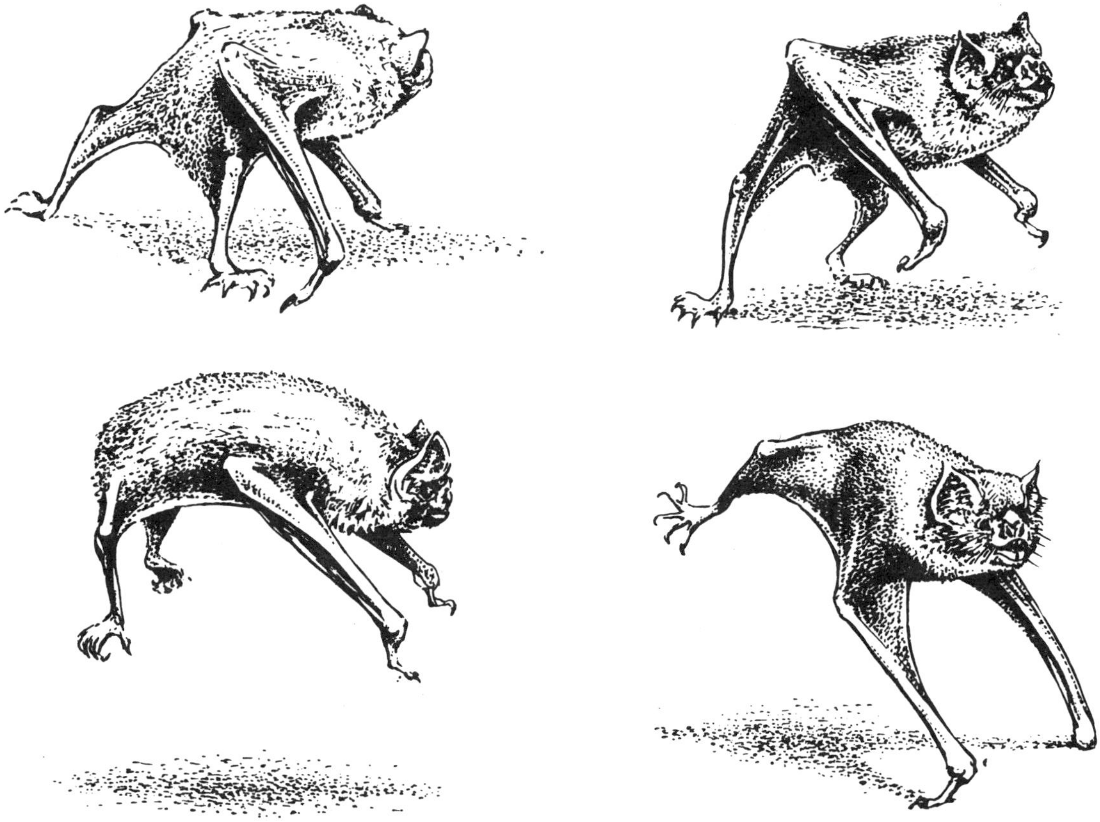

Figure 6-1. The characteristic locomotor capacity of vampire bats is unique among the Chiroptera. They can hop sideways, forward, or backward with great agility. In this way, they are able to approach victims stealthily, or skillfully evade them. (From Schober, W. *The Lives of Bats*. Edition Leipzig. Leipzig, Germany, 1984. Drafted by Michael Lissmann. Reproduced with permission.)

the pool decays, it releases ammonia, which, according to Greenhall (1985), can be detected as much as a quarter of a mile away. Numerous invertebrates live in and about the pool, which is strongly alkaline (pH 13). The excretory pools formed by *Diaemus* are smaller than those of *Desmodus*, and *Diphylla* leaves only small drops of bloody feces (Greenhall, 1991).

Distribution and Energetics of the Vampire Bat

Discounting folklore of Transylvanian vampires of the genus *Dracula* (*Nosferatu*), vampire bats are found only in tropical America, which includes Mexico, and Central and South America (Figure 6-3). Their northern limits in Mexico extend to the state of Tamaulipas on the Atlantic coast and the state of Sonora on the Pacific coast. The southern limits of their range extend to the coasts of Chile, central Argentina, and the coasts of Uruguay. They range from sea level to over 2,000 meters above sea level (Flores-Crespo and Arellano-Sota, 1991). Vampires are not found among the islands of the Caribbean, but are present on the islands of Trinidad and Margarita (along the northern coast of Venezuela). They are not common deep in the rainforests or in other undisturbed habitats, but have expanded their range with the introduction of livestock into new areas.

Vampire bats are limited in both their northern and southernmost ranges to regions with a minimal mean temperature of 10° C (50° F). In the United States, this condition is met in Browns-

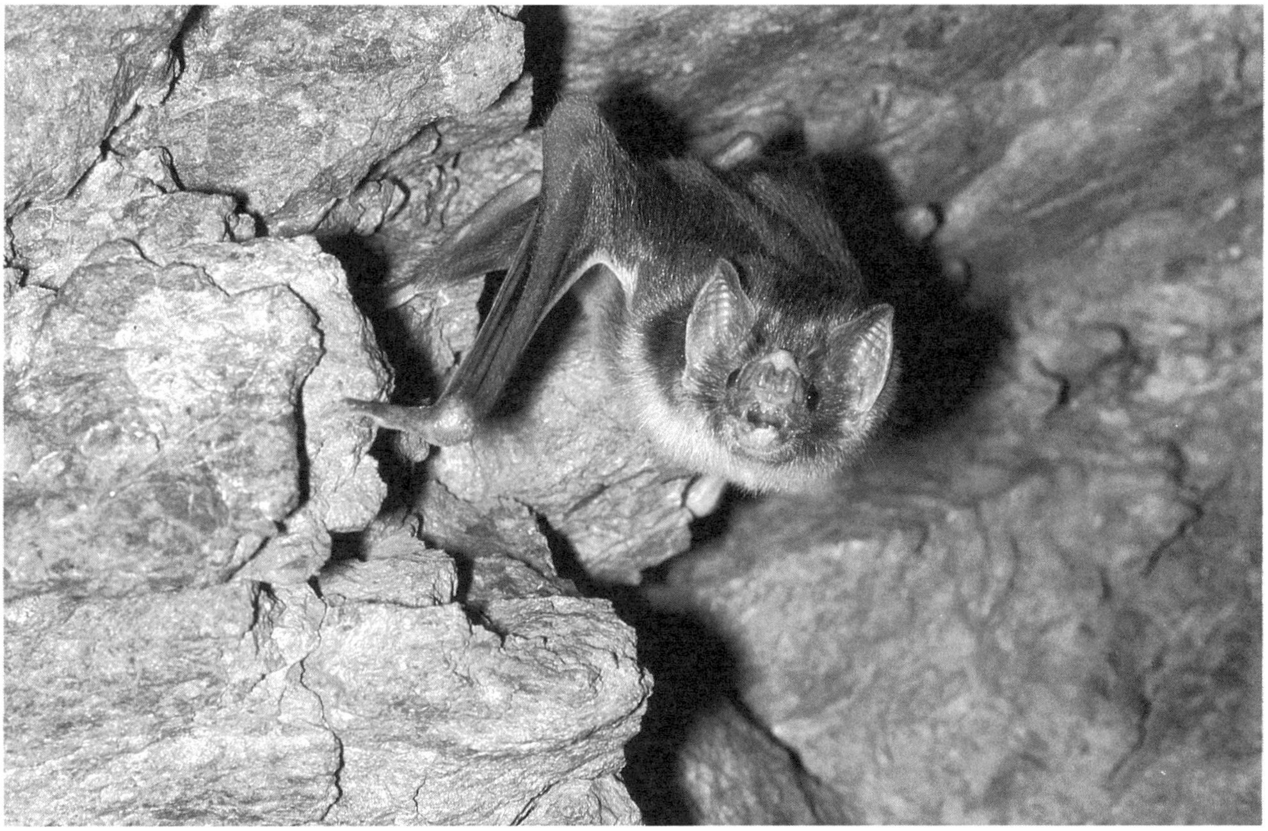

Figure 6-2. Within their roosts, vampires can be distinguished from other bats by their characteristic rodent-like locomotion. Photo © Randall D. Babb.

ville, Texas and in Florida, south of Tampa Bay (McNab, 1973). In areas where caves are present, however, the average annual cave temperature is slightly lower than in tropical regions.

Based on his laboratory studies of energy metabolism, McNab (1973) concluded that the lower temperatures in caves north of the vampire's current tropical distribution would strain the limits of the bat's metabolic capabilities, requiring a higher expenditure of energy for maintenance of normal body temperature than the bat could afford. Their capacity for thermoregulation is marginal, accounting, in part, for their restricted distribution (Lyman and Wimsatt, 1966; McNab, 1969).

Due to evaporative water loss during flight, vampire bats may be limited in the amount of time they can spend foraging for food in the course of an evening. In a temperate-zone environment, therefore, the vampire's typical nightly feeding (limited in duration by the bat's flight capacity) might not be sufficient to sustain it. Captive vampires will increase both their food consumption and muscular activity when maintained in a cold environment (Wimsatt, 1962).

Diphylla reportedly ranges from southern Tamaulipas south through eastern Mexico and Central America. It has not been reported west of the Andes, but ranges along the eastern Andes as far south as northern Bolivia and then across south central Brazil to the east coast of South America. It has not been reported from most of the Amazon basin and is not found on the islands of either Margarita or Trinidad (Koopman, 1988).

The respective ranges of *Diaemus* and *Diphylla* are believed to overlap throughout Central America, but *Diaemus* appears to have a more extensive range throughout South America. South of Colombia, *Diaemus* is not found west of the Andes. It may be confined to the lowlands. *Diaemus* ranges across the Amazon basin and Guianas as far south as northern Argentina and southeastern Brazil. It has been reported from both Margarita and Trinidad (Koopman, 1988).

Fossil Remains of Vampire Bats in the Americas

Although vampire-bat populations today are closely tied to tropical livestock-rearing areas, the bats did, at one time, inhabit what is now the continental United States (Figure 6-3). Fossil remains of vampire bats in portions of what is now the United States suggest that warmer temperatures may have characterized these regions in the distant past (although it is also possible that extinct populations of vampire bats may have been able to withstand cooler temperatures than modern, extant populations). Vampire remains have been found in pleistocene deposits in Texas (Cockerell, 1930), Florida (Gut, 1959; Olsen, 1960), Arizona (Mead, 1981), New Mexico (Harris, 1985, 1987), California (Hutchison, 1967), and West Virginia (Grady, 1987). Koopman (1958) reported that they also inhabited Cuba in pleistocene times.

It has been suggested that pleistocene vampire bats fed principally on large, flightless birds and on ground sloths, which may have inhabited the same caves (Koopman, 1958; Olsen, 1960). Olsen speculated on the contribution of vampire bats to the eventual mass extinction of Florida's pleistocene mammal population. Dobson (cited by Malaga-Alba, 1966) suggested that vampire bats may have been responsible for the disappearance of other large mammal species in the New World. With the extinction of the ground sloth and the absence of other large native mammals, these vampire bats may have been unable to adapt to alternate food sources. There is no evidence to indicate that this is true and these ideas remain purely speculative. However, modern examples of this type of linked population decline are known, particularly in species that have become so specialized as to feed exclusively on one type of food.

In view of the apparent willingness of vampire bats to subsist on blood from diverse host populations, Ray et al (1988) suggested that the decline in vampire populations in what is now the United States was not likely to have been due to the extinction of ground sloths. Greenhall (1991) speculated that prehistoric vampires may have fed on several other hosts, including deer, capybara, and humans.

Hunting and Feeding Characteristics

Vampire bats are creatures of the night, taking their blood meal during the darkest part of the evening, before the moon rises or after it has set (Wimsatt, 1969; Flores-Crespo et al, 1972; Turner, 1975). In selecting herds of cattle to feed upon, Gilyard (1945) believed that the bats do not fly any farther than needed to find a blood meal. According to Linhart (1975), however, vampires do not necessarily feed on cattle nearest to their diurnal roosts. There is no general consensus as to whether vampires feed once or twice during the night, but they are believed to feed at least once each night, if possible. Failure to obtain a blood meal on any given evening severely presses the limits of their endurance (McFarland and Wimsatt, 1969; McNab, 1973; Wilkinson, 1984, 1990).

It is believed that the vampire bat hunts in small groups and that these groups may form a social structure within the roost (Schmidt et al, 1980). Greenhall et al (1971) observed them to arrive at hosts in groups of 2 to 6. Turner (1975) suggested that territorial aggression in vampire bats may be a means whereby males maintain control over an animal while females feed. In view of the presence of large cattle herds, this type of activity might be an evolutionary throwback to a time when exclusive domination of a small animal by a social unit of vampires may have been critical to their survival.

Diphylla and *Diaemus* both appear to prefer avian blood (Villa-Ramirez, 1969; Gardner, 1977 [cited by Sazima and Uieda, 1980]; Goodwin and Greenhall, 1961; Hoyt and Altenbach, 1981; Uieda, 1982; Kaplan, 1985). Even in captivity, *Diphylla* has refused nonavian sources of food. McCarthy (1987) reported a weak precipitin reaction for mammalian blood in one blood meal obtained from a specimen of *Diphylla* in southern Belize.

Host Selection

Captive vampire bats are known to feed on snakes (including rattlesnakes), lizards, crocodiles, turtles, and marine toads. In addition to various reptiles and amphibians, vampires in cap-

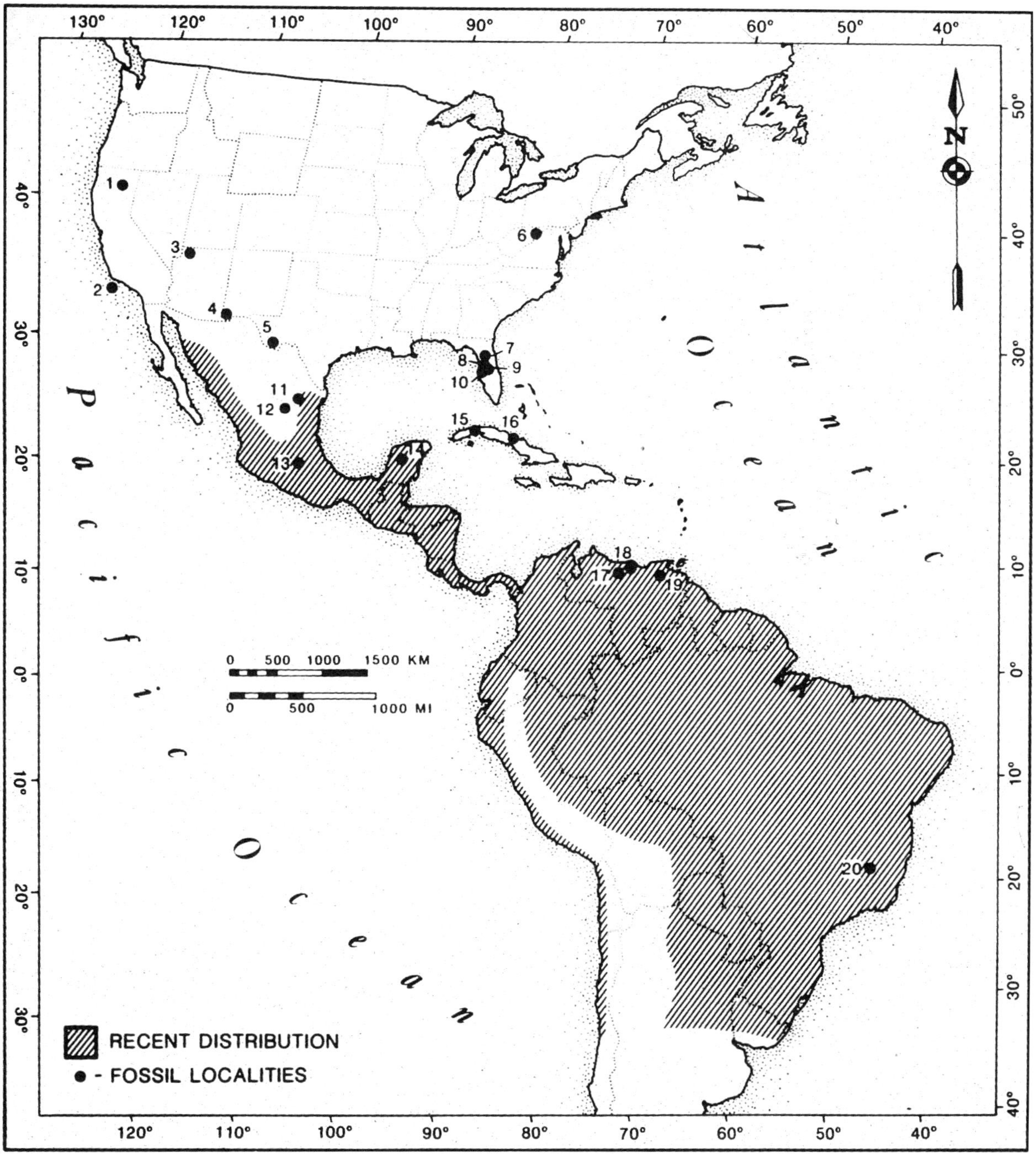

Figure 6-3. Recent distribution and fossil localities for vampire bats. Shaded area represents modern distribution of *Desmodus rotundus.* Numbers correspond to the following location of fossil findings: 1) Potter Creek Cave, Shasta County, California; 2) San Miguel Island, Santa Barbara County, California; 3) Rampart Cave, Mohave County, Arizona; 4) U-Bar Cave, Hidalgo County, New Mexico; 5) Little Thirty-eight Mine, Brewster County, Texas; 6) New Trout Cave, Pendleton County, West Virginia; 7) Haile, Alachua County, Florida; 8) Arredondo, Alachua County, Florida; 9) Reddick, Marion County, Florida; 10) Inglis, Citrus County, Florida; 11) Cueva de San Josecito, Nuevo Leon, Mexico; 12) Matehuala, San Luis Potosi, Mexico; 13) Cerro de Tlapacoya, Mexico; 14) Loltun, Yucatan, Mexico; 15) Cueva Lamas, Cuba; 16) Cueva Centenario de Lenin, Cuba; 17) Cueva de Quebrada, Venezuela; 18) Cueva de la Brujula, Venezuela; 19) Cueva del Guacharo, Venezuela; 20) Lapa da Lagoa do Sumidouro, Brazil. (From Ray, C. E., Linares, J., and G. S. Morgan. Paleontology. In A. M. Greenhall and U. Schmidt (eds.) *Natural History of Vampire Bats.* © CRC Press, Inc. Boca Raton, Florida, 1988. Reproduced with permission.)

Table 6-1

Percentage of Wild-Caught Vampire Bats in Costa Rica (La Pacifica and Palo Verde) Feeding on Domestic Livestock, Based on Results of Precipitin and Hemagglutination Tests on Vampire Blood-Meal Samples

Conditions of Capture	Number of Bats Sacrificed	Number of Feedings	Percentage Feeding on Domestic Stock
Wet Season	9	27	100
Dry Season	5	15	100
New Moon	6	18	100
Full Mooon	3	9	100
Male bats	5	15	100
Females[a]	6	18	100
Females[b]	4	12	100
Palo Verde Cave Bats	20	60	100

[a]Inactive females; [b]Pregnant or lactating females.

From Turner, D. C. *The Vampire Bat—A Field Study in Behavior and Ecology.* The Johns Hopkins University Press. Baltimore, 1975. Reproduced with permission.

tivity have been observed to feed upon a variety of other wild animals, including armadillos, porcupines, water buffalo, seals, coati, ocelots, opossums, raccoons, skunks, cave rats, coyotes, and hawks and other birds (Acha, 1981). Captive vampire bats have also been observed to feed on other species of bats (Constantine et al, 1968; Lord et al, 1973) and Lord et al (1973) reported capturing a yellow-shouldered bat (*Sturnira lilium*) with a distinctive vampire-bat bite wound on its back. Although long-term maintenance studies have not yet been done, Breidenstein (1984) discussed the merits of feeding captive vampire bats freeze-dried blood.

In the wild state, vampires are believed to take meals only from "warm-blooded" animals. As shown in Table 6-1, domestic livestock, if available, are much preferred over wild species (Greenhall, 1970; Turner, 1975). Those most commonly fed upon include cattle, horses, goats, swine, poultry, sheep, dogs, and humans, reportedly in this order of preference (Goodwin and Greenhall, 1961). Arellano et al (1971) suggested that docile breeds of cattle are preferentially attacked. In a study in Mexico, percentages of bitten cattle breeds (723 head out of a herd of 2,482) were as follows: Holsteins - 38%, Hereford - 35%, Santa Gertrudis - 32%, Angus - 30%, Charolais - 25%, and Zebu (or Brahman) - 15% (Arellano et al, 1971). Host availability may have influenced these results.

A variety of factors may influence the dietary preferences shown by the vampire bat (Thompson et al, 1982). These include availability; vulnerability; accessibility; abundance; degree of domestication; or some unique feature of size, odor, or color of a particular host species. Thompson et al (1982) did not believe taste to be an important factor in host selection by vampire bats.

Delpietro et al (1993) suggested that apparent feeding preferences of vampire bats are not related to qualitative differences among potential host species, but are proportional to the biomass available, with a strict order of preference for the most abundant host species. This feeding preference may enable the vampire to better adapt to its host, favoring an increase in vampire populations in areas containing a livestock ecosystem.

Campos and Arellano (1971 [cited by Baer, 1991]) reported finding human blood in 15.7% of the stomach contents of 70 vampire bats collected in Colima, Mexico. This suggests that the bats may bite humans fairly frequently. Dogs are reportedly rarely victimized. Gilyard (1945) believed this to be due to their "natural alertness." Although vampire bats have been observed attempting to attack dogs, and feeding from dogs has been observed, attacks are often unsuccessful. Possibly, this is due to the inherent difficulty the bat would face in "sneaking up" on a potential victim who could hear its ultrasonic echolocative cries (Malaga-Alba, 1954; Fenton, 1983). However, recent work suggests that host-generated noise may be more important to vampire bats for detecting suitable food sources (Schmidt et al, 1991).

In observing vampire bats in Costa Rica, Turner (1975) observed that calves were preferred over adult cattle. Arellano et al (1971) observed similar preferences among vampires in Mexico. Turner noted that when calves were present in a herd, the mean distance between animals was greater than when adults alone were present. Calves also spent more time during the night asleep than did adults. These features increased the probability of calves being exposed to attacking vampires and may have been significant factors in host selection by the bats. Relative docileness and thinner skin of calves may also be important.

Vampires may also demonstrate a predilection for cows over bulls. In studying facets of host selection in a limited population, Turner (1975) found that vampire bats preferentially attacked females in estrus. When they are in heat, cows are hyperactive, even at night. Turner thought that this might make these individuals more visible targets for the bats. The hyperactivity could distract the cows from the presence of the bats and they might be less inclined to shake their heads and swish their tails in response to attack.

In considering this observed preference of vampire bats to feed on estrus cows, Turner theorized a relationship between steroid levels in the cow's blood and the potential for these hormones to exert neuroendocrine feedback effects in the vampire bat. Notable in the short (about 15 hours) estrus phase of the bovine estrous cycle are the minimal levels of progesterone and the rapidly falling estrogen levels (McDonald, 1980; Knickerbocker et al, 1986). Thus, minimal levels of these hormones would be ingested by the bat and any potential effects that they might exert on the bat's own physiology would be marginal. Turner cited an interesting parasitic relationship between rabbits and fleas that lends some measure of plausibility to this hypothesis. The rabbit flea (*Spilopsyllus cuniculi*) feeds on blood from rabbit hosts. Both male and female fleas are dependent on the steroid hormones of a pregnant host to initiate and maintain their own reproductive cycles (Rothschild, 1955; Rothschild and Ford, 1964; Rothschild et al, 1970). Foster (1969) reported a similar relationship between birds and certain Mallophagan lice (*Ricinus picturatus* and *Menacanthus sp.*). The potential for ingested hormones to affect the vampire's physiology remains unproven and Turner's hypothesis regarding the possibility of ingested steroids affecting the vampire's reproductive status remains purely speculative.

Turner (1975) believed that the host preferences shown by the Costa Rican population of vampires may have been a reflection of an evolutionary adjustment to prevent excessive parasitism of host stock. In areas where the populations of bats and livestock are not so well balanced, this type of feeding adaptation may not be practical and bats would be forced to feed on all cattle. In support of this interpretation, Turner cited the work of MacArthur and Pianka (1966), Emlen (1966), and MacArthur (1972) who reasoned that predators are more selective in their feeding habits when food is abundant and less discriminating when suitable hosts are not plentiful.

Detection and Tracking of Hosts

A variety of senses may play a role in the detection and tracking of host species by vampire bats. Vampire bats have relatively large olfactory bulbs (Mann, 1960 [cited by Baer, 1975]) and an acute sense of smell (Schmidt, 1973). It has been postulated that vampires rely heavily on olfactory cues in detecting hosts (Schmidt, 1973; Turner, 1975). Researchers at the Denver Wildlife Research Center (1969) discussed the importance of olfactory attraction in the capture of bats. Baer (1975) suggested that olfaction may play a role in attracting bats to specific hosts again and again. This phenomenon has been taken advantage of in trapping vampire bats by a process called baiting

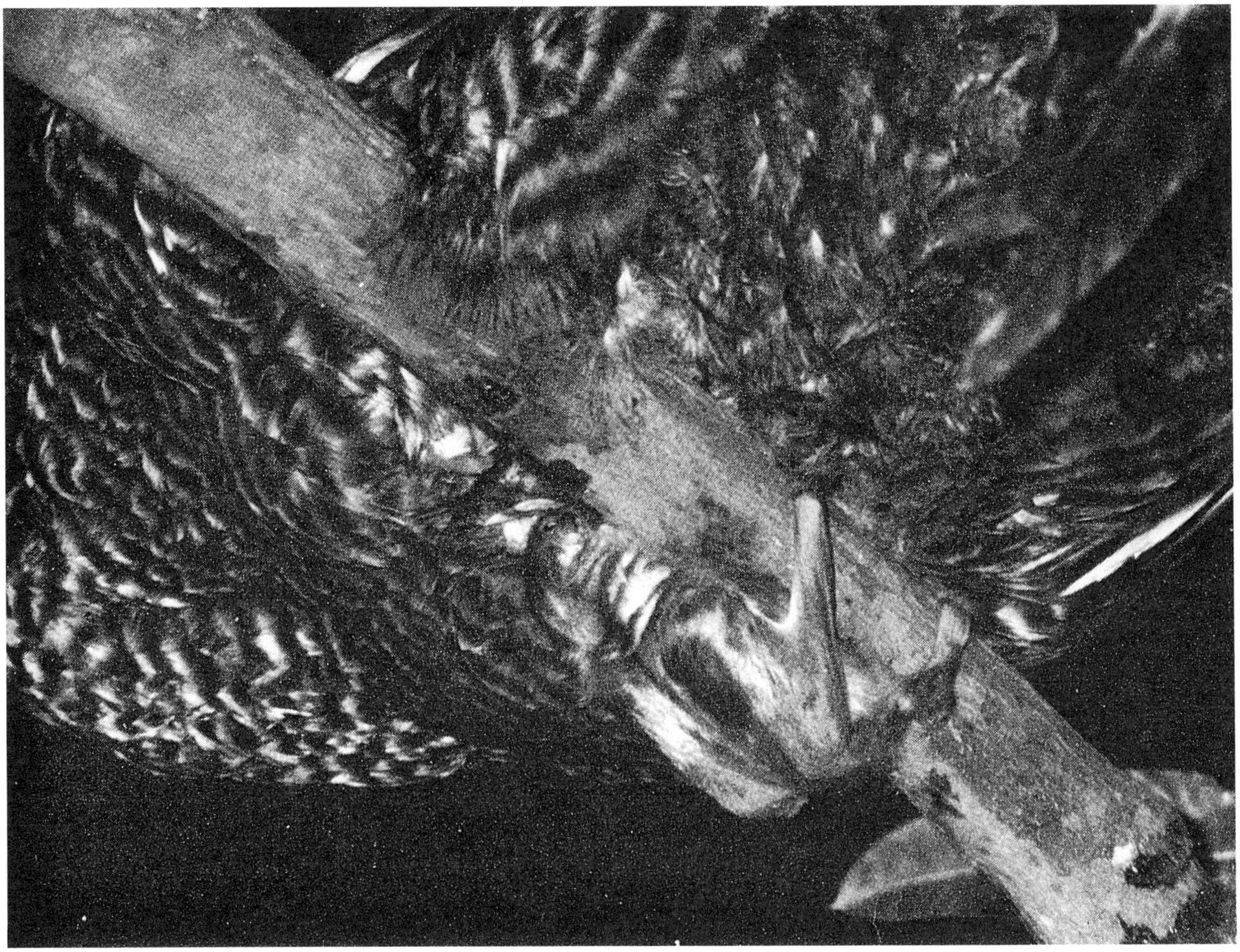

Figure 6-4. White-winged vampire bat feeding on the toes of a chicken. (From Sazima, I. and W. Uieda. Feeding behavior of the white-winged vampire bat, *Diaemus youngii*, on poultry. *J. Mammal*. 61(1): 102, 1980. Reproduced with permission.)

(see page 118).

Schmidt et al (1970 [cited by Schmidt, 1973]) suggested that vampire bats may be preferentially attracted to certain cattle breeds because of a more favorable odor. Perhaps olfactory cues were instrumental in guiding vampire bats to estrus cows in Turner's (1975) Costa Rican study. Even though the wounds inflicted by the bats continue to drip blood for quite some time, Turner believed that blood itself was not the olfactory determinant attracting bats, but considered it possible that the odor of bat urine may have played a role as an attractant (vampire bats urinate copiously during or immediately after feeding [see page 76]). Greenhall (1991) suggested that the odor of urine might serve both to help vampires locate host species as well as to identify previous feeding sites, and may contribute to the repeated attacks that some horses, cows, or humans may experience.

Uieda (1982) suggested that bird excrement may serve as an olfactory attractant for *Diphylla* and *Diaemus*. The daily return of birds to favored roosting sites may make detection by hematophagous bats easier. The presence of foliage may hinder feeding and Uieda (1982) reported that birds roosting on leafless branches were preferentially attacked.

Recently, Schmidt et al (1991) discussed the role of audition in host detection and tracking. Accordingly, they suggested that vampire bats might not rely on echolocation as a means of detecting hosts. Having possibly evolved to feed

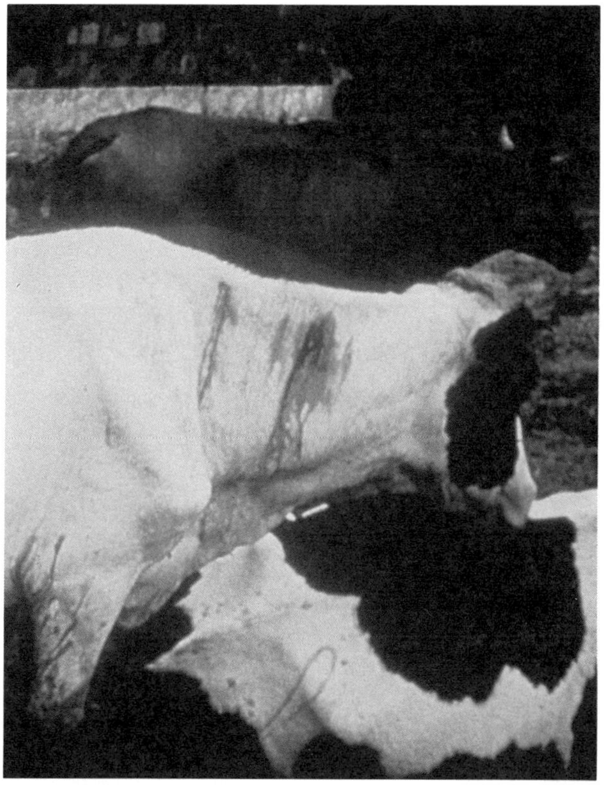

Figure 6-5. Bite wounds on the neck of victimized cow. Photo courtesy of Dr. G. Clay Mitchell. Denver Wildlife Research Center.

on host mammals hiding under cover at night, it is unlikely that echolocation would be of significant value in identification of food sources. Rather, it is possible that they have developed an auditory mechanism sensitive to frequencies below those of an echolocative nature, but capable of detecting the breathing noises of host species. The authors suggested that animal-generated noises be considered among the possible cues that vampire bats use for detection of potential hosts. In this respect, they reported the identification of brain stem neurons in the medial aspect of the rostral inferior colliculus which responded to human breathing noises.

Vampire bats have an ability to detect infrared heat emissions (Kurten and Schmidt, 1982). Apart from vision, olfaction, and echolocation (or other auditory cues), this thermal sense may be critical for providing the vampire bat with short-range information about its host. In particular, thermal perception may enable the bat to select a suitable site (i.e., presence of surface vessels) to feed from (Schmidt, 1988). Bats will, for example, preferentially select the warmer of two rabbit ears to feed upon (Schmidt and Manske, 1982 [cited by Schmidt, 1988]).

Kurten and Schmidt (1982) described the gross and histologic structure of facial pit organs in the vampire bat, similar to the heat-detecting systems known in certain snakes. Kishida et al (1984) identified a nuclear structure in the brain stem of vampire bats that may be intimately associated with thermal sensation. They have called this nucleus the vampire DLV (nucleus of the descending lateral trigeminal tract). With the exception of vampire bats and a few species of reptiles, heat-sensing organs are unknown in vertebrates (Kurten and Schmidt, 1982). A similar nuclear structure has been identified in the brains of pigeons, but no peripheral sensory structure has yet been found.

Distribution of Bites on Animal Hosts

Greenhall et al (1971) observed vampires to approach cattle from a height of 0.5 to 1.5 meters, circle for a few minutes, and either alight on the backs of the animals or on the ground nearby. Vampires often stalk their hosts by following them on the ground.

Typically, the vampire selects particular sites on its victim to bite (de Verteuil and Urich, 1936). When biting poultry, cocks are often bitten on the comb, whereas hens are commonly bitten on the legs. When approaching poultry, bats are very cautious to avoid the bill (Ditmars and Greenhall, 1935, 1960). *Diphylla* frequently bites chickens in the cloacal region (Hoyt and Altenbach, 1981; Uieda, 1982), interrupting their meal when the bird defecates. *Diaemus* reportedly prefers the toes and tarsi of chickens and Guinea fowl (Figure 6-4). Turkeys are bitten more commonly between the feather tracts of the lower breast, possibly because of the thicker skin of the turkey's legs and feet. Ducks were not observed to be attacked by *Diaemus* (Sazima and Uieda, 1980).

Cattle, horses, sheep, and goats are often bitten on the shoulders and neck and, less commonly, on the flanks and legs (Figures 6-5 and 6-6). According to researchers at the Denver Wildlife Research Center (1969), captive vam-

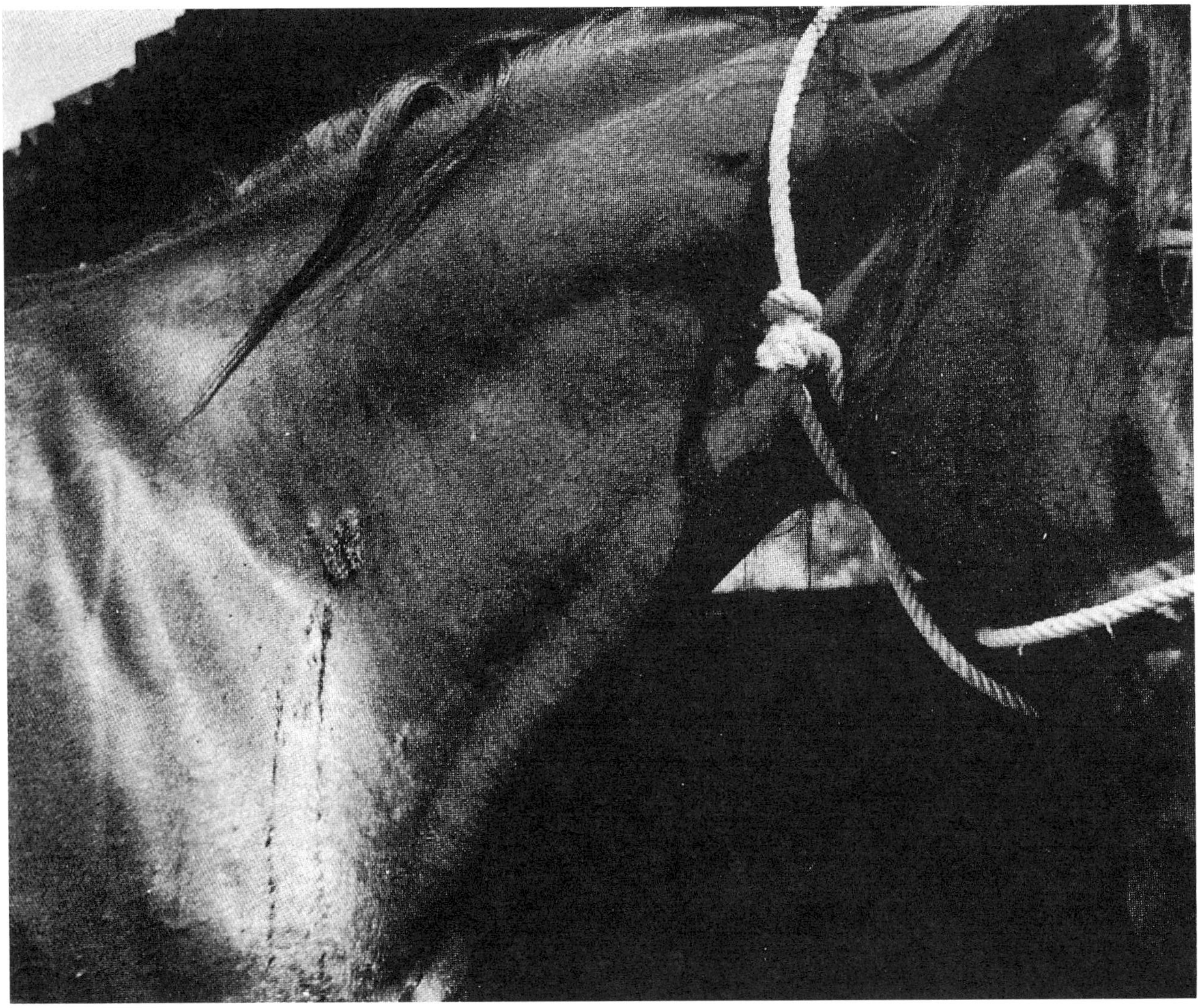

Figure 6-6. Fresh vampire-bat bite on the neck of a horse. (From Kverno, N. B. and G. C. Mitchell. Vampire bats and their effect on cattle production in Latin America. *Wld. Anim. Rev.* (Food and Agriculture Organization of the United Nations). 17: 1, 1976. Reproduced with permission.)

pires preferred biting cattle at the hoof and preferred feeding on recumbent animals without climbing upon them. Piccinini et al (1985) found vampires to feed on all regions of a cow's body, but with distinct preference for the legs, withers, and other dorsal regions. Water buffalo, immersed in water, are commonly bitten about the nose, and seals are often bitten about the ears.

Of 24 human deaths in Peru during 1989, 66.6% of the victims were bitten on the toes (75% of these on the great toe), 17% on the head, 13% on the head and feet, and 4% on the forearm (Lopez, 1991). Of 29 human deaths reported in Peru during 1990, Lopez et al (1992) reported that 73% of victims were bitten on the head, 22% on the nose, 14% on the toes, and 14% on the fingers (Figure 6-7). Dalquest (1955) reported that vampire bats in Mexico primarily bit humans on the face and rarely on the toes.

Wounds incurred by livestock may impair function to a varying extent. Bites about the neck may interfere with placement of yokes on beasts of burden (Greenhall, 1985). Wounds on the withers of horses may interfere with placement of saddles (Malaga-Alba, 1954). Sows are often bitten on the teats and may have subsequent dif-

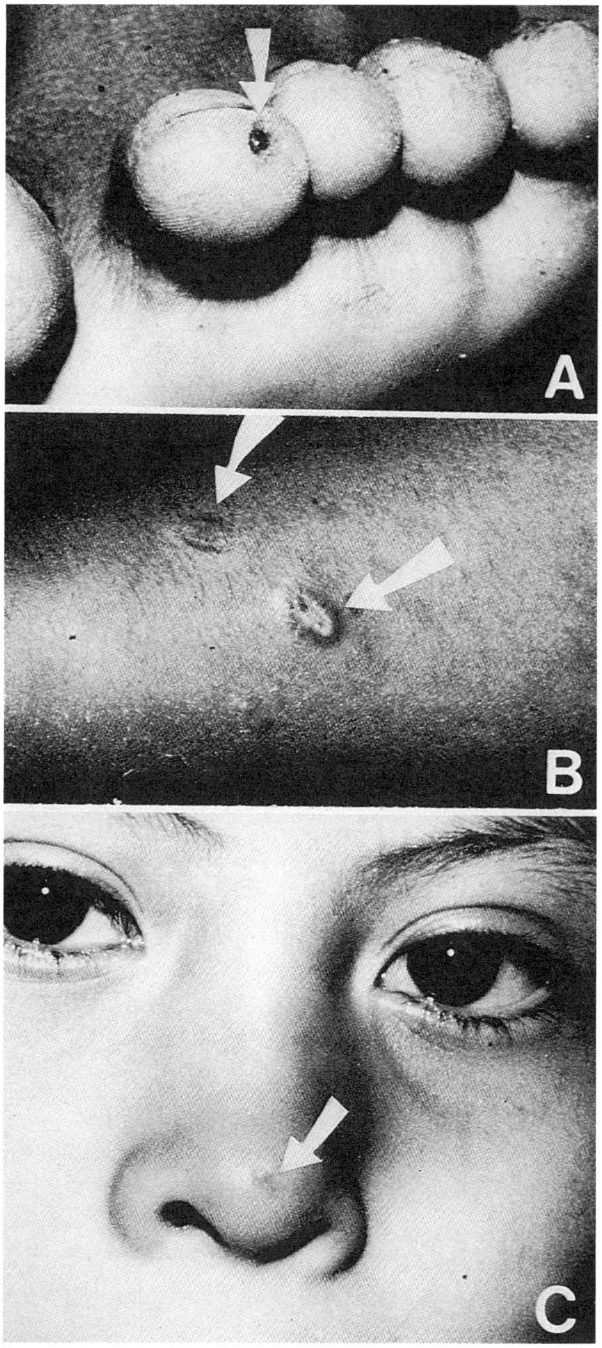

Figure 6-7. Examples of wounds on toe (A), arm (B), and nose (C) inflicted by vampire bats in the village of San Miguel, Belize. (From McCarthy, T. J. Human depredation by vampire bats (*Desmodus rotundus*) following a hog cholera campaign. *Am. J. Trop. Med. Hyg.* 40(3): 320, 1989. Reproduced with permission.)

ficulty nursing young due to fibrotic induration (Gilyard, 1945). In fact, during one year, 350 piglets died of starvation in one swinery in Brazil which was regularly visited by vampire bats (McCarthy, 1993).

Many researchers have observed that dark-colored animals are preferentially attacked. Animals that are mixed black and white in color tend to be bitten on the darker-colored patches. Unless no other domesticated livestock are available, the zebu cattle, which are completely white, are almost never bitten. However, when no other breeds are available for predation, the zebu cattle may be severely attacked. To the extent that skin and hair coloration alter infrared emissivity, the vampire's apparent preference for dark-colored animals may be related to its thermal sense. No evidence exists to support such a correlation and the relationship remains purely speculative. Its validation, therefore, awaits future study.

Cases of paralytic rabies among humans in Trinidad have involved only black individuals, but bats are not known to discriminate among human races (Hurst and Pawan, 1932; Cutright, 1940). The colored natives of the laboring class, being of a generally lower socioeconomic class and frequently sleeping out of doors, are more readily exposed to the nightly forays of vampires (see page 101). Turner (1975) did not believe host color to have been highly significant in his Costa Rican study.

The Vampire-Bat Bite

Once on an animal, the bat may meander back and forth in crab-like fashion until it finds a suitable site to make a bite. Its thermal sense may play a role in identifying the location of surface vessels. It has often been reported that the "stealthily inflicted" wound is not felt, nor does it waken human victims (Gilyard, 1945; Bush, 1961). Beebe (1925) described a vampire's "light-footedness" as it crawled upon his naked chest. Accordingly, he wrote,

> *Now and then a small body touched the sheet for an instant; and then, with a soft little tap, a vampire alighted on my chest. I was half-sitting up, yet I could not see him, for I had found that the least hint of light ended any possibility of a visit. I breathed as quietly as I could, and made sure both hands were clear. For a long time there was no move-*

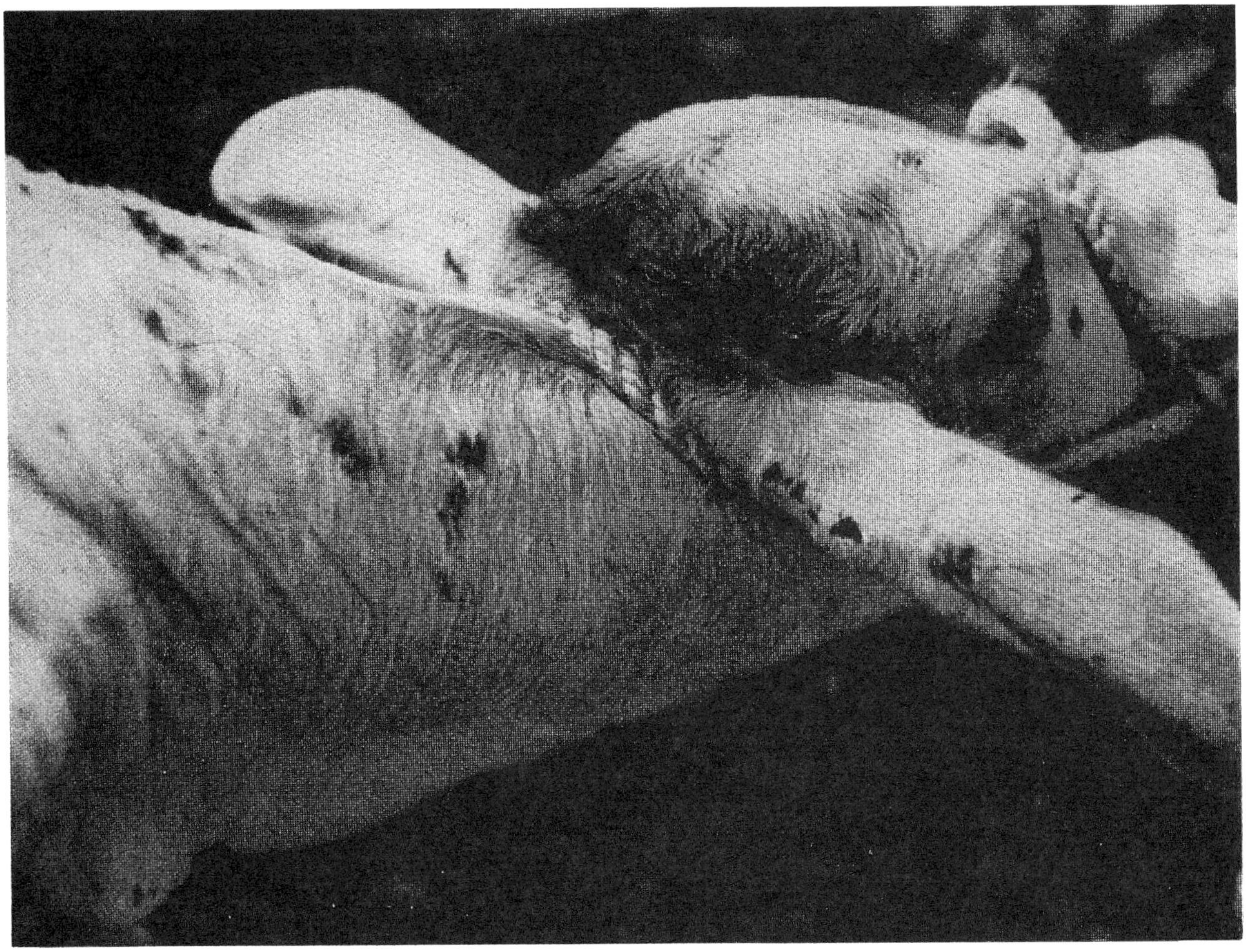

Figure 6-8. Calf with multiple vampire-bat bites on face, ears, and neck. (From Kverno, N. B. and G. C. Mitchell. Vampire bats and their effect on cattle production in Latin America. *Wld. Anim. Rev.* (Food and Agriculture Organization of the United Nations). 17: 1, 1976. Reproduced with permission.)

ment, and the renewed swishes [of wings] made me suspect that the bat had again taken flight. Not until I felt a tickling on my wrist did I know that my visitor had shifted, and, unerringly, was making for the arm which I had exposed. Slowly it crept forward, but I hardly felt the pushing of the feet and pulling of the thumbs as it crawled along. If I had been asleep, I should not have awakened. It continued up my forearm and came to rest at my elbow. Here another long period of rest, and then several short, quick shifts of body. With my whole attention concentrated on my elbow, I began to imagine various sensations as my mind pictured the long, lancet tooth sinking deep into the skin, and the blood pumping up. I even began to feel the hot rush of my vital fluid over my arm, and then found that I had dozed for a moment and that all my sensations were imaginary. But soon a gentle tickling became apparent and, in spite of putting this out of my mind and with increasing doubts as to the bat being still there, the tickling continued. It changed to a tingling, rather pleasant than otherwise, like the first stage of having one's hand asleep. It really seemed as if this were the critical time. Somehow or other the vampire bat was at work with no pain or even inconvenience to me, and now was the moment to seize him, call for a lantern, and solve his supersurgical skill, the exact method of this vespertilial anaesthetist. Slowly, very slowly, I lifted the other hand, always thinking of my elbow, so

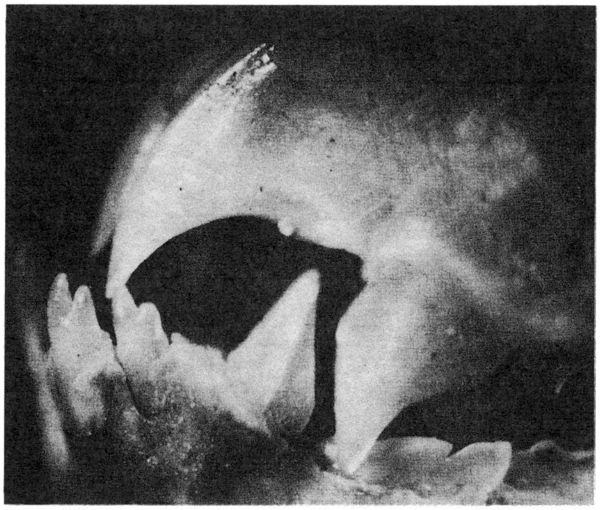

Figure 6-9. Tooth-sharpening system (thegosis) of the vampire bat. It has been suggested that the anterior edges of the upper canines hone against the posterior edges of the lower ones. The posterior edges of the upper canines and oblique lower premolars sharpen each other as they cross. (From Greenhall, A. M. The biting and feeding habits of the vampire bat, *Desmodus rotundus*. *J. Zool. (Lond.)*. 168: 451, 1972. Reproduced with permission.)

> *that I might keep all the muscles relaxed. Very slowly it approached, and with as swift a motion as I could achieve, I grasped at the vampire. I felt a touch of fur and I gripped a struggling, skinny wing: there came a nip of teeth, and the wing tip slipped through my fingers. I could detect no trace of blood by feeling, so turned over and went to sleep. In the morning I found a tiny scratch, with the skin barely broken; and, heartily disappointed, I realized that my tickling and tingling had been the preliminary symptoms of the operation.*

With a quick and decisive bite, the incisor teeth deftly puncture the skin, scooping out tissue until blood flows freely. Greenhall (1972a) described seven different types of bites that vampires inflict (typical, scraping, shaving, shearing, rasping, bore, and defensive).

In studying attack patterns of vampires feeding on captive cows, Piccinini et al (1985) found that bats returned to previously made wounds with an index of repetition of 60%, but still made new wounds almost daily. A bite wound might be abandoned for as much as six days and subsequently returned to or abandoned completely (Figure 6-8). When feeding from a recently made wound, the bat merely reopens the scab (Greenhall, 1972a).

The vampire's striking dentition, adapted for cutting into flesh, is a diagnostic characteristic. The dental formula for *Desmodus* is I1/2 C1/1 P1/2 M1/1; for *Diphylla*, it is I2/2 C1/1 P1/2 M2/2; and for *Diaemus*, it is I1/2 C1/1 P1/2 M2/1 (Bhatnagar, 1988). A space between the lower two incisors permits extension of the tongue during feeding.

With constant usage the vampire's teeth would dull rapidly if no mechanism to sharpen them existed. Even elderly vampires have razor-sharp teeth. Greenhall (1972a, 1988) described a tooth-sharpening system in the vampire called thegosis (Figure 6-9). Reportedly lacking in enamel, the vampire's teeth might be sharpened when the cutting edge of one crosses that of another. Vierhaus (1983 [cited by Griffiths and Criley, 1989]) suggested that large, horny papillae at the tip of the tongue may be used to sharpen the incisor teeth. Contrary to earlier reports, Bhatnagar and Wimsatt (1989) reported the presence of enamel on the teeth of vampire bats, necessitating a reevaluation of the mechanisms of tooth sharpening.

The depth of the vampire's bite is generally constant and the layers of skin pierced are dependent upon the skin thickness of the bat's victim (King and Saphir, 1937). In guinea pigs, for example, histological examination of bite wounds has shown them to extend only through the dermis, whereas in the more thin-skinned pigeon, bites extend through the panniculus adiposus, sometimes penetrating into the underlying superficial musculature. Dalquest (1955) reported the depth to be about 1 mm. Greenhall (1972a) indicated it could be as much as 5 mm. The wound appears as a shallow, crater-like depression 2 to 6 mm wide, 1 to 5 mm deep, and 6 to 10 mm long (Greenhall, 1972a; Thomas and Harlan, 1981). The bite of a vampire bat can usually be easily recognized by its characteristic shape and location (Malaga-Alba, 1954), although the shape of a bite may vary with its location and the character of the underlying tissues (Thomas and

Harlan, 1981). The wound may be mistaken for that made by the screw-worm (Greenhall, 1991).

In general, animals show little reaction of pain to the actual bite. In instances where bites have evoked a painful response, it has been suggested that this was due to the inexperience of less skilled, younger bats (Ditmars and Greenhall, 1935). Various observers have not substantiated the old myth that vampire bats hover above their victims, slowly fanning them with their wings to keep them comfortably asleep. However, Greenhall et al (1971) postulated that the myth might have arisen from the vampire's practice of circling about a victim for several minutes prior to alighting. In an earlier report, Greenhall (1965) described captive bats fanning themselves with their wings.

In the course of detailed observations of captive vampire bats, Ditmars and Greenhall (1935, 1960) referred to the keen awareness that the bats maintain of their surroundings while feeding. When drinking blood from the backs of animals, bats would deftly crawl out of harm's way to avoid being struck by obstacles as the victim moved about. Facial tactile hairs are in constant contact with the victim and may serve to warn the bat of any sudden, potentially dangerous movements made by the victim during feeding (Schmidt, 1988).

Although the actual bite might not evoke a significant response in most victims, Delpietro (1989) reported that cattle and horses sometimes reacted to approaching bats by scattering from a group onto open prairie. Because the bats seem to prefer feeding on recumbent animals, this may afford livestock some measure of protection against attack.

The Feeding Process

Perhaps the most remarkable observation of vampire bat feeding is that they do not, as commonly believed, suck blood at all (Dunn, 1932; Ditmars, 1934; Ditmars and Greenhall, 1935). Rather, the bats "lap" blood from a freely flowing wound, using their rapidly darting tongue (Figure 6-10). Ditmars (1934) reported that a captive vampire "lapping" blood from a dish would dart its tongue in and out at a rate of four times per second. Except when making the initial wound, the lips of the bat never contact the host animal. The lateral edges of the tongue are turned downward and grooves on its ventral surface act as straws. As it is alternately protruded and retracted, the tongue's intrinsic musculature is believed to initiate peristaltic waves. This produces a partial vacuum in the mouth which facilitates the flow of blood (Mann, 1950 and Villa-Ramirez, 1958 [cited by Greenhall, 1972a]; Glass, 1970).[2] Blood passes to the mouth along the ventral surface of the tongue, while saliva simultaneously flows down its dorsal aspect.

The vampire bat is, therefore, more correctly referred to as a "blood-lapper," rather than a blood-sucker, although the "lapping" mechanism should not be confused with that displayed by dogs and cats when drinking water from a bowl. It has also been suggested that blood is drawn up principally through capillary action (Griffiths and Criley, 1989).

Investigators have been impressed by the prodigious appetite of the vampire. It generally feeds for about 9 to 40 minutes, in the course of which it swells into a small sphere (hence the specific name *rotundus*). Although blood is the major component of the stomach contents of all vampire bats, Arata et al (1967) reported that chunks of muscle (sometimes larger than 5 mm in size) could occasionally be found. In addition to these pieces of flesh, remains of large insects have also been found.

Greenhall (1965) reported that captive vampire bats consume an average of 10 to 25 ml of blood each evening, but suggested that with two feedings per night and adequate room for exercise, a single vampire might consume as much as 45 ml per night. Wimsatt and Guerriere (1962) observed captive bats to ingest as much as 52 ml of blood while feeding and Busch (1988) reported that vampire bats in captivity consumed an average of 60% of their body weight in blood over 30 minutes (Table 6-2). Pawan (1936) reported that a captive vampire bat could bleed a rabbit to death

[2]According to de La Torre and Bedford (1964 [cited by Greenhall, 1985]), this suction mechanism does not exist in *Diaemus* and *Diphylla*.

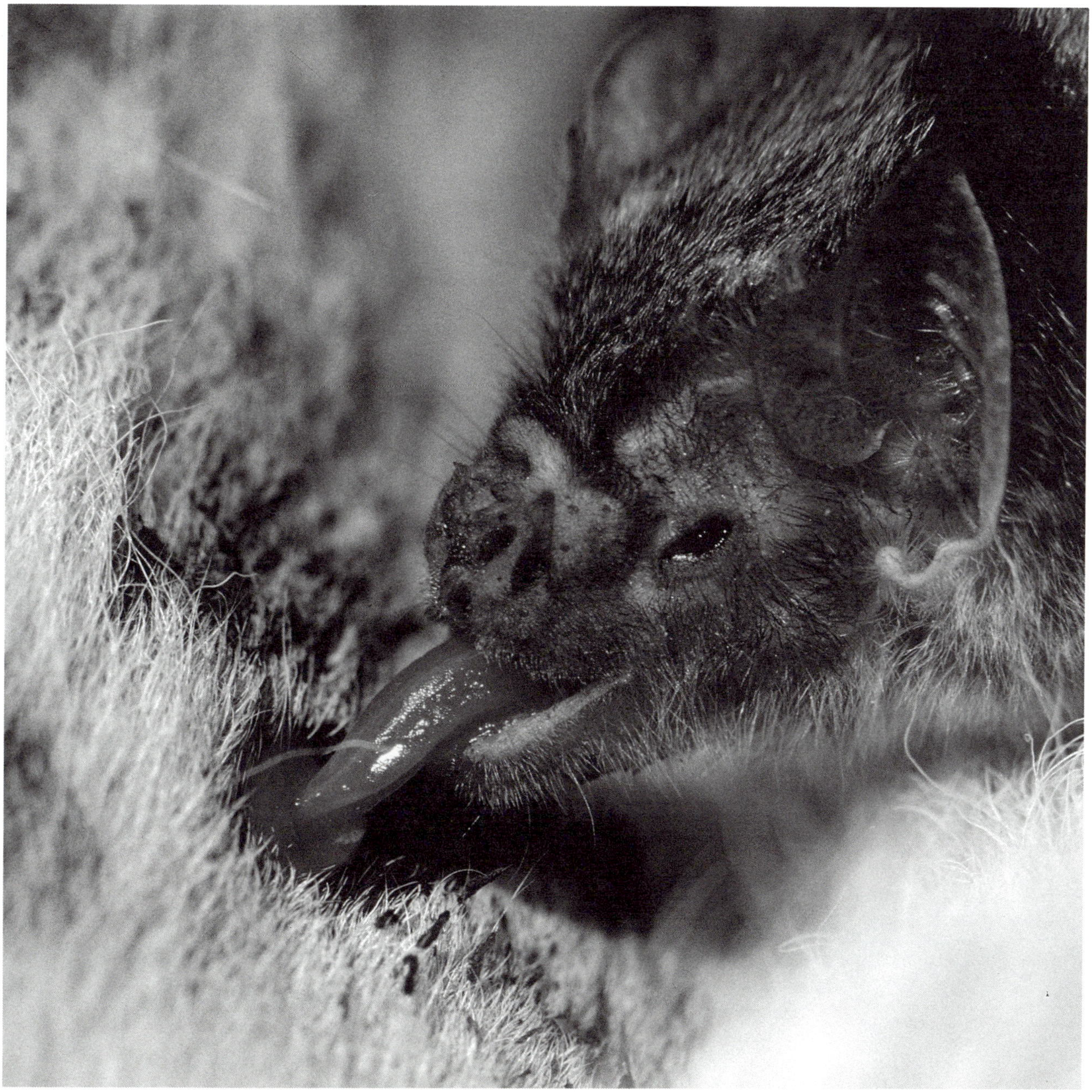

Figure 6-10. Vampire bats do not suck blood from their victims. Their lips never touch the host except during the initial bite. They "lap" blood from a freely flowing wound. Blood passes to the mouth along the ventral surface of the tongue, while saliva simultaneously flows down its dorsal aspect. During the course of their lengthy feeding, rabid vampire bats may inoculate victims with large doses of virus. Photo by Bruce Dale, © National Geographic Society.

in a single evening.

Anticoagulation and Fibrinolysis

In order to subsist on a diet of fluid blood, the vampire bat requires a means of overcoming the normal blood-clotting mechanisms of its host. Adaptations must exist that enable the vampire to inhibit blood clotting at the site of vascular injury, thereby allowing continuous flow of blood during feeding, as well as keeping the blood in a liquid state during the course of feeding. That such mechanisms exist is attested to by the prolonged bleeding of vampire-inflicted wounds (Figure 6-5). Wounds which would normally clot within a

Table 6-2

Blood Consumption by Captive Vampire Bats

Body Weight (grams)	Mean Blood Consumed in 2 Hours as % of Initial Body Weight[a]
25.0	78.7 (8)
26.3	42.9 (5)
26.4	51.7 (5)
28.6	58.8 (5)
29.6	52.9 (7)
30.3	58.6 (5)
32.4	72.9 (8)
36.0	67.8 (7)
36.2	51.8 (8)
Mean	
30.1+/-1.4 (SE)	59.5+/-4.1 (SE)

[a]Days of measurement in parentheses

From Busch, C. Consumption of blood, renal function and utilization of free water by the vampire bat, *Desmodus rotundus*. *Comp. Biochem. Physiol.* 90A(1): 141, 1988. © Pergamon Press Ltd, Headington Hill Hall, Oxford OX3 OBW, UK. Reproduced with permission.

matter of minutes may continue to bleed for several hours after feeding (Bier, 1932 [cited by Cutright, 1940]; Hawkey, 1966, 1967; Cartwright, 1974).

Adaptations to prevent blood coagulation during feeding are both mechanical and chemical (anticoagulants) in nature. Mechanical considerations include the razor-sharp teeth of the vampire and the physical action of the tongue (which the bat uses to probe the wound during ingestion of blood). The sharp teeth minimize tissue trauma at the site of the bite wound, diminishing the relative stimulus for local aggregation of platelets (the first step in the blood-clotting process). Mechanical action of the tongue will further aid anticoagulation by preventing the formation of a stable clot or by dislodging clots that do form.

Potent anticoagulant substances are present in vampire-bat saliva. One substance inhibits the formation of a platelet plug by retarding the aggregation of platelets at the site of vessel damage. A second factor appears to inhibit the coagulation cascade at the stage encompassing activation of factor XI to XIA (Figure 6-11). Lastly, a family of four known potent fibrinolytic substances function to break down any fibrin clots that do form. The vampire plasminogen activators are collectively referred to as desmokinase (also called vampire bat salivary plasminogen activator [Bat-Pa] or *Desmodus* salivary plasminogen activator [DSPA]).

The plasminogen activators of *Desmodus* are specific in action to fibrin clots of mammalian blood. A similar substance isolated from the saliva of *Diaemus* is effective in avian blood, as well, suggesting a correlation to host preference (Cartwright and Hawkey, 1969). Reactivity of vampire-bat saliva with mammalian plasminogen also indicates species specificity, reacting with human, bovine, and equine blood, but not with ovine or canine blood. This provides further support of major host dietary preferences (Hawkey, 1988).

Because of certain unique biological properties, synthetic vampire-bat salivary plasminogen activators hold therapeutic promise for the treatment of various thrombotic complications in certain human patients (Gardell et al, 1990; Bang, 1991; Kratzschmar et al, 1991; Bergum and Gardell, 1992; Hare and Gardell, 1992; Mellott et al, 1992; Witt et al, 1992). Plasminogen activators unique to the vampire bat are distinct from other currently known plasminogen activators in their fastidious requirement of fibrin for activity. Because of this strict dependence, the vampire-bat salivary plasminogen activators are much less likely to activate plasminogen that isn't already bound to fibrin (i.e., that which is free in the circulation). Use of presently available plasminogen activators to dissolve blood clots is complicated by potentially life-threatening hemorrhage, as plasminogen throughout the circulation is nonselectively activated, causing a plasminemia.

The remarkable properties of the vampire-bat salivary plasminogen activators are of enormous therapeutic significance, and may provide a means for antithrombotic therapy without signifi-

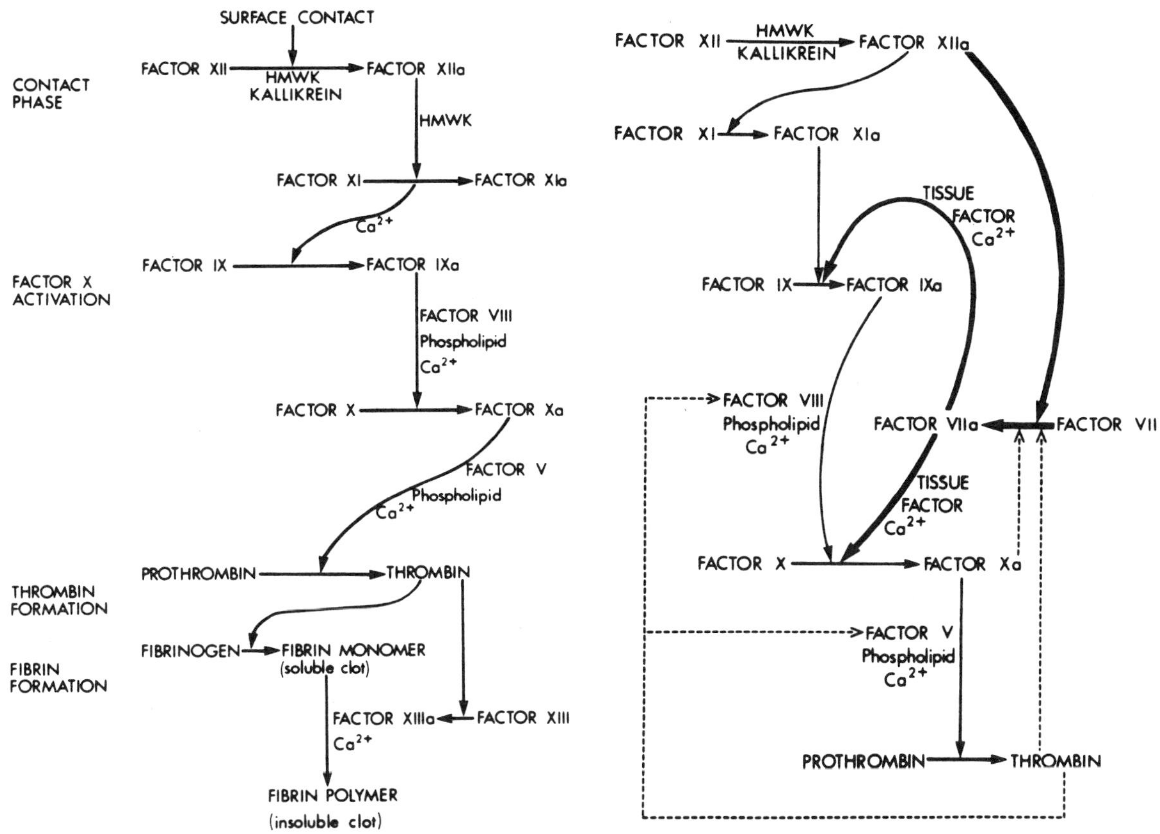

Figure 6-11. Intrinsic (left) and extrinsic (right) coagulation cascades. (From Gentry, P. A. and H. G. Downie. Blood Coagulation. In M. J. Swenson (ed.) *Duke's Physiology of Domestic Animals*. 10th Edition. © Comstock Publishing Associates, Cornell University Press. Ithaca, New York, 1984. Reproduced with permission.)

cant risk of bleeding. Limited availability of these substances has hindered in-depth study; however, recently perfected techniques have allowed researchers to mass synthesize vampire-bat salivary plasminogen activators (Kratzschmar et al, 1992). Witt et al (1992) demonstrated that rD-SPα_1, a recombinant protein corresponding to one of the two larger natural plasminogen activators of *Desmodus*, is an effective thrombolytic agent in vivo (experimental pulmonary embolism in rats) and may lyse blood clots even faster than t-PA (human tissue-type plasminogen activator).

Flight After Feeding

Several investigators have commented on the vampire bat's flitting down to the ground after feeding, the gluttonous bats engorging themselves to the point of being unable to launch themselves into the air without first climbing up a wall (Ditmars and Greenhall, 1935, 1960; de Verteuil and Urich, 1936; Wimsatt, 1969). Engorged vampire bats reportedly fly with difficulty (de Verteuil and Urich, 1936). In 1969, researchers at the Denver Wildlife Research Center reported that "vampires were reluctant to fly after feeding and preferred to rest for a period of time." Fasted vampire bats have no difficulty in taking flight from the ground (McFarland and Wimsatt, 1969).

In his comprehensive study of terrestrial locomotion, jumping behavior, and flight in vampire bats, Altenbach (1979) suggested that their characteristic leaping behavior serves to launch them into the air after partaking of a heavy blood meal. Greenhall et al (1971), on the other hand, did not observe satiated bats to have any difficulty either taking off or flying and Flores-Crespo et al (1970) reported that most vampires could fly without difficulty carrying up to 33% of their body weight (and one up to 50%).

Roosts and Digestion

The duration of foraging flights has been reported to be about two hours (McFarland and Wimsatt, 1969). After feeding, the bats may seek out a nearby location for quietly digesting their meal (Goodwin and Greenhall, 1961). Their tarry excrement marks these digesting places, which include such sites as stables, abandoned rooms, and beneath bridges. The bats remain inactive in their roost until their next meal the following evening (McFarland and Wimsatt, 1969).

In contrast to earlier reports, Wimsatt (1969) maintained that vampires did not use temporary digesting places, but returned directly to their diurnal roosts following feeding. Turner (1975) was of the opinion that bats selected a herd to feed on for the night and then retreated to the nearest available roost site. This would be related to herd movement. Return to the nearest roost would be strictly dependent upon the conservation of limited metabolic resources.

Villa-Ramirez (1969) reported that vampires changed roosts nightly and the population makeup of colonies he studied was in a continual state of flux. Lopez-Forment et al (1971) reported that vampires remained within a particular area, visiting the same roosts on a regular basis. However, they might change roosts daily or even travel to distant roosts periodically. Burns and Flores-Crespo (1975) also observed movement of bats between roosts separated by less than 3 km. According to Horst (1972), if all bats within a particular cave were collected in an evening, the cave would be repopulated the next day, indicating continual movement of bats throughout their home range. However, others have observed that repopulation of roosts may take months (Arellano-Sota, 1991; Rupprecht, 1993) and vampire bats have been captured in the same roost where they had been banded as much as 12 years earlier (Flores-Crespo and Arellano-Sota, 1991), although this does not necessarily imply that they had remained within the same roost the entire time.

Table 6-3

Mean Blood Consumption of Three Vampire Bats With and Without Water for One-Week Periods

Grams of Blood Consumed	
Water Present	Water Not Present
9.0	13.7
12.8	18.0
8.6	10.4
Mean	
10.1 +/- 1.3 (SE)	14.0 +/- 2.2 (SE)

From Busch, C. Consumption of blood, renal function and utilization of free water by the vampire bat, *Desmodus rotundus. Comp. Biochem. Physiol.* 90A(1): 141, 1988. © Pergamon Press Ltd, Headington Hill Hall, Oxford OX3 OBW, UK. Reproduced with permission.

Metabolic Waste and Water Consumption

Vampires generally urinate either while feeding or within minutes after (Wimsatt and Guerriere, 1962; Horst, 1969; McFarland and Wimsatt, 1969; Greenhall et al, 1971; Breidenstein, 1982; Busch, 1988). Copious diuresis of a nearly isotonic urine with a low urea content continues for 1 or 2 hours. On a body-weight-per-minute basis, the vampire bat has the highest urine flow rate of any known mammal. This may be an adaptation for reducing flight weight after a heavy blood meal (bats also lose considerable water through evaporation during flight). Several investigators have discussed the possibility that the odor of bat urine on cattle may serve as an olfactory attractant for the bats. There is no evidence to suggest that urinary excrtion of virus is a means of transmitting rabies to cattle.

In feeding exclusively on blood, vampire bats subsist on a protein-rich diet. The nitrogenous wastes (urea) from protein breakdown are typically eliminated from the body in the urine. However, virtually all of the urea excreted in the urine appears after the feeding diuresis (McFarland and Wimsatt, 1969). Thus, vampires have little water available for urinary excretion of the nitrogenous wastes of protein metabolism. These facts are made even more remarkable by the observation that vampire bats may not drink free water in the wild. This has been a point of controversy. The vampire's ability to concentrate its urine to very high levels is consistent with a lack of free-water intake.

Results of investigations of the vampire's water requirements have been variable. Although they may drink free water in captivity, they might not require it. Greenhall (1965) reported that free water is essential to bats in captivity and Greenhall et al (1971) observed vampires drinking water in the wild. Busch (1988) reported that vampire bats in captivity may drink less blood when provided with a source of water (Table 6-3). Hoyt and Altenbach (1981) reported that captive specimens of *Diphylla* drank no water in captivity during the course of 261 days of observation and Wimsatt and Guerriere (1961) observed captive vampire bats (*Desmodus*) to drink little free water. In fact, they maintained bats in healthy condition without offering water for as long as two years. It is unknown whether or not vampires regularly consume free water in the wild state. They may be forced into consumption of free water to rehydrate if hunting has not been successful (Busch, 1988).

The vampire bat may live in a delicate water balance, similar to animals living in the desert. They solve the problem by excreting a very concentrated urine (as high as 4,650 mOsm/L, approximate specific gravity of 1.155). In this regard, McFarland and Wimsatt (1969) suggested that "the vampire bat can be considered to inhabit a desert in the midst of the tropics."

References

Acha, P. N. (1981). *A Review of Rabies Prevention and Control in the Americas 1970 to 1980—Overall Status of Rabies*. Presented at the Joint C.N.E.R.-WHO Scientific Meeting on Animal Rabies. Nancy and Malzeville, France. June 3-5, 1981

Altenbach, J. S. (1979). *Locomotor Morphology of the Vampire Bat, Desmodus rotundus*. Special Publication No. 6. The American Society of Mammalogists.

Anderson, B. A. (1990). *The Vampire Bat: An Extreme in Evolutionary Morphology?* M.S. Thesis. University of Calgary. Calgary, Alberta. Courtesy of B. A. Anderson.

Arata, A. A., Vaughn, J. B., and M. E. Thomas (1967). Food habits of certain Colombian bats. *J. Mammal.* 48(4): 653

Arellano-Sota, C. (1991). Regional Officer on Animal Production and Health. Food and Agriculture Organization of the United Nations. Santiago, Chile. Personal communication.

Arellano-Sota, C., Sureau, P-., and A. M. Greenhall (1971). Preferencia de la predacion del vampiro en relacion a la edad y raza del ganado y a la epoca del anno (Preferences for age and breed of cattle and for the time of year, in predation by the vampire bat). *Tec. Pec. (Mex.)*. 17: 23 (English abstract) in *Vet. Bull.* (1972). 42(5): 276

Babb, R. D. (1993). Information Specialist. Arizona Game and Fish Department. Mesa, Arizona. Personal communication.

Baer, G. M. (1975). Bovine Paralytic Rabies and Rabies in the Vampire Bat. In G. M. Baer (ed.) *The Natural History of Rabies*. Vol. II. Academic Press. New York.

Baer, G. M. (1991). Vampire Bat and Bovine Paralytic Rabies. In G. M. Baer (ed.) *The Natural History of Rabies*. 2nd Edition. CRC Press, Inc. Boca Raton, Florida.

Baker, R. J., Honeycutt, R. L., and R. A. Bass (1988). Genetics. In A. M. Greenhall and U. Schmidt (eds.) *The Natural History of Vampire Bats*. CRC Press, Inc. Boca Raton, Florida.

Bang, N. V. (1991). Leeches, snakes, ticks, and vampire bats in today's cardiovascular drug development. *Circulation*. 84(1): 436

Banziger, H. (1968). Preliminary observations on a skin-piercing blood-sucking moth (*Calyptra eustrigata* (HMPS.) (LEP., Noctuidae)) in Malaya. *Bull. Ent. Res.* 58(1): 159

Beebe, W. (1925). *Edge of the Jungle*. Garden City Publishing Co. New York.

Bergum, P. W. and S. J. Gardell (1992). Vampire bat salivary plasminogen activator exhibits a strict and fastidious requirement for polymeric fibrin as its cofactor, unlike human tissue-type plasminogen activator. A kinetic analysis. *J. Biol. Chem.* 267(25): 17726

Bhatnagar, K. P. (1988). Anatomy. In A. M. Greenhall and U. Schmidt (eds.) *The Natural History of Vampire Bats*. CRC Press, Inc. Boca Raton, Florida.

Bhatnagar, K. P. and W. A. Wimsatt (1989). Vampire bats do have fully developed enamle. Abstracts—AAA 102nd Meeting. *Anat. Rec.* 223(4): 14A

Bier, O. G. (1932). Action anticoagulante et fibrinolytique de l'extrait des glandes salivaires d'une chauvesouris hematophage (*Desmodus rufus*). *C. R. Soc. Biol.* (Paris). Vol. 110

Breidenstein, C. P. (1982). Digestion and assimilation

of bovine blood by a vampire bat (*Desmodus rotundus*). *J. Mammal.* 63(3): 482

Breidenstein, C. P. (1984). The palatability of reconstituted freeze-dried blood when used as a food supply for vampire bats (*Desmodus rotundus*). *Bat Res. News.* 25(1): 3

Brown, J. H. (1968). Activity patterns of some neotropical bats. *J. Mammal.* 49(4): 754

Brown, D. E. (1993). Department of Biology. Arizona State University. Tempe, Arizona. Personal communication.

Brown, D. E. (1994). *Vampiro: The Vampire Bat in Fact and Fantasy.* High-Lonesome Press. Silver City, New Mexico.

Burns, R. J. and R. Flores-Crespo (1975). Notes on local movement and reproduction of vampire bats in Colima, Mexico. *SW Nat.* 19: 446

Busch, C. (1988). Consumption of blood, renal function and utilization of free water by the vampire bat, *Desmodus rotundus*. *Comp. Biochem. Physiol.* 90A(1): 141

Bush, D. L. (1961). Epizootic bat rabies in Surinam—Effectiveness of a mass field immunization program. *J. Am. Vet. Med. Assoc.* 138(7): 363

Campos, J. and C. Arellano (1971). *Resum. Octava Reun. An. Inst. Nac. Invest. Pec. Mex.* p. 36

Cartwright, T. (1974). The plasminogen activator of vampire bat saliva. *Blood.* 43(3): 317

Cartwright, T. and C. Hawkey (1969). Activation of the blood fibrinolytic mechanism by saliva of the vampire bat (*Diaemus youngi*). *J. Physiol.* 201: 45P

Cockerell, T. T. A. (1930). An apparently extinct Euglandina from Texas. *Proc. Colo. Mus. Natur. Hist.* 9: 52

Constantine, D. G., Tierkel, E. S., Kleckner, M. D., and D. M. Hawkins (1968). Rabies in New Mexico cavern bats. *Pub. Hlth. Repts.* 83(4): 303

Cutright, P. R. (1940). *The Great Naturalists Explore South America.* Essay Index Reprint Series. Books for Libraries Press. The Macmillan Company. New York.

Dalquest, W. W. (1955). Natural history of the vampire bats of eastern Mexico. *Am. Midl. Nat.* 53(1): 79

de La Torre, L. and D. E. Bedford (1964). The microanatomy of the tongue of the vampire bat, *Desmodus rotundus*. *Bat Res. News.* 5: 32

Delpietro, H. A. (1989). Case reports on defensive behaviour in equine and bovine subjects in response to vocalization of the common vampire bat (*Desmodus rotundus*). *Appl. Anim. Behav. Sci.* 22(3-4): 377

Delpietro, H. A., Marchevsky, N., and E. Simonetti (1993). Relative population densities and predation of the common vampire bat (*Desmodus rotundus*) in natural and cattle-raising areas in north-east Argentina. *Prev. Vet. Med.* 14: 13

Denver Wildlife Research Center (1969). Annual Report. *Vampire Bats—Rabies Transmission and Livestock Production in Latin America.* U. S. Bureau of Sport Fisheries and Wildlife. Field Station. Palo Alto, Mexico.

de Oviedo, G. F. (1526). *Natural History of the West Indies.* Translated and edited by S. A. Stoudemire. University of North Carolina Studies in the Romance Languages and Literature. Number 32, 1959. The University of North Carolina Press. Chapel Hill, North Carolina.

de Verteuil, E. and F. W. Urich (1936). The study and control of paralytic rabies transmitted by bats in Trinidad, British West Indies. *Trans. Roy. Soc. Trop. Med. Hyg.* XXIX(4): 317

Ditmars, R. L. (1934). *Confessions of a Scientist.* The Macmillan Company. New York.

Ditmars, R. L. and A. M. Greenhall (1935). The vampire bat. A presentation of undescribed habits and review of its history. *Zoologica.* XIX(2): 53

Ditmars, R. L. and A. M. Greenhall (1960). The vampire bat. *Smithsonian Treas. Sci.* 2: 571

Dunn, L. H. (1932). Experiments in the transmission of *Trypanosoma Hippicum Darling* with the vampire bat, *Desmodus rotundus murinus* Wagner, as a vector in Panama. *J. Prev. Med.* 6(5): 415

Emlen, J. M. (1966). The role of time and energy in food preference. *Am. Nat.* 100(916): 611

Fenton, M. B. (1983). *Just Bats.* University of Toronto Press. Toronto.

Fenton, M. B. (1992a). *Bats.* Facts on File, Inc. New York.

Fenton, M. B. (1992b). Wounds and the origin of blood-feeding in bats. *Biol. J. Linn. Soc.* 47: 161

Flores-Crespo, R. and C. Arellano-Sota (1991). Biology and Control of the Vampire Bat. In G. M. Baer (ed.) *The Natural History of Rabies.* 2nd Edition. CRC Press, Inc. Boca Raton, Florida.

Flores-Crespo, R., Burns, R. J., and S. B. Linhart (1970). Load-lifting capacity of the vampire bat. *J. Mammal.* 51(3): 627

Flores-Crespo, R., Linhart, S. B., Burns, R. J., and G. C. Mitchell (1972). Foraging behavior of the common vampire bat related to moonlight. *J. Mammal.* 53(2): 366

Foster, M. S. (1969). Synchronized life cycles in the orange-crowned warbler and its Mallophagan parasites. *Ecology.* 50(2): 315

Gardell, S. J., Hare, T. R., Bergum, P. W., Cuca, G. C., O'Neill-Palladino, L., and S. M. Zavodny (1990). Vampire bat plasminogen activator is quiescent in human plasma in the absence of fibrin unlike human tissue plasminogen activator. *Blood.* 76(12): 2560

Gardner, A. L. (1977). Feeding Habits. In R. J. Baker, J. K. Jones, and D. C. Carter (eds.) *Biology of Bats* *of the New World Family Phyllostomatidae*. Part II. Spec. Publ. Mus., Texas Tech Univ. 13: 1

Gentry, P. A. and H. G. Downie (1984). Blood Coagulation. In M. J. Swenson (ed.) *Duke's Physiology of Domestic Animals*. 10th Edition. Comstock Publishing Associates, Cornell University Press. Ithaca, New York.

Gillette, D. D. (1975). Evaluation of feeding strategies in bats. *Tebiwa*. 18: 39

Gilyard, R. T. (1945). Bat transmitted paralytic rabies. *Cornell Vet*. XXXV(3): 195

Glass, B. P. (1970). Feeding Mechanisms of Bats. In B. H. Slaughter and D. W. Walton (eds.) *About Bats*. Southern Methodist University Press. Dallas, Texas.

Goodwin, G. C. and A. M. Greenhall (1961). A review of the bats of Trinidad and Tobago. *Bull. Am. Mus. Nat. Hist*. 122: 187

Grady, F. (1987). In Dyas digest. *NSS (Natl. Speleol. Soc.) News*. 45(10): 351

Greenhall, A. M. (1959). The ecological role of Trinidad bats, especially the vampire, and bat rabies. *Vet. Rec*. 71(10): 188

Greenhall, A. M. (1965). Notes on behavior of captive vampire bats. *Mammalia*. 29(4): 441

Greenhall, A. M. (1970). The use of a precipitin test to determine host preferences of the vampire bats, *Desmodus rotundus* and *Diaemus youngi*. *Bijdragen tot de Dierkunde*. 40(1): 36

Greenhall, A. M. (1972a). The biting and feeding habits of the vampire bat, *Desmodus rotundus*. *J. Zool. (Lond.)*. 168: 451

Greenhall, A. M. (1972b). Identification of the vampire bat. *Wld. Anim. Rev*. (FAO). 2: 44

Greenhall, A. M. (1974). Vampire bat control in the Americas: A review and proposed program for action. *Bull. Pan Am. Hlth. Org*. 8(1): 30

Greenhall, A. M. (1985). Effects of Vampire Bats and Paralytic Rabies on Livestock Production. In S. M. Gaafar, W. E. Howard, and R. E. Marsh (eds.) *Parasites, Pests and Predators*. Elsevior Science Publishing Co., Inc. New York.

Greenhall, A. M. (1988). Feeding Behavior. In A. M. Greenhall and U. Schmidt (eds.) *The Natural History of Vampire Bats*. CRC Press, Inc. Boca Raton, Florida.

Greenhall, A. M. (1991). Ethology and Ecology of Vampire Bats. In *Expert Consultation on the Care of Persons Exposed to Rabies Transmitted by Vampire Bats*. PAHO/WHO. Programs for Veterinary Public Health. Washington, D.C. April 1-5, 1991

Greenhall, A. M., Schmidt, U., and W. Lopez-Foment (1971). Attacking behavior of the vampire bat, *Desmodus rotundus*, under field conditions in Mexico. *Biotropica*. 3(2): 136

Griffiths, T. A. and B. B. Criley (1989). Comparative lingual anatomy of the bats *Desmodus rotundus* and *Lonchophylla robusta* (Chiroptera: Phyllostomidae). *J. Mammal*. 70(3): 608

Gut, H. J. (1959). A pleistocene vampire bat from Florida. *J. Mammal*. 40(4): 534

Handley, Jr., C. O. (1980). Inconsistencies in Formation of Family-Group and Subfamily-Group Names in Chiroptera. In D. E. Wilson and A. L. Gardner (eds.) *Proceedings of the 5th International Bat Research Conference*. Texas Tech Press. Lubbock, Texas.

Hare, T. R. and S. J. Gardell (1992). Vampire bat salivary plasminogen activator promotes robust lysis of plasma clots in a plasma milieu without causing fluid phase plasminogen activation. *Thrombosis and Haemostasis*. 68(2): 165

Harris, A. H. (1985). Preliminary report on the vertebrate fauna of U-bar Cave, Hidalgo County, New Mexico. *New Mex. Geol*. 7: 74

Harris, A. H. (1987). Reconstruction of Mid-Wisconsin environments in southern New Mexico. *Nat. Geogr. Res*. 3: 142

Hawkey, C. (1966). Plasminogen activator in saliva of the vampire bat *Desmodus rotundus*. *Nature*. 211: 434

Hawkey, C. (1967). Inhibitor of platelet aggregation present in saliva of the vampire bat *Desmodus rotundus*. *Br. J. Haematol*. 13: 1014

Hawkey, C. M. (1988). Salivary Antihemostatic Factors. In A. M. Greenhall and U. Schmidt (eds.) *The Natural History of Vampire Bats*. CRC Press, Inc. Boca Raton, Florida.

Heick, A. (1992). Prince Dracula, rabies, and the vampire legend. *Ann. Int. Med*. 117(2): 172

Hemphill, R. E. and T. Zabow (1983). Clinical vampirism: A presentation of 3 cases and a re-evaluation of Haigh, the "acid-bath murderer." *S. Afr. Med. J*. 63(8): 278

Horst, R. (1969). Observations on the Structure and function of the Kidneys of the Vampire Bat (*Desmodus rotundus murinus*). In C. C. Hoff and M. L. Riedesel (eds.) *Physiological Systems in Semiarid Environments*. University of New Mexico Press. Albuquerque.

Horst, R. (1972). Discussion. In Cave Bats: Their Ecology, Physiology, Behavior, and Future Survival. A Symposium with Recommendations. *Bull. Natl. Speleol. Soc*. 34(2): 71

Hoyt, R. A. and J. S. Altenbach (1981). Observations on *Diphylla ecaudata* in captivity. *J. Mammal*. 62(1): 215

Hurst, E. W. and J. L. Pawan (1932). A further account of the Trinidad outbreak of acute rabic myelitis: Histology of the experimental disease. *J. Path. Bact*. XXXV(3): 301

Hutchison, J. H. (1967). A pleistocene vampire bat

(*Desmodus stocki*) from Potter Creek Cave, Shasta County, California. *Paleobios (Berkeley)*. 3: 1

Kaplan, C. (1985). Rabies: A Worldwide Disease. In P. J. Bacon (ed.) *Population Dynamics of Rabies in Wildlife*. Academic Press. New York.

King, B. G. and R. Saphir (1937). Some observations on the feeding methods of the vampire bat. *Zoologica*. XXII(18): 281

Kishida, R., Goris, R. C., Terashima, S., and J. L. Dubbeldam (1984). A suspected infrared-recipient nucleus in the brain stem of the vampire bat, *Desmodus rotundus*. *Brain Res.* 322: 351

Knickerbocker, J. J., Drost, M., and W. W. Thatcher (1986). Endocrine Patterns During the Initiation of Puberty, the Estrous Cycle, Pregnancy and Parturition in Cattle. In D. A. Morrow (ed.) *Current Therapy in Theriogenology 2—Diagnosis, Treatment and Prevention of Reproductive Diseases in Small and Large Animals*. W. B. Saunders. Philadelphia.

Koopman, K. F. (1958). A fossil vampire bat from Cuba. *Breviora*. 90: 1

Koopman, K. F. (1988). Systematics and Distribution. In A. M. Greenhall and U. Schmidt (eds.) *The Natural History of Vampire Bats*. CRC Press, Inc. Boca Raton, Florida.

Kratzschmar, J., Haendler, B., Langer, G., Boidol, W., Bringmann, P., Alagon, A., Donner, P., and W.-D. Schleuning (1991). The plasminogen activator family from the salivary gland of the vampire bat, *Desmodus rotundus*: Cloning and expression. *Gene*. 105: 229

Kratzschmar, J., Haendler, B., Bringmann, P., Dinter, H., Hess, H., Donner, P., and W.-D. Schleuning (1992). High-level secretion of the four salivary plasminogen activators from the vampire bat, *Desmodus rotundus*, by stably transfected baby hamster kidney cells. *Gene*. 116: 281

Kurten, L. and U. Schmidt (1982). Thermoperception in the common vampire bat (*Desmodus rotundus*). *J. Comp. Physiol.* 146: 233

Kverno, N. B. and G. C. Mitchell (1976). Vampire bats and their effect on cattle production in Latin America. *Wld. Anim. Rev.* (Food and Agriculture Organization of the United Nations). 17: 1

Linhart, S. B. (1975). The Biology and Control of Vampire Bats. In G. M. Baer (ed.) *The Natural History of Rabies*. Vol. II. Academic Press. New York.

Lopez-Forment, W., Schmidt, U., and A. M. Greenhall (1971). Movement and population studies of the vampire bat (*Desmodus rotundus*) in Mexico. *J. Mammal.* 52(1): 227

Lopez-R., A. (1991). Report of the Outbreaks of Human Rabies in Peru. In *Expert Consultation on the Care of Persons Exposed to Rabies Transmitted by Vampire Bats*. PAHO/WHO. Programs for Veterinary Public Health. Washington, D.C. April 1-5, 1991

Lopez-R., A., Miranda-P., P., Tejada-V., E., and D. B. Fishbein (1992). Outbreak of human rabies in the Peruvian jungle. *The Lancet*. 339: 408

Lord, R. D., Delpietro, H., and L. Lazaro (1973). Vampiros que se alimentan de murcielagos (Vampire predation on bats). *Physis. Secc. C. Cont. Org. Terr.* 32(84): 255 (English abstract in *Biol. Abstr.* (1974) 57(2): 754

Lyman, C. P. and W. A. Wimsatt (1966). Temperature regulation in the vampire bat. *Physiol. Zool.* 39: 101

MacArthur, R. H. (1972). *Geographical Ecology—Patterns in the Distribution of Species*. Harper and Row. New York.

MacArthur, R. H. and E. Pianka (1966). An optimal use of a patchy environment. *Am. Nat.* 100(916): 603

Malaga-Alba, A. (1954). Vampire bat as a carrier of rabies. *Am. J. Pub. Hlth.* 44: 909

Malaga-Alba, A. (1966). Ecological Relationship of Rabies in Wildlife. *International Symposium on Rabies*. Symp. Series Immunobiol. Standard. Vol. I. Karger, Basel. New York. Talloires, 1965

Mann-F., G. (1950). Succion de sangre en el vampiro. *Investnes Zool. Chil.* 2: 7

Mann-F., G. (1960). *Investnes Zool. Chil.* 6: 79

McCarthy, T. J. (1987). Distributional Records of Bats from the Caribbean Lowlands of Belize and Adjacent Guatemala and Mexico. In B. D. Patterson and R. M. Timm (eds.) *Studies in Neotropical Mammalogy: Essays in Honor of Philip Hershkovitz. Fieldiana: Zoology*, n.s., No. 39

McCarthy, T. J. (1989). Human depredation by vampire bats (*Desmodus rotundus*) following a hog cholera campaign. *Am. J. Trop. Med. Hyg.* 40(3): 320

McCarthy, T. J. (1993). Advisor, The Vampire Bat Education and Control Programme, Ministry of Agriculture and Fisheries, Belize. Section of Mammals. Carnegie Museum of Natural History. Pittsburgh, Pennsylvania. Personal communication.

McDonald, L. E. (1980). Reproductive Patterns of Cattle. In L. E. McDonald (ed.) *Veterinary Endocrinology and Reproduction*. Lea and Febiger. Philadelphia.

McFarland, W. N. and W. A. Wimsatt (1969). Renal function and its relation to the ecology of the vampire bat, *Desmodus rotundus*. *Comp. Biochem. Physiol.* 28: 985

McNab, B. K. (1969). The economics of temperature regulation in neotropical bats. *Comp. Biochem. Physiol.* 31: 227

McNab, B. K. (1973). Energetics and the distribution of vampires. *J. Mammal.* 54(1): 131

Mead, J. I. (1981). The last 30,000 years of faunal history within the Grand Canyon, Arizona. *Quat. Res.* 15: 311

Mellott, M. J., Stabilito, I. I., Holahan, M. A., Cuca, G. C., Wang, S., Li, P., Barrett, J. S., Lynch, J. J., and S. J. Gardell (1992). Vampire bat salivary plasminogen activator promotes rapid and sustained reperfusion without concomitant systemic plasminogen activation in a canine model of arterial thrombosis. *Arteriosclerosis and Thrombosis.* 12: 212

Mills, R. S. (1980). Parturition and social interaction among captive vampire bats, *Desmodus rotundus. J. Mammal.* 61(2): 336

Mitchell, G. C. (1986). Vampire Bat Control in Latin America. In D. Policansky (ed.). *Ecological Knowledge and Problem-Solving.* National Academy Press. Washington, D. C.

Morgan, G. S. (1991). Neotropical chiroptera from the pliocene and pleistocene of Florida. *Bull. Am Mus. Nat. Hist.* No. 206: 176

Olsen, S. J. (1960). Additional remains of Florida's pleistocene vampire. *J. Mammal.* 41: 458

Pawan, J. L. (1936). Rabies in the vampire bat of Trinidad, with special reference to the clinical course and the latency of infection. *Ann. Trop. Med. Parasitol.* 30: 401

Piccinini, R. S., Peracchi, A. L., Souza, J. C. P., Albuquerque, S. T., Raimundo, S. D. L., Tannure, A. M., and L. L. Furtado (1985). Comportamento do morcego hematofago *Desmodus rotundus* (Chiroptera) relacionado com a taxa de attaque a bovinos em cativeiro. *Pesq. Vet. Bras.* 5(4): 111

Ray, C. E., Linares, O. J., and G. S. Morgan (1988). Paleontology. In A. M. Greenhall and U. Schmidt (eds.) *The Natural History of Vampire Bats.* CRC Press, Inc. Boca Raton, Florida.

Rosenthal, J. E. (1972). *AID (Agency for International Development) Finds Ways to Control Vampire Bat.* War on Hunger, Agency for International Development.

Rothschild, M. (1955). Fleas. *Sci. Amer.* 213: 44

Rothschild, M. and B. Ford (1964). Breeding of the Rabbit flea (*Spilopsyllus cuniculi* Dale), controlled by the reproductive hormones of the host. *Proc. Roy. Ent. Soc. Lond.* 29(1): 1

Rothschild, M., Ford, B., and M. Hughes (1970). Maturation of the male rabbit flea (*Spilopsyllus cuniculi*) and the oriental rat flea (*Xenopsylla cheopis*): Some effects of mammalian hormones on development and impregnation. *Trans. Zool. Soc. Lond.* 32: 105

Rupprecht, C. E. (1993). Associate Professor. Department of Microbiology and Immunology, Center for Neurovirology, Thomas Jefferson University, Jefferson Medical College. Philadelphia, Pennsylvania. Personal communication

Sazima, I. and W. Uieda (1980). Feeding behavior of the white-winged vampire bat, *Diaemus youngii*, on poultry. *J. Mammal.* 61(1): 102

Schmidt, U. (1973). Olfactory threshold and odour discrimination of the vampire bat (*Desmodus rotundus*). *Period. Biol.* 75: 89

Schmidt, U. (1988). Orientation and Sensory Functions in *Desmodus rotundus.* In A. M. Greenhall and U. Schmidt (eds.) *The Natural History of Vampire Bats.* CRC Press, Inc. Boca Raton, Florida.

Schmidt U. and U. Manske (1982). Thermopraferenz bei der Gemeinen Vampirfledermaus *Desmodus rotundus. Z. Saugetierkunde.* 47: 118

Schmidt, U., Greenhall, A. M., and W. Lopez-Forment (1970). Vampire bat control in Mexico. *Bijdragen tot de Dierkunde.* 40: 74

Schmidt, C., Schmidt, U., and U. Manske (1980). Observations of the behavior of orphaned juveniles in the common vampire bat (*Desmodus rotundus*). In D. E. Wilson and A. L. Gardner (eds.) *Proceedings of the 5th International Bat Research Conference.* Texas Tech Press. Lubbock, Texas.

Schmidt, U., Schlegal, P., Schweizer, H., and G. Neuweiler (1991). Audition in vampire bats, *Desmodus rotundus. J. Comp. Physiol. A.* 168: 45

Schober, W. (1984). *The Lives of Bats.* Edition Leipzig. Leipzig, Germany.

Thomas, J. G. and H. J. Harlan (1981). Vampire bat bites seen in humans in Panama: Their characterization, recognition, and management. *Military Medicine.* 146: 410

Thompson, R. D., Elias, D. J., Shumake, S. A., and S. E. Gaddis (1982). Taste preferences of the common vampire bat (*Desmodus rotundus*). *J. Ecol. Chem.* 8(4): 715

Timson, J. (1993). How vampire bats acquired a taste for blood. *New Scientist.* 137(1855): 18

Trapido, H. (1946). Observations on the vampire bat with special reference to longevity in captivity. *J. Mammal.* 27(3): 217

Turner, D. C. (1975). *The Vampire Bat—A Field Study in Behavior and Ecology.* The Johns Hopkins University Press. Baltimore.

Uieda, W. (1982). *Aspectos do Comportamento Alimentar das Tres Especies do Morcegos Hematofagos (Chiroptera, Phyllostomidae).* Master's Thesis (English summary). Instituto de Biologia da Universidade Estadual de Campinas, Brazil.

Vierhaus, H. (1983). Wie Vampirfledermause (*Desmodus rotundus*) ihre Zahne sharfen. *Z. Saugetierk.* 48: 269

Villa-C., B. and M. Canela-R. (1988). Man, Gods, and Legendary Vampire Bats. In A. M. Greenhall and U. Schmidt (eds.) *The Natural History of Vampire Bats.* CRC Press, Inc. Boca Raton, Florida.

Villa-Ramirez, B. (1958). El acto de tomar la sangre en los murcielagos hematofagos (familia Desmodontidae). *An. Inst. Biol. Univ. Mex.* 28: 339

Villa-Ramirez, B. (1969). *The Ecology and Biology of*

Vampire Bats and Their Relationship to Paralytic Rabies. Report to the Government of Brazil. United Nations Development Programme/Food and Agriculture Organization. FAO No. TA2656. Rome, 1969

Wilkinson, G. S. (1984). Reciprocal food sharing in the vampire bat. *Nature*. 308(8): 181

Wilkinson, G. S. (1990). Food sharing in vampire bats. *Sci. Amer*. 262(2): 76

Williams, H. E. (1960). Bat transmitted rabies in Trinidad. *Can. Vet. J.* 1(1): 20

Wimsatt, W. A. (1962). Responses of captive common vampires to cold and warm environments. *J. Mammal.* 43(2): 185

Wimsatt, W. A. (1969). Transient behavior, nocturnal activity patterns, and feeding efficiency of vampire bats (*Desmodus rotundus*) under natural conditions. *J. Mammal.* 50(2): 233

Wimsatt, W. A. and A. Guerriere (1961). Care and maintenance of the common vampire bat in captivity. *J. Mammal.* 42(4): 449

Wimsatt, W. A. and A. Guerriere (1962). Observations on the feeding capacities and excretory functions of captive vampire bats. *J. Mammal.* 43(1): 17

Witt, W., Baldus, B., Bringmann, P., Cashion, L., Donner, P., and W.-D. Schleuning (1992). Thrombolytic properties of *Desmodus rotundus* (vampire bat) salivary plasminogen activator in experimental pulmonary embolism in rats. *Blood*. 79(5): 1213

Chapter 7:
CLINICAL MANIFESTATIONS OF RABIES IN THE VAMPIRE BAT

Early Descriptions of Clinical Disease

In his studies of clinical disease, Pawan (1936) described six separate manifestations of rabies infection in the vampire bat, as follows:

1) Classical furious form, with fury being the predominant stage and followed by paralysis and death.
2) Classical paralytic form, with the dumb form of rabies being the predominant stage, fury not being present. Paralysis is followed directly by death.
3) Furious form, in which a paralytic stage does not exist. Fury is followed directly by death.
4) Complete absence of signs, marked by sudden and unexpected death.
5) Furious form, in which the stage of fury is followed by recovery.
6) Subclinical form of infection, in which the bat continues living without any signs of abnormality, but still capable of transmitting disease (so-called asymptomatic salivary carrier state).

The incubation period in experimentally infected bats has ranged from 7 to 171 days. No abnormalities are noted during this time. A prodromal stage, usually 12 to 24 hours in duration, may sometimes be evident. It is characterized by restlessness and irritability, or apathy and reluctance to eat. In the furious phase, bats become increasingly excited and restless. In captivity, they may fly violently about their cage and are actively aggressive, losing all traces of the shyness exhibited by normal vampire bats. While healthy individuals will withdraw from a prodding stick, rabid vampires will snap at it. Horst and Langworthy (1972) observed naturally infected individuals in a colony of captive vampires. They reported intense fighting in response to minimally disruptive stimuli, bats screaming and biting each other viciously. The furious stage generally lasts from 1 to 5 days.

In the paralytic phase, initial paralysis may involve the legs, wings, neck, eyelids, head, or jaws. Neural impairment may extend to the urinary bladder, with resulting urinary incontinence. Fecal incontinence may also be a feature. Paralysis spreads throughout the body until, in terminal stages, the bat lies helpless on the ground. Death usually ensues within a few days.

Asymptomatic Salivary Carrier State

The purported ability of vampire bats to regularly recover from rabies infection, while remaining infectious themselves (asymptomatic salivary carrier state), is a widely reported, but mistaken concept. This belief can probably trace its origins to the limited laboratory technology available to researchers in the early part of this century (Johnson, 1971; Constantine, 1988).

More recently, it has been shown that vampire bats inoculated intracerebrally with rabies of vampire origin, all died of rabies (Moreno and Baer, 1980). Intramuscular or subcutaneous inoculation (as might occur in the wild from bites) was less lethal. Virus was found in the saliva of all bats that became sick, with the longest period of shedding prior to the onset of clinical signs being eight days. No bat that remained healthy secreted virus in its saliva and no animal that showed clinical signs was observed to recover. This is in agreement with the findings of Johnson

(1971), who studied more than 150 vampire bats captured in areas of epizootic cattle rabies.

The finding of virus in saliva in the absence of concomitant brain infection has not been supported by modern virologic techniques. Early reports to the contrary may have been based on the mistaken identification of other bat salivary-gland viruses (see page 154). These may have included Rio Bravo virus, Tamana bat virus, Tacaribe virus, or others (Price, 1978a, 1978b).

Modern evidence is consistent with the fact that vampire bats die of rabies. Acha and Arambulo, III (1985) wrote,

> *Vampire bats appear to react to rabies in the same fashion as do other animals, with variable incubation periods and some excretion of virus in the saliva; but no prolonged excretion (or carrier state). After a variable incubation period vampire bats ultimately die, but asymptomatic transmission does not occur.*

References

Acha, P. N. and P. V. Arambulo, III (1985). Rabies in the Tropics—History and Current Status. In E. Kuwert, C. Merieux, H. Koprowski, and K. Bogel (eds.) *Rabies in the Tropics*. Springer-Verlag. New York.

Constantine, D. G. (1988). Transmission of Pathogenic Microorganisms by Vampire Bats. In A. M. Greenhall and U. Schmidt (eds.) *The Natural History of Vampire Bats*. CRC Press, Inc. Boca Raton, Florida.

Horst, R. and M. Langworthy (1972). Rabies in a colony of vampire bats. *J. Mammal.* 53(4): 903

Johnson, H. N. (1971). General Epizootiology of Rabies. In Y. Nagano and F. M. Davenport (eds.) *Rabies*. Proceedings of Working Conference of Rabies. Sponsored by the Japan-United States Cooperative Medical Science Program. University Park Press. Baltimore.

Moreno, J. A. and G. M. Baer (1980). Experimental rabies in the vampire bat. *Am. J. Trop. Med. Hyg.* 29(2): 254

Pawan, J. L. (1936). Rabies in the vampire bat of Trinidad, with special reference to the clinical course and latency of infection. *Ann. Trop. Med. Parasit.* 30: 401

Price, J. L. (1978a). Isolation of Rio Bravo and a hitherto undescribed agent, Tamana bat virus, from insectivorous bats in Trinidad, with serological evidence of infection in bats and man. *Am. J. Trop. Med. Hyg.* 27(1): 153

Price, J. L. (1978b). Serological evidence of infection of Tacaribe virus and arboviruses in Trinidadian bats. *Am. J. Trop. Med. Hyg.* 27(1): 162

Chapter 8:
EPIZOOTIOLOGY OF VAMPIRE-BAT RABIES

Economic Impact of Bovine Paralytic Rabies

Dependent on nightly meals of blood for nourishment, it is apparent how the rabid vampire bat may readily infect victimized livestock. Depending on the nature of the disease in the bat population of a particular locale at any given time, the incidence of bovine paralytic rabies among area livestock may be nonexistent or may periodically reach epizootic proportion.[1] Subsisting solely on blood, the vampire bat serves in an almost ideal capacity for the transmission of rabies to its hosts. In the span of its rather lengthy feeding time, the bat may inoculate a host with heavy doses of virus. Other blood-borne diseases and parasites might also be transmitted from animal to animal during the feeding process, or invade the wound at a later time (Gilyard, 1945; Sulkin, 1962; Constantine, 1970; Prieto and Baer, 1972; Rawlins, 1985).

An estimated population of approximately 70 million head of cattle exist within the range of the vampire bat (Acha, 1986 [cited by Acha and Malaga-Alba, 1988]). In the 1960's, several studies reported that vampire-bat rabies was responsible for approximately 500,000 cattle deaths annually throughout the American tropics (Malaga-Alba, 1962 and UNDP/FAO/WHO, 1966 [cited by Acha and Malaga-Alba, 1988]; Acha, 1967). The economic impact of these losses reportedly approached 50 million U. S. dollars. Acha (1967) tabulated vampire-inflicted losses of cattle and dollars throughout Latin America (Table 8-1). Steele (1966, 1969) reported that the economic impact of bovine paralytic rabies exceeded 100 million dollars in direct loss, and approached a quarter of a billion dollars in indirect losses (including malnutrition, myiasis, and blood loss).

It has been suggested by some that early reports documenting the economic impact of bovine paralytic rabies may have been grossly inaccurate due to incomplete reporting by livestock producers, a lack of adequate diagnostic facilities, or the death of most cattle in the field without subsequent laboratory investigation (Malaga-Alba, 1966; Kaplan, 1985; Centro Panamericano de Zoonosis, 1980 and 1985 [cited by Acha and Malaga-Alba, 1988]). Others have suggested that individual countries may have inflated their estimates of cattle deaths in order to impress the United Nations Preparatory Assistance Mission on Paralytic Rabies in Latin America (Greenhall, 1985).

More recently, it has been reported that an average of 100,000 head of cattle die from rabies annually, representing an economic loss of about 30 million dollars (Acha and Arambulo, 1985). Acha (1986 [unpublished data cited by Acha and Malaga-Alba, 1988]) studied cattle losses due to vampire-induced disease between 1983 and 1984 and reported annual economic losses of approximately 44 and 42 million dollars, respectively (Table 8-2). Both the number of clinically diagnosed and laboratory-confirmed cases were considered to be under-reported (Acha and Malaga-Alba, 1988). Greenhall (1991) reported that "Throughout Latin America the extent of the losses of livestock from rabies transmitted by vampire bats remains unknown but is dramatic." Revised estimates are needed.

[1]All bovine rabies in Latin America is not of vampire-bat origin. Livestock may also be infected by terrestrial sources, including skunks, foxes, dogs, etc. (Lord et al, 1975).

Table 8-1

Bovine Paralytic Rabies in the Americas

Reporting Country	Number of Cases Annually	Estimated Annual Mortality	Number of Cattle Vaccinated Annually	Annual Loss (U.S. Currency Equivalent)
Argentina	18,000 (1964)	50,000	100,000 (1965)	$10,000,000 (1964)
Bolivia	20,000 (1965)	50,000	5,000 (1965)	15,000,000 (1965)
Brazil	32,200 (1965)	200,000	1,300,000 (1965)	22,000,000 (1965-66)
British Honduras	815 (1962)	2,000	200 (1962)	100,000 (1961)
Colombia	5,300 (1964)	50,000	150,000 (1963)	1,260,000 (1964)
Costa Rica	132 (1964)	10,000	18,000 (1963)	365,000 (1962)
Ecuador	930 (1962)	5,000	4,500 (1962)	850,000 (1963)
El Salvador	1,080 (1961)	3,000	7,000 (1964)	108,000 (1961)
French Guiana	600 (1958)	1,000	Not Available	60,000 (1958)
Guatemala	1,120 (1964)	12,000	8,000 (1964)	168,000 (1964)
Guyana	2,000 (1957)	3,000	30,000 (1963)	43,000 (1959)
Honduras	348 (1960)	6,000	5,000 (1963)	87,000 (1960)
Mexico	1,502 (1963)	90,000	1,000,000 (1963)	10,400,000 (1964)
Nicaragua	831 (1962)	10,000	8,000 (1964)	200,000 (1962)
Panama	218 (1962)	8,000	5,000 (1963)	115,000 (1962)
Paraguay	320 (1963)	5,000	2,000 (1964)	94,000 (1963)
Suriname	733 (1963)	2,000	5,013 (1963)	55,000 (1963)
Trinidad	2 (1965)	500	24,047 (1963)	5,000 (1961)
Uruguay	83 (1965)	2,000	Not Available	63,000 (1965)
Venezuela	215 (1965)	5,000	53,032 (1963)	119,000 (1960)
Total	86,439	514,500	2,724,792	$47,592,000

From Acha, P. N. Epidemiology of paralytic bovine rabies and bat rabies. *Bol. Of. Int. Epiz.* 67: 343, 1967. Reproduced with permission.

The Pan American Zoonoses Center (Pan American Health Organization) has maintained a rabies surveillance program throughout Latin America. Officially reported cases of bovine paralytic rabies throughout the range of the vampire bat from 1970 to 1991 are shown in Table 8-3. Although not all cases of bovine rabies are of vampire origin, the vast majority are. The official figures provided represent an "extreme understatement" of the true extent of bovine rabies (Lord, 1993). Accordingly, while respective Ministries of Agriculture report only one or a few cases during an outbreak, local authorities may report 6 or 7 cases, whereas cattle owners may report as many as 70 to 80 cattle deaths if queried (Lord, 1993).

Between 1970 and 1979, countries reporting the most cattle deaths due to paralytic rabies were Brazil, Argentina, Mexico, Venezuela, and Colombia. Between 1980 and 1992, countries reporting the most cattle deaths were Brazil, Bolivia, Colombia, Venezuela, and Mexico.

As shown in Figure 8-1, the very large number of bovine rabies cases officially reported from Brazil in the early 1980's obscures annual trends throughout Latin America. Figure 8-2 (which excludes data from Brazil) reveals that the large increase in the number of cases in Brazil was not manifest elsewhere. The downward trends in all countries (especially as shown in Figure 8-3 for Venezuela) probably reflect increasing use of anticoagulants to control vampire populations (Lord, 1993).

In considering the epidemiology and epizootiology of vampire-bat rabies, principal concerns have focused on several areas, including:

1) Mechanisms by which rabies is maintained within vampire populations.

Table 8-2

Rabies in Cattle, Frequency of Animals Bitten by Vampire Bats, and Estimated Economic Losses in Some Countries in Latin America, 1983-1984

1983					
Reporting Country	**Cattle Population at Risk[a]**	**Frequency of Bitten Animals[b]**	**Clinical Cases Reported**	**Cases Confirmed by Lab Diagnosis**	**Estimated Losses U.S.$[c]**
Argentina	3,650,000	+	326	18	260,800
Bolivia	450,500	+	120	82	1,252,800
Brazil	42,000,000	+++	7,959	854	33,922,000
Colombia	3,000,000	+	146	60	2,524,240
Costa Rica	450,000	+	No Cases	No Cases	182,290
Ecuador	185,500	No Information	31	31	No Information
Guatemala	2,500,000	+	43	26	448,920
Honduras	230,000	++(44)	35	26	271,440
Mexico	7,451,530	++(6,588)	921	921	3,925,037
Nicaragua	360,000	+	16	9	130,200
Panama	328,000	++(36)	18	18	187,920
Paraguay	2,500,000	+	50	23	522,000
Peru	1,880,556	+	No Information	32	334,080
Venezuela	4,669,034	+	239	75	783,000
Total	69,655,120		9,904	2,175	44,744,727

1984					
Reporting Country	**Cattle Population at Risk[a]**	**Frequency of Bitten Animals[b]**	**Clinical Cases Reported**	**Cases Confirmed by Lab Diagnosis**	**Estimated Losses U.S.$[c]**
Argentina	3,500,000	+	115	24	250,560
Bolivia	450,000	+	83	28	866,520
Brazil	42,000,000	+++	2,557	1,146	30,898,000
Colombia	3,000,000	+	193	128	2,950,000
Costa Rica	465,000	++(475)	4	0	182,680
Ecuador	180,000	No Information	35	35	No Information
Guatemala	2,580,000	+	49	24	511,560
Honduras	250,000	++(46)	42	36	375,840
Mexico	7,681,990	++(7,320)	1,104	1,104	4,166,430
Nicaragua	360,000	+	No Cases	No Cases	115,300
Panama	350,000	++(76)	6	6	145,600
Paraguay	2,500,000	+	32	17	334,100
Peru	1,342,142	+	No Information	28	292,320
Venezuela	4,717,065	+	354	123	1,284,120
Total	69,376,197		4,574	2,699	42,373,030

Parenthesis = number of bitten animals observed in recent outbreaks.

[a] Number of cattle in the enzootic areas where bovine paralytic rabies has been reported in the past 10 years.

[b] Frequency of bitten animals in the enzootic areas: (+) = less than 5%; (++) = between 5 - 10%; (+++) = above 10%

[c] Economic losses calculated by estimated loss of weight (average 15%) in vampire-bitten animals—compared to market price of ton of beef; and number of total cattle deaths from rabies—considering average cost per head of cattle in each country.

From Acha, P. N. and A. Malaga-Alba. Economic Losses Due to *Desmodus rotundus*. In A. M. Greenhall and U. Schmidt (eds.). *Natural History of Vampire Bats*. © CRC Press, Inc. Boca Raton, Florida, 1988. Reproduced with permission.

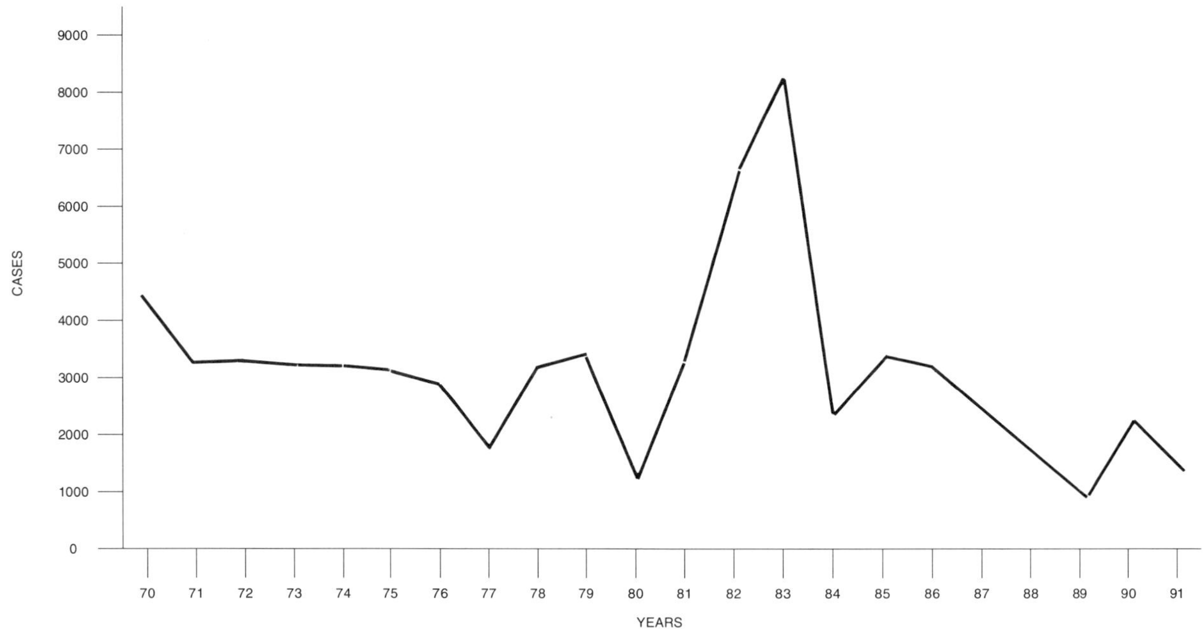

Figure 8-1. Reported cases of bovine paralytic rabies in 21 Latin American countries, 1970-1991. (Data from *Epidemiological Surveillance of Rabies for the Americas*. Pan American Zoonoses Center, Pan American Health Organization.)

2) Extent and significance of viral transmission to human and animal hosts, especially livestock.

3) Potential for virus to spread to bats in areas outside of the tropical focus of disease, as well as the implications that this might have for human and animal health.

4) Methods of control.

Social Grooming

Hanging in close contact with its neighbors, the vampire bat roosts in colonies varying in size from 6 to 200 individuals (Figure 8-4). Most colonies comprise about 100 bats (Dalquest, 1955; Kverno and Mitchell, 1976). Rarely, a colony with as many as 2,000 individuals may be found (Linhart, 1975; Flores-Crespo and Arellano-Sota, 1991). Aspects of colony organization are discussed on page 97.

Closed-circuit television monitoring of bats within their roosts has revealed that vampire bats spend as much as three hours a day grooming each other. At any one time, as much as 30% to 50% of a captive colony may be involved in grooming (Linhart [cited by Rosenthal, 1972]). Researchers at the Denver Wildlife Research Center (1969) reported that five captive vampire bats spent as much as 19% of their day in grooming, with a potential of 1,040 mouth-to-body contacts in a 24-hour period. Flores-Crespo et al (1972) observed five captive vampire bats to spend 9.4% (34 minutes) of a six-hour observation period grooming. Mills (1980) reported that members of a colony of captive vampire bats clustered about and groomed a mother and her newborn offspring.

Social grooming may serve as a means of transferring infectious saliva from one bat to another and thereby play a role in the intraspecific transmission of virus. Aspects of social grooming have also proven to be highly significant in developing strategies for controlling populations of vampire bats. Material on the body of one bat would quickly be spread through the colony and ingested by others (see page 118). Anticoagulant warfare, in particular, has taken advantage of the vampire's propensity for social grooming.

Table 8-3

Reported Cases of Bovine Paralytic Rabies in 21 Latin American Countries, 1970-1991

Country	1970	1971	1972	1973	1974	1975	1976	1977	1978	1979	1980	1981	1982	1983	1984	1985	1986	1987	1988	1989	1990	1991	Total
Argentina	221	496	671	136	112	150	1360	131	296	144	68	78	92	18	3	3	5	1	-	0	-	0	3985
Belize	14	2	-	-	-	5	-	3	2	-	8	3	0	3	4[a]	2	4	3	1	1	2	0	57
Bolivia	82	-	31	110	174	17	2	2	6	20	0	332	159	82	9[a]	151	8	65	82	24	0	0	1356
Brazil	2572	1290	1540	1706	1938	2037	682	1076	2467	2801	537	2407	5900	7959	1875	2990	2740	1825	1311	501	883	1205	48242
Colombia	168	136	37	18	54	26	31	34	58	73	38	161	139	-	105	93	76	46	75	42	44	28	1482
Costa Rica	7	-	1	-	-	-	2	5	10	7	1	1	0	0	0	15[a]	6	0	0	2	1	3	61
Chile	2	3	8	8	1	-	2	4	3	-	0	0	0	1	0	0	0	1	0	2	0	0	35
Ecuador	21	35	35	-	7	10	10	26	5	38	36	44	45	31	29[a]	12[a]	7	14	-	20	27	36	488
El Salvador	13	47	110	162	81	68	32	34	22	29	3	22	7	20[a]	11[a]	-	29[a]	33	25	7	8	18	781
Fr. Guiana	-	-	-	9	-	-	-	1	-	-	0	4	0	0	0	2	-	-	0[a]	0	-	-	16
Guatemala	7	14	7	10	6	9	7	13	21	3	12	24	22	6	14[a]	16	14[a]	8	46	28	20	24	331
Guyana	-	-	-	-	-	-	-	112	3	-	9	12	0	9	0	-	-	-	0	0	-	0	145
Honduras	54	27	31	32	4	10	223	12	7	33	16	26	19	26	36	20[a]	32[a]	4[a]	34	39	1	3	689
Mexico	979	435	210	335	264	265	329	312	211	201	371	25	35	43	66[a]	27[a]	-	-	-	-	898[b]	0	5006
Nicaragua	2	19	2	1	6	4	75	6	14	9	8	1	1	1[a]	0[a]	1	3	3	0[a]	1	2	1	160
Panama	37	2	-	6	11	23	18	4	4	7	10	2	8	3[a]	1[a]	0	9	-	-	63	13	4	225
Paraguay	132	4	28	99	15	10	4	6	1	2	4	8	9	23	17	17	17	18	18	13	121	50	616
Peru	53	5	6	15	15	54	16	12	30	23	9	29	32	32	30	44	18	11	16	7	30	18	505
Suriname	-	1	-	2	-	-	-	-	16	6	1	1	0	0	0	0	0	40	0	0	0	1	68
Trinidad	-	5	20	3	15	7	4	22	20	16	3	0	2	2[a]	0	0	-	1[a]	0	4	0	0	124
Venezuela	54	656	732	656	548	379	114	18	21	40	23	71	54	50	60	90	112	67	80	36	51	26	3938
Total	4418	3177	3469	3308	3251	3074	2911	1833	3217	3452	1157	3251	6524	8309	2260	3483	3080	2140	1688	790	2101	1417	68310

[a]Information incomplete

[b]The figures given for Mexico in 1990 were reported as "others" and arbitrarily assigned to cattle, but may include cases in foxes and vampire bats.

Data from *Epidemiological Surveillance of Rabies for the Americas*. Pan American Zoonoses Center, Pan American Health Organization.

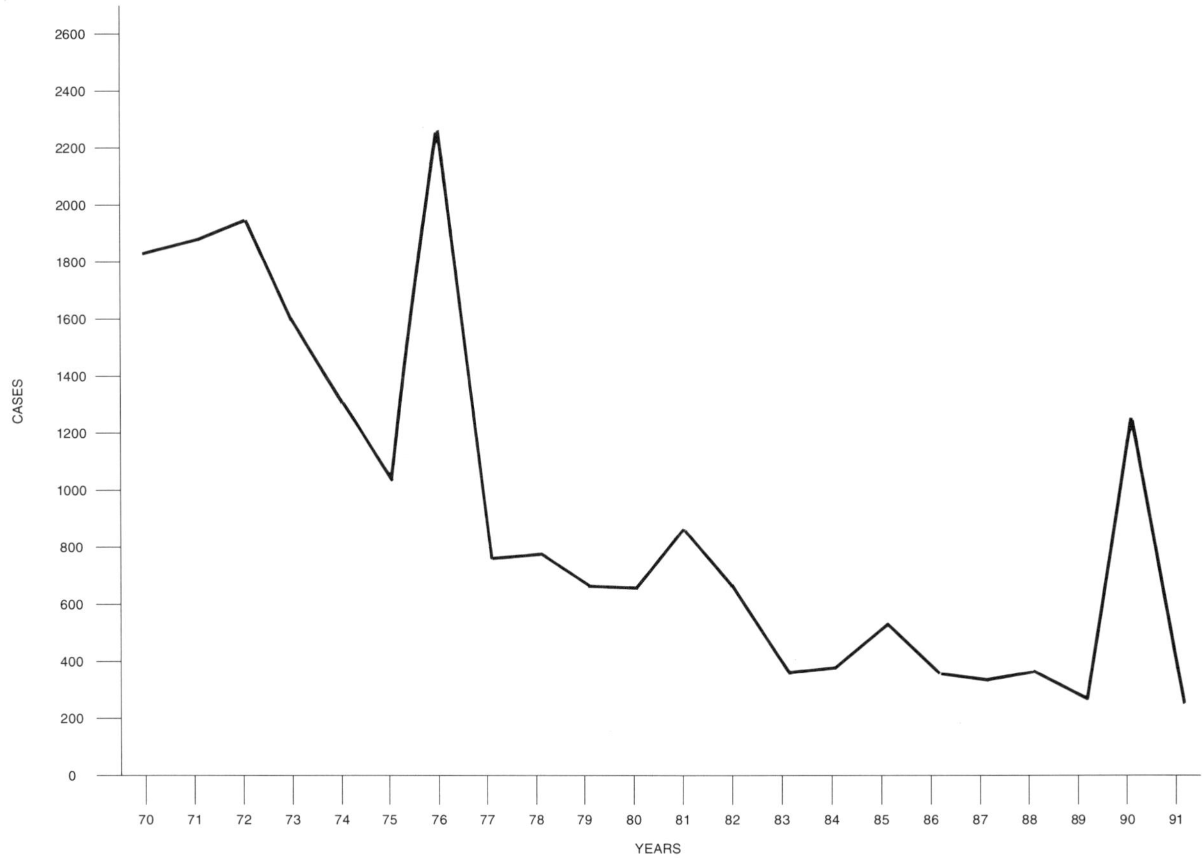

Figure 8-2. Reported cases of bovine paralytic rabies in 21 Latin American countries, excluding Brazil, 1970-1991. (Data from *Epidemiological Surveillance of Rabies for the Americas*. Pan American Zoonoses Center, Pan American Health Organization.)

Reciprocal Food Sharing

Vampires have a very long period of juvenile development. Young are nursed for about 300 days. Mouth-to-mouth regurgitation of blood from mother to offspring usually begins by the second month. Young begin to drink blood on their own at about four months of age; however, the mother will continue to nurse and regurgitate blood until the young bat is about ten months old. Should a young bat become orphaned, other lactating mothers in the social group will both suckle it and feed it blood (Schmidt et al, 1980). Schmidt and Manske (1973 [cited by Turner, 1975]) observed submissive behavior in juvenile vampires when approaching adults. This behavior entailed lifting one folded wing, while bending the body sideways. Mills (1980) reported captive female vampires regurgitating blood to another female who had just given birth. He also observed the mother regurgitating blood into the mouth of her offspring when it was only one week of age. Young vampires may receive their first taste of blood in this manner.

In addition to the large colonies of vampire bats sometimes observed in caves, smaller social groups are often formed. Long-term nonrandom associations among small groups (8 to 12 individuals) of related and unrelated adult females and their dependent offspring have been observed (Wilkinson, 1984, 1985a, 1985b, 1986, 1987, 1988a, 1988b, 1990; Park, 1991). Wilkinson (1987) reported that these groups maintained nonoverlapping foraging ranges. In considering the benefits that might be derived from such an association, Wilkinson (1985a) discussed the following possibilities:

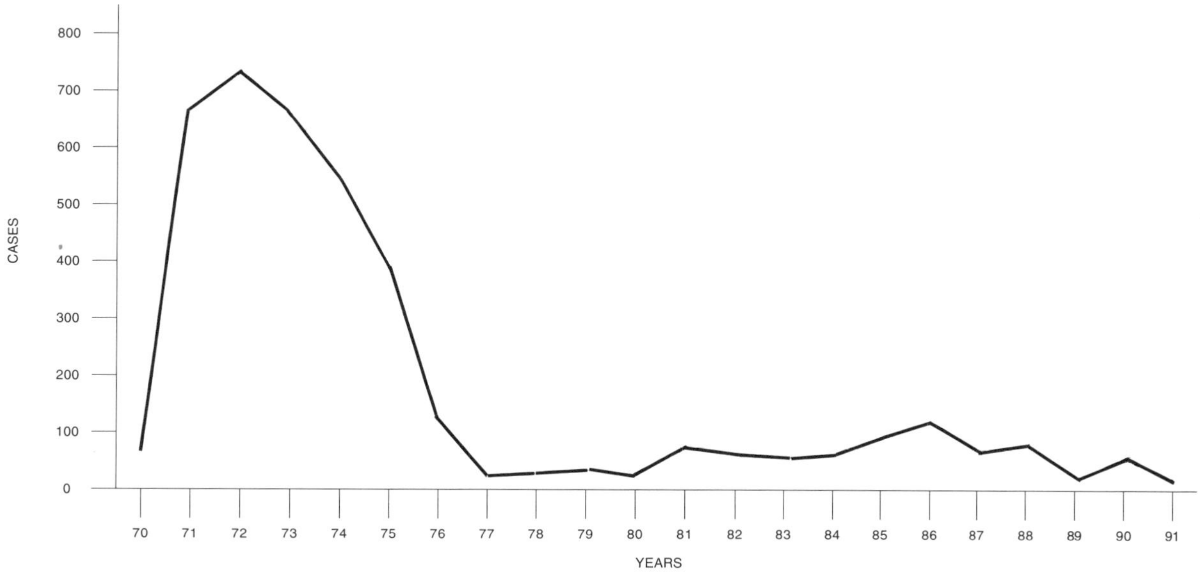

Figure 8-3. Reported cases of bovine paralytic rabies in Venezuela, 1970-1991. (Data from *Epidemiological Surveillance of Rabies for the Americas*. Pan American Zoonoses Center, Pan American Health Organization.)

1) Share a suitable microclimate.
2) Avoid predators.
3) Avoid ectoparasite infestations.
4) Minimize travel to animal hosts.
5) Respond to coercive males.
6) Feed simultaneously from a bite.
7) Remove ectoparasites by mutual grooming (allogrooming).
8) Share food by regurgitating blood to other bats within the roost.

Wilkinson's studies suggested that the primary benefit to be derived from the association was one of reciprocal food sharing. He found that regurgitation and subsequent sharing of blood occurs between mothers and their offspring, as well as between related and unrelated individuals. A starved bat is preferentially fed by one to which the recipient had recently donated blood. Thus, the feeding is reciprocated (Wilkinson, 1985a). Maintenance of reciprocal food sharing requires:

1) Sufficient number of interactions.
2) Overall benefit to reciprocal interactions.
3) Recognition and punishment (fighting?) of nonreciprocating individuals.

Wilkinson (1986) suggested a relationship between reciprocal food sharing and social grooming. In this regard, social grooming might be of value not only in identifying group members but also in determining their relative degree of abdominal swelling. He reported that much of the social grooming occurs beneath the wings in the area of the stomach. The latter determination could help roostmates assess each other's potential status (donor or recipient) regarding blood regurgitation (Figure 8-5). Females were never observed to either groom or regurgitate blood to an adult male (Wilkinson, 1985a). Wilkinson (1988a, 1988b) defined the following criteria to categorize a behavior as one of reciprocal altruism:

1) The behavior must reduce a donor's fitness relative to the selfish alternative.
2) The fitness of the recipient must be elevated relative to a nonrecipient.
3) Performance of the behavior must not depend on receipt of immediate benefit.
4) A mechanism for detecting individuals

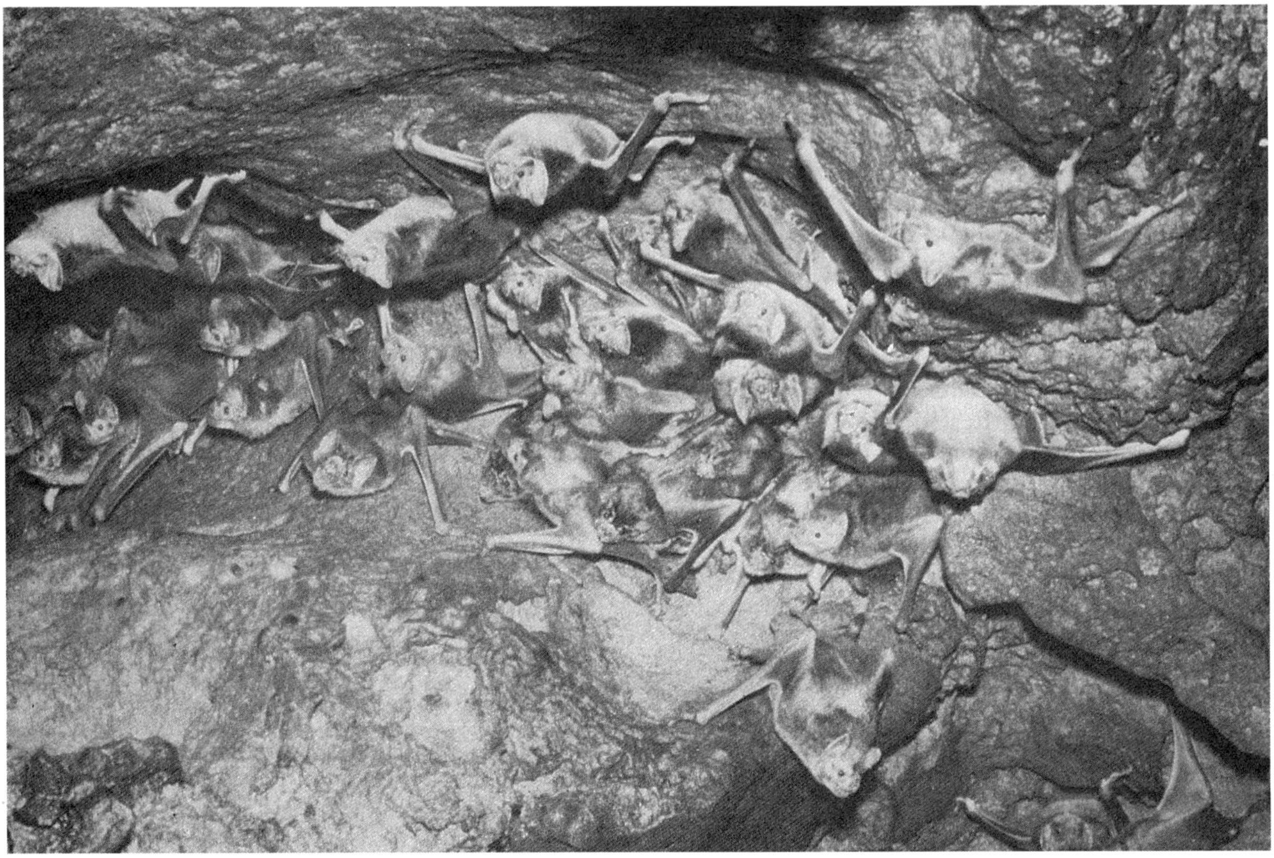

Figure 8-4. A tightly packed cluster of vampire bats roosting in a cave. (From Kverno, N. B. and G. C. Mitchell. Vampire bats and their effect on cattle production in Latin America. *Wld. Anim. Rev.* (Food and Agriculture Organization of the United Nations). 17: 1, 1976. Reproduced with permission.)

who receive benefits but never pay altruistic costs has to exist.

5) A large, but indefinite, number of opportunities to exchange aid must exist within each individual's lifetime.

A vampire bat is likely to die if it fails to feed for two consecutive evenings, losing as much as 25% of its body weight after 60 hours without food (McNab [cited by Wilkinson, 1990]). Unlike most mammals, the vampire bat does not seem to have an ability to store energy as fat for future use (Breidenstein, 1982). Between 7% to 30% of a population of vampires will not successfully feed each evening (Wilkinson, 1990). Reciprocal food sharing will permit survival of a starved individual for another evening. A starving individual can gain as much as 12 to 18 hours of additional life following reciprocal feeding, with comparable loss of less than 12 hours of life from a recently fed donor. This leaves an additional 36 hours of life before the donor reaches a critical state.

Reciprocity theory suggests and Wilkinson (1990) has shown that the only bats to be fed by roostmates are those with less than 24 hours of life remaining. Wilkinson's analysis of field data indicated that there should be an annual mortality of 82% among adult vampire bats in the absence of reciprocal food sharing. Actual mortality is only 24%, documenting the value of altruistic food sharing. Both reciprocity and kin selection are significant in food sharing among vampire bats (Wilkinson, 1990).

Any social interaction involving exchange of saliva among individual vampire bats in a colony may foster spread of disease (e.g., rabies) through the population. Thus, reciprocal food sharing may play an important role in the intraspecific transmission of disease.

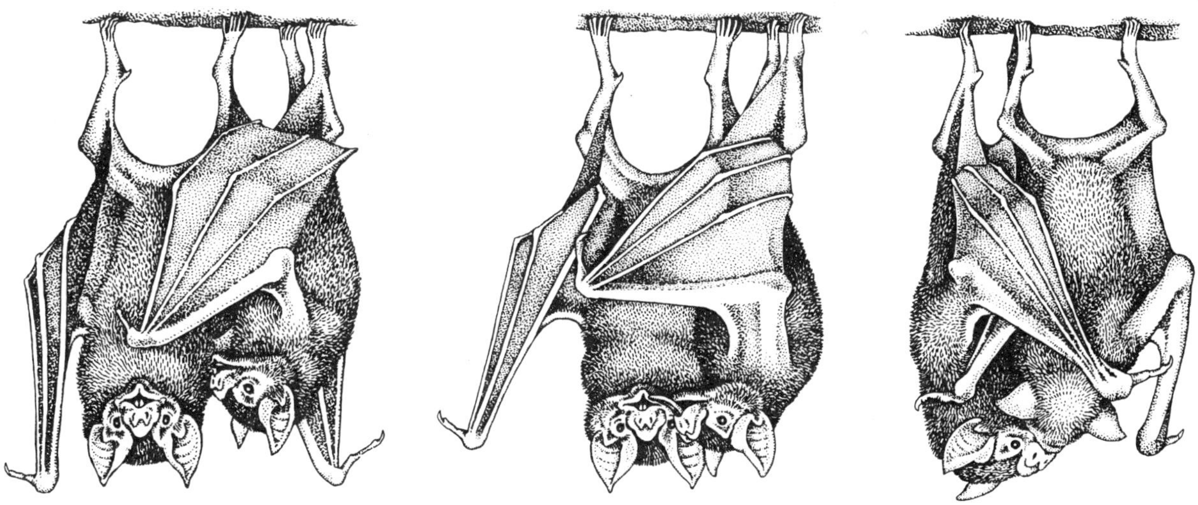

Figure 8-5. A hungry bat solicits regurgitated blood from a roostmate first by grooming, which consists of licking the potential donor under her wing, and then by licking the donor's lips. If the donor is receptive, she responds by regurgitating blood. Only bats who are close relatives or who have had a long-term association give blood to each other. (From Wilkinson, G. S. Food sharing in vampire bats. *Sci. Amer.* 262(2): 76, 1990. Reproduced with permission.)

Intraspecific Aggression Among Vampire Bats

A large number of bats captured by de Verteuil and Urich (1936) had numerous scars about the head and body. In captivity, vampires frequently attack one another when hungry (Wimsatt, 1959a, 1959b; Greenhall, 1959a, 1965a; Villa-Ramirez, 1969). Greenhall (1972) reported that clusters of males frequently nip at mating pairs. Biting also occurs during fighting over roosting sites and during sexual play. Malaga-Alba (1959) reported that captured vampires frequently have ear wounds and that the bats may bite each other through the skull. Such observations attest to the possible transmission of virus among members of a colony of vampire bats. Bats sustaining skull wounds may die as a direct result of the wound trauma or secondary infection, or they may become intracranially infected with rabies.

In support of bite-induced transmission as a mechanism of maintaining rabies virus within a vampire population, Moreno and Baer (1980) showed that vampires would develop rabies following intramuscular inoculation of virus of homologous origin (virus isolated from a naturally infected member of the same species).

It is also possible, however unlikely, that aerosol (Constantine, 1970, 1971), transplacental (Adams and Baer, 1966; Baer, 1975; Steece and Calisher, 1989), or transmammary transmission of virus may be involved in the maintenance of disease in vampire-bat populations.

Interactions Among Vampires at Feeding Sites

Bats might infect each other through salivary contact at wound sites or by biting each other during encounters on the backs of animal hosts. Bats tend to revisit old wounds repeatedly and this might increase the likelihood of chance encounters.

Greenhall et al (1971) and Schmidt and Greenhall (1973) discussed some aspects of social interaction at feeding sites on cattle. They observed instances of pushing, jumping, screaming, fighting amongst themselves, and territorial aggression. Although some bats were seen to feed simultaneously from a single wound, sequential feeding was the most commonly observed event.

In one case, a single bleeding wound on the neck of a cow was used by seven bats in succession over a three-hour period. Schmidt and Van de Flierdt (1973 [cited by Turner, 1975]) described stereotypic patterns of aggression in captive vampire bats, but noted that actual biting was rare.

In *Diaemus*, agonistic displays by bats feeding on birds have been observed when other bats approached (Sazima and Uieda, 1980). This may be related to the fact that a bird is too small to support more than one vampire at a time or to the possibility that more than one bat on so small an animal might disturb it to the point of making feeding impossible.

Propagation of the Vampire Rabies Epizootic

Following the appearance of bovine paralytic rabies in Brazil, outbreaks were reported throughout much of Latin America (Schroeder et al, 1952; Malaga-Alba, 1957; Greenhall, 1959b; Verlinde et al, 1970, 1975; de Diego and Valotta, 1973). Recognition of widely dispersed outbreaks was related, in part, to "migration" of vampire epizootics and, in part, to an increased public awareness of the disease. Vampire bats of Chile and coastal areas of Peru have apparently remained free of rabies infection (Steele, 1973; Beran, 1981).[2]

From the coastline of Venezuela, the epizootic of vampire-bat rabies might have spread to Trinidad. Van Rooyen and Rhodes (1948 [cited by Martin, 1959]) considered the possibility that rabid vampire bats may have been transported to Trinidad by ship (this has also been suggested as an unlikely means whereby European bats may have become infected with an African-like variant of rabies-related virus). The distance from the Venezuelan coastline to Trinidad is well within the vampire's flight range. Vampire bats were known to exist on Chacachacare, an island midway between Venezuela and Trinidad, and bats have been observed flying across the Gulf of Paria from the Venezuelan coastline towards Trinidad (Pawan, 1936). Gilyard (1945) suggested that such flights may have been caused by "rabic hallucinations" and Sulkin (1962) stated that deranged, rabid bats may lose their "homing instinct" and stray from their usual homesite.

Pawan (1936, 1939) postulated that the outbreaks in Trinidad may have arisen from a local source of virus, already present on the island prior to recognition of its economic and public-health significance. As evidence, he cited the following three prominent examples. In 1889, a local chemist who was dissecting a vampire bat was stricken with a fatal acute ascending paralysis (Constantine [1988] recommended that biologists wear gloves when dissecting bats because of the possibility of contamination of wounds with virus). In 1919, a peasant girl and a woman were bitten by a "strange, mad cat." Within six weeks, they both developed a fatal ascending paralysis, with symptoms of extreme thirst and inability to swallow. Pawan also mentioned the difficulty of early villagers in Siparia to successfully rear livestock, due to "the ravages of bats." Siparia, on the southernmost part of the island, was the site of the first human case of paralytic rabies in 1929. These incidents were suggestive of a viral presence already on the island as early as the late 19th century.

In areas littered with caves or other suitable roosting sites, many distinct populations of vampire bats exist, which may freely communicate with each other. This may allow for the transmission of virus from colony to colony within a district and, gradually, from one district to another (Lord et al 1975). Based on their studies of vampire-bat rabies in Argentina, Lopez et al (1969 [cited by Lord et al, 1975]) and de Diego and Valotta (1973) reported that a "migrating" epizootic of vampire-bat rabies moved at a rate of about 40 to 50 km annually.

Lord et al (1975) captured vampires during

[2]In 1985, 13 rabid Brazilian free-tailed bats (*Tadarida brasiliensis*) were found in Chile (Favi and Catalan, 1986; Nunez et al, 1987). These were the first published reports of bat rabies in Chile. Monoclonal antibody analysis of rabies isolates from eight of these bats (as well as from a rabid cat found in Chile) revealed reactivity patterns distinct from those of both vampire bats and dogs in enzootic areas (Smith, 1989). By 1988, 50 free-tailed bats had been reported positive for rabies in Chile (Favi and Duran, 1991).

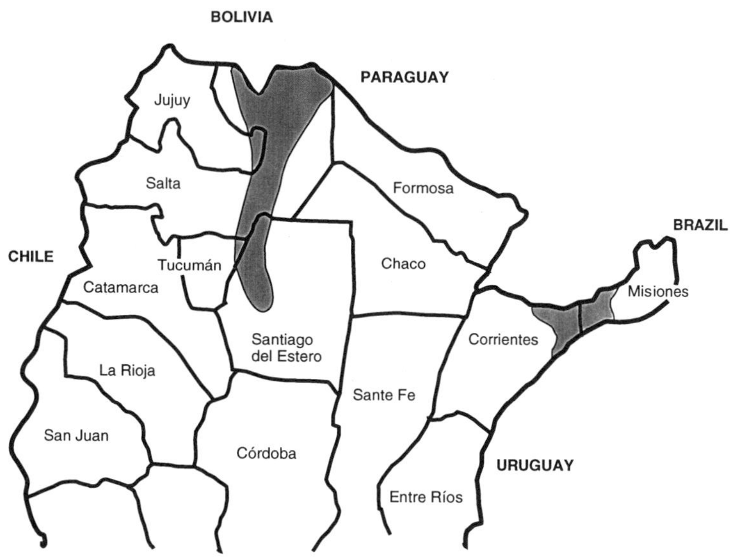

Figure 8-6. A map of northern Argentina showing regions (shaded sectors) where two widely separated epizootics of vampire-transmitted bovine rabies occurred. (From Lord, R. D., Fuenzalida, E., Delpietro, H., Larghi, O. P., de Diaz, A. M. O., and L. Lazaro. Observations on the epizootiology of vampire bat rabies. *Bull. Pan Am. Hlth. Org.* IX(3): 189, 1975. © Pan American Health Organization. Washington, D.C. Redrawn with permission.)

1971 and 1972 from the provinces of Corrientes, Santiago del Estero, and Tucaman in connection with the study of two widely separated outbreaks of bovine paralytic rabies in Argentina (Figure 8-6). Table 8-4 categorizes 877 captured bats with respect to site of capture, time between capture and the presence of a rabies outbreak in local cattle, and the presence or absence of serum neutralizing antibodies against the rabies virus. With only one exception (Piedrabuena, Tucaman), the presence of rabies-neutralizing antibodies was not commonly detected in vampires captured prior to the presence of a rabies outbreak in local cattle. A slightly higher percentage of individuals with rabies-neutralizing antibodies was found in bats captured in the midst of a rabies outbreak in local cattle. The highest percentage of bats with detectable neutralizing antibodies was found in animals captured seven months after the rabies outbreak in cattle.

Rabies virus could be isolated only from bats captured during or just prior to an outbreak of disease in cattle. Eleven of 83 (13.3%) vampire bats captured just a few weeks prior to onset of disease in cattle were found to be rabies positive. Nine of 50 (18%) bats captured during an epizootic of cattle rabies were found to be rabies positive (Fornes et al, 1974; Lord et al, 1975). Delpietro et al (1972) reported isolation of rabies virus from 8 of 31 (25.8%) vampires captured in the midst of an outbreak of bovine paralytic rabies. No virus could be isolated from any of 99 bats captured from an area one year after an outbreak, although rabies-neutralizing antibodies could be detected in 24 of them (24.2%). Similar findings were reported by Delpietro and Konolsaisen (1991) during study of an 18-month-long outbreak of bovine paralytic rabies in the province of Misiones, Argentina.

Consistent with these findings, onset of rabies in a vampire population is characterized by infection of a significant portion of the population. Some of the bats succumb to the disease, whereas others are immunized and do not sicken. As the number of bats susceptible to illness decreases to a level below the threshold required to maintain the epizootic, the outbreak either subsides or "migrates" to nearby susceptible populations.

The epizootic in vampires arises abruptly and is short-lived in an area. It is marked by outbreaks of bovine paralytic rabies, which usually last between 3 and 6 months. By the time disease

Table 8-4

Rabies-Neutralizing Antibody in Vampire Sera, Grouped According to the Capture Site and the Time Between Capture and Occurrence of a Local Bovine Rabies Outbreak

Locality	Months Before (-) or After (+) Outbreak	Presence of Neutralizing Antibody	
		No. Positive/Tested	Percent Positive
		Specimens Bled Prior to Outbreak	
Retiro, Santiago del Estero	23 (-)	0/7	0
Las Cejas, Santiago del Estero	8 (-)	1/92	1
San Felix, Santiago del Estero	8 (-)	0/98	0
San Ramon, Santiago del Estero	8 (-)	0/6	0
Timbo Viejo, Tucuman	8 (-)	0/6	0
El Naranjo, Tucuman	8 (-)	0/139	0
Talo Pozo, Tucuman	7 (-)	3/40	8
Arenales, Santiago del Estero	7 (-)	0/43	0
San Felix, Santiago del Estero	5 (-)	0/6	0
Piedrabuena, Tucuman	5 (-)	16/110	15
Bobadal, Santiago del Estero	4 (-)	0/16	0
El Rincon, Santiago del Estero	2 (-)	1/65	2
El Azul, Santiago del Estero	2 (-)	0/66	0
	Subtotal:	21/694	3.1
		Specimens Bled During Outbreak	
Siete Arboles, Santiago del Estero	0	1/31	3
San Pedro, Santiago del Estero	0	2/14	14
San Jose, Tucuman	0	0/18	0
Ita Ibaté, Corrientes	0	2/13	15
	Subtotal:	5/76	6.6
		Specimens Bled After Outbreak	
San Vicente, Santiago del Estero	1 (+)	1/32	3
San Antonio, Santiago del Estero	2 (+)	5/21	24
San Miguel, Santiago del Estero	4 (+)	1/6	17
Las Lajas, Santiago del Estero	5 (+)	3/23	13
Virasoro, Corrientes	5 (+)	7/12	58
Las Lajas, Santiago del Estero	7 (+)	1/13	8
	Subtotal:	18/107	16.8
		Specimens Bled From 6 months to 4 Years After Outbreak (exact interval unknown)	
Teyu Cuaré, San Ignacio, Misiones	? (+)	2/7	29
Almafuerte, Misiones	? (+)	2/8	25
Santa Ana, Misiones	? (+)	2/11	18
Candelaria, Misiones	? (+)	0/60	0
Rincon Chico, San Carlos, Misiones	? (+)	7/61	11
	Subtotal:	13/147	8.9

From Lord, R. D., Fuenzalida, E., Delpietro, H., Larghi, O. P., de Diaz, A. M. O., and L. Lazaro. Observations on the epizootiology of vampire bat rabies. *Bull. Pan Am. Hlth. Org.* IX(3): 189, 1975.

is recognized in livestock, the infected vampire bats have died and the majority of cattle exposures have occurred (Johnson, 1971). After several years and several generations of bats, waning herd immunity may increase the susceptibility of the population enough to make them susceptible to another epizootic.

Seasonal Influences on the Incidence of Bovine Paralytic Rabies

Many vampire bats prefer to roost in river caves (Constantine, 1970). With the coming of the rainy season, however, the swelling underground rivers drive the bats to seek more hospitable habitats in other regions. Vampires roosting in hollow trees may also seek drier sites at this time (Greenhall, 1965b [cited by Constantine, 1970]). Movement of bats with the onset of the rainy season has been correlated with an increased frequency of bovine paralytic rabies in Mexico, Venezuela, Paraguay, Argentina, Trinidad, and Costa Rica. Concomitant relocation of cattle into drier country may contribute to the increased incidence of cattle disease often observed at this time (Enright, 1956; Constantine, 1970).

Turner (1975) suggested that increased transmission of rabies during the rainy season may be due to a change in feeding habits of the vampires. At this time, fewer bats seem to revisit wounds and so, many more cattle may be attacked.

Lord (1992) reported an increased probability of viral transmission to young male vampires during the wet season. Accordingly, young males within a colony may be driven out by the dominant male at this time. Joining satellite colonies of other bachelor males, in-fighting and biting may lead to an increased transmission of disease among these bats.[3] This corresponds to reported increases in bovine paralytic rabies during the wet season (Lord, 1992). Seasonal occurrence of vampire bat rabies may also be related to climatic factors such as El Niño[4] (Acha and Malaga-Alba, 1988).

References

Acha, P. N. (1967). Epidemiologia de la rabia bovina parlitica y de la rabia del murcielago. In: *Primer Seminario Internacional sobre rabia par las Americas.* Buenos Aires, 1967. Pan American Sanitary Bureau (Sci. Publ. 169), Washington, D.C.

Acha, P. N. (1986). Informacion epidemiologica sobre rabia bovina en Latinoamerica, anos 1983-1984, segun pais. Unpublished data.

Acha, P. N. and P. V. Arambulo, III (1985). Rabies in the Tropics—History and Current Status. In E. Kuwert, C. Merieux, H. Koprowski, and K. Bogel (eds.) *Rabies in the Tropics.* Springer-Verlag. New York.

Acha, P. N. and A. Malaga-Alba (1988). Economic Losses Due to *Desmodus rotundus.* In A. M. Greenhall and U. Schmidt (eds.) *The Natural History of Vampire Bats.* CRC Press, Inc. Boca Raton, Florida.

Adams, D. B. and G. M. Baer (1966). Cesarian section and artificial feeding device for suckling bats. *J. Mammal.* 47(3): 524

Baer, G. M. (1975). Bovine Paralytic Rabies and Rabies in the Vampire Bat. In G. M. Baer (ed.) *The Natural History of Rabies.* Vol. II. Academic Press. New York.

Beran, G. W. (1981). Rabies and Infections by Rabies-Related Viruses. In G. W. Beran (section ed.) *CRC Handbook Series in Zoonoses. Section B: Viral Zoonoses.* Volume II. CRC Press, Inc. Boca Raton, Florida.

Breidenstein, C. P. (1982). Digestion and assimilation of bovine blood by a vampire bat (*Desmodus rotundus*). *J. Mammal.* 63(3): 482

Burns, R. J. and R. W. Bullard (1979). Diphacinone residue from whole bodies of vampire bats: A laboratory study. *Bull. Pan Am. Hlth. Org.* 13(4): 365 (Author's translation) in *Bol. Of. Sanit. Panam.*

[3]The social structure observed in small colonies of vampire bats is of a harem nature, with the dominant (alpha) male roosting near the main group (consisting of females and their infants), a second (beta) male roosting in an area used by the females as a temporary residence, and a third (beta) male roosting some distance away. Only the alpha male demonstrates territorial behavior (Park, 1991). Fights often result in bites. Adolescent females remain within the main group. However, adolescent males leave the group at 12 to 18 months of age (Wilkinson, 1985b) or 20 to 27 months of age (Park, 1991), forming temporary bachelor colonies.

[4]Periodic warming trend of the normally cold water currents in the Pacific Ocean originating off the coasts of Chile, Peru, and Ecuador.

88(5): 396

Centro Panamericano de Zoonosis (1980). *Vigilancia Epidemiologica de la Rabia.* Supplemento Especial Vol. XII, December.

Centro Panamericano de Zoonosis (1985). *Epidemiological Surveillance of Rabies for the Americas.* Third and Fourth Quarters. Vol. 16, No. 7-12, November.

Constantine, D. G. (1970). Bats in Relation to the Health, Welfare, and Economy of Man. In W. Wimsatt (ed.) *Biology of Bats.* Vol. II. Academic Press. New York.

Constantine, D. G. (1971). Bat Rabies: Current Knowledge and Future Research. In Y. Nagano and F. M. Davenport (eds.) *Rabies.* Sponsored by the Japan-United States Cooperative Medical Science Program. University Park Press. Baltimore.

Constantine, D. G. (1988). Transmission of Pathogenic Microorganisms by Vampire Bats. In A. M. Greenhall and U. Schmidt (eds.) *The Natural History of Vampire Bats.* CRC Press, Inc. Boca Raton, Florida.

Dalquest, W. W. (1955). Natural history of the vampire bats of eastern Mexico. *Am. Midl. Nat.* 53(1): 79

de Diego, A. and J. R. Valotta (1973). Rabia transmitida por murcielagos. Situacion en la Republica Argentina. (Bat-transmitted rabies. Situation in Argentina.) *Revista de Medicina Veterinaria, Argentina.* 54(4): 275 (English abstract) in *Vet. Bull.* (1974). 44(4): 217

Delpietro, H. A. and J. F. Konolsaisen (1991). Dinamica da raiva em uma populacao de morcegos hematofagos (*Desmodus rotundus*) no nordeste Argentino, e sua relacao com a raiva paralitica dos herbivoros. *Arq. Biol. Tecnol.* 34(3/4): 381

Delpietro, H., de Diaz, A. M. C., Fuenzalida, E., and J. F. Bell (1972). Determinacion de la tasa de ataque de rabia en murcielagos (Determination of the frequency of rabies in vampire bats). *Bol. Of. Sanit. Panam.* 73(3): 222 (English abstract) in *Vet. Bull.* (1973). 43(8): 415

Denver Wildlife Research Center (1969). Annual Report. *Vampire Bats—Rabies Transmission and Livestock Production in Latin America.* U. S. Bureau of Sport Fisheries and Wildlife. Field Station. Palo Alto, Mexico.

de Verteuil, E. and F. W. Urich (1936). The study and control of paralytic rabies transmitted by bats in Trinidad, British West Indies. *Trans. Roy. Soc. Trop. Med. Hyg.* XXIX(4): 317

Enright, J. B. (1956). Bats and their relation to rabies. *Ann. Rev. Microbiol.* 10: 369

Favi, C. M. and G. R. Catalan (1986). Rabia en murcielagos en Chile (Rabies in bats in Chile). *Avances en Ciencias Veterinarias.* 1(2): 73 (English abstract) in *Vet. Bull.* (1988). 58(2): 97

Favi, C. M. and R. J. C. Duran (1991). Epidemiologia de la rabia en Chile (1929-88) y perspectivas en mamiferos silvestres (Epidemiology of rabies in Chile 1929-88 and prospects in wild animals). *Avances en Ciencias Veterinarias.* 6(1): 13 (English abstract) in *Vet. Bull.* (1992). 62(9): 929

Flores-Crespo, R. and C. Arellano-Sota (1991). Biology and Control of the Vampire Bat. In G. M. Baer (ed.) *The Natural History of Rabies.* 2nd Edition. CRC Press, Inc. Boca Raton, Florida.

Flores-Crespo, R., Linhart, S. B., and R. J. Burns (1972). Comportamiento del vampiro (*Desmodus rotundus*) en cautiverio. (English abstract) *SW Nat.* 17(2): 139

Fornes, A., Lord, R. D., Kuns, M. L., Larghi, O. P., Fuenzalida, E., and L. Lazara (1974). Control of bovine rabies through vampire bat control. *J. Wildl. Dis.* 10: 310

Gilyard, R. T. (1945). Bat transmitted paralytic rabies. *Cornell Vet.* XXXV(3): 195

Greenhall, A. M. (1959a). Discussion. In *Proceedings of Conference on Research in Bat Rabies.* July 10-11. National Institutes of Health. Bethesda, Maryland. p. 134

Greenhall, A. M. (1959b). The ecological role of Trinidad bats, especially the vampire, and bat rabies. *Vet. Rec.* 71(10): 188

Greenhall, A. M. (1965a). Notes on behavior of captive vampire bats. *Mammalia.* 29(4): 441

Greenhall, A. M. (1965b). Aspects of ecology in vampire bat control in Trinidad. *Ann. 2nd Congr. Latino-Amer. Zool.* 1962, pp. 321-325

Greenhall, A. M. (1972). The biting and feeding habits of the vampire bat, *Desmodus rotundus. J. Zool. (London).* 168: 451

Greenhall, A. M. (1985). Effects of Vampire Bats and Paralytic Rabies on Livestock Production. In S. M. Gaafar, W. E. Howard, and R. E. Marsh (eds.) *Parasites, Pests and Predators.* Elsevior Science Publishing Co., Inc. New York.

Greenhall, A. M. (1991). Ethology and ecology of vampire bats. In *Expert Consultation on the Care of Persons Exposed to Rabies Transmitted by Vampire Bats.* PAHO/WHO. Programs for Veterinary Public Health. Washington, D.C. April 1-5, 1991

Greenhall, A. M., Schmidt, U., and W. Lopez-Foment (1971). Attacking behavior of the vampire bat, *Desmodus rotundus*, under field conditions in Mexico. *Biotropica.* 3(2): 136

Horst, R. and M. Langworthy (1972). Rabies in a colony of vampire bats. *J. Mammal.* 53(4): 903

Johnson, H. N. (1971). General Epizootiology of Rabies. In Y. Nagano and F. M. Davenport (eds.) *Rabies.* Proceedings of Working Conference of Rabies. Sponsored by the Japan-United States Cooperative Medical Science Program. University Park

Press. Baltimore.

Kaplan, C. (1985). Rabies: A Worldwide Disease. In P. J. Bacon (ed.) *Population Dynamics of Rabies in Wildlife*. Academic Press. New York.

Kverno, N. B. and G. C. Mitchell (1976). Vampire bats and their effect on cattle production in Latin America. *Wld. Anim. Rev.* (FAO). 17: 1

Linhart, S. B. (1975). The Biology and Control of Vampire Bats. In G. M. Baer (ed.) *The Natural History of Rabies*. Vol. II. Academic Press. New York.

Lopez, A., Silva, M., and M. LaMata (1969). Rabia paralitica en el Norte Argentino. In: *Seminario sobre Rabia par los Paises de la Zona IV—Bolivia, Colombia, Ecuador, Peru*. pp. 161-203. Washington, D.C. Pan American Health Organization. October 6-11, 1969

Lord, R. D. (1992). Seasonal reproduction of vampire bats and its relation to seasonality of bovine rabies. *J. Wildl. Dis.* 28(2): 292

Lord, R. D. (1993). The History of Vampire Bat Transmitted Bovine Rabies in the Americas. *Proceedings of the Fourth Annual International Meeting on Rabies Control in the Americas*. Thomas Jefferson University. Philadelphia, Pennsylvania. October 28-30, 1993

Lord, R. D., Fuenzalida, E., Delpietro, H., Larghi, O. P., de Diaz, A. M. O., and L. Lazaro (1975). Observations on the epizootiology of vampire bat rabies. *Bull. Pan Am. Hlth. Org.* IX(3): 189

Malaga-Alba, A. (1957). Rabies in wildlife in Middle America. *J. Am. Vet. Med. Assoc.* 130: 386

Malaga-Alba, A. (1959). Pathogenesis of Rabies in Bats—Vampires. In *Proceedings of Conference on Research in Bat Rabies*. p. 85. National Institutes of Health. Bethesda, Maryland. July 10-11, 1959

Malaga-Alba, A. (1962). The vampire bat problem in Latin America. *A Report to the UN Food and Agriculture Organization (FAO)*. Rome.

Malaga-Alba, A. (1966). Ecological Relationship of Rabies in Wildlife. *International Symposium on Rabies*. Symp. Series Immunobiol. Standard. Vol. I. Karger, Basel. New York. Talloires, 1965

Martin, R. L. (1959). A history of chiropteran rabies with special reference to occurrence and importance in the United States. *Wildl. Dis.* 3: 1

Mills, R. S. (1980). Parturition and social interaction among captive vampire bats, *Desmodus rotundus*. *J. Mammal.* 61(2): 336

Moreno, J. A. and G. M. Baer (1980). Experimental rabies in the vampire bat. *Am. J. Trop. Med. Hyg.* 29(2): 254

Nunez, S. F., Favi, C. M., Urcelay, V. S., Sepulveda, C. C., and G. F. Fabrega (1987). Wild rabies in insectivorous bats in Chile. *Bol. Of. Sanit. Panam.* 103(2): 140. (English translation) in *Wildl. Dis. Rev.* VI(2): 88-2003

Park, S.-R. (1991). Development of social structure in a captive colony of the common vampire bat, *Desmodus rotundus*. *Ethology*. 89: 335

Pawan, J. L. (1936). The transmission of paralytic rabies in Trinidad by the vampire bat (*Desmodus rotundus murinus* Wagner, 1840). *Ann. Trop. Med. Parasit.* 30: 101

Pawan, J. L. (1939). Paralysis as a clinical manifestation in human rabies. *Ann. Trop. Med. Parasit.* 33: 21

Prieto, J. F. and G. M. Baer (1972). An outbreak of bovine paralytic rabies in Tuxtepec, Oaxaca, Mexico. *Am. J. Trop. Med. Hyg.* 21(2): 219

Rawlins, S. C. (1985). Current trends in screwworm myiasis in the Caribbean region. *Vet. Parasitol.* 18(3): 241

Rosenthal, J. E. (1972). *AID (Agency for International Development) Finds Ways to Control Vampire Bat.* War on Hunger, Agency for International Development.

Sazima, I. and W. Uieda (1980). Feeding behavior of the white-winged vampire bat, *Diaemus youngi*, on poultry. *J. Mammal.* 61(1): 102

Schmidt, U. and A. M. Greenhall (1973). Preliminary studies of the interactions between feeding vampire bats, *Desmodus rotundus*, under natural and laboratory conditions. *Mammalia.* 36(2): 241

Schmidt, U. and U. Manske (1973). Die jugendenwicklung der vampirfledermause (*Desmodus rotundus*). *Z. f. Saugetierkunde*. 38: 14

Schmidt, U. and K. van de Flierdt (1973). Innerartliche aggression bei vampirfledermausen (*Desmodus rotundus*) am futterplatz. *Z. Tierpsychol.* 32: 139

Schmidt, C., Schmidt U., and U. Manske (1980). Observations of the behavior of orphaned juveniles in the common vampire bat (*Desmodus rotundus*). In D. E. Wilson and A. L. Gardner (eds.) *Proceedings of the 5th International Bat Research Conference.* Texas Tech Press. Lubbock, Texas.

Schroeder, C. R., Black, J., Burkhart, R. L., and H. Koprowski (1952). Rabies in cattle. I. Prevention of vampire bat paralytic rabies, derriengue, by vaccination with chick-embryo-adapted rabies virus. *Vet. Med.* 47: 502

Smith, J. S. (1989). Rabies virus epitopic variation: Use in ecologic studies. *Advances in Virus Research.* 36: 215

Steece, R. S. and C. H. Calisher (1989). Evidence for prenatal transfer of rabies virus in the Mexican free-tailed bat (*Tadarida brasiliensis mexicana*). *J. Wildl. Dis.* 25(3): 329

Steele, J. H. (1966). International aspects of veterinary medicine and its relation to health, nutrition, and human welfare. *Mil. Med.* 131: 765

Steele, J. H. (1969). Understanding the disease is vital to rabies control. *J. Environ. Hlth.* 31: 473

Steele, J. H. (1973). The epidemiology and control of

rabies. *Scand. J. Infect. Dis.* 5: 312

Sulkin, S. E. (1962). The bat as a reservoir of viruses in nature. *Prog. Med. Virol.* 4: 157

Turner, D. C. (1975). *The Vampire Bat—A Field Study in Behavior and Ecology.* The Johns Hopkins University Press. Baltimore.

UNDP/FAO/WHO (1966). *Preparatory Assistance Mission on Paralytic Rabies in Latin America.* Document. United Nations Development Programme, Food and Agriculture Organization and the World Health Organization.

Van Rooyen, C. E. and A. J. Rhodes (1948). *Virus Diseases of Man.* Thomas Nelson and Sons. New York.

Verlinde, J. D., Kooij, P., and J. Versteeg (1970). Vampire-bat transmitted rabies virus from Surinam. Comparison of properties with European street virus and fixed virus. *Trop. Geogr. Med.* 22: 119

Verlinde, J. D., Li-Fo-Sjoe, E., Veersteeg, J., and S. M. Decker (1975). A local outbreak of paralytic rabies in Surinam children. *Trop. Geogr. Med.* 27: 137

Villa-Ramirez, B. (1969). *The Ecology and Biology of Vampire Bats and Their Relationship to Paralytic Rabies.* Report to the Government of Brazil. United Nations Development Programme/Food and Agriculture Organization. FAO No. TA2656. Rome, 1969

Wilkinson, G. S. (1984). Reciprocal food sharing in the vampire bat. *Nature.* 308(8): 181

Wilkinson, G. S. (1985a). The social organization of the common vampire bat. I. Pattern and cause of association. *Behav. Ecol. Sociobiol.* 17: 111

Wilkinson, G. S. (1985b). The social organization of the common vampire bat. II. Mating system, genetic structure, and relatedness. *Behav. Ecol. Sociobiol.* 17: 123

Wilkinson, G. S. (1986). Social grooming in the common vampire bat, *Desmodus rotundus. Anim. Behav.* 34: 1880

Wilkinson, G. S. (1987). Altruism and Co-Operation in Bats. In M. Brock Fenton, P. Racey, and J. M. V. Rayner (eds.) *Recent Advances in the Study of Bats.* Cambridge University Press.

Wilkinson, G. S. (1988a). Social Organization and Behavior. In A. M. Greenhall and U. Schmidt (eds.) *The Natural History of Vampire Bats.* CRC Press, Inc. Boca Raton, Florida.

Wilkinson, G. S. (1988b). Reciprocal altruism in bats and other mammals. *Ethol. and Sociobiol.* 9: 85

Wilkinson, G. S. (1990). Food sharing in vampire bats. *Sci. Amer.* 262(2): 76

Wimsatt, W. A. (1959a). Attempted "cannibalism" among captive vampire bats. *J. Mammal.* 40(3): 439

Wimsatt, W. A. (1959b). Discussion. In *Proceedings of Conference on Research in Bat Rabies.* National Institutes of Health. Bethesda, Maryland. p. 134. July 10-11, 1959

Chapter 9:
HUMAN EXPOSURE TO RABIES OF VAMPIRE-BAT ORIGIN

Reports of Vampire-Inflicted Human Rabies in Latin America

In noting the occurrence of human paralytic rabies in the apparent absence of any animal bite, Hurst and Pawan (1931) suggested that individuals in Trinidad may have been bitten by an animal leaving so small a wound as to have gone virtually unnoticed by the victim. In expressing the opinion that vampire bats may have served to vector the virus, investigators offered a means of explaining two oddities of the human disease: the often focal nature of initial clinical signs and the frequent lack of a known source of exposure. When bitten during their sleep, people were frequently unaware of the occurrence. Many were not awakened and those that were may not have had a full awareness of the attack. Only the dried blood in the morning remained to mark the event. Moreover, bites in humans were commonly received on a toe, thereby explaining the initial occurrence of localized symptoms. Thus, the vampire-bat hypothesis would simultaneously provide an explanation for the localized symptomatology often reported and the apparent lack of known history of animal bite.

Early in the course of Trinidad's human epidemic, inquiries with respect to animal bites had been made of friends and relatives long after the patients' death. Those questioned were not likely to have been aware of or taken notice of a bat bite in the middle of the night. Bites by vampire bats were not uncommon. In later cases, however, inquiries were made of patients before death. All but one person questioned before death reported that a bat had inflicted a bite, generally within 3 to 4 weeks of the onset of symptoms. Details of these cases can be found in the work by Pawan (1936).

According to Hurst and Pawan (1931), human rabies in Trinidad was confined to the laboring classes. It did not exist among the well-to-do natives or among Europeans. This was probably due to the greater exposure afforded vampires by the less affluent laborers. In 1932, Hurst and Pawan wrote,

> *In Trinidad the houses are built with a space between the eaves and the walls for purposes of ventilation; this gap is usually packed with spiny branches to prevent entry of bats. At night the windows are kept closed and the better classes usually burn a night-light, consisting of a cup containing coconut oil and wick floating in a basin of water to obviate risk of fire. Among the labouring classes these precautions are frequently omitted. A very common site for bat-bite is the toes, apparently because here during sleep the bat is less disturbed by movement, e.g. of respiration, than on any other part of the body. The bite is often accompanied by profuse haemorrhage, but the victim does not experience much pain, and has, during the process, a rather happy and soothed feeling.*

A medical history, typical of those reported by Hurst and Pawan (1932) from the human outbreaks in Trinidad, is recounted. On July 6, 1931, a 28-year-old East Indian housewife felt something "sting" her while sleeping. She woke her husband, who observed blood on her feet and saw a bat flying from the foot of the bed. An elliptical wound less than a quarter of an inch long was present on the second toe of her left foot. Her two children had similar wounds; however, they remained well. The timing of this bite coincided with an outbreak of disease, thought to be botulism, in district cattle. A burning sensation and

Table 9-1

Clinical Features of Rabies in 29 Human Patients During an Outbreak of Vampire-Induced Rabies in the Peruvian Jungle[a]

Feature	Number (%) of Cases
Hydrophobia	25(86)
Fever	24(83)
Headache	22(76)
Hypersalivation	20(69)
Malaise	19(66)
Dysphagia	19(66)
Abdominal pain	17(59)
Paresthesia	16(55)
Restlessness	16(55)
Psychomotor excitation	13(45)
Vomiting	13(45)
Delirium	9(31)
Hallucinations	6(21)
Aerophobia	6(21)
Photophobia	3(10)

[a] Symptoms present in less than 10% of patients included paraplegia and constipation.

From Lopez-R., A., Miranda-P., P., Tejada-V., E., and D. B. Fishbein. Outbreak of human rabies in the Peruvian jungle. *The Lancet*. 339: 408, 1992. Reproduced with permission.

periodic cramps in her left foot were noted by August 2. She described the foot as "feeling dead" and was unable to flex her ankle. An increasing weakness spread to her leg and by August 4, paresthesia was present in her other foot. On admission to the hospital on August 7, there was a flaccid paralysis and loss of all reflexes in her left lower limb. The woman complained of inability to urinate freely and a urinary catheter was inserted. Loss of feeling extended over her trunk to the level of the eighth or ninth rib. Later that evening, weakness and a growing area of anesthesia were observed in her right leg. By the next day, a mild respiratory distress was observed and her arms became increasingly incoordinated. Her condition rapidly deteriorated and, by the following day, her respiration was labored. She became semi-conscious and died on August 8.

Clinical manifestations present in 29 cases of human rabies transmitted by vampire bats during a recent outbreak that occurred in Peru are shown in Table 9-1.

Human disease had not been a recognized feature of the early Brazilian epizootics of bovine paralytic rabies. It was first reported in Trinidad in 1929 and over the next eight years, 89 human deaths were reported from Trinidad (Hurst and Pawan, 1931; Pawan, 1936; Butcher, 1959; Waterman, 1959). Since 1937, no additional human cases have been reported from Trinidad and no new cases were reported from Latin America until 1951.

Children less than 16 years of age have been over-represented in the reports of humans sustaining vampire attacks (although not necessarily in mining communities) as well as those who have died due to vampire-inflicted rabies (Hurst and Pawan, 1931, 1932; de Verteuil and Urich, 1936; Nehaul and Dyrting, 1965; Verlinde et al, 1975; McCarthy, 1989; Flores-Crespo, 1991; Lopez et al, 1992). Some of the suggested reasons for the bias towards schoolage children include the following:

1) Children may be less likely to use mosquito netting while sleeping.
2) Children may be less resistant to vampire-induced rabies.
3) Children may sleep longer and be less easily aroused than adults.
4) Children may be more likely to sleep in the darker regions of a dwelling, making them more vulnerable to vampire attacks.

Many historical accounts have documented human depredation by vampire bats. Johnson (1948), for example, cited the observations of Guillon (1910) in French Guiana of patients in the leprosarium of Acarouany and of convicts in the penal colony of Saint Jean du Maroni being regularly bitten by vampire bats while they slept.

Cutright (1940) cited numerous accounts of early explorers being attacked by vampires while asleep. Despite numerous accounts of human depredation by bats, there have been relatively few reports of human fatalities across Latin America during the 20th century. In 1931, Lyon, Jr. wrote,

> *No instance is recalled in which their [vampire bats'] attacks on human beings have resulted in more than trifling annoyances... Although the vampire bats must be regarded as among the free-living or temporary ectoparasites of man and other mammals, they can scarcely be regarded as more than curiosities in the field of human medicine. They are very much more easy to secure protection from than are mosquitoes and bedbugs. It has never been shown that they are carriers of any infection. In the field of animal husbandry they may at times be of more than passing interest.*

De Oviedo (1526), however, did record human fatalities among early explorers that were associated with vampire bites. Nevertheless, it is curious that more cases of human deaths have not been recorded. Disease continues to ravage livestock, particularly in areas where cattle immunizations are not routine, and people continue to be bitten by bats. In the face of these facts, it is difficult to completely understand the apparent lack of reported human disease. Suggested reasons include the following:

1) Misdiagnosis of early cases.
2) Biased reporting due to concern for the negative impact that such reports might have on tourism.
3) Alteration in the pathogenicity of virus during passage through countless generations of vampire bats.
4) Relatively low susceptibility of humans to the variant of rabies virus found in vampire bats.
5) Inadequacies in surveillance and reporting systems.

After an apparent hiatus of almost 15 years, reports of human rabies inflicted by vampire bats began to surface again in the 1950's. Many of these reports involved multiple deaths. In 1951, a vampire bat in El Platanito, in the state of Sinaloa, Mexico, attacked nine sleeping children (ages 2 to 12 years) in two neighboring families. The father of one of the families was bitten while killing the bat. The father and four children died with clinical signs of paralytic rabies (Landa, 1951 [cited by Malaga-Alba, 1954]). This was the first report of human death from vampire-induced rabies since the outbreaks in Trinidad (1929-1937). Later in the same year, seven individuals in the state of Jalisco, Mexico sustained bites from vampire bats. Three of these victims died with clinical signs of rabies (Mendez, 1951 [cited by Malaga-Alba, 1954]).

In 1955, Nehaul reported the deaths of nine miners two years earlier in what was formerly British Guiana (now Guyana). Clinical signs were those of acute ascending myelitis, with initial symptoms of "pins and needles" referable to toes and fingers. Brain smears made from five of these men revealed the presence of Negri bodies. Vampire-bat bites were confirmed in five of the victims. Eight additional cases were reported between 1960 and 1961, with laboratory confirmation of rabies in four of them (Nehaul and Dyrting, 1965). The people involved usually slept outside, unprotected from bats, and claimed to have been bitten by bats. Rabies in the local canine population was unknown.

The rivers and mountain streams of many isolated regions of Peru and Brazil are rich in gold, and prospectors are attracted to these areas in large numbers (Ruiz and Diaz, 1990; Schneider, 1991). The miners usually sleep in temporary housing. A plastic roof is available for protection against the rain but open sides leave the miners vulnerable to vampire attacks.

In 1989, a severe outbreak of vampire-induced rabies was reported from Peru, in the community of Choque (District of Madre de Dios, Province of Manú, Department of Madre de Dios). Between May and October of 1989, 24 cases of human rabies were reported from the gold-washing camps in this community (Lopez, 1991). Confirmation of vampire-inflicted rabies was based on clinical history and results of studies

Host	Country	Hybridoma Number																			
		1	2	3	4	5	6	7	8	9	10	11	12	13	14	15	16	17	18	19	20
Cattle	Paraguay	■							■							■	■		■		
	Venezuela	■							■							■	■		■		
Vampire bat	Standard	■							■							■	■		■		
	Brazil	■							■							■	■		■		
	Argentina	■							■							■	■		■		
	Venezuela	■							■							■	■		■		
Human	Peru	■							■							■	■		■		
Dog	Caribbean																		■		
	Mexico																		■		
ERA virus	-																				

□ Positive reaction ■ Negative reaction

Figure 9-1. Antigenic characterization of rabies variants isolated from different hosts and from vampire bats in South America. Note the identical reactivity pattern to a panel of 20 monoclonal antibodies of viral isolates obtained from naturally infected vampire bats in several Latin American countries and those from human and bovine victims of vampire-inflicted rabies. The reactivity pattern of the ERA vaccine strain of virus (originally isolated from the brain of a rabid dog), as well as that of naturally infected dogs in various regions of enzootic canine rabies, are distinct from vampire isolates (additional information on the use of monoclonal antibodies in rabies epidemiology and research can be found in Chapter 16). (From Diaz, A. M., Areito, J. C., and A. E. Nebel. Monoclonal antibody characterization of vampire bat rabies virus isolates in South America. In *Expert Consultation on the Care of Persons Exposed to Rabies Transmitted by Vampire Bats*. PAHO/WHO. Programs for Veterinary Public Health. Washington, D.C. April 1-5, 1991. Reproduced with permission.)

on brain samples obtained from nine patients at autopsy. Monoclonal antibody analysis of viral isolates from brain specimens of five of the victims showed a reactivity pattern identical to that found in vampire bats (Figure 9-1).

Although human rabies was not a reported feature of the early epizootics of vampire-induced rabies in Brazil, as many as 62 human deaths have subsequently been reported since 1960. The largest number of deaths occurred in 1990, when an outbreak occurred in a mining camp near the town of Apiacás in the state of Mato Grosso. The economy of the area is based on gold mining and petty trading, although some regions of the state support extensive cattle-raising operations (Schneider, 1991). Between December of 1989 and February of 1990, human depredations by vampire bats were numerous. All of the residents of the camp were bitten, with reports of as many as 25 bites on a single person. Residents were bitten through mosquito netting and in spite of the presence of burning lights at night. Seven deaths were reported from the Piauí mining site, which comprised 40 people in nine encampments. Several lines of evidence pointed to vampire-induced rabies as the cause of death in at least five of the cases, principally including: clinical signs and symptoms which were consistent with paralytic rabies, reports that all victims had been bitten multiple times by bats, no preventative treatment among members of the community, presence of clinical cases of rabies in domestic animals in the area, and no evidence of any other disease that could result in a similar clinical spectrum (Schneider, 1991).

As was the case in the Choque (Peru) outbreak of 1989, the miners of Apiacás slept in huts with open sides, leaving them exposed to vampire attacks at night. The combination of demanding physical labor and frequent drinking binges left them exceptionally vulnerable to attack when deep asleep.

Human deaths from vampire-inflicted rabies have been reported from 11 Latin American countries (Trinidad, Mexico, Guyana, Brazil, Suriname, Colombia, Argentina, Bolivia, Peru, El Salvador, and Venezuela). At present, several hundred human deaths in the Americas have been attributed to bites from rabid vampire bats (Table 9-2). The recorded figures are only approximations because of the great difficulty involved in accumulating accurate information from Latin America, where many cases of human rabies occur in isolated regions remote from any medical facilities. Furthermore, marked discrepancies exist in the published literature and confirmation of their validity is virtually impossible. The published records of human deaths due to vampire-bat rabies (varying between 275 and 471) are probably incomplete. A small percentage of reported cases are believed to have been due to nonhematophagous bats. However, an accurate assessment is not available.

Availability of Animal Food Sources and Human Depredation by Vampire Bats

As the reality of bovine paralytic rabies dawned on the population of Trinidad and its possible connection with vampire bats was recognized, livestock producers began to take steps to protect their animals from attack by bats. These included batproofing animal enclosures and/or removal of animals from potential problem areas. With their normal avenues of feeding thus cut off, the bats may have sought other readily available sources of blood, thereby accounting for increased attacks on human populations and the subsequent epidemics of human paralytic rabies. This may, in part, explain the relative restriction of human cases to limited localities.

Consistent with this theory, de Verteuil and Urich (1936) reported on two separate areas of Trinidad (Monos and Gasparee) where livestock were not present and where vampires fed primarily on poultry and humans. In those regions where poultry were better protected, humans reportedly sustained more bites.

In Suriname, Verlinde et al (1975) reported the deaths of seven children due to paralytic rabies between December of 1973 and January of 1974. About one month prior to the onset of this epidemic, the villagers had slaughtered a number of white-lipped peccaries around the village. This might have played a role in increasing the number of vampire bites among villagers.

In Belize, McCarthy (1989) reported an increase in the number of vampire attacks on humans following slaughter of pigs to control an outbreak of hog cholera. The pigs had been a staple component of the vampires' diet in this region prior to the cholera outbreak.

Similarly, Lopez et al (1992) reported an outbreak of human rabies of vampire origin in two rural Aguarunas Indian communities (Tutino and Mamayaque in the Department of Amazonas) in the high jungle of Peru, following elimination of their respective pig populations. Inhabitants reported that the local vampire populations had increased several months prior to the outbreak in connection with the development of a swine-raising program. Over the course of several months, however, the pigs were gradually eliminated from both communities after they began to devour the village crops. Despite eradication of the swine population, the numbers of vampire bats appeared to remain stable, and the number of bites sustained by villagers seemed to increase.[1] Twenty-nine of 636 (4.6%) people living in the two communities died between January 1 and April 30, 1990 (5 of 311 or 1.6% in Tutino and 24 of 325 or 7.4% in Mamayaque). Interviews with 23 of the patients or their families documented a history of bat bite in 22 (96%) of the cases.

In Tutino, the homes were completely enclosed and residents were more likely to use mosquito nets at night. In Mamayaque, the homes were open-sided, providing vampire bats with greater ease of access. These differences may

[1]The authors also considered the possibility that the outbreak of disease was not related to destruction of the pigs, but rather to the invasion of the area by a "wave" of infected vampires.

Table 9-2

Countries Reporting Human Rabies Cases Following the Bite of a Vampire Bat, 1929-1990[a]

Country	Number of Cases	Year	Reference
Trinidad	89	1929-1937	Butcher, 1959
Guyana	8	-	Baer, 1991
Guyana	9	1953	Nehaul, 1955
Guyana	8	1960-1961	Nehaul and Dyrting, 1965
Colombia	5	1980-1981	Constantine, 1988
Colombia	9	1987-1989	PAHO/WHO, 1991a
Mexico	5	1951	Landa, 1951
Mexico	3	1951	Mendez, 1951
Mexico	24	1951-1963	Ornelas and Aranalde, 1964
Mexico	87	1970-1986	Flores-Crespo, 1991
Mexico	18	1987-1990	PAHO/WHO, 1991a
Suriname	7	1973-1974	Verlinde et al, 1975
Brazil	8	1960	Constantine, 1988
Brazil	54	1975-1990	Schneider, 1991
Bolivia	1	1960	Constantine, 1988
Argentina	5	1965	Constantine, 1988
Argentina	1	1984	PAHO/WHO, 1991a
El Salvador	6	1980-1990	PAHO/WHO, 1991a
Venezuela	4	1980-1989	PAHO/WHO, 1991a
Peru	17	1971-1976	Lopez, 1991
Peru	11	1982	PAHO/WHO, 1991a
Peru	17	1984	Ruiz and Diaz, 1990
Peru	7	1987	Ruiz and Diaz, 1990
Peru	39	1989	Ruiz and Diaz, 1990
Peru	29	1990	Lopez et al, 1992
Total	471		

[a] Numbers are approximate due to widespread discrepancies in reporting and to the fact that not all cases are confirmed by laboratory study. A small percentage of these cases (exact number unknown) are believed to have been due to nonhematophagous bats.

have accounted for the fact that the number of human cases was almost five times greater in Mamayaque.

An autopsy was performed on one of the victims and rabies was confirmed as the cause of death. Monoclonal antibody analysis of the viral isolate obtained from this patient revealed a reactivity pattern identical to that found in infected vampire bats throughout Latin America.

In the last several years, there has been a marked increase in the number of persons bitten by vampire bats in Latin America, particularly in Peru and Brazil. Schneider (1991) attributed this, in part, to the fact that local clearing of forests may result in significant ecological disruption of resident wildlife populations. Major disturbances in the vampire ecosystem may reduce availability of animal hosts, ultimately favoring depredation of the resident human population. Some activities which may cause significant ecological disruption and lead to an increase in human exposure to vampire attacks, include: mining, deforestation, road and dam construction, development of human settlements, and military and guerilla activity (Ruiz and Diaz, 1990).

Batista-da-Costa et al (1993) reported a sudden outbreak of vampire bites in the Brazilian village of Honorópolis. They reported a temporal relationship between the onset of human bites and the initial use of a pyrethroid insecticide to control horn flies (*Haematobia irritans*) in village cattle. The authors hypothesized that the vampire bats may have avoided treated cattle, forcing the bats to seek an alternate food source. Further investigation was recommended.

Risks Associated with Handling and Ingestion of Infected Cattle

Initial abnormalities of locomotion in afflicted cattle were so characteristic that ranchers readily recognized rabid individuals. Fearing the death of entire herds, livestock producers would often sell their cattle at the first signs of disease (Prieto and Baer, 1972). At some slaughterhouses, even clinically normal cattle were found to be rabies positive. Martell and Del Valle (1971 [cited by Baer, 1975]) reported that in 1970, 4% (40 of 1,000) of randomly selected and apparently healthy head of cattle at the Ferrería Slaughterhouse in Mexico City were confirmed rabies positive by fluorescent antibody test.

There have been no reported cases of human rabies following consumption of meat from infected cattle (Baer, 1975). Nevertheless, the possibility of oral transmission of rabies virus has been demonstrated and the potential for this form of transmission to man, however remote, does exist. Alexander (1936) and Camargo Nunez et al (1953 [cited by Constantine, 1988]) reported deaths, with rabies-like signs, of Mexican dogs within a month of consuming meat (presumably raw) from livestock that had died of clinically diagnosed (as opposed to laboratory confirmed) rabies.

Meat from rabid animals (i.e., livestock) is not considered fit for human or animal consumption in the United States and is condemned. However, within seven days of being bitten by a rabid animal, meat of exposed livestock may be eaten locally on the farm of origin, provided that liberal portions of the bitten area are removed. Federal meat inspectors reject for slaughter any animal with a known exposure to rabies within the preceding eight months (National Association of State Public Health Veterinarians, 1992, 1993, 1994).

In China, two human deaths from rabies resulted from the handling of rabid dog carcasses being prepared for human consumption (Kureishi et al, 1992). In one of these cases, the patient killed, skinned, and cooked his dog after it began behaving abnormally. The entire family participated in the meal; however, no other family members became ill. In the other case, a stray dog was captured and prepared for consumption. In this instance, the victim had an open wound on his hand that may have served as the portal of viral entry. Mexican Indians have reportedly developed a nonfatal paraplegia after butchering animals with clinically diagnosed rabies (Tellez Giron, 1945 [cited by Constantine, 1988]). Tariq et al (1991) reported the case of a Pakistani butcher who died of rabies two and a half months after skinning a calf that had died of clinically diagnosed rabies. The calf had been bitten by a rabid dog three months earlier. These various reports suggest that butchers and slaughterhouse workers in areas of enzootic rabies may be at increased risk of infection (Constantine, 1988).

Risk Assessment and the Implementation of Public-Health Programs

Historically, cases of human rabies transmitted by vampire bats have been relatively few in number; those reported frequently involved ranchers carving out an existence on land usurped from the surrounding jungle. Typically, the area was occupied by an increased population of vampire bats secondary to the introduction of domesticated livestock.

Outbreaks of human rabies have recently been noted in remote jungle regions supporting mining, timbering, or agrarian activities (Schneider, 1991). In fact, both human and animal deaths from vampire-induced rabies have sharply increased in regions of Central and South America from which similar reports had previously been uncommon (Greenhall, 1991). Widespread clearing of local vegetation by slashing and burning is a common feature of both agrarian and nonagrarian jungle communities. Continued human encroachment into the jungle has resulted in man's becoming incorporated into the vampire bat's ecosystem. Once integrated into the bat's staple diet, resident human populations are likely to experience a continued increase in the number of bites inflicted by regional vampire populations.

Recent outbreaks of human rabies attributed to vampire bats, such as those in Brazil and Peru, have necessitated a careful reassessment of existing public-health programs, including the initiation of feasibility studies designed to assess the practicality of implementing preventative health measures for populations perceived to be at increased risk.

The Immunization Practices Advisory Committee (Centers for Disease Control, 1991) has defined a number of discrete human populations considered to be at increased risk of exposure to rabies and in whom pre-exposure rabies prophylaxis is justified (see page 31).[2] In reality, although these populations are at increased risk of exposure to rabies, they are really not at significantly increased risk of developing clinical disease. This is because exposures are generally recognized and efficacious post-exposure rabies prophylaxis is readily available and usually promptly administered when warranted.

The inhabitants of isolated communities in the jungles of Latin America constitute a unique, geographically dispersed population. Frequent (and perhaps unrecognized) exposure to vampire attacks, combined with a lack of adequate medical care (including availability of efficacious biologicals for post-exposure rabies prophylaxis), establish the basis for a truly high-risk population. Members of these communities are at increased risk not only of exposure to rabies, but to development of clinical disease as well. As such, the practicality of pre-exposure immunization of these populations merits serious consideration (Fishbein, 1991; PAHO/WHO, 1991a; Lopez et al, 1992).

Because of their extreme isolation from public-health facilities, there is very little likelihood that the inhabitants of these communities could obtain post-exposure rabies prophylaxis if needed (even in the face of confirmed exposure to one or more vampire attacks). For example, the local residents of Mamayaque and Tutino not only lacked access to post-exposure rabies prophylaxis, they were completely ignorant of it. These isolated populations constitute a truly high-risk group and intervention (i.e., pre-exposure rabies prophylaxis) may be required to help safeguard their safety in near-wilderness surroundings (Fishbein, 1991).

Many of these communities are far removed from even the most basic of medical care and access to such isolated locations is extremely limited. Extensive pre-exposure immunization of these jungle communities would be very difficult and costly to implement, severely taxing already overburdened health-care systems. Moreover, the efficacy of pre-exposure rabies prophylaxis alone to protect exposed individuals who are not likely to obtain post-exposure treatment or periodic booster inoculations, if needed, is questionable.

Continued investigation will be necessary not

[2] In recommending pre-exposure immunization, it is tacitly understood that an abbreviated post-exposure protocol is still required in the face of an exposure.

only to evaluate the efficacy of pre-exposure immunization alone to protect individuals at high risk, but also to assess the cost-effectiveness of implementing long-range plans for protecting inhabitants of isolated jungle communities (Fishbein, 1991). At a recent meeting sponsored by the Pan American Health Organization, strategies for implementation of long-range public-health programs in communities at high risk were discussed (PAHO/WHO, 1991b). Major recommendations of the participants included:

1) Delineation of risk factors that would allow identification of human populations at high risk. Some of the known risk factors include: presence of a limited livestock population in the area, presence of increased vampire populations in the area, identification of vampire-bat bites in humans and animals in the region, development of disease in human and animal populations, and utilization of unprotected dwellings by local inhabitants.
2) Establishment of a surveillance program in order to systematize the application of pre-exposure rabies prophylaxis in those populations believed to be at high risk.
3) Investigation of cost/benefit and cost/efficiency models of public health assistance.
4) Evaluation of the efficacy of pre- and post-exposure rabies prophylaxis in populations identified as being at high risk.
5) Ongoing study of vampire-bat ecology to help identify human populations at high risk.
6) Development of educational programs and investigation of means to disseminate information to isolated communities.
7) Development of educational programs for health-care workers.

References

Acha, P. N. and B. Szyfres (1987). Rabies. In *Zoonoses and Communicable Diseases Common to Man and Animals*. 2nd Edition. Pan American Health Organization, Pan American Sanitary Bureau, Regional Office of the World Health Organization. Scientific Publication No. 503

Alexander, H. A. (1936). *Contribucion al estudo del derriengue, Tesis*. Escuela Nacional de Medicina Veterinaria, Coyoacan. D. F., Mexico.

Baer, G. M. (1975). Bovine Paralytic Rabies and Rabies in the Vampire Bat. In G. M. Baer (ed.) *The Natural History of Rabies*. Vol. II. Academic Press. New York.

Baer, G. M. (1991). Vampire Bat and Bovine Paralytic Rabies. In G. M. Baer (ed.) *The Natural History of Rabies*. 2nd Edition. CRC Press, Inc. Boca Raton, Florida.

Batista-da-Costa, M., Bonito, R. F., and S. Nishioka (1993). An outbreak of vampire bat bite in a Brazilian village. *Trop. Med. Parasitol.* 44: 219

Butcher, L. V. (1959). The present status of paralytic rabies (bat-transmitted) in Trinidad. *Carib. Med. J.* XXI (1-4): 166

Camargo Nunez, F., Velazquez, E. A., and Ramirez Valenzuela, M. (1953). Historia del derriengue en Mexico (1881 a 1950), *Memoria del Congreso Cientifico Mexicana, Mexico*. 9: 265

Centers for Disease Control (1991). Rabies Prevention—United States, 1991. Recommendations of the Immunization Practices Advisory Committee (ACIP). *MMWR*. 49(RR-3): 1

Constantine, D. G. (1988). Transmission of Pathogenic Microorganisms by Vampire Bats. In A. M. Greenhall and U. Schmidt (eds.) *The Natural History of Vampire Bats*. CRC Press, Inc. Boca Raton, Florida.

Cutright, P. R. (1940). *The Great Naturalists Explore South America*. Essay Index Reprint Series. Books for Libraries Press. The Macmillan Company. New York.

Dalquest, W. W. (1955). Natural history of the vampire bats of eastern Mexico. *Am. Midl. Nat.* 53(1): 79

de Oviedo, G. F. (1526). *Natural History of the West Indies*. Translated and edited by S. A. Stoudemire. University of North Carolina Studies in the Romance Languages and Literature. Number 32, 1959. The University of North Carolina Press. Chapel Hill, North Carolina.

de Verteuil, E. and F. W. Urich (1936). The study and control of paralytic rabies transmitted by bats in Trinidad, British West Indies. *Trans. Roy. Soc. Trop. Med. Hyg.* XXIX(4): 317

Diaz, A. M., Areito, J. C., and A. E. Nebel (1991). Monoclonal antibody characterization of vampire bat rabies virus isolates in South America. In *Expert Consultation on the Care of Persons Exposed to Rabies Transmitted by Vampire Bats*. PAHO/WHO. Programs for Veterinary Public Health. Washington, D.C. April 1-5, 1991

Fishbein, D. B. (1991). Community wide rabies preexposure prophylaxis for isolated human populations at risk of exposure to rabid vampire bats: Target populations, economics, and immunologic considerations. In *Expert Consultation on the Care of Persons Exposed to Rabies Transmitted by Vampire Bats*. PAHO/WHO. Programs for Veterinary Public Health. Washington, D.C. April 1-5, 1991

Flores-Crespo, R. (1991). Techniques to control vampire bats. In *Expert Consultation on the Care of Persons Exposed to Rabies Transmitted by Vampire Bats*. PAHO/WHO. Programs for Veterinary Public Health. Washington, D.C. April 1-5, 1991

Greenhall, A. M. (1991). Ethology and ecology of vampire bats. In *Expert Consultation on the Care of Persons Exposed to Rabies Transmitted by Vampire Bats*. PAHO/WHO. Programs for Veterinary Public Health. Washington, D.C. April 1-5, 1991

Guillon, A. (1910). Les vampires. *La Clinique*. 5: 433

Hurst, E. W. and J. L. Pawan (1931). An outbreak of rabies in Trinidad without history of bites, and with the symptoms of acute ascending myelitis. *The Lancet*. 221: 622

Hurst, E. W. and J. L. Pawan (1932). A further account of the Trinidad outbreak of acute rabic myelitis: Histology of the experimental disease. *J. Path. Bact.* XXXV(3): 301

Johnson, H. N. (1948). Derriengue: Vampire bat rabies in Mexico. *Am. J. Hyg*. 47: 189

Kureishi, A., Xu, L. Z., Wu, H., and H. G. Stiver (1992). Rabies in China: Recommendations for control. *Bull. Wld. Hlth. Org*. 70(4): 443

Landa-Larin, H. (1951). Medical Report to the Servicios Coordinados of the State of Sinaloa, Mexico.

Lopez-R., A. (1991). Report of the outbreaks of human rabies in Peru. In *Expert Consultation on the Care of Persons Exposed to Rabies Transmitted by Vampire Bats*. PAHO/WHO. Programs for Veterinary Public Health. Washington, D.C. April 1-5, 1991

Lopez-R., A., Miranda-P., P., Tejada-V., E., and D. B. Fishbein (1992). Outbreak of human rabies in the Peruvian jungle. *The Lancet*. 339: 408

Lyon, Jr., M. W. (1931). The vampire bat. *Science*. 73(1883): 124

Malaga-Alba, A. (1954). Vampire bat as a carrier of rabies. *Am. J. Pub. Hlth*. 44: 909

Martell, M. A. and P. Del Valle (1971). *Proceedings of the 11th World Veterinary Congress*, short communication.

McCarthy, T. J. (1989). Human depredation by vampire bats (*Desmodus rotundus*) following a hog cholera campaign. *Am. J. Trop. Med. Hyg*. 40(3): 320

Mendez-Martinez, O. (1951). *Reporte de Labores Epidemiologicas. Contra la Rabia (Ep. 14)*. Departamento de Epidemiologia General. Secretaria de Salud y Asistencia Publica, Mexico.

National Association of State Public Health Veterinarians (1992). Compendium of Animal Rabies Control. *J. Am. Vet. Med. Assoc*. 200(2): 145

National Association of State Public Health Veterinarians (1993). Compendium of Animal Rabies Control. *J. Am. Vet. Med. Assoc*. 202(2): 199

National Association of State Public Health Veterinarians (1994). Compendium of Animal Rabies Control. *J. Am. Vet. Med. Assoc*. 204(2): 173

Nehaul, B. B. G. (1955). Rabies transmitted by bats in British Guiana. *Am. J. Trop. Med. Hyg*. 4: 550

Nehaul, B. B. G. and A. E. Dyrting (1965). An outbreak of rabies in man in British Guiana. *Am. J. Trop. Med. Hyg*. 14: 295

PAHO/WHO (1991a). Consideration on the prevention, control and epidemiologic surveillance of vampire bat-transmitted rabies in man in the Americas. In *Expert Consultation on the Care of Persons Exposed to Rabies Transmitted by Vampire Bats*. PAHO/WHO. Programs for Veterinary Public Health. Washington, D.C. April 1-5, 1991

PAHO/WHO (1991b). Expert consultation on the care of persons exposed to rabies transmitted by vampire bats—Final Report. In *Expert Consultation on the Care of Persons Exposed to Rabies Transmitted by Vampire Bats*. PAHO/WHO. Programs for Veterinary Public Health. Washington, D.C. April 1-5, 1991

Pawan, J. L. (1936). The transmission of paralytic rabies in Trinidad by the vampire bat (*Desmodus rotundus murinus* Wagner, 1840). *Ann. Trop. Med. Parasit*. 30: 101

Prieto, J. F. and G. M. Baer (1972). An outbreak of bovine paralytic rabies in Tuxtepec, Oaxaca, Mexico. *Am. J. Trop. Med. Hyg*. 21(2): 219

Ruiz, A. and A. M. Diaz (1990). *Epidemiology of Rabies Transmitted by Vampire Bats*. Subject 3.8. Pan American Health Organization, Pan American Sanitary Bureau, Regional Office of the World Health Organization, WHO Seminar on Wildlife Rabies Control. Geneva. July 2-5, 1990

Schneider, M. C. (1991). Epidemiological Situation of Human Rabies Transmitted by Bats in Brazil. In *Expert Consultation on the Care of Persons Exposed to Rabies Transmitted by Vampire Bats*. PAHO/WHO. Programs for Veterinary Public Health. Washington, D.C. April 1-5, 1991

Tariq, W. U. Z., Shafi, M. S., Jamal, S., and M. Ahmad. (1991). Rabies in man handling infected calf. *The Lancet*. 337: 1224

Tellez-Giron, A. (1945). Relacion immunologica entre los virus del derriengue (cepa *Desmodus*) y el de la rabia. *Rev. Soc. Mex. Hist. Nat*. 6: 179

Verlinde, J. D., Li-Fo-Sjoe, E., Veersteeg, J., and S. M. Decker (1975). A local outbreak of paralytic rabies in Surinam children. *Trop. Geogr. Med*. 27: 137

Waterman, J. A. (1959). Acute ascending rabic myelitis: Rabies—transmitted by bats to human beings and animals. *Carib. Med. J*. XXI (1-4): 46

Chapter 10:
METHODS IN THE CONTROL OF VAMPIRE-BAT RABIES

Prevention of Bat Bites

In the years following the initial outbreaks of bovine paralytic rabies, several approaches to eradication and control of the disease have been implemented, with varying degrees of success. Programs have generally included protective measures to prevent vampire bites, pre-exposure immunization in the case of animals, post-exposure rabies prophylaxis in the case of humans, and destruction of bats in the wild (both in their natural habitats as well as in the vicinity of livestock). An elaborate set of directives (*The Paralytic Rabies Regulations*, 1956) was instituted in Trinidad in an attempt to regulate handling of infected livestock (Boos and Farrell, 1956).

In Trinidad, post-exposure rabies prophylaxis was recommended for humans bitten by bats. According to the Office of the Surgeon General (1935), it was "exceptionally difficult to persuade persons bitten by bats to undergo this prophylactic treatment, but every effort has been made by means of public lectures and other forms of propaganda to instil into the minds of the people the importance and necessity of early treatment." Recommendations were made for protection of humans against bat bites (Wise, 1932; de Verteuil and Urich, 1936). These included:

1) Use of mosquito nets over beds.
2) Use of wire screening to cover all openings.
3) Use of lights at night.
4) Hanging spiky branches in upper parts of rooms or galleries.

Early attempts were also made to protect animals by using bat deterrents or by batproofing stables. Sanborn (1931) reported that gasoline-burning lanterns hung from trees would ward off marauding bats, although Greenhall (1965 [cited by Constantine, 1970]) reported this method to be ineffective against vampires in Trinidad. According to Marcaída (1960 [cited by Constantine, 1970]), the presence of pigeons was a vampire deterrent and ranchers sometimes utilized pigeon roosts to drive away vampires. Delpietro et al (1989) mentioned the use of a cat in a goat corral and Bush (1961) described the use of swinging "scarecrows" to frighten away bats.

Batproofing barns was never completely successful. Pawan (1936) reported instances of vampire bats actually crawling beneath barn doors in attempts to reach stabled livestock. Doors needed to be virtually flush with the ground because vampire bats can easily pass through openings as small as 1/2" x 1" wide.

Protective screening has been utilized successfully in Mexico to cover cenotes (natural wells used as roosts), preventing bats from colonizing them. Mesh openings were no larger than half an inch. Screening has also been used extensively in swine and poultry production units. Delpietro et al (1989) described the use of an underground tunnel, covered with netting, for protection of goats against bat attack. Corrals could also be covered to protect valuable livestock. Protective screening, however, is very expensive and not economically feasible with the livestock operations generally in use throughout Latin America (Greenhall, 1970).

During early studies of vampire-bat ecology, Turner (1975) recommended a means of protecting cattle by taking advantage of the vampire's reluctance to fly on moonlit nights. He suggested that in the four-day stretch around the calendar new moon, cattle should be moved to foraging areas away from known vampire roosts. During

Table 10-1

Duration of Immunity and Protection Against Viral Challenge in Cattle Given Different Antirabies Vaccines

Vaccine	Months Duration of Immunity	Percentage of Animals Protected
ERA strain in pig kidney cells	72	100
V.319 (Acatlán) strain in BHK cells[a]	33 45	100 87
Pitman-Moore strain in Nil II cells (inactivated)	36	100
Roxane strain in pig kidney cells	12	100
IB strain in pig kidney cells	12	80
Flury (HEP) strain in dog kidney cells	6	20

[a] There were two trials of this vaccine.

From Arellano-Sota, C. Vampire bat-transmitted rabies in cattle. *Rev. Infect. Dis.* 10(Suppl. 4): S707, 1988.

this time, vampires will be extremely stressed. With their normal avenues of feeding cut off, Turner postulated that the bats would starve during this critical time. Such an approach would require the cooperative action of all local ranchers. A very serious drawback to implementation of such a program is that a marked increase in the number of attacks on human populations may be sustained as vampires search for other available food sources.

Prophylactic Vaccination of Livestock

Early in the history of rabies epizootics, prophylactic vaccination of livestock was recommended. In Trinidad, vaccine had been made available free of charge for immunization of animals belonging to "peasant farmers." Estate proprietors were charged one shilling per dose (Director of Agriculture, 1932). A variety of vaccines have since been made available for immunizing cattle (Abelseth, 1964; Ornelas and Aranalde, 1964; Arnold et al, 1973; Bijlenga and Hernandez-Baumgarten, 1984). In Mexico, the Instituto Nacional de Investigaciones Pecuarias (National Institute of Livestock Research) evaluated the efficacy of many vaccines in the early to mid-1970's. Several of the vaccines tested protected greater than 80% of immunized cattle against lethal challenge with a known strain of vampire rabies one year after vaccination (Table 10-1). Some of the vaccines protected 100% of immunized cattle three years after vaccination (Arellano-Sota, 1988a). Inactivated vaccines may be preferable to attenuated ones due to their greater stability, particularly in instances when delays in shipping or actual use may be expected (Baer, 1991; Barrat et al, 1991).

While Greenhall (1974) suggested that cost should not be the primary factor upon which a control program is based, Fornes et al (1974) stressed the expense and labor involved in capturing pastured animals for individual vaccination. According to Williams (1960), many "peasant farmers" were reluctant to incur the expense (perhaps as much as a full day's wages) of rounding up cattle and they exhibited a marked tendency to forego prophylactic vaccinations at times between outbreaks of disease. When outbreaks did occur, they clamored for vaccinations and grew disappointed with the fact that vaccines were not effective in treating animals already in-

Table 10-2

Reduction in Vampire Bat Attacks When Cattle at Three Mexican Ranches Were Given Single Intraruminal Injections of Diphenadione (1 mg/kg)

	Immediately Before Treatment		After Treatment			
Ranch	Number of Animals Examined	Number of Fresh Bites	Days After Treatment	Number of Cattle Examined	Number of Fresh Bites	Reduction in Bites (%)
1	93	80	13	84	5	93.8
2	71	88	14	77	9	89.8
3	43	46	12	49	1	97.8
Totals and Mean	207	214		210	15	93.0

From Thompson, R. D., Mitchell, G. C., and R. J. Burns. Vampire bat control by systemic treatment of livestock with an anticoagulant. *Science*. 177: 806, 1972. © by the American Association for the Advancement of Science. Reproduced with permission.

fected and incubating disease (Metivier, 1935; Delpietro and Nader, 1989).

In the course of epizootics of vampire-bat rabies, the disease appears abruptly in vampire populations, spills over into the bovine population, and then migrates to another area, generally within about six months. Once disease has been identified in cattle herds, the majority of cattle exposures have already occurred and the infected bats have died. Destruction of bats or vaccination of cattle at this time will have no beneficial effect. Cattle will succumb for the duration of the incubation period, which may be as long as several months (Johnson, 1971).

Although many livestock producers refused to take advantage of Trinidad's free government service (Butcher, 1958), the livestock vaccination program conducted by the Department of Agriculture significantly minimized cattle losses in the country (Greenhall, 1959).

Since cattle themselves do not play a role in the transmission cycle of rabies, disease among vampire populations remained undiminished by livestock vaccination (Fornes et al, 1974).[1] Unvaccinated livestock remained at risk. Additionally, vaccination programs did not alleviate the burden of vampire attacks. Cattle remained susceptible to blood loss, parasite attack, and potential transmission of other vampire-borne diseases. Therefore, an integrated approach, combining livestock vaccination with vampire population-reduction programs, was suggested (Greenhall, 1970; de Diego and Valotta, 1973; Bijlenga and Hernandez-Baumgarten, 1984) and recommendations for the widespread destruction of vampires bats continued.

Vampire Population Control

Reduction in vampire populations has been approached in one of two principal fashions. These have centered either on the destruction of bats in their wild environment or on poisoning bats in the vicinity of cattle. Population reduction takes advantage of the low reproductive potential of the vampire bat. With a gestation period of about seven months duration and delivery of only one offspring each year, recovery of vampire populations following reduction programs is very slow (Wimsatt and Trapido, 1952; Burns, 1970; Mitchell, 1986; Schmidt, 1988; Ruiz and Diaz, 1990; Lord, 1992).

In considering the ecological ramifications of

[1]Bijlenga (1975) suggested immunizing cattle with tissue preparations of vampire-bat origin, so that appropriate titers of bovine anti-vampire antibodies would be present in ingested blood.

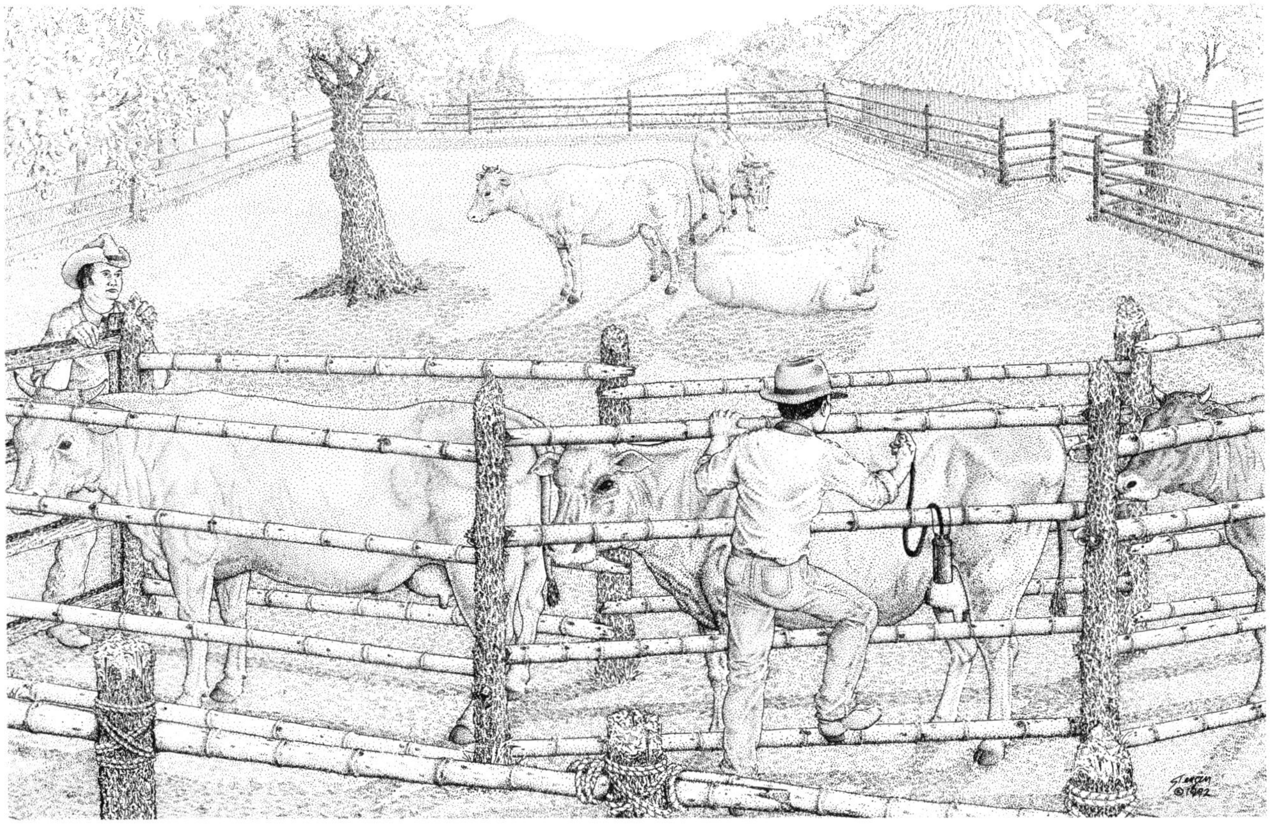

Figure 10-1. Intraruminal injection of anticoagulants renders the blood of cattle lethal to vampire bats for several days.

vampire-bat control, Greenhall (1970, 1972) noted that the balance of nature regarding vampire-bat ecology had already been upset. Expansion of the livestock industry favored the continued population increase of the bats, disturbing prior biological equilibriums. Only in remote ecosystems, such as Amazonian rain forests, where the bats continue to subsist on native fauna, is it likely that balanced vampire-bat populations still exist (Greenhall, 1970). While they endure, these regions may provide unique living laboratories for studying natural cycles of vampire-bat rabies and population ecology (Greenhall, 1988).

Portions of the Amazon basin are continually being cleared for livestock production. This will almost certainly lead to increases in local vampire populations. Selective control of vampire bats in the vicinity of cattle-raising operations might help to drive remaining populations back towards the original native animals upon which they fed before the natural balance was upset by introduction of livestock (Arellano-Sota, 1991).

The day-time roosting and night-time digesting places of vampire bats had been identified and this was followed by the systematic decimation of their populations. A variety of techniques, some more effective than others, had been adopted to kill vampires (see reviews by Greenhall, 1963, 1970, 1974, 1985; Linhart, 1975) and included the following:

1) Firearms - including use of scatter-shot cartridges.

2) Electrocution - devised to kill bats within caves.

3) Smoke and Fire - often effective in driving bats from hollow trees. During World War II, American armed forces used flame throwers to kill cave-dwelling bats in Trinidad.

4) Dynamite, Gasoline Bombs, and Poison Gas - especially Rhodiatrox (a phosphorous-base compound) and cyanide gas. One scientist died while inspecting a gassed well (Fornes et al, 1974).

Table 10-3

Results of Intramuscular Treatment of Cattle at Four Ranches With Vampirinip III (5 mg/kg Warfarin)

	San Carlos		San Pedro		Kanto		Ojo De Agua	
	At Time of Treatment	17 Days After Treatment	At Time of Treatment	16 Days After Treatment	At Time of Treatment	14 Days After Treatment	At Time of Treatment	14 Days After Treatment
No. Cattle Examined	40[a]	49[b]	25[b]	25[b]	392	276	40[b]	40[b]
No. Cattle Bitten	33	8	25	4	302	21	38	9
No. Vampire Bites	81	10	52	5	890	23	178	12
Avg. No. Bites/Bovine	1.7	0.2	2.1	0.2	2.3	0.08	4.5	0.3
% Cattle Bitten	67.3	16.3	100	16.0	77	7.6	95	22.5
% Reduction Cattle Bitten	-	75.8	-	84.0	-	90.1	-	76.3
% Reduction No. Bites	-	87.7	-	90.4	-	96.5	-	93.2

[a] There were 49 cattle in the San Carlos herd, but nine escaped from the chute at the time of the first visit and could not be examined or treated.
[b] All the cattle at the ranch.

From Flores-Crespo, R. F., Fernandez, S. S., De Anda, L. D., Velarde, F. I., and R. M. Anaya D. G. Intramuscular inoculation of cattle with warfarin: A new technique for the control of vampire bats. *Bull. Pan Am. Hlth. Org.* 13(2): 147, 1979. © Pan American Health Organization. Washington, D.C. Reproduced with permission.

5) Biological Warfare - Abello-Fernandez (1966 [cited by Constantine, 1970]) reported the destruction of 5,000 vampire bats in Colombia by infecting them with Newcastle disease via airborne instillation of atomized virus. Not only is such an approach highly indiscriminate, but it is potentially dangerous to humans as well as poultry.

One may also envision a host of less imaginative, if not more personalized, techniques involving hand-held implements. Linhart (cited by Rosenthal, 1972) mentioned discussions of such inventive ideas as strapping small bombs to captive bats that would explode later in the cave,[2] or even applying slow-release poison-gas capsules that would poison other bats in the roost.

The methods described above share the common disadvantage of being nonselective in the species of bats that were trapped or killed. Greenhall (1970) identified several species of bats that roost in association with vampires. The random and needless destruction of these species might have far-ranging ecological and public-health ramifications.

Other methods were designed primarily to selectively kill vampire bats while in the process of attacking cattle. These principally included use of poisons (such as strychnine and arsenic) and

[2]As farfetched as this might sound, a similar proposal was studied intently by the United States Armed Forces during World War II. Over the course of several years, investigators studied the feasibility of attaching small incendiary bombs to Mexican free-tailed bats. The bats could then be dropped in great numbers over various enemy installations. It was hoped that they would then fly into the various buildings to roost, whereupon the small bombs would set the sites ablaze. The program, known as Project X-Ray, was abandoned shortly before development of the atomic bomb, but not before a number of test bats had escaped and set fire to the project's headquarters.

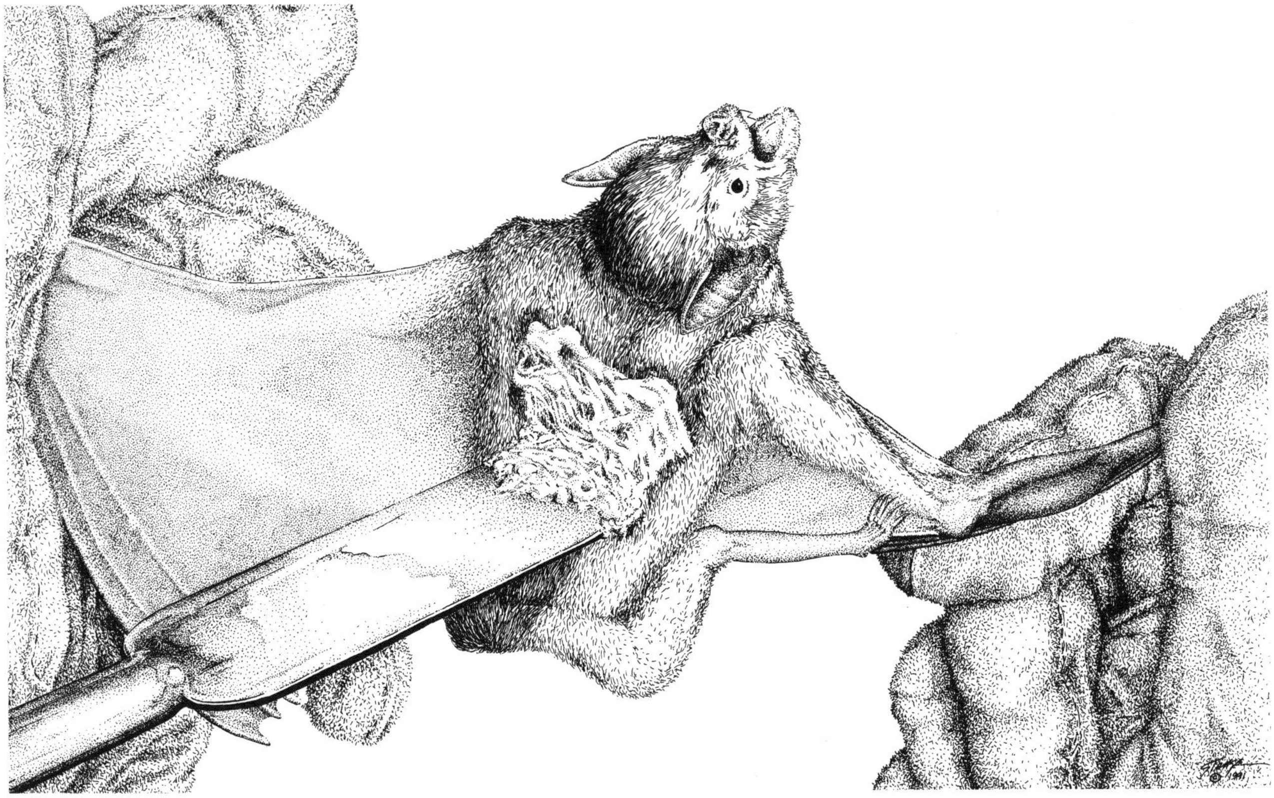

Figure 10-2. Application of topical anticoagulants to the backs of captured vampire bats plays an important role in the control of vampire-bat rabies.

various anticoagulants.

1) **Strychnine** - When properly applied to an open wound, a vampire lapping the poison will die within moments. This method takes advantage of the vampire's tendency to revisit old wounds. Strychnine has been effectively used on cattle, goats, sheep, mules, donkeys, and poultry (de Verteuil and Urich, 1936; Greenhall, 1963). Arsenic has also been used in similar fashion.

   These materials may present a significant health hazard to people applying them and to livestock, if applied in an area where it could be licked (Flores-Crespo and Arellano-Sota, 1991). Although the technique is basically effective, it has been recommended that substances less toxic to both cattle and human handlers should be investigated (Flores-Crespo, 1991).

2) **Anticoagulants** - The vampire bat is sensitive to low levels of anticoagulants, and these have been the mainstay in man's battle against the ravages of vampire bats. Drugs such as diphenadione (Table 10-2), when injected directly into the rumen of cattle, render their blood lethal to vampires for three days (Figure 10-1). Thompson et al (1972), reported that the dose needed to kill bats is considerably less than that which has an observable effect on cattle, although Elias et al (1978) reported that calves may be susceptible to diphenadione poisoning at the dosages employed. At 1 mg/kg, calves were not affected by suckling and preliminary studies indicated no residue problems with respect to human consumption. In one large herd in Nicaragua, intraruminal administration of anticoagulant reduced the number of bites sustained by a herd of 212 head of cattle by more than 99%, from 1,560 to 7 per day (Mitchell, 1993). Ac-

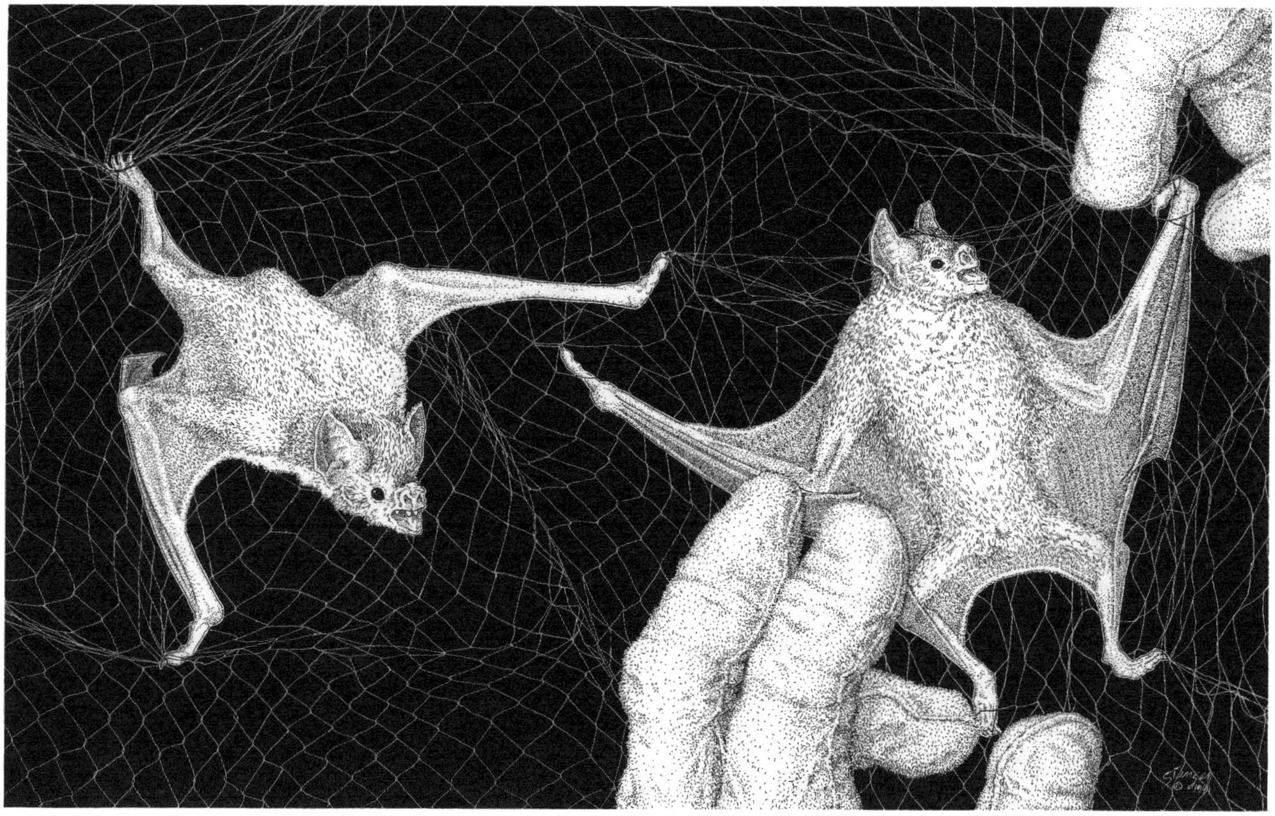

Figure 10-3. Bats can be captured using mist nets set up along known flight paths or in the vicinity of livestock.

cording to Flores-Crespo (1991), the technique has not been in popular use for several years. Three disadvantages to intraruminal anticoagulants include:

1) Inability to regulate absorption, accounting for the short period of effectiveness (three days).
2) The fact that it cannot be used in calves less then one year old because of toxicity.
3) Only ruminants can be treated, leaving other species unprotected from local vampire populations if the bats do not feed on treated ruminants as well.

Said-Fernandez and Flores-Crespo (1991) reported that intramuscular administration of the anticoagulant, diphacinone, resulted in 100% efficacy for up to two days following administration. This decreased to 67% by day five. A drawback to the procedure, however, was the large volume of carrier vehicle required. The authors recommended use of drugs soluble in smaller volumes of diluent.

Warfarin, a potent anticoagulant found in many rat poisons, has also proven effective. A single intramuscular injection in cattle at risk induced 100% mortality in feeding vampires for four days. Flores-Crespo et al (1979) studied the efficacy of this treatment at four different ranches in Mexico. As Table 10-3 shows, reduction in the number of vampire bites was significant. Calves were not affected by consuming milk from treated cows, although due to their relatively low intrinsic levels of vitamin K, treatment of calves is not recommended before one year of age.

The longer-lasting action of intramuscular warfarin, compared to intraruminal diphenadione, may be advantageous under field conditions. Intramuscular injections also require less technical knowledge of farm workers than intraruminal administration. Because of its ease of administration, it may be the most practical method of con-

Table 10-4

Dead Vampires in a Captive Colony After Topical Treatment with Warfarin[a]

Days After Treatment	Numbr of Dead Vampires	Cumulative Percentage of Dead Vampires
1-2	0	0
3	8	40
4	10	90
5	2	100
Totals	20	100

[a] 0.0234 g warfarin suspended in 2 ml of vaseline.

From Flores-Crespo, R. and C. Arellano-Sota. Biology and Control of the Vampire Bat. In G. M. Baer (ed.) *The Natural History of Rabies*. 2nd Edition. © CRC Press, Inc. Boca Raton, Florida, 1991. Reproduced with permission.

Table 10-5

Reduction of Vampire Bats Biting Cattle after the Topical Application of Anticoagulant[a] to 20 Vampires at the Huichi Ranch, San Luis Potosí, Mexico

	Before Treatment	14 Days After Treatment
Number of Bovines Observed	90	90
Number of Bovines with Recent Bites	45	3
Number of Recent Bites	82	3
% Reduction of Recent Bites	-	96.4

[a] 0.0234 g warfarin suspended in 2 ml of vaseline.

From Flores-Crespo, R. and C. Arellano-Sota. Biology and Control of the Vampire Bat. In G. M. Baer (ed.) *The Natural History of Rabies*. 2nd Edition. © CRC Press, Inc. Boca Raton, Florida, 1991. Reproduced with permission.

trol. According to Flores-Crespo (1991), intramuscular injection of warfarin is the only systemic technique still widely used throughout much of Latin America.

Anticoagulants may be applied to the surfaces of vampire roosts. The bats die following contact with and ingestion of the substance, which is readily spread through the colony by grooming activity. Chlorophacinone, diphenadione, and warfarin have all proven effective when applied in this fashion; however, it is probably not a practical approach to vampire population control and significant ecological concerns for nontarget species attend its use (Flores-Crespo et al, 1974). At the First International Symposium of Vampire Bat Control in Managua, Nicaragua in 1976, Flores-Crespo presented evidence demonstrating the indiscriminate killing of other bat species using this method and recommended that its use be discontinued (McCarthy, 1993).

Anticoagulants contained in a paste may also be applied to open wounds on cattle or to the backs of captured bats (Figure 10-2, Tables 10-4 and 10-5). Following their return to the roost, treated bats will contaminate others which may come into physical contact with them during grooming and roosting (Linhart et al, 1972; Linhart, 1975).

Application of anticoagulant paste to bats requires the capture of individual vampires and various techniques have been developed for this purpose. Netting has proven to be quite effective (Figure 10-3). Mist, sieve, and trammel nets have been effective in capturing bats at entrances of caves, mines, hollow trees, etc., as well as along established flyways and near barns and corrals.

Baiting took advantage of an unexplained natural attraction that vampire bats may have for certain individual animals, leading to preferential attack. Hundreds of vampire bats, for example, had been captured around one particular bull in Trinidad over the course of several years (Greenhall, 1970). Even de Oviedo (1526), as early as the 16th century, noted that vampire bats would often seek out preferential victims. At that time he wrote, "They [the vampire bats] have another peculiarity, and this is that if among one hundred men they bite one man, they will return to the same man on successive nights even though he

Table 10-6

Effect of Topical Treatment with Warfarin[a] on Cattle Injuries Caused by Vampire Bites in a Captive Colony

Day	Treatment	Number of Dead Vampires	Cumulative Percentage
1	yes	0	0
2	yes	0	0
3	yes	0	0
4	-	1	10
5	-	5	60
6	-	3	90
7	-	1	100
Total		10	100

[a] 0.0117 g of warfarin suspended in 1 ml of vaseline.

From Flores-Crespo, R. and C. Arellano-Sota. Biology and Control of the Vampire Bat. In G. M. Baer (ed.) *The Natural History of Rabies*. 2nd Edition. © CRC Press, Inc. Boca Raton, Florida, 1991. Reproduced with permission.

be among a great number."

Application of anticoagulants to previously made wounds on cattle takes advantage of the propensity of vampire bats for revisiting old wounds, repeatedly opening scabs to feed. Anticoagulants (warfarin) suspended in vaseline have been very efficacious, although tedious and possibly only useful for ranchers with small herds (Flores-Crespo, 1991).

Flores-Crespo et al (1976 [cited by Flores-Crespo and Arellano-Sota, 1991]) studied the efficacy of topically applied warfarin in a controlled environment. Ten vampires were allowed to feed at will on two Hereford cattle housed in a covered corral. Cattle wounds were treated for three consecutive days, after which vampire bats began to die. All ten bats were dead within seven days (Table 10-6). Under field conditions, these authors observed this method to significantly reduce the number of vampire bites sustained by cattle in three heavily attacked herds after 15 days (Table 10-7).

Delpietro et al (1991) reported the successful use of a warfarin pour-on technique for control of vampire bats. It has been used effectively to protect cattle, horses, goats, and pigs.

Each method of anticoagulant application has its advantages and disadvantages (Mitchell and Burns, 1973).

Advantages of treating the bats directly include:

- All domestic animals are equally protected.
- It is faster and more effective than other methods in establishing control.
- It is less expensive than treating cattle directly since there is no need to round up pastured cattle and no requirement for chute facilities.
- No need to know location of vampire roosts.
- Simultaneous destruction of several colonies.

Disadvantages of treating the bats directly include:

- Special equipment, especially mist nets, is required. Mist nets, which are currently manufactured only in Japan, are presently at the heart of a unique international trade dispute and continued supply is seriously threatened (Miller, 1992).
- A team trained in bat identification is required.
- Team members suffer the threat of bites. They must, therefore, be pre-exposure immunized against rabies and wear gloves when handling bats.
- Anticoagulant residues may be left on roost walls or contaminate water in well roosts, posing a potential threat to humans and wildlife.
- Consumption of poisoned bats may pose a threat to other wildlife.
- Requirement for working at night.

Table 10-7

Effect of Topical Treatment with Warfarin[a] on Cattle Injuries Caused by Vampire Bites Under Field Conditions

Ranch/ Number of Cattle	During Treatment			15 Days After Treatment			
	Average of Treated Bovines	Average of Treated Bites	Average Bites per Bovine	Number of Bovines Observed	Number of Bites Observed	Average of Bites per Bovine	Percentage of Bite Reduction
San Isidro/183	58	413	7.0	112	40	0.3	94.9
Habano/45	29	104	3.6	45	23	0.5	85.6
Aguada Chucum/40	19	71	3.7	40	28	0.7	81.1

[a] 0.0117 g of warfarin suspended in 1 ml of vaseline.

From Flores-Crespo, R. and C. Arellano-Sota. Biology and Control of the Vampire Bat. In G. M. Baer (ed.) *The Natural History of Rabies*. 2nd Edition. © CRC Press, Inc. Boca Raton, Florida, 1991. Reproduced with permission.

Advantages of treating the cattle directly include:

- No need to handle bats.
- No requirement for specialized capture equipment.
- No need to selectively identify bat species.
- No need to know location of vampire roosts.
- No need to work at night.

Disadvantages of treating the cattle directly include:

- Facilities required for cattle restraint.
- More expensive and time consuming than other methods.
- Often impractical to capture free-ranging livestock.
- Smaller number of bats killed.
- Protects only treated cattle.
- 30-day drug-withdrawal time for slaughter and milk.
- May require veterinary assistance.

Following reduction of the local vampire population, a decrease in the number of attacks sustained by livestock will persist for a varying period of time, dependent upon repopulation of local roosts. This may occur following renewal of the existing population through natural reproductive processes or as a result of the entry of migrant populations from surrounding locales. Kverno and Mitchell (1976) reported that vampire populations generally remained diminished for extended periods of time (Table 10-8).

Economic Significance of Vampire Population Control

In cattle-raising areas where no evidence of rabies infection in the local vampire populations exists, the value of population control may be variable. In studying the effects of vampire population reduction on bovine milk production, Thompson et al (1977) found that a 99% reduction in daily vampire bites sustained by a healthy, well-managed, parasite-free herd had no significant influence on milk production. In a poorly managed, parasite-infested herd in generally poor condition, a 100% reduction in the number of daily vampire bites resulted in a 16% increase in milk production. Under controlled conditions, no effects of vampire bites on milk production were found (de La Rosa Pedraza et al, 1977).

De Anda et al (1976 [cited by Flores-Crespo

Table 10-8

Results of Topical Application of Diphenadione to Vampire Bats at Three Cattle Ranches in Two Areas of Brazil

Ranch	Habitat	Time Checked, in Relation to Treatment	No. of Cattle Checked	No. of Fresh Bites	No. of Vampires Treated	% Reduction in Bites After Control
Engenho Santo Estava, near Cabo	Coastal, humid	Before	44	73	33	
		14 days after	44	0		100.0
		1 year after	45	4		94.5
		18 months after	45	4		94.5
		27 months after	42	14		80.8
Engenho Velho, near Cabo	Coastal, humid	Before	60	67	54	
		1 year after	60	3		95.5
		14 days after	60	6		91.0
		18 months after	60	6		91.0
		27 months after	67	5		92.5
Fazenda Barra Nova, near Aguas Belas	Inland, arid	Before	195	74	80	
		11 days after	195	0		100.0
		1 year after	260	0		100.0

From Kverno, N. B. and G. C. Mitchell. Vampire bats and their effect on cattle production in Latin America. *Wld. Anim. Rev.* (Food and Agriculture Organization of the United Nations). 17: 1, 1976. Reproduced with permission.

and Arellano-Sota, 1991]) measured weights of 976 calves at birth, weaning, and at 1 to 2 years of age on a cattle ranch in San Luis Potosí, Mexico which was subject to heavy vampire attacks. They compared these figures to those of 159 animals measured after implementation of a successful program for controlling the population of local vampire bats. No statistical differences in weight gain were observed.

Thus, blood loss due to vampire parasitism may not be particularly debilitating in healthy herds and control efforts in these instances are not likely to yield significant benefit with respect to weight gain and milk production. In herds that are subject to physical stress associated with poor management practices (such as improper diet, extremes of climate, external or internal parasitism, or various infectious or other medical conditions), alleviation of blood loss due to vampire attacks may be of economic benefit (Thompson et al, 1977). Cattle deaths due to vampire-induced paralytic rabies remains significant regardless of overall herd health. Management practices should include implementation of a vampire control program if a "migrating" epizootic threatens the area.

Efficacy of Available Control Methods

The use of topical anticoagulants applied to a bat's back is very efficacious in reducing vampire-bat populations. When treated bats return to their roosts, the anticoagulant will be ingested by roostmates as the bats groom one another. Depending on various circumstances, between 20 and 40 bats may be killed for each one treated (Linhart et al, 1972; Kverno and Mitchell, 1976; World Health Organization, 1984; Lewin, 1986; Mitchell, 1986). Reduction in vampire populations will occur in several colonies simultaneously. McCarthy (1993) recommends the concurrent use of both topical and systemic treatments.

The key to a successful vampire control program lies in accurately predicting the path of a

Table 10-9

Changes in the Incidence of Bovine Paralytic Rabies in the Americas, 1968-1985

Country	1968	1978	1985	Overall Result
Argentina	C	C	L	I
Belize	-	L	L	S
Bolivia	H	H	M	R
Brazil	H	H	M	R
Colombia	C	C	C	S
Costa Rica	C	C	L	I
Ecuador	L	L	L	S
El Salvador	L	M	H	I
Guatemala	C	M	L	R
Guyana	C	M	M	S
Honduras	C	L	L	S
Mexico	C	H	M	R
Nicaragua	H	L	L	R
Panama	H	L	M	R
Paraguay	M	C	C	R
Suriname	U	L	L	S
Trinidad	L	L	L	S
Venezuela	C	C	L	I

(U) = unlikely to be present in the country; (L) = low sporadic incidence; (M) = moderate incidence; (H) = high incidence; (C) = confined to certain regions; (S) = same situation since 1968; (R) = reduction in incidence since 1968; and (I) = increase in incidence since 1968.

From Arellano-Sota, C. Vampire bat-transmitted rabies in cattle. *Rev. Infect. Dis.* 10(Suppl. 4): S707, 1988.

"migrating" epizootic of vampire-bat rabies. Random application of control methods will be of limited value in curtailing further outbreaks. Lord (1980) suggested an ecological strategy for controlling bovine paralytic rabies in Latin America. Accordingly, this takes advantage of the relatively predictable movement of "migrating" epizootics, which frequently move along a path dictated by particular ecologic, topographic, and geologic features. Once its course of "migration" is understood, propagation of the vampire epizootic can be interrupted by selective destruction of vampire bats between 10 to 20 km (depending on the rate of "migration") ahead of the last known case of bovine paralytic rabies. According to Lord (1988), the depth of the control area should be 15 km and its width should extend beyond the outbreak by 15 km on each side. The method has been successfully implemented in several countries, notably Brazil and Venezuela.

As shown in Tables 10-9 and 10-10, the currently used methods of vampire-bat control have proven very effective in various trials (Thompson et al, 1972; Kverno and Mitchell, 1976; Piccinini et al, 1982, 1985; Flores-Crespo and Arellano-Sota, 1991). Bites sustained by cattle have been reduced between 85% and 95% in many herds. Various international organizations (especially the Agency for International Development and the Pan American Health Organization) have instituted training programs in 18 countries suffering from vampire-bat rabies (Lord, 1980; World Health Organization, 1984). Unfortunately, the success of anticoagulant control methods in ameliorating the vampire bat's impact on livestock economy has led to drastic reductions in available funding for continued vampire-bat research. Nevertheless, rabies of vampire-bat origin continues to be a problem in many areas.

Control methods using anticoagulants have proven very effective in reducing vampire populations. Anticoagulant control tends to target only vampire bats and several investigators have found little evidence of significant deleterious effects on other species within roosts. However, topically applied anticoagulant paste can rub off on cave walls and persist in active form for extended periods. Furthermore, since vampires always occupy the highest points within a roost, secretions or excretions from poisoned vampire bats may flow down walls or rain onto nonhematophagous bats below them, with unpredictable effects. Lord (1988) emphasized the need for comprehensive long-term studies of the potential impact that topical anticoagulant control of vam-

Table 10-10

Effectiveness of Various Uses of Anticoagulants in Reducing Vampire Bat Populations

Control Method	% Reduction in Number of Bites
Topical Treatment of Vampires	95
Topical Treatment of Bites on Victims	81-95
Systemic Treatment of Cattle	
Intraruminal (diphenadione)	93-98
Intramuscular (warfarin)	88-96

From Arellano-Sota, C. Biology, ecology, and control of the vampire bat. *Rev. Infect. Dis.* 10(Suppl. 4): S615, 1988.

pire bats may have on populations of nontarget species. Species at potential risk include other bats, as well as terrestrial and avian predators of bats.

Future Trends in Vampire Control

Recently, the technology of genetic engineering has been brought to bear on rabies vaccine production (see page 252). The development of recombinant viral vaccines may prove highly promising in the continued protection of cattle in Latin America.

The possibility of immunizing vampires against rabies has also been investigated (Rupprecht et al, 1987, 1988; Rupprecht, 1991). Development of orally effective vaccines for immunization of vampire bats needs to be thoroughly investigated (Lord, 1988; Charlton, 1992). If an orally effective vaccine can be developed, delivery should be relatively straightforward. Topical treatment of both cattle and captured vampires with anticoagulants has already proven to be highly effective as a means of delivering orally active agents to vampire populations. A variety of safe and efficacious vaccines of potential value already exist. Their application merely awaits efficacy testing in vampire bats.

Lord (1993) has also suggested the possibility of using mosquitos to act as vectors of a rabies vaccine. If released into caves or other roosts harboring vampire colonies, mosquitos may feed upon the bats, inoculating them with a vaccine product in the process. Determination of the efficacy of such a program awaits further research.

Impact of Random Bat Destruction

In the years between 1950 and 1959, an average of 1,350 vampire bats were killed annually in Trinidad (Williams, 1960). Hundreds, and perhaps thousands, of caves in Brazil were destroyed by dynamiting, indiscriminately killing vampires and other species of bats (Fitter, 1968; Bouliere, 1968 [cited by Constantine, 1970]; Villa-Ramirez, 1969), and an estimated 900,000 bats of various species were gassed annually in Venezuela from 1964 to 1966 (Dumith Arteaga et al, 1967 [cited by Constantine, 1970]). Pint (1994) reported that the entrances of various caves in Mexico which harbored populations of nonhematophagous bats had been barricaded with chicken wire in attempts to seal in and destroy vampire bats presumed to be inside. McCarthy (1978a) reported that anticoagulant paste was indiscriminately smeared on randomly collected bats of many beneficial species by untrained personnel in Belize, resulting in the needless deaths of many bats of significant ecological value. Such misidentification attests to the importance of proper training in the use of these materials.

The widespread and random destruction of bat populations has ramifications of economic, ecologic, moral/ethical, and public-health significance. As Linhart (1975) pointed out, our understanding of the ecology of tropical bats and the impact that their wholesale destruction may have on local ecosystems is fragmentary.

Villa-Ramirez (1969), Greenhall (1968, 1970), and McCarthy (1978b, 1981) urged caution in indiscriminate decimation of bat populations and this cannot be stressed enough. Insectivorous bats are extremely important in controlling insect pests and frugivorous species play valuable roles in pollination, seed dispersal, and reforestation. Thus, nonhematophagous bats provide important agricultural and public-health benefits that require careful consideration when developing control programs that might target

Chiropteran species other than just vampires. As McCarthy (1981) observed, "Appreciation for the richness of bat faunas in the tropics cannot be established by two sentences in a training manual." Greenhall (1968) quoted Howard (1965) as stating,

> *...the primary objective of all control methods should be to accomplish the desired effect with a maximum of safety to man and to forms of life useful or of neutral value to him, and that they be carried out with a minimum of disturbance to the biotic community.*

In stressing the ecological aspects of rabies control, Greenhall (1968) described two major aims:

1) Regulation of population levels of the offending species, rather than indiscriminate destruction of individuals.
2) Protection of nontarget species.

In controlling vampire populations, it is imperative that restraint and caution be applied, recognizing the ease with which species may be driven to extinction (IUCN, 1968). According to the Expert Committee on Rabies (World Health Organization, 1984),

> *...the objective of wildlife population reduction should be to lower the population density of the main rabies reservoir species below the threshold necessary for maintenance of the disease in that population; eradication of the population is not an appropriate objective.*

Continued investigations will be of inestimable value in assessing the efficacy and long-term safety of ongoing control programs. This will provide the basis for a rational and conservative long-range approach to rabies control. Such studies should be of priority importance in the war against vampire-bat rabies. As the National Geographic Society (1973) has observed,

> *No creature seems more repulsive than one who thrives on blood and lives by night. But, [the vampire bat] is neither good nor evil. He is just another creature trying to survive.*

References

Abello-Fernandez, C. (1966). Intento de erradicacion de murcielagos hematophagos. *5th Cong. Panamer. Med. Vet. Zootec.* 1966 Doc. 51

Abelseth, M. K. (1964). An attenuated rabies vaccine for domestic animals produced in tissue culture. *Can. Vet. J.* 5: 279

Arellano-Sota, C. (1988a). Vampire bat-transmitted rabies in cattle. *Rev. Infect. Dis.* 10(Suppl. 4): S707

Arellano-Sota, C. (1988b). Biology, ecology, and control of the vampire bat. *Rev. Infect. Dis.* 10(Suppl. 4): S615

Arellano-Sota, C. (1991). Regional Officer on Animal Production and Health. Food and Agriculture Organization of the United Nations. Santiago, Chile. Personal communication.

Arnold, R. M., Stouraitis, P., and J. Salvatierra (1973). Immunity against paralytic rabies in cattle following vaccination with ERA vaccine under ranch conditions in Bolivia: III. The influence of maternal antibody on the success of vaccination of calves at different ages. *Trop. Anim. Hlth. Prod.* 5: 167

Baer, G. M. (1991). The current status of rabies vaccines in Latin America. In *Expert Consultation on the Care of Persons Exposed to Rabies Transmitted by Vampire Bats.* PAHO/WHO. Programs for Veterinary Public Health. Washington, D.C. April 1-5, 1991

Barrat, J., Guillemin, F., Brun, A., Lacoste, F., and P. Precausta (1991). Cattle vaccination against rabies—Immunity duration and challenge three years after vaccination. In *Expert Consultation on the Care of Persons Exposed to Rabies Transmitted by Vampire Bats.* PAHO/WHO. Programs for Veterinary Public Health. Washington, D.C. April 1-5, 1991

Bijlenga, G. (1975). Une methode immunobiologique de controle des populations de vampires (*Desmodus rotundus*). Vaccination anti-espece vampire des proies. (An immunological method of controlling vampire bat populations. Anti-vampire bat tissue vaccination of prey.) *Bull. Soc. Sci. Vet. Med. Comp. (Lyon).* 77(3): 171 (English abstract) in *Vet. Bull.* (1975). 45(11): 811

Bijlenga, G. and M. Hernandez-Baumgarten (1984). A plaque-purified rabies virus (strain V-319) derived from a vampire bat (*Desmodus rotundus*) in Mexico: Vaccine potential. *Cornell Vet.* 74: 155

Boos, W. J. and T. F. Farrell (1956). *The Paralytic Rabies Regulations, 1956.* Government Notice No. 50. The Animals (Diseases and Importation) Ordinance, 1954 (No. 19 of 1954). Regulations. Made by the Governor in Council Under Section 13 of the Animals (Diseases and Importation) Ordinance, 1954. Reported in *Carib. Med. J.* (1959). XXI (1-4): 183

Bouliere, F. (1968). Discussion. *Int. Union Conser. Nature Natur. Resour. Publ. [N.S.].* 13: 86

Burns, R. J. (1970). Twin vampire bats born in captivity. *J. Mammal.* 51: 391

Bush, D. L. (1961). Epizootic bat rabies in Surinam—Effectiveness of a mass field immunization program. *J. Am. Vet. Med. Assoc.* 138(7): 363

Butcher, L. V. (1958). The present status of paralytic rabies (bat-transmitted) in Trinidad. *West Ind. Med. J.* 7: 17

Charlton, K. M. (1992). Report of the meeting "Control of Rabies in the Americas." Animal Diseases Research Institute. September 11-13, 1991. *Can. Vet. J.* 33: 98

Constantine, D. G. (1970). Bats in Relation to the Health, Welfare, and Economy of Man. In W. Wimsatt (ed.) *Biology of Bats.* Vol. II. Academic Press. New York.

de Diego, A. I. and J. R. Valotta (1973). Rabia transmitida por murcielagos. *Bol. Of. Sanit. Panam.* 86(6): 495

de La Rosa Pedraza, R., Flores-Crespo, R., and V. J. M. Berruecos (1977). La influencia de los vampiros en la produccion lactea del ganado bovino (Influence of vampire bats on milk production from cattle). *Tecnia Pecuaria en Mexico.* No. 33: 53 (English abstract) in *Vet. Bull.* (1979). 49(8): 644

Delpietro, H. A. and A. J. Nader (1989). Rabies of herbivores transmitted by vampire bats in north-eastern Argentina. *Revue Scientifique et Technique.* 8(1): 177 (English abstract) in *Vet. Bull.* (1990). 60(1): 20

Delpietro, H. A., Patire, J., and A. Callon (1989). Dos curiosas formas de defender los caprinos del ataque de los vampiros: Un corral con "tunel subterraneo" y un "gato pastor" (Two unusual methods of protecting goats from vampire attack: A corral with an underground tunnel, and a resident cat). *Veterinaria Argentina.* 6(57): 467 (English abstract) in *Vet. Bull.* (1990). 60(4): 453

Delpietro, H. A., Russo, G., Alli, C., and J. Patire (1991). Una nueva forma de combatir vampiros (A new method of controlling vampire bats). *Veterinaria Argentina.* 8(77): 455 (English abstract) in *Vet. Bull.* (1992). 62(4): 334

de Oviedo, G. F. (1526). *Natural History of the West Indies.* Translated and edited by S. A. Stoudemire. University of North Carolina Studies in the Romance Languages and Literature. Number 32, 1959. The University of North Carolina Press. Chapel Hill, North Carolina.

de Verteuil, E. and F. W. Urich (1936). The study and control of paralytic rabies transmitted by bats in Trinidad, British West Indies. *Trans. Roy. Soc. Trop. Med. Hyg.* XXIX(4): 317

Director of Agriculture (1932). *Administration Reports of the Director of Agriculture (Trinidad) for the Year 1932.* Reported in *Carib. Med. J.* (1959). XXI (1-4): 172

Dumith Arteaga, G., Lopez Adaros, H., and H. Rosales Gill (1967). Venezuela. *1st Semin. Int. Rabis Amer.*, Ramos Mejia, 1967 p. 416

Elias, D. J., Thompson, R. D., and P. J. Savarie (1978). Effects of the anticoagulant diphenadione on suckling calves. *Bull. Environ. Contam. Toxicol.* 20(1): 71

Fitter, M. (1968). How not to control vampire bats. *Oryx.* 9: 248

Fleming, T. H., Hooper, E. T., and D. E. Wilson (1972). Three Central American bat communities: Structure, reproductive cycles and movement patterns. *Ecology.* 53(4): 557

Flores-Crespo, R. (1978). La rabia, los murcielagos y el control de los hematofagos. In R. Moreno-Chan (ed.) *Cienci Veterinaria.* Vol 2. Mexico City. Universidad Nacional Automoma de Mexico.

Flores-Crespo, R. (1991). Techniques to control vampire bats. In *Expert Consultation on the Care of Persons Exposed to Rabies Transmitted by Vampire Bats.* PAHO/WHO. Programs for Veterinary Public Health. Washington, D.C. April 1-5, 1991

Flores-Crespo, R. and S. Said-Fernandez (1972). Reduccion de la dosis de anitcoagulantes (difenadione) para el control de los vampiros. *Tecnica Pecuaria en Mexico.* 23: 19

Flores-Crespo, R. and C. Arellano-Sota (1991). Biology and Control of the Vampire Bat. In G. M. Baer (ed.) *The Natural History of Rabies.* 2nd Edition. CRC Press, Inc. Boca Raton, Florida.

Flores-Crespo, R., Linhart, S. B., and R. J. Burns (1971). Comportamiento del vampiro (*Desmodus rotundus*) durante su alimentacion en ganado bovino en cautiverio. *Tecnica Pecuaria en Mexico.* 18: 40

Flores-Crespo, R., Linhart, S. B., and R. J. Burns (1972). Comportamiento del vampiro (*Desmodus rotundus*) en cautiverio. (English abstract.) *SW Nat.* 17: 139

Flores-Crespo, R., Burns, R. J., and S. Said-Fernandez (1974). Evaluacion de una tecnica para combatir los vampiros en sus refugios. *Bol. Of. Sanit. Panam.* 76(5): 427

Flores-Crespo, R., Ibarra, F., and D. De Anda-Lopez (1976). Vampirinys II, un procducto utilizable en tres metodos para el control del murcielago hematofago. *Tecnica Pecuaria en Mexico.* 30: 67

Flores-Crespo, R., Said-Fernandez, S., De Anda-Lopez, D., Velarde, F. I., and R. M. Anaya D. G. (1979). Intramuscular inoculation of cattle with warfarin: A new technique for the control of vampire bats. *Bull. Pan Am. Hlth. Org.* 13(2): 147

Fornes, A., Lord, R. D., Kuns, M. L., Larghi, O. P., Fuenzalida, E., and L. Lazara (1974). Control of bovine rabies through vampire bat control. *J. Wildl. Dis.* 10: 310

Greenhall, A. M. (1959). The ecological role of Trinidad bats, especially the vampire, and bat rabies. *Vet. Rec.* 71(10): 188

Greenhall, A. M. (1963). Use of mist nets and strychnine for vampire control in Trinidad. *J. Mammal.* 44(3): 396

Greenhall, A. M. (1965). Aspects of ecology in vampire bat control in Trinidad. *Ann. 2nd Congr. Latino-Amer. Zool.* 1962, p. 321

Greenhall, A. M. (1968). Bats, rabies and control problems. *Oryx.* 9: 263

Greenhall, A. M. (1970). Vampire Bat Control: A Review and Proposed Programme for Latin America. In R. H. Dana (ed.) *Proceedings of the Fourth Vertebrate Pest Conference.* California Vertebrate Pest Committee. West Sacramento, California. March 3-5, 1970

Greenhall, A. M. (1972). The problem of bat rabies, migratory bats, livestock and wildlife. *Transactions of the North American Wildlife and Natural Resources Conference*—No. 37. Mexico City, Mexico. March 12-15, 1972

Greenhall, A. M. (1974). Vampire bat control in the Americas: A review and proposed program for action. *Bull. Pan Am. Hlth. Org.* 8(1): 30

Greenhall, A. M. (1985). Effects of Vampire Bats and Paralytic Rabies on Livestock Production. In S. M. Gaafar, W. E. Howard, and R. E. Marsh (eds.) *Parasites, Pests and Predators.* Elsevior Science Publishing Co., Inc. New York.

Greenhall, A. M. (1988). Feeding Behavior. In A. M. Greenhall and U. Schmidt (eds.) *The Natural History of Vampire Bats.* CRC Press, Inc. Boca Raton, Florida.

Howard, W. E. (1965). *Principles of Vertebrate Animal Control.* Congres de la Protection des Cultures Tropicales. Marseille, France. March, 1965

International Union for the Conservation of Nature and Natural Resources (1968). *Latin American Regional Conference on Conservation of Renewable Natural Resources.* San Carlos de Bariloche, Argentina. April 2, 1968

Johnson, H. N. (1971). General Epizootiology of Rabies. In Y. Nagano and F. M. Davenport (eds.) *Rabies.* Proceedings of Working Conference of Rabies. Sponsored by the Japan-United States Cooperative Medical Science Program. University Park Press. Baltimore.

Koprowski, H., Celis, E., Curtis, P., Dietzschold, B., Rupprecht, C., Tollis, M., and W. Wunner (1987). Rabies experiment. *Nature (Lond.).* 326: 636

Kverno, N. B. and G. C. Mitchell (1976). Vampire bats and their effect on cattle production in Latin America. *Wld. Anim. Rev.* (FAO). 17: 1

Lewin, R. (1986). Why dynamiting vampire bats is wrong. *Science.* 232: 24

Linhart, S. B. (1975). The Biology and Control of Vampire Bats. In G. M. Baer (ed.) *The Natural History of Rabies.* Vol. II. Academic Press. New York.

Linhart, S. B., Flores-Crespo, R., and G. C. Mitchell (1972). Control of vampire bats by topical application of anticoagulant. *Bol. Of. Sanit. Panam.* 6: 31

Lord, R. D. (1980). An ecological strategy for controlling rabies through elimination of vampire bats. In J. P. Clark and R. E. Marsh (eds.) *Proceedings of the 9th Vertebrate Pest Conference.* Fresno, California. p. 170, March 4-6, 1980

Lord, R. D. (1988). Control of Vampire Bats. In A. M. Greenhall and U. Schmidt (eds.) *Natural History of Vampire Bats.* CRC Press, Inc. Boca Raton, Florida.

Lord, R. D. (1992). Seasonal reproduction of vampire bats and its relation to seasonality of bovine rabies. *J. Wildl. Dis.* 28(2): 170

Lord, R. D. (1993). Professor of Biology. Department of Biology. Indiana University of Pennsylvania. Indiana, Pennsylvania. Personal communication.

Marcaída, A. (1960). El murcielago vampiro un enemigo de las explotaciones porcinas. *Rev. Protinal (Caracas).* 7: 61, chapter 10

McCarthy, T. J. (1978a). Comments on paralytic rabies in Belize. *Contribution of the Vampire Bat Education and Control Program, Belize.* Unpublished document. Courtesy of T. J. McCarthy.

McCarthy, T. J. (1978b). Vampire Bat Control in Belize. Comments on Ecology and a Program of Education, Research and Control. *Proceedings of the First International Symposium on Vampire Bat Control.* Managua, Nicaragua. June 29-30, 1976

McCarthy, T. J. (1981). Comments on vampire bat catching: Status of control and programming in Belize. *American Society of Mammalogists.* Miami University. Oxford, Ohio. June 7-11, 1981

McCarthy, T. J. (1993). Advisor, The Vampire Bat Education and Control Programme, Ministry of Agriculture and Fisheries, Belize. Section of Mammals. The Carnegie Museum of Natural History. Pittsburgh, Pennsylvania. Personal communication.

Metivier, H. V. M. (1935). Paralytic rabies in livestock. *J. Comp. Path. Ther.* 48: 245

Miller, M. (1992). Endangered product: What Japan won't sell us—Trade dispute has net result of threat to bird studies. *The San Diego Union-Tribune.* December 6, I-1

Mitchell, G. C. (1986). Vampire Bat Control in Latin America. In D. Policansky (ed.). *Ecological Knowledge and Problem-Solving.* National Academy Press. Washington, D. C.

Mitchell, G. C. (1993). Denver Wildlife Research Center. Denver, Colorado. Personal communication.

Mitchell, G. C. and R. J. Burns (1973). *Chemical Control of Vampire Bats.* Denver Wildlife Research Center, U. S. Bureau of Sport Fisheries and Wildlife. Denver, Colorado.

Montano, J. A., Polack, G. W., and E. F. Mora (1987). Rabies in vaccinated cattle. II. Epidemiological situation in the State of Parana, Brazil - 1984 (English abstract) in *Vet. Bull.* (1988). 58(1): 18

National Geographic Society (1973). *Strange Creatures of the Night.* Product No. 51376. Washington, D. C.

Office of the Surgeon General (1935). *Administration Report of the Surgeon General (Trinidad) for the Year 1935.* Reported in *Carib. Med. J.* (1959). XXI (1-4): 230

Ornelas, O. and G. Aranalde (1964). Bat rabies in Mexico. *Southern Vet.* 1: 13

Pawan, J. L. (1936). The transmission of paralytic rabies in Trinidad by the vampire bat (*Desmodus rotundus murinus* Wagner, 1840). *Ann. Trop. Med. Parasit.* 30: 101

Pawan, J. L. (1948). Fruit-eating bats and paralytic rabies in Trinidad. *Ann. Trop. Med. Parasit.* 42: 173

Pawan, J. L. (1955). Rabies in bats. *Vet. Bull.* 14(4): 52

Piccinini, R. S., Jorge, M. A., Cavalcanti, R. J., Tabosa, A. G., and V. T. Curvelo (1982). O uso de difenadiona (2-difenilacetil-1,2 indandiona) para o controle de vampiros em areas endemicas de raiva, Nordeste do Brasil (Use of the anticoagulant diphenadione for vampire bat control in endemic rabies areas in northeastern Brazil). *Arquivos da escola de Veterinaria da Universidade Federal de Minas Gerais.* 34(2): 289 (English abstract) in *Vet. Bull.* (1983). 53(2): 164

Piccinini, R. S., Freitas, C. E. A., and J. C. P. De Souza (1985). Vampiricidas de uso topico em animais domesticos e em morcegos hematofagos (Vampiricides for topical use on domestic animals and vampire bats). *Pesquisa Veterinaria Brasileira.* 5(3): 97 (English abstract) in *Vet. Bull.* (1986). 56(8): 729

Pint, J. J. (1994). Who cares about Mexican bats? *NSS (Natl. Speleol. Soc.) News.* 52(3): 94

Romero, S. C., Ruiz, J. M., Campero, D. B., Hernandez-Baumgarten, E., and G. C. Viladomat (1991). Evaluacion de la vacuna antirrabica inactivada cepa Pasteur RIV en bovinos, mediante desafio con la cepa patogena de virus rabico CASS-88 (Evaluation of the inactivated Pasteur-RIV rabies vaccine in cattle by challenge with the pathogenic bat virus strain (CASS-88). *Tecnica Pecuaria en Mexico.* 29(1): 1 (English abstract) in *Vet. Bull.* (1992). 62(7): 670

Rosenthal, J. E. (1972). *AID (Agency for International Development) Finds Ways to Control Vampire Bat.* War on Hunger, Agency for International Development.

Ruiz, A. and A. M. Diaz (1990). *Epidemiology of Rabies Transmitted by Vampire Bats.* Subject 3.8. Pan American Health Organization, Pan American Sanitary Bureau, Regional Office of the World Health Organization, WHO Seminar on Wildlife Rabies Control. Geneva. July 2-5, 1990

Rupprecht, C. E. (1991). Associate Professor. Department of Microbiology and Immunology, Center for Neurovirology, Thomas Jefferson University, Jefferson Medical College. Philadelphia, Pennsylvania. Personal communication.

Rupprecht, C. E., Lord, R., Papo, S., Dietzschold, B., and A. M. Greenhall (1987). Bovine paralytic rabies control: Immunization of vampire bats with an inactivated oral rabies vaccine (abstract). *17th Annual North American Symposium on Bat Research.* Toronto, Canada.

Rupprecht, C. E., Papo, S., Deresienski, D., Lord, R., and B. Dietzschold (1988). Investigations on vampire bat rabies (abstract). *18th Annual North American Symposium on Bat Research.* Calgary, Canada.

Said-Fernandez, S. and R. Flores-Crespo (1991). Control of the common vampire bat (*Desmodus rotundus*) using intramuscular administration of diphacinone in cattle (English abstract). *Veterinaria* (Mexico City). 22(2): 165

Sanborn, C. C. (1931). Protection against vampire bats. *J. Mammal.* 12: 312

Schmidt, C. (1988). Reproduction. In A. M. Greenhall and U. Schmidt (eds.) *The Natural History of Vampire Bats.* CRC Press, Inc. Boca Raton, Florida.

Thompson, R. D., Mitchell, G. C., and R. J. Burns (1972). Vampire bat control by systemic treatment of livestock with an anticoagulant. *Science.* 177: 806

Thompson, R. D., Elias, D. J., and G. C. Mitchell (1977). Effects of vampire bat control on bovine milk production. *J. Wildl. Manage.* 41(4): 736

Thornton, H. (1980). An ingenious method of destroying the vampire bats which transmit rabies to cattle. *Centr. Afr. J. Med.* 26(9): 207

Turner, D. C. (1975). *The Vampire Bat—A Field Study in Behavior and Ecology.* The Johns Hopkins University Press. Baltimore.

Villa-Ramirez, B. (1969). *The Ecology and Biology of Vampire Bats and Their Relationship to Paralytic Rabies.* Report to the Government of Brazil. United Nations Development Programme/Food and Agriculture Organization. FAO No. TA2656. Rome, 1969

Williams, H. E. (1960). Bat transmitted rabies in Trinidad. *Can. Vet. J.* 1(1): 20

Wimsatt, W. A. and H. Trapido (1952). Reproduction and the female reproductive cycle in the tropical American vampire bat (*Desmodus rotundus murinus*). *Am. J. Anat.* 91(3): 414

Wise, K. S. (1932). *Administration Report of the Surgeon General (Trinidad) for the Year 1932.* Reported in *Carib. Med. J.* XXI (1-4): 224

World Health Organization (1984). *Expert Committee on Rabies. Seventh Report.* WHO Tech. Rpt. No. 709. Geneva.

SECTION III

Insectivorous Bats and Rabies in North America

Chapter 11: PREVALENCE AND DISTRIBUTION OF RABIES IN INSECTIVOROUS BATS

Compartmentalization of Rabies Virus

Of concern in the formulation of rabies control programs is the relative importance of different animal species in spreading the disease. In developing nations, an urban rabies cycle is particularly important, dogs being the most significant viral reservoir. Monies are oftentimes not available to finance adequate vaccination and control programs. The large number of free-roaming rabid dogs (community or neighborhood dogs) in these countries may engender considerable fear among the local populace. On a worldwide basis, the urban rabies cycle has earned this disease a prominent position as one of the most dreaded zoonoses known to mankind. Historically, many cultures have regarded rabies with extraordinary fear, due principally to the image of a blindly furious animal biting all in its path, but also because of the panic and terror so characteristic of the human disease (Tsiang, 1993).

Urban rabies involving domestic animals is no longer conspicuous in most of the United States, although a significant urban rabies problem involving raccoons is emerging in the eastern part of the country. Widespread vaccination of dogs has markedly reduced their importance as reservoirs of virus, although problems may periodically occur in regions adjacent to areas of enzootic rabies in neighboring countries (such as at the United States/Mexico border). With the decline in the extent of urban rabies (especially canine), a corresponding decrease was observed in human rabies cases (Parker, 1969).

During the years in which urban rabies cycles were paramount, attention of public-health officials was focused primarily on rabies in dogs and less so on wildlife. In the late 1950's, reported cases of rabies in wildlife began to overtake those in domestic species (see Figure 2-1). In the United States at present, the number of reported cases of wildlife rabies far surpasses those in domesticated animals.

As the focus of attention shifted to wildlife, it became apparent that foci of rabies were compartmentalized in both geographic and species-specific fashion. In this regard, the significance of different species in sylvatic (wildlife) rabies cycles were observed to vary from one area of the country to another. It is now known that in a particular region of enzootic animal rabies, cases will predominate in a single reservoir species (single-species involvement), with low numbers of cases in other species in the same area and low numbers of cases in this reservoiring species in different areas (Figure 11-1).

Sporadic cases of rabies in nonreservoir species are regarded as spillover from infection in the geographic reservoir, although the occurrence of small, independent enzootics in other species within a particular zone may be possible (Smith and Baer, 1988; Smith, 1989). Maintenance of virus in natural "compartments" suggests that eradication of disease in a local area may follow from elimination of disease in the primary reservoir species (Smith et al, 1990).

One or more unique combinations of virus, host, and environment must be present in order to account for compartmentalization (Tinline, 1988). One possible reason for the compartmentalization of infection involves a differential species sensitivity to virus (Sikes, 1962). Foxes, for example, are more susceptible to virus of fox origin than are skunks. In an area of enzootic fox rabies, rabid foxes may shed a sufficient amount of virus in their saliva to infect other foxes, but not skunks. On the other hand, the higher viral

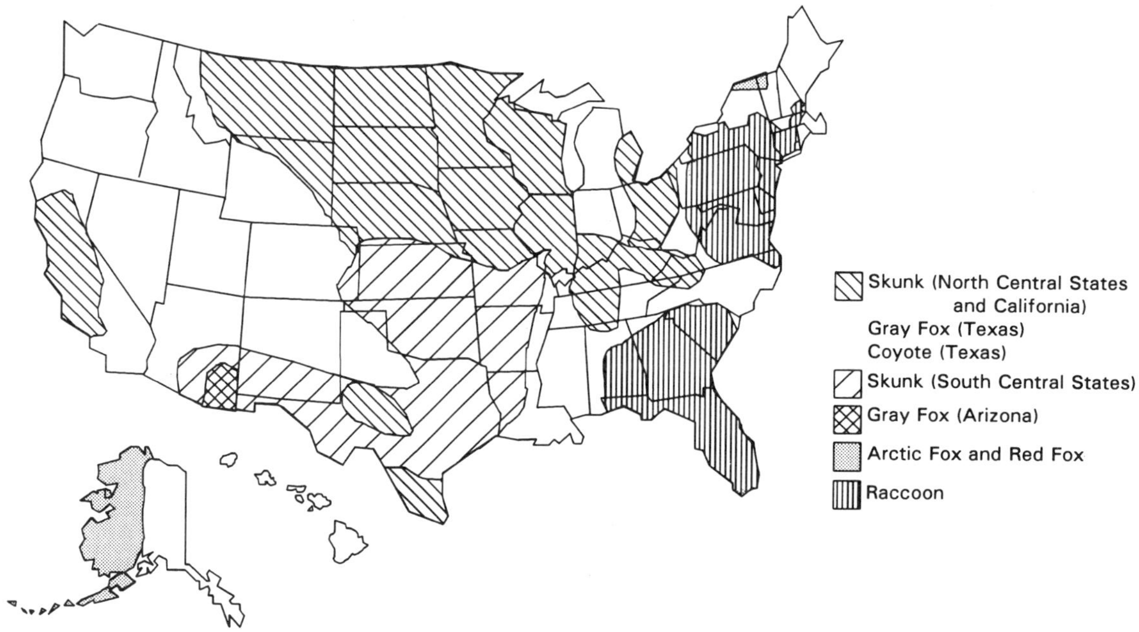

Figure 11-1. Distribution of five antigenically distinct ecotypes of rabies virus and the predominant wildlife species affected in the United States during 1992. (From Krebs, Strine, T. W., and J. E. Childs. Rabies surveillance in the United States during 1992. *J. Am. Vet. Med. Assoc.* 203(12): 1718, 1993. Reproduced with permission.)

titers in salivary secretions of rabid skunks may kill an infected fox before salivary secretion of virus begins (see discussion by Smith and Baer, 1988). Skunks have also been shown to be susceptible to a lower dosage of a skunk variant of virus than raccoons (Hill and Beran, 1992). Other mechanisms that may account for viral compartmentalization include a lack of interspecies contact because of behavioral or ecological isolation, and failure of small animals to survive the transmission wound of larger animals. Low population density of respective species does not appear to be a factor (Smith, 1989).

Relationship Between Terrestrial and Nonterrestrial Rabies

Nationwide, important terrestrial wildlife reservoirs of sylvatic rabies have included skunks, raccoons, and foxes. Superimposed on this terrestrial sylvatic cycle is a largely independent (nonterrestrial) cycle in insectivorous bats. The nature of the interrelationship between terrestrial (sylvatic and urban) and nonterrestrial (bat) rabies cycles is not fully understood. That they intimately overlap one another has been suggested repeatedly. Time and time again, bats have been implicated as a fundamental reservoir of virus, from which wildlife infection continually emanates. This is now known not to be the case (see Figure 15-1).

In considering the role of bats in sylvatic rabies cycles, it becomes evident that a complexity of only partially understood factors act in concert to maintain wildlife disease. Significant species differences exist among bats that may influence their relationship to terrestrial rabies cycles. These include features related to their ability to transmit disease, as well as to their ability to disperse disease. Differences related to habitat preference, seasonal behavior, and clinical manifestations of rabid individuals may all affect vector competence and virus dispersal. Rabies cycles may be entirely different in hematophagous vampire bats, frugivorous bats, and various insectivorous species (Constantine and Woodall, 1966; Constantine et al, 1968a; Trimarchi and Debbie, 1980). Colonial versus solitary and migratory versus nonmigratory habits may also lead to vastly different potential roles in transmission and dispersal of disease. Migratory behavior, for example, is significant in that a bat that can carry virus several hundred or even several thousand miles (and thereby act as a possible migrating vector) presents a different problem than a nonmigratory bat, which remains a local resident at its roost (Glass, 1959; Constantine and Woodall, 1966; Beauregard, 1969; Schowalter, 1980; Brosset, 1990; Rupprecht et al, 1991).

Suggestions of different degrees of bat involvement in sylvatic cycles may necessitate a variety of approaches to controlling disease. This, in turn, may manifest as a need for regionally distinct public-health programs. One such comprehensive program is that found in New York State (Figure 11-2), where a holistic approach (Frantz, 1989) to management of bat rabies should serve as an example for public-health departments nationwide.

In considering the possible importance of insectivorous bats in the epidemiology of rabies in the United States, three significant concerns include:

1) What is the prevalence and distribution of enzootic rabies in insectivorous bats?

2) What is the relationship of bat rabies to rabies in other animal species, both wild and domestic?

3) What is the public-health significance of rabies in bats?

Early Reports of Rabies in Bats

On June 23, 1953 at 10:30 a.m., a seven-year-old boy in Hillsborough County (Tampa), Florida was bitten by a lactating Florida yellow bat (*Lasiurus intermedius*) while looking for a ball lost in some shrubbery. The yellow bat is an insectivorous, solitary species, living in shrubs and moss. The bat flew out at the boy in an apparently unprovoked attack and remained firmly attached to his chest until knocked off by the child's mother. The owner of the ranch where the boy's father was employed was familiar with rabies in vampire bats. Predominantly at his urging, the bat was sent to the Tampa Regional Laboratory of the Florida Board of Health, where it was confirmed as rabid. Post-exposure rabies prophylaxis was administered. Despite grave concern over developing shock, no signs of rabies developed and the boy recovered. This finding was the first reported case of rabies in an insectivorous bat in the United States (Venters et al, 1954; Scatterday, 1954; Scatterday and Galton, 1954). It also appears to have been the first bat submitted for rabies testing in this country.

Three months later (6:00 p.m. on September 29), a 39-year-old woman watching her husband feed waterfowl along a lake in Boiling Springs, Pennsylvania was suddenly attacked by what is believed to have been a hoary bat (*Lasiurus cinereus*). The bat landed on her left arm and bit her without any apparent provocation. It clung to her arm tenaciously until she pulled it off and hurled it against a fence. Before its death, the bat was retained by the Pennsylvania Game Commission, where it was observed to be in the throes of what appeared to be a form of furious rabies, repeatedly hurling itself against its cage (Kough, 1954). The bat was sent to the laboratory of the Pennsylvania Bureau of Animal Industry where it was confirmed as rabid. Routine post-exposure rabies prophylaxis was administered and the woman suffered only local symptoms from the bite itself (Witte, 1954).

These early reports of rabies in insectivorous bats pointed to a potential viral reservoir heretofore unrecognized. The significance of rabies in bats was unknown and early investigators began survey studies in attempts to define the extent of the disease among bat populations. Of 385 healthy-appearing bats captured at the Hillsborough County ranch, from other areas within a 40-mile radius of the ranch, and from regions of northwest Florida and south Georgia, five were confirmed as rabid (Venters et al, 1954; Scatterday, 1954; Scatterday and Galton, 1954). These included four yellow bats and one Seminole bat (*Lasiurus seminola*).

On August 2, 1958, a 53-year-old woman in Magalia Butte County, California was bitten on the finger by an apparently injured silver-haired bat (*Lasionycteris noctivagans*) while trying to pick it up. The bat was later confirmed as rabid. Post-exposure rabies prophylaxis was administered from September 2 until September 26, but the woman died on November 4 (additional details of this case can be found on page 236). This

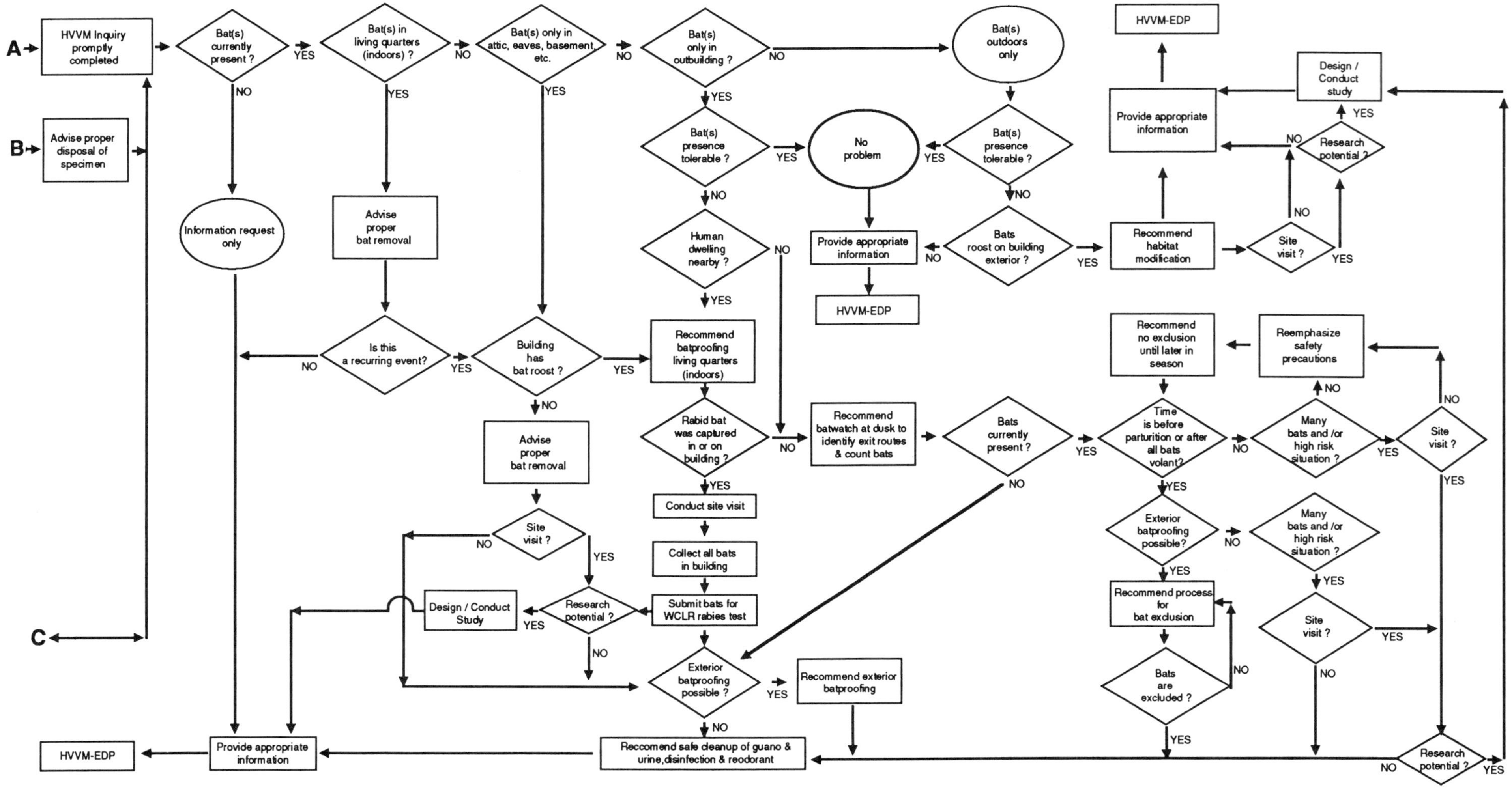

Figure 11-2. Comprehensive program for management of bats and bat-related health concerns, New York State. (From Frantz, S. C. Bat rabies management: New York State's holistic approach. *Fifth International Theriological Congress.* Rome, Italy. August 29, 1989. Reproduced with permission.)

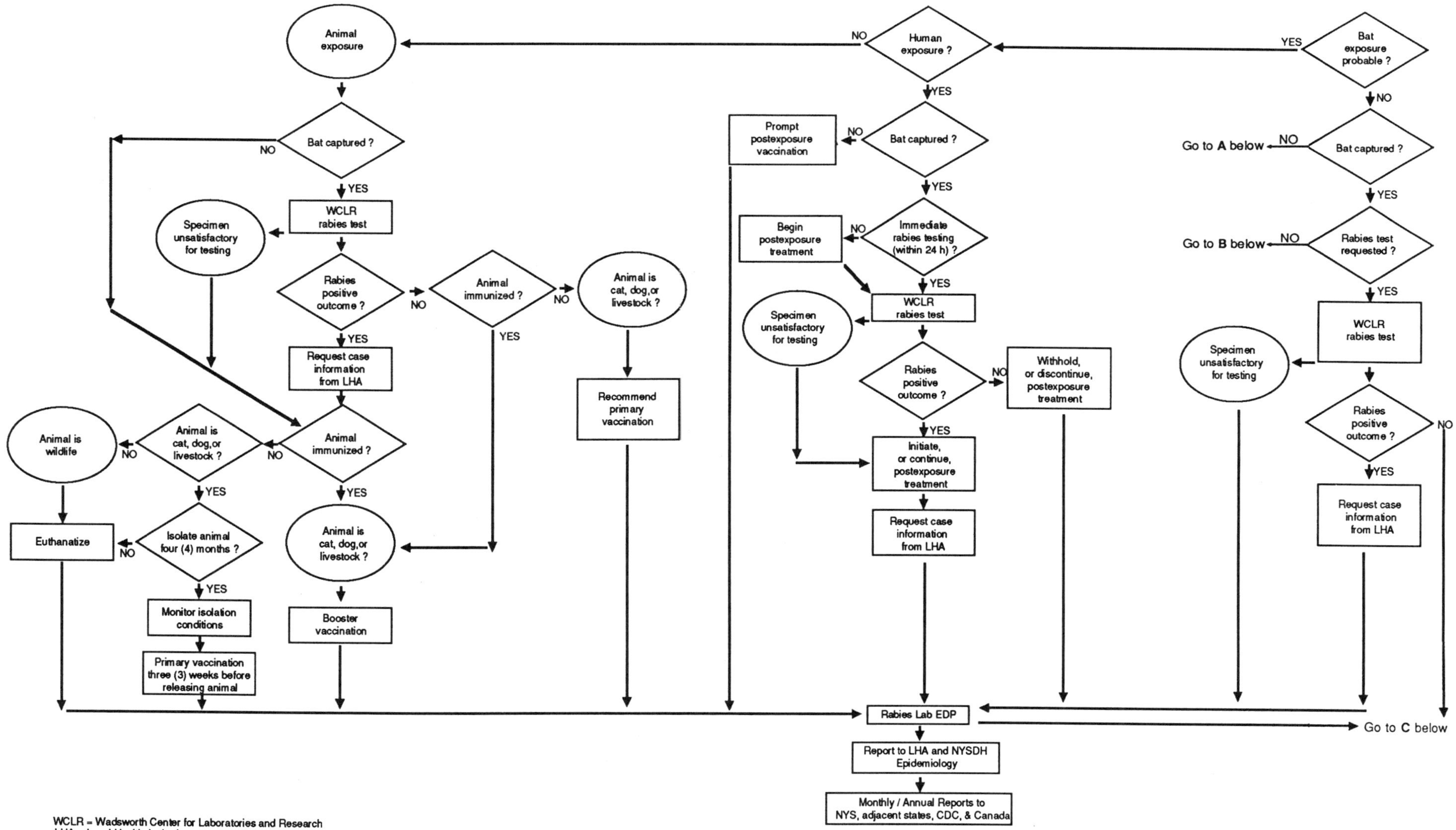

WCLR = Wadsworth Center for Laboratories and Research
LHA = Local Health Authority
Rabies Lab EDP = WCLR Rabies Laboratory Electronic Data Processing
HVVM = WCLR Holistic Vertebrate Vector Management Program
CDC = Centers for Disease Control, US Public Health Service, Atlanta, GA

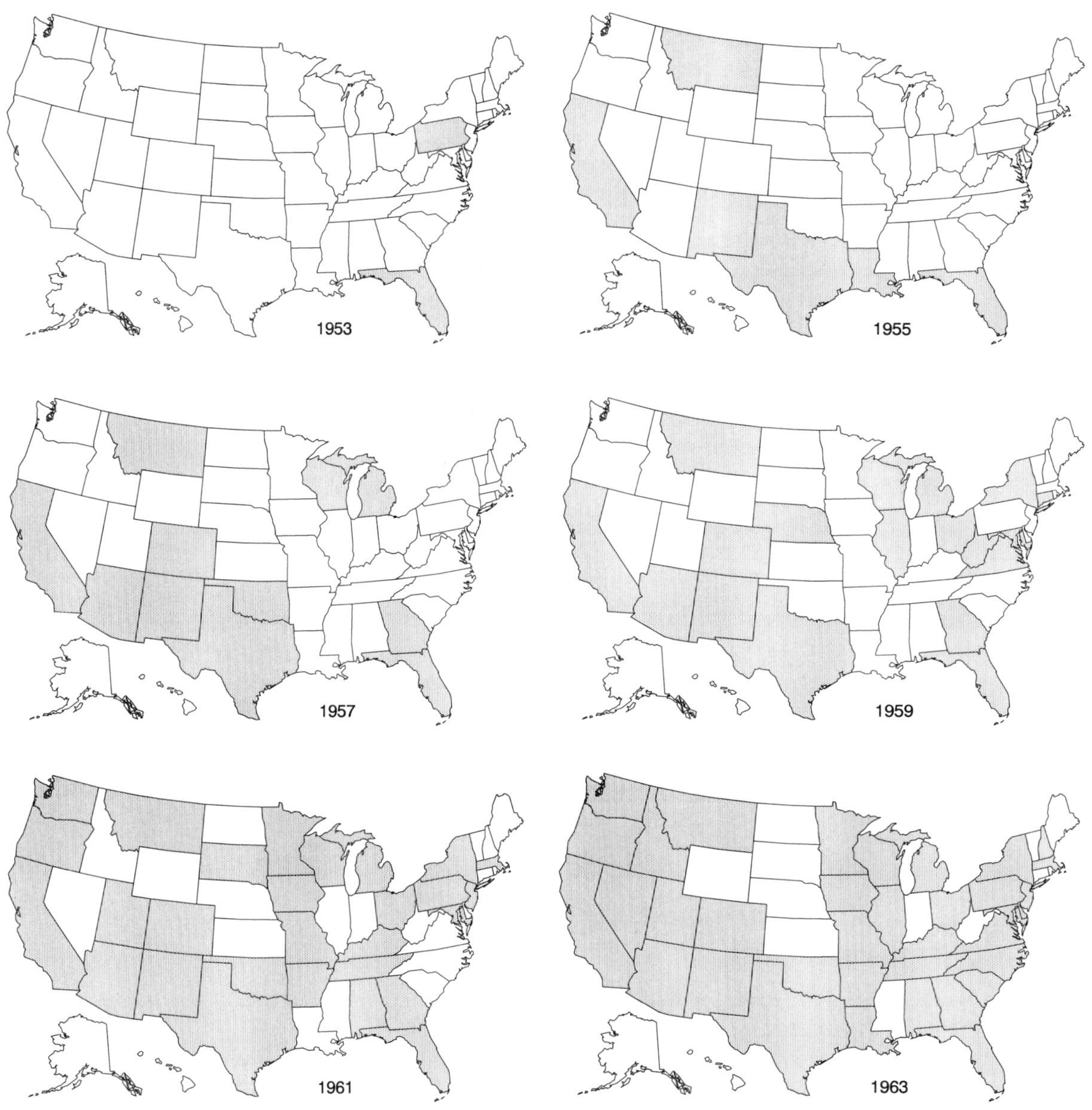

Figure 11-3. Rapid progression in the distribution of bats reported rabid in the United States, 1953-1963. (Data compiled from *Annual Rabies Surveillance Reports*. Centers for Disease Control, U. S. Department of Health and Human Services, Public Health Service. Atlanta, Georgia.)

is considered by many to be the first fully documented human death due to bat-inflicted rabies in the United States (Martin, 1959; Humphrey et al, 1960; Lennette et al, 1960).

Although the presence of rabies in insectivorous bats was undiagnosed in the United States prior to 1953, the recognition of infection in bats prompted the realization that human exposure may have occurred previously. Sulkin and Greve (1954) reported the case of a woman who, in October of 1951, was bitten on the arm by an unidentified sick bat that she had picked up along a road in Parkland County, Texas. Sixteen days later, she became ill and had pain in the bitten arm. This was followed by paralysis of the arm, inability to swallow, coma, and death. Negri bodies were demonstrated in her brain and, although the bat was not available for examination, a retrospective diagnosis of bat-transmitted rabies was made (additional details of this case can be found on page 237).

Distribution of Bat Rabies in the United States

Rabies in North American bats was probably widely distributed before its initial discovery in 1953. In fact, early reports confirming the presence of rabies in various species of insectivorous bats lent new significance to an ancient Pima Indian belief. The Pima Indians feared bats, claiming that, "If a bat bites you, you will go crazy and die." (Maddy et al, 1958). In the decades following this initial discovery, bat rabies has been reported from all 48 contiguous states and the District of Columbia (Figures 11-3 and 11-4) and, as shown in Table 11-1, in most species that have been adequately sampled (Constantine, 1979). Among the major reservoirs of rabies virus in North America, the geographic distribution of infected individuals is greatest among the bats.

Hawaii is the only rabies-free state in the United States (rabies exists in Alaska, but bat rabies has not been reported). On March 27, 1991, a big brown bat, subsequently confirmed as rabid, was discovered by stevedores during unloading of the container ship *Sea Land Hawaii* while docked at Honolulu Harbor, Sand Island. The bat had been found in a container of automobiles newly arrived from the mainland. The three automobiles within the container had originated at a General Motors plant in Detroit, Michigan. From there, they had been driven to Oakland, California, where they had been loaded onto the container ship. One stop had been made by the ship in Long Beach, California prior to its arrival in Hawaii (Sasaki et al, 1992).

Although this incident was quickly contained by local health authorities before the bat could escape into the wild, it does point out the fragility

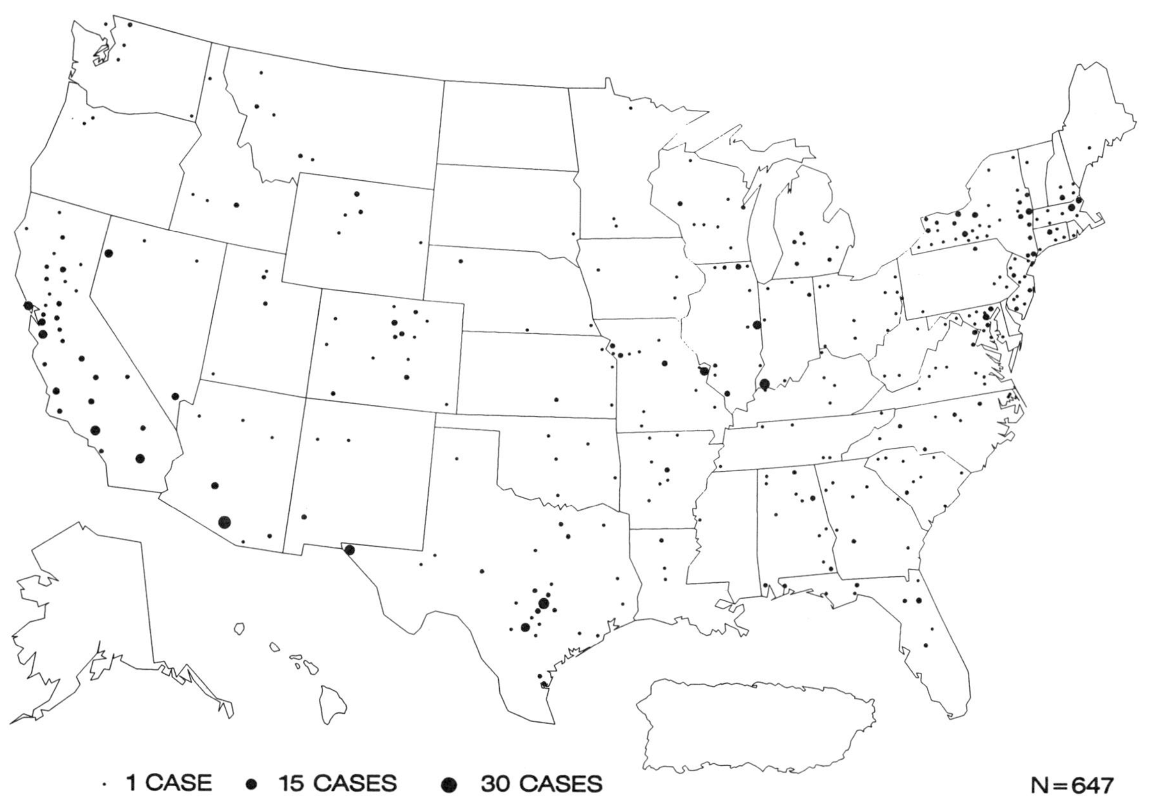

Figure 11-4. Reported cases of rabies in bats, by county, 1992. Dot size is proportional to the number of cases in the county. (From Krebs, J. W., Strine, T. W., and J. E. Childs. Rabies surveillance in the United States during 1992. *J. Am. Vet. Med. Assoc.* 203(12): 1718, 1993. Reproduced with permission.)

Table 11-1

Rabies Status (+/-) of North American Bats North of Mexico

Family	Genus and Species[a]	Status
Phyllostomidae	*Macrotus californicus*	+
	Choeronycteris mexicana	+
	Leptonycteris nivalis	+[b]
	Leptonycteris sanborni	+
Vespertilionidae	*Myotis lucifugus*	+
	Myotis yumanensis	+
	Myotis grisescens	+
	Myotis velifer	+
	Myotis keenii	+
	Myotis evotis	+
	Myotis auriculus	+
	Myotis thysanodes	+
	Myotis sodalis	+
	Myotis volans	+
	Myotis californicus	+
	Myotis leibii	+
	Lasionycteris noctivagans	+
	Pipistrellus hesperus	+
	Pipistrellus subflavus	+
	Eptesicus fuscus	+
	Lasiurus borealis	+
	Lasiurus seminolus	+
	Lasiurus cinereus	+
	Lasiurus intermedius	+
	Lasiurus ega	+
	Nycticeius humeralis	+
	Euderma maculatum	+
	Plecotus townsendii	+
	Plecotus rafinesquii	+
	Idionycteris phyllotis	+
	Antrozous pallidus	+
Molossidae	*Tadarida brasiliensis*	+
	Tadarida femorosacca	+
	Tadarida macrotis	+
	Eumops perotis	+
	Eumops underwoodi	+
	Eumops glaucinus	+
Mormoopidae	*Moormoops megalophyla*	+

[a] Excludes three species, single individuals of which have been reported and may have been accidently transported from more southerly, tropical areas: *Artibeus jamaicensis*, from Key West, Florida; *Diphylla ecaudata*, from near Comstock, Texas; *Enchisthenes hartii*, from Tuscon, Arizona.
[b] Reported rabies-infected only in Mexico.

From Constantine, D. G. An updated list of rabies-infected bats in North America. *J. Wildl. Dis.* 15: 347, 1979. Reproduced with permission.

of a rabies-free status and the need for constant vigilance on the part of public-health officials to prevent, or at least quickly contain, cases of imported rabies. Hawaii has maintained a four-month quarantine on all arriving dogs and cats since 1912. The only animals allowed to bypass the existing quarantine are those shipped directly from the United Kingdom, Australia, or New Zealand—other countries currently enjoying a rabies-free status.[1]

Rabies in insectivorous bats is widespread in the United States and Canada and infection with the European bat lyssavirus (rabies-related virus) has recently become more prevalent in Europe. Only limited reports exist from Africa and Asia (see Chapters 22 and 23).

Inherent Difficulties in Studying Wildlife Disease

Of concern to public-health officials is the prevalence and distribution of rabies infection in various bat populations. Unfortunately, the information-gathering process in this respect suffers from assorted sampling biases and these must be clearly recognized before adequate interpretations can be made (Constantine, 1988). Some of the problems intrinsic in data collection are unique to rabies surveillance studies, whereas others pertain to studies of wildlife biology in general (Constantine, 1988; Brass, 1991).

Study of wildlife health suffers from an inherent inability to sample animals in a truly random fashion. In extracting individuals from a wild population, researchers may actually sample in a selective fashion and do not necessarily obtain a representative cross-section of that population. This is particularly true when considering the incidence of a debilitating disease, such as rabies. Under certain collecting conditions, for example, animals in a weakened or behaviorally altered state may be more easily captured than healthy ones. Using a different collection protocol, however, a debilitated or behaviorally isolated animal, in not "traveling with the pack," may be lost to collection. In either case, a representative sample may not be procured and results might be biased to an unknown degree.

In discussing the relationship of sampling technique to reported disease prevalence, Constantine (1988) wrote,

> *Survey of bats to determine rabies prevalence can be misleading, depending on collection techniques and collection sites. Ill bats are easily collected from their roosts in contrast to healthy bats, which escape more readily. A day roost that also serves as a popular night roost may accumulate sick bats during nightly visits of hundreds or thousands of bats. Thus, a popular night roost may contain only incapacitated bats by day, i.e., bats that fell ill during a nighttime visit and could not leave, conveying the impression that a rabies "outbreak" is in progress. Multiple births by an infected female can result in all litter members becoming infected, skewing survey samples and creating the impression that a small "outbreak" is in progress. But nothing resembling an "outbreak" or large-scale rabies destruction of a bat colony has been detected, despite careful seeking.*

Investigations carried out in conjunction with public-health facilities (passive rabies surveil-

[1]Not subject to the quarantine periods required of domestic animals, rabies-free counties have no specific safeguards against imported human rabies (Bucens and O'Connor, 1988). Australia is an example of a rabies-free country in which two cases of imported human rabies have recently been reported. In August 1987, a ten-year-old boy died of rabies in Australia. This was the first confirmed report of rabies being present in either human or animal populations in Australia. It is believed that the child was infected by the bite of a wild monkey, sustained 16 months earlier at a marketplace in northern India (Faoagali et al, 1988). In November 1990, a second case of human rabies in Australia occurred, also with a long incubation period. Investigations pointed to a probable exposure over six years earlier in North Vietnam (Bek et al, 1992; Smith et al, 1992; Grattan-Smith et al, 1992; McColl et al, 1993; Smith and Seidel, 1993). Australia currently enjoys a rabies-free status, but a limited serological survey of bats has been undertaken in Queensland (Dunn et al, 1988). Forman (1993) reported that considerable mingling occurs among the migrant bats of northeast Australia, the neighboring islands of the Torres Strait, and those of New Guinea, although he pointed out that no evidence of rabies-positive bats in these locales exists.

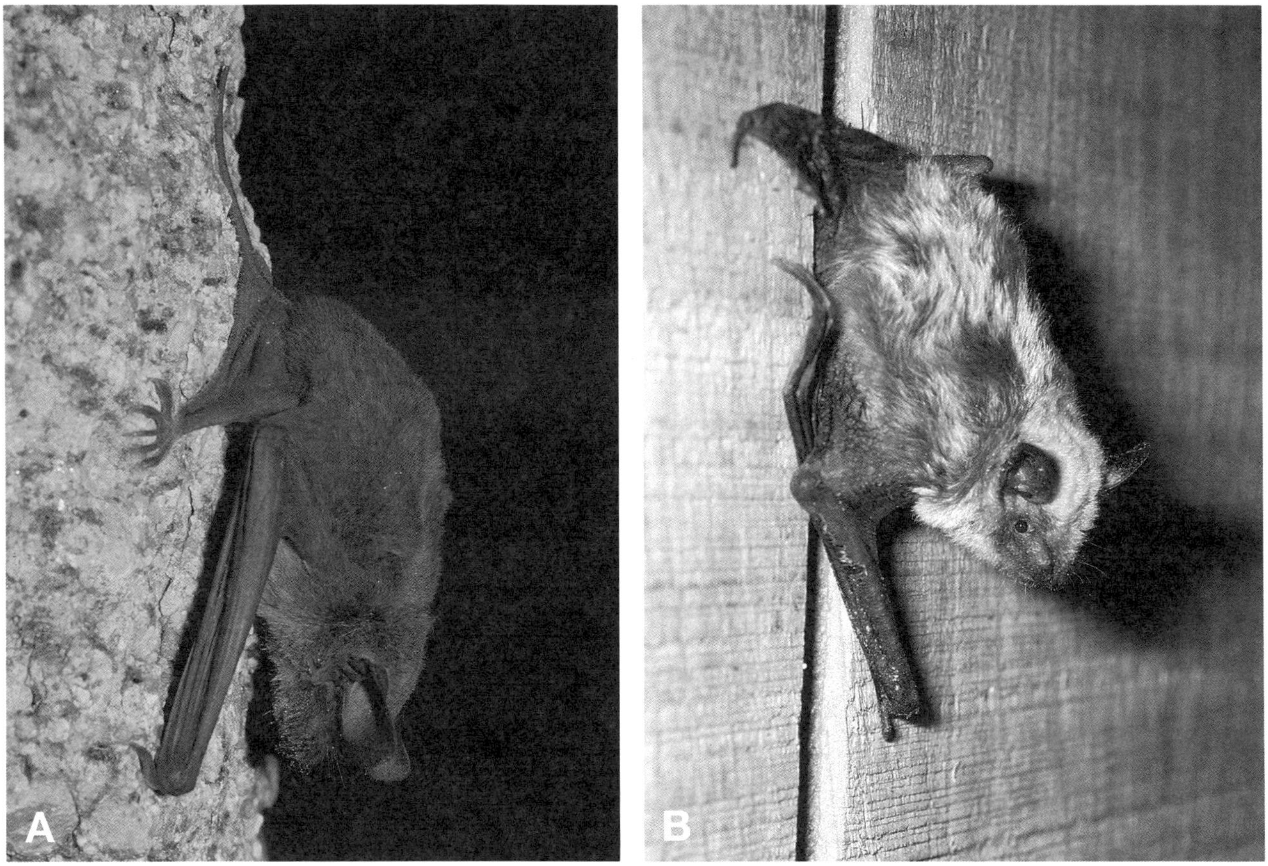

Figure 11-5. Among the colonial bats, those most commonly reported rabid include A) the Mexican free-tailed bat and B) the big brown bat. Photos © Randall D. Babb.

lance) provide yet another means of sampling bat populations. Bats presented to diagnostic laboratories for rabies testing include specimens that are dead, moribund, found in association with a human dwelling, or those which have physically interacted with a person or pet. Clearly, these specimens also do not represent a randomly selected sample of the population, debilitated bats encountered by humans generally considered as being in a higher risk group for rabies infection.

Furthermore, not all bats submitted to rabies diagnostic laboratories are necessarily tested. Some facilities, for example, will test only those specimens for which there is a history of human exposure (Girard et al, 1965; Constantine et al, 1979; Steece et al, 1982). Such bats are much more likely to be rabid than randomly captured specimens and, while economic justifications may certainly validate such an approach to testing, the inherent bias of these reports must be clearly identified before meaningful interpretations can be made.

Finally, there has been a longstanding failure of many laboratories to accurately identify submitted bat specimens (Kurta, 1979; Wampler II and Kirkland, Jr., 1981). These laboratories have merely reported that so many bats are positive or negative for rabies virus, but without speciating them. This has probably been a reflection of limited interest and training of laboratory personnel. In the absence of species-specific data, however, it has been difficult to define precise parameters in our approach to understanding the role of bats in rabies epidemiology. Fortunately, this trend in laboratories is changing and many more have begun to speciate submitted specimens.

Species-specific data may still be prejudiced, especially with respect to population density and distribution of individual bat species. Thus, it is not altogether unusual to find that the most commonly reported rabid species are also among the most predominant (and, hence, easily collected)

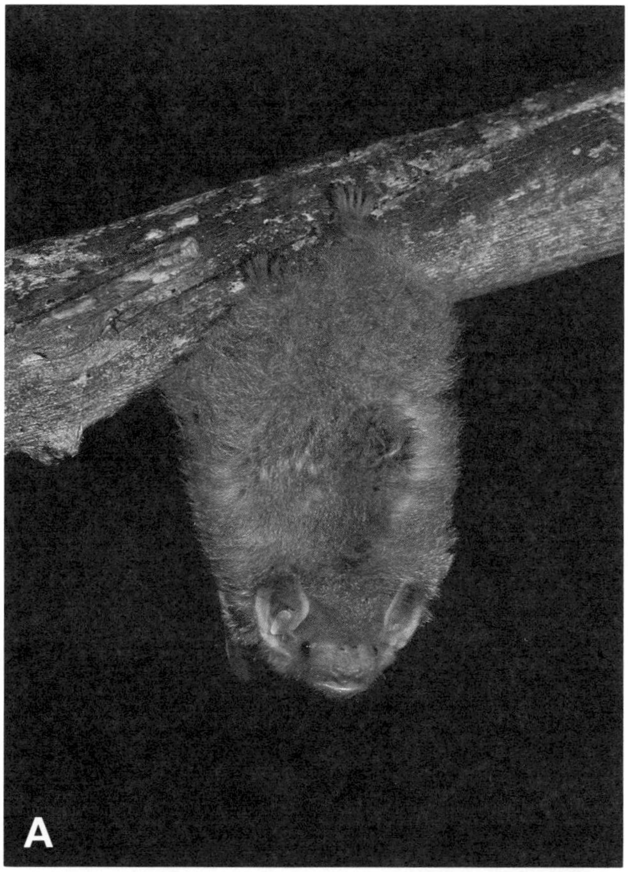

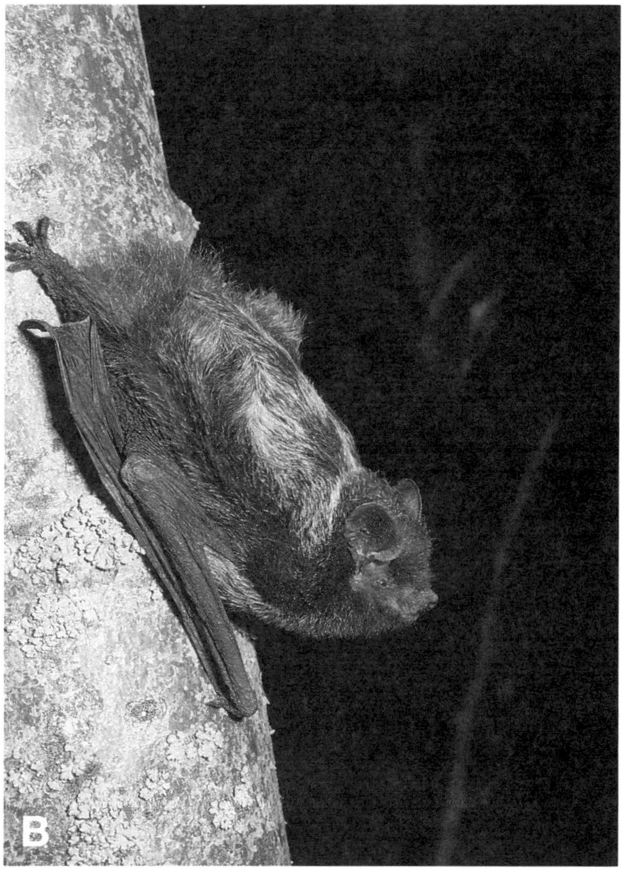

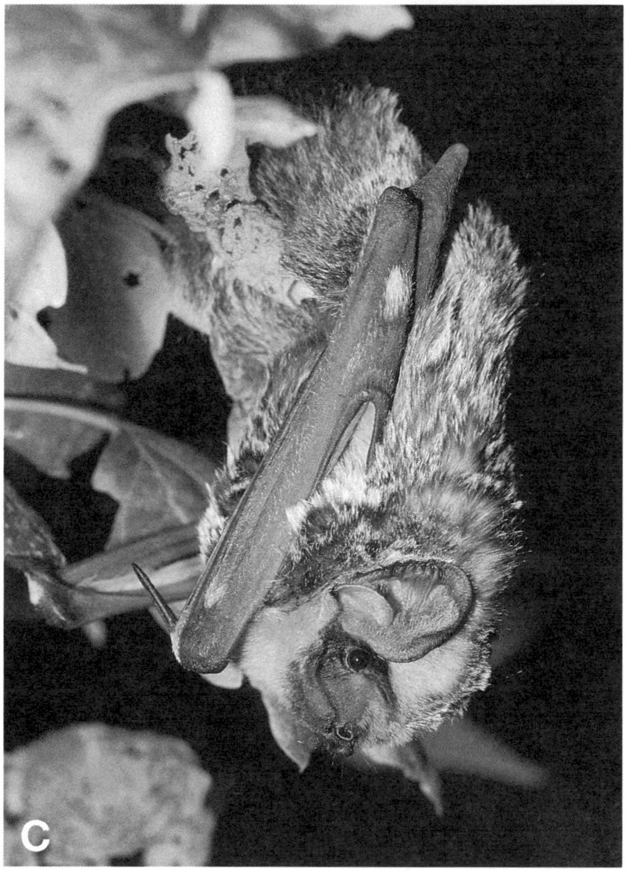

Figure 11-6. Among the solitary bats, those most commonly reported rabid include A) the red bat, B) the silver-haired bat, and C) the hoary bat. These are migratory species that typically roost singly or in small groups in trees, shrubs, or under loose bark. They are less commonly encountered by man than colonial species. Because of sampling biases inherent in surveillance studies, the reported prevalence of infection in suspect submissions is relatively high. Due principally to sampling difficulties, no good estimates of overall disease prevalence in wild populations of solitary bats exist, although they are believed to be low.

Photo credits: Red bat, Laura Riley © Bruce Coleman, Inc., N.Y.; Silver-haired bat, Edgar T. Jones © Bruce Coleman, Inc., N.Y.; Hoary bat, © Randall D. Babb.

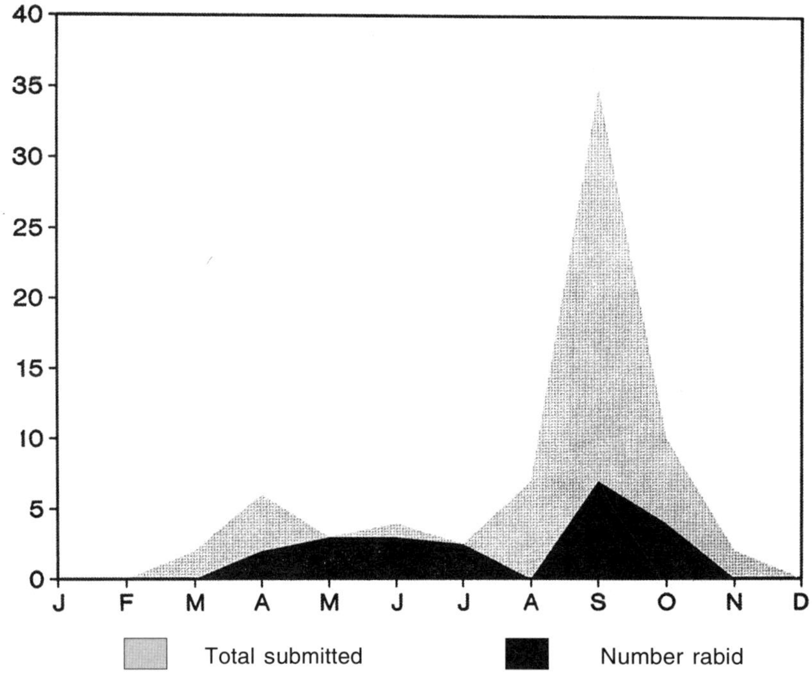

Figure 11-7. Mexican free-tailed bats submitted and those found rabid in New Mexico, by month, 1958-1964. (From Baer, G. M. and J. S. Smith. Rabies in Nonhematophagous Bats. In G. M. Baer (ed.) *The Natural History of Rabies.* 2nd Edition. © CRC Press, Inc. Boca Raton, Florida, 1991. Reproduced with permission.) Original data from Constantine, D. G. *Pub. Hlth. Repts.* 82(10): 867, 1967

in the area, while the highest prevalence of rabies may occur among the more rarely encountered species. A good correlation between reported and actual disease prevalence may not exist. There is, perhaps, little that can be done to completely eliminate these problems. However, recognition of the limitations inherent in sampling studies is important. Sampling biases notwithstanding, "random" collection of healthy-appearing individuals must serve as our first and best approximation of disease prevalence in natural populations.

Prevalence of Rabies in Colonial versus Solitary Species

The colonial bats congregate en masse in various protected areas, such as in caves, under bridges, or within buildings. They are more common than solitary species and relatively easily collected. They may be local residents at their roosts or migratory in nature. Solitary species, on the other hand, are usually found alone (or with a few others of the same species). They live in wooded areas and are often found in trees or shrubs. They are typically migratory, relatively uncommon, and difficult to capture.

In view of the suggested mechanisms whereby rabies is thought to cycle through bat populations, it would seem likely that prevalence would be higher among the colonial species of bats. Unfortunately, due to the very different habits of colonial and solitary bats and the inherent difficulty in sampling from populations of solitary species, this issue has not been thoroughly assessed.

In terms of absolute numbers, more cases of rabies are diagnosed annually in colonial species. Since colonial bats are oftentimes found in close association with human populations and because sampling from a large colony is relatively easy, more colonial species are tested annually. Therefore, a greater number of rabid colonial bats is not an unexpected finding. Among colonial species, those most commonly reported infected include the Mexican free-tailed bat and the big brown bat (Figure 11-5).

Although rabies is diagnosed more commonly

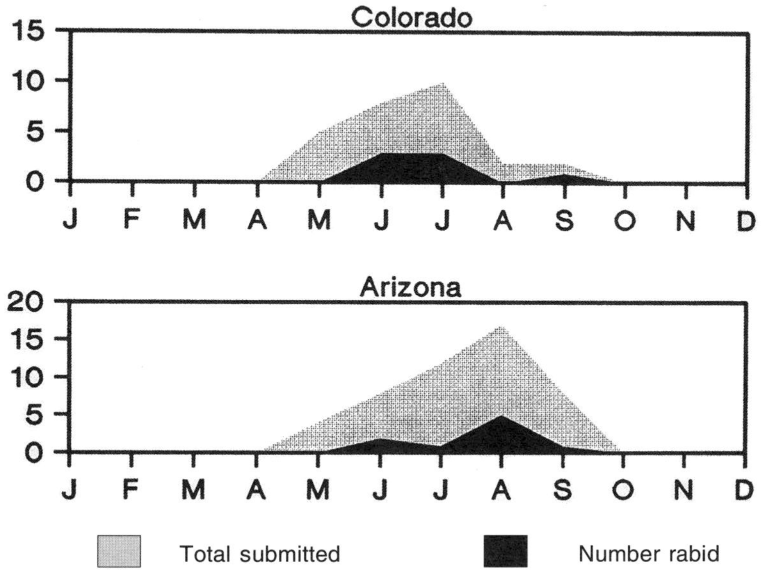

Figure 11-8. Big brown bats submitted and those found rabid in Colorado and Arizona, by month, 1959-1963. (From Baer, G. M. and J. S. Smith. Rabies in Nonhematophagous Bats. In G. M. Baer (ed.) *The Natural History of Rabies*. 2nd Edition. © CRC Press, Inc. Boca Raton, Florida, 1991. Reproduced with permission.) Original data from Constantine, D. G. *Pub. Hlth. Repts.* 82(10): 867, 1967

among colonial bats, the actual percentage of rabies-positive specimens is generally greater among solitary species. This probably reflects the relative rarity of human encounters with healthy solitary bats. Unlike their colonial counterparts, detection and capture of healthy solitary bats is difficult (Daniels et al, 1960; Trimarchi, 1978; Wampler, II and Kirkland, Jr., 1981). The sampling bias built into the collection of solitary species accounts for an apparent higher prevalence of infection. No good estimates really exist of rabies prevalence in wild populations of solitary bats. Solitary bats most commonly reported infected include the red bat (*Lasiurus borealis*), silver-haired bat, and hoary bat (Figure 11-6). These are also the most common of the arboreal solitary bats.

The best estimates of rabies prevalence in randomly collected individuals from a given wild population of colonial species has been obtained from sampling Mexican free-tailed bats captured during emergence flights from caves. Results of large-scale survey studies have shown that generally less than 1% of apparently healthy bats are infected with rabies (Constantine, 1967; Constantine et al, 1968b). A slightly higher prevalence (as much as 2% to 3%) has been found during migration and may be related to the stresses imposed by migratory activity (Constantine, 1967; Constantine et al, 1968b; Burnett, 1989). Similar findings have been reported in migratory Lasiurine bats as well. Extensive sampling studies of healthy-appearing big brown bats have revealed a higher prevalence (1.6% to 4.1%) than expected in a nonmigratory colonial species (Dean et al, 1960; Schnurrenberger et al, 1964; Girard et al, 1965; Constantine, 1967).

In not accounting for behavioral abnormalities, such as roosting apart from a colony or flying during daylight hours (which may cause rabid bats to be away from their roost during collections and possibly too debilitated to find their way back), random sampling studies may actually underestimate disease prevalence to an unknown degree. Those bats in the early stages of disease incubation may also test falsely negative.

Mexican free-tailed bats are most commonly reported rabid between April and November (Figure 11-7). Two distinct peaks are believed to be related to their seasonal migration, one in June during their migration to the United States from Mexico and Central America, and a second in September when they fly south (Constantine, 1967; Constantine et al, 1968b; Baer and Adams,

Table 11-2
Confirmed Cases of Bat Rabies in the United States, by State, 1953-1972

State	1953	1954	1955	1956	1957	1958	1959	1960	1961	1962	1963	1964	1965	1966	1967	1968	1969	1970	1971	1972
Alabama	0	0	0	2	0	0	0	0	2	0	1	0	2	3	3	2	1	6	4	1
Alaska	0	0	0	0	0	0	0	0	0	0	0	0	0	0	0	0	0	0	0	0
Arizona	0	0	0	0	5	0	2	3	6	6	26	17	14	17	16	20	9	13	10	14
Arkansas	0	0	0	0	0	0	0	0	1	0	16	13	7	4	12	5	4	4	8	7
California	0	1	2	4	2	8	18	12	34	28	54	53	71	54	41	50	45	55	106	94
Colorado	0	0	0	0	2	0	5	4	3	4*	12	8	10	13	10	8	31	23	18	14
Connecticut	0	0	0	0	0	0	1	0	0	0	0	0	2	0	0	1*	12*	4*	17*	7*
Delaware	0	0	0	0	0	0	0	0	0	0	2*	0	0	0	0	1*	0	0	4*	7*
Dist. Columbia	0	0	0	0	0	0	0	0	0	0	0	0	0	0	2	3*	0	0	0	0
Florida	8	3	9	11	7	7	7	4	7	14	12	45	38	21	14	18	21	9	17	20
Georgia	0	0	0	6	1	2	1	1	2	5	3	2	15	16	27	13	5	7	9	4
Hawaii	0	0	0	0	0	0	0	0	0	0	0	0	0	0	0	0	0	0	0	0
Idaho	0	0	0	0	0	0	0	0	0	1	3*	2*	15*	7*	3	3	3*	4*	4*	1*
Illinois	0	0	0	0	0	0	2	0	0	1	2	1	13	6	2	2	2	2	8	7
Indiana	0	0	0	0	0	0	0	2	0	0	0	0	2	10	25	10	3	16	7	3
Iowa	0	0	0	0	0	0	0	2	2	2	3	0	6	3	7	4	8	5	8	5
Kansas	0	0	0	0	0	0	0	1	0	0	0	0	5	8	2	2	0	1	2	12
Kentucky	0	0	0	0	0	0	0	0	2	1	3	0	2	0	3	5	1	3	2	5
Louisiana	0	0	1	0	0	0	0	0	0	1	1	1	5	4	16	2	4	5	1	10
Maine	0	0	0	0	0	0	0	0	0	0	0	4	1	0	0	1	0	1	4	4
Maryland	0	0	0	0	0	0	1	0	3	0	2*	1	22	5	5*	4	3*	3*	3*	19
Massachusetts	0	0	0	0	0	0	0	0	1*	3*	6*	1*	3*	4*	5*	6*	3*	4*	6*	6*
Michigan	0	0	0	1	1	0	1	1	2	4	3	4	3	4	3	5	5	4	9	6
Minnesota	0	0	0	1	0	0	0	0	3	3	1	0	4	2	5	4	7	2	9	7
Mississippi	0	0	0	0	0	0	0	0	0	0	0	67*	42*	22*	11*	7*	6*	3*	5*	4*
Missouri	0	0	0	0	0	0	0	2	6	0	3	1	2	3	2	2	1	2	5	6
Montana	0	1	4	0	3	2	9	3	1	1*	1*	8	4	1	5	5	5	2	2	2
Nebraska	0	0	0	0	0	2	2	1	0	0	0	0	0	1	1	1	0	1	0	2
Nevada	0	0	0	0	0	0	0	0	0	0	11*	14	0	10*	9	2*	13*	11*	2	2*
New Hampshire	0	0	0	0	0	0	0	0	0	0	1	1*	1	4	4	1	0	1	3	4*
New Jersey	0	0	0	0	0	0	0	1	7	9	16*	18*	21*	22	21*	14*	16*	11*	19	21*
New Mexico	0	0	1	0	3	3	3	0	1	1	18	2	10	4	2	7	5	6	1	9
New York	0	0	0	1	0	2	2	2	14	8	8	11	14	12	16	8	10	12	29	20
North Carolina	0	0	0	0	0	0	0	0	0	0	9	2	2	3	2	8	1	2	5*	4*
North Dakota	0	0	0	0	0	0	0	0	0	0	0	0	1	0	1	0	0	0	2	1
Ohio	0	0	0	2	0	1	3	1	4	3	4	5	6	9	7	2	8	6	6	2
Oklahoma	0	0	0	2	1	0	0	0	1	1	1	1	36	13	31	6	3	1	6	6
Oregon	0	0	0	0	0	0	0	7	14	17	15	10	8	4	2	6*	4*	4*	9*	4*
Pennsylvania	1	0	0	0	0	1	0	0	8	1	3	6	5	1	5	5	7	4*	10	18
Puerto Rico	0	0	0	0	0	0	0	0	0	0	0	0	0	0	0	0	0	0	0	0
Rhode Island	0	0	0	0	0	0	0	0	0	0	0	0	0	0	2*	0	0	3*	1*	2*
South Carolina	0	0	0	0	0	0	0	0	0	0	5	2*	2	1*	2*	0	0	0	20*	12
South Dakota	0	0	0	0	0	0	0	0	1	0	0	0	1	0	0	1	1	3	4	4
Tennessee	0	0	0	0	0	0	0	0	2	3	5	13	30	26	18	10	8	10	9	20
Texas	0	2	1	11	4	42	24	22	45	31	22	20	29	36	54	14	44	24	38	63
Utah	0	0	0	1	0	0	0	0	7	0	2	1	2*	3*	3*	2	4	2*	7	9*
Vermont	0	0	0	0	0	0	0	0	0	0	0	1	0	1	6	2	0	1	4	1
Virginia	0	0	0	0	0	0	2	0	0	2	4	2	3	3	4	9	5	2	1	17
Washington	0	0	0	0	0	0	0	0	5*	0	20*	6*	22*	15*	2*	2*	4	7	5	9*
West Virginia	0	0	0	0	0	0	1	0	0	1	0	3	1	1	1	1	5	1	1	1
Wisconsin	0	0	0	0	6	3	1	0	2	6	5	6	1	1	2	7	4	4	11	8
Wyoming	0	0	0	0	0	0	0	0	0	0	0	0	1	0	0	0	0	2	4	0
Annual Total	9	7	18	42	35	73	85	69	186	157	303	352	484	377	414	291	321	296	465	504

*Indicates that bats were the only animal reported rabid in the state during that year.

Table 11-2 (Cont'd)
Confirmed Cases of Bat Rabies in the United States, by State, 1973-1992

State	1973	1974	1975	1976	1977	1978	1979	1980	1981	1982	1983	1984	1985	1986	1987	1988	1989	1990	1991	1992
Alabama	2	3	4	7	2	4	14	8	33	66	30	43	27	45	21	19	19	8	15	17
Alaska	0	0	0	0	0	0	0	0	0	0	0	0	0	0	0	0	0	0	0	0
Arizona	11	23	19	17	22	14	17	19	21	32	19	31	29	28	22	0	22	25	32	31
Arkansas	7	5	14	15	10	6	14	11	18	19	16	16	13	14	2	0	9	9	12	9
California	141	108	99	128	166	114	142	151	142	198	148	211	136	135	116	129	117	105	106	104
Colorado	6	20	26	37	56*	37*	51*	51*	38	47*	36*	44*	25	30	30	27	33	23*	27	24
Connecticut	5*	6	8*	2	8*	6	2*	10*	6*	5*	6*	8*	7*	2*	3*	8*	3*	3*	7	7
Delaware	6*	1*	6*	22*	2*	3*	2*	4*	3*	2*	5	5	1*	1*	1	8	9	0	2	0
Dist. Columbia	0	0	0	0	0	0	0	0	0	0	1	0	1	0	0	0	0	0	0	0
Florida	10	5	2	38	16	8	10	0	17	18	69	48	21	34	22	32	32	19	14	16
Georgia	6	10	7	6	12	16	19	16	25	13	22	5	10	17	13	6	5	8	6	9
Hawaii	0	0	0	0	0	0	0	0	0	0	0	0	0	0	0	0	0	0	1*	0
Idaho	1*	3*	0	8*	4*	6	0	2*	7*	11*	17*	11	10*	9*	10*	11	11*	7*	5	6
Illinois	7	20	15	7	11	17	10	20	12	26	38	16	23	9	12	11	16	11	11	27
Indiana	4	2	6	5	3	4	6	6	27	10	7	8	11	5	12	8	16	12	29*	19*
Iowa	3	0	7	2	2	2	8	7	25	7	5	8	17	6	12	5	4	11	7	3
Kansas	3	4	0	9	0	2	6	6	6	7	3	3	4	6	3	3	3	5	6	5
Kentucky	4	1	3	4	0	2	2	11	18	9	5	7	9	8	2	2	2	4	4	5
Louisiana	3	4	4	3	5	2	7	3	14	10	7	15	10	4	1	4	7	1	1	4
Maine	1	1	1	1	4	3	4	3	0	3	7	0	1*	1*	3*	0	2*	1*	4	1*
Maryland	14	26	15*	39	16*	20	39*	37*	34	17	43	46	34	27	18	21	26	14	13	17
Massachusetts	6	4*	11	26*	10*	7*	9*	14	10	9*	15	14*	14	8*	5*	3*	5*	10*	12	15
Michigan	9	5	5	6	5	6	1	7	11	2	17	20	17	18	24	21	24	46	32	10
Minnesota	4	10	10	7	9	3	3	5	4	9	9	8	5	5	3	7	9	17	14	3
Mississippi	1*	3*	1*	2*	1*	6*	7*	4*	4*	13*	9*	15*	10*	9*	9*	9*	4*	3*	4*	1*
Missouri	0	8	6	6	4	4	7	8	8	10	11	13	20	10	15	12	22	12	15	28
Montana	4	1	6	10	11	11	14	17	27	32	15	0	12	14	14	16	10	16	15	7
Nebraska	3	1	1	3	0	1	0	6	8	2	1	3	1	3	1	4	3	0	4	4
Nevada	4*	4*	5	17*	7*	7*	6*	1*	6*	6*	38*	23*	15*	12	15*	20	9*	17	11*	16
New Hampshire	7	2	2*	1*	2*	3*	5*	6*	6*	1*	3	16	1*	1*	0	3	2*	2	4*	6
New Jersey	18*	22	22	27*	28*	14*	12*	18*	24*	16*	24*	35*	38*	17*	18*	15	26	9	11	14
New Mexico	5	30	18	8	14	10	13	15	18	13	7	2	9	3	3*	4	4	7	5	5
New York	17	17	26	24	33	39	34	39	41	41	29	72	43	46	48	38	54*	84	79	61
North Carolina	14*	26*	11	15	14*	16	25	18*	18*	38	17	25	12*	10*	8*	3	7	6	10	13
North Dakota	1	3	0	0	4	3	0	2	4	2	0	1	2	0	1	1	3	0	1	0
Ohio	3	5	8	23	9	11	13	10	13	14	25	17	15	12	11	6*	10	8	15	10
Oklahoma	4	3	4	5	5	1	8	4	4	6	3	4	6	5	4	0	6	1	5	5
Oregon	8*	5	6*	11*	16*	13	16	4*	11	5*	3*	6	6*	5*	5*	6*	5	1*	4	2*
Pennsylvania	18	16	16	24	14	21	16	19*	7	25	33	35	44	17	16	11	25	19	14	6
Puerto Rico	0	0	0	0	0	0	0	0	0	0	0	0	0	0	0	0	0	0	0	0
Rhode Island	1*	4*	4*	5	0	0	2*	1*	2*	0	0	0	0	2	2*	0	1*	0	0	1*
South Carolina	5	6*	8	2	16	26	19	15	14	13	9	17	11	15	4	9	9	4	7	10
South Dakota	1	2	0	1	2	2	2	1	4	1	4	1	6	0	3	3	1	6	2	1
Tennessee	5	7	6	11	6	7	8	11	16	16	5	13	10	14	7	10	9	6	5	6
Texas	21	76	68	71	51	46	115	95	79	120	88	118	99	132	66	57	72	45	59	69
Utah	3*	1*	3*	21	10	6	10	10*	11	18*	10	6*	4*	6*	7*	10*	9*	15	16	6*
Vermont	0	1*	0	0	0	1	1*	0	0	2*	2*	0	1*	2*	0	0	1*	0	1*	1
Virginia	14	16	5	23	3	8	10	7	8	9	17	11	16	2	6	11	14	6	8	12
Washington	10*	2*	10	13	6	5*	20	3*	15*	8*	10*	3*	5*	8	10	4*	9*	4*	9*	6
West Virginia	3	5	0	3	5	10	1	3	1	10	7	6	0	4	4	7	5	5	6	6
Wisconsin	9	9	7	11	5	10	9	9	12	11	5	12	13	10	7	3	4	12	7	11
Wyoming	0	8	9	11	8	10	7	9	26	25	10*	17	6	17	10	13	22	6	12	8
Annual Total	432	544	514	737	637	567	756	726	858	975	910	1038	830	788	629	600	720	637	690	647

Data compiled from Annual Rabies Surveillance Reports. Centers for Disease Control, U. S. Department of Health and Human Services, Public Health Service. Atlanta, Georgia.

Table 11-3

Confirmed Cases of Wildlife Rabies in the United States, by Animal, as a Percentage of the Total Number of Wildlife Cases, 1961-1992

	Year															
Animal	**1961**	**1962**	**1963**	**1964**	**1965**	**1966**	**1967**	**1968**	**1969**	**1970**	**1971**	**1972**	**1973**	**1974**	**1975**	**1976**
Raccoon	2.7	2.7	6.2	4.9	3.0	4.5	4.5	5.7	9.5	7.1	5.5	4.8	3.9	6.9	8.6	10.2
Bat	8.5	6.8	11.6	9.9	14.9	12.8	12.9	10.8	12.0	11.6	13.5	14.6	14.7	21.6	22.9	27.1
Fox	28.2	25.7	23.8	29.8	31.9	29.3	30.5	29.6	33.2	30.2	19.5	18.5	16.1	11.9	12.4	6.9
Skunk	57.5	62.6	55.9	53.6	48.6	51.7	48.8	51.8	43.3	48.4	58.5	60.5	63.2	56.8	54.7	53.9

	Year															
Animal	**1977**	**1978**	**1979**	**1980**	**1981**	**1982**	**1983**	**1984**	**1985**	**1986**	**1987**	**1988**	**1989**	**1990**	**1991**	**1992**
Raccoon	10.3	14.3	12.0	7.1	7.9	20.9	36.0	35.2	29.1	28.4	31.4	35.1	36.6	42.1	48.5	54.5
Bat	23.3	20.1	16.8	13.1	14.0	17.6	17.2	20.1	16.2	14.2	15.1	15.3	17.0	14.7	10.9	8.2
Fox	4.5	5.2	3.2	3.9	3.2	4.0	2.1	2.7	3.5	3.7	2.9	4.4	4.9	4.6	5.0	5.0
Skunk	59.6	58.7	67.2	74.2	73.1	55.8	43.2	40.2	49.1	42.9	48.8	42.9	39.2	36.5	32.6	29.5

Data compiled from *Annual Rabies Surveillance Reports*. Centers for Disease Control, U. S. Department of Health and Human Services, Public Health Service. Atlanta, Georgia.

1970). In the big brown bat, a nonmigratory, colonial species that hibernates from November through March, most rabid specimens are reported from June to August, when they are most commonly encountered (Figure 11-8). However, suspect submissions may be submitted throughout the year in some regions (Evans, 1987).

Rabies prevalence in suspect specimens submitted to diagnostic laboratories for testing is somewhat higher, as much as 4% to 10% (Wiseman et al, 1962; Richardson et al, 1966; Birney and Rising, 1967; Whitaker and Miller, 1974; Trimarchi and Debbie, 1977; Girard, 1978; Kurta, 1979; Schowalter, 1980; Steece et al, 1982; Pybus, 1986; Burnett, 1989; Trimarchi, 1980, 1991, 1992, 1993). An even higher prevalence is sometimes reported in suspect submissions. However, these are usually associated with small sample sizes. Actual prevalence in wild populations may vary from time to time, species to species, and region to region. In selecting for unhealthy individuals, sampling of submission suspects certainly overestimates disease prevalence in the entire wild population.

Since the early reports of rabid insectivorous bats in the United States, the reported number of rabies-positive specimens has dramatically increased. The percentage of positive bats, however, has remained essentially unchanged. Rabies in bat populations is not on the rise. The reported increases from year to year are actually artifacts of the reporting system. The number of bats collected and tested for rabies, and consequently the number of rabies-positive findings, is a manifestation of both public interest and human population density. The publicity associated with bat rabies leads to heightened public interest, more widespread testing, and, inevitably, to the finding of more positive bats (Constantine, 1967, 1971, 1988; Baer and Adams, 1970; Bigler et al, 1975; Lewis, 1972; Dorward et al, 1977; Kurta, 1979; Wampler, II and Kirkland, Jr., 1981; Steece et al, 1982; Trimarchi, 1980, 1983; Baer, 1983; Rosatte, 1985).

In its annual rabies surveillance reports, the Centers for Disease Control summarizes the number of cases of rabies in the United States, by species and state. Table 11-2 shows the number of reported cases of rabies in bats, by state, since 1953. Starred (*) numbers indicate that bats were the only species found to be positive for rabies in the state during that year. Table 11-3 shows the percentage of rabies in wildlife accounted for by bats for the same time frame.

In depending upon individual states to submit data, passive surveillance studies may underestimate the number of rabid individuals. Without a knowledge of the total number of bats tested or the circumstances leading to their having been tested, these numbers are of limited value, representing dangling numerators.

Biased Perspectives

Although different perspectives are emphasized by various sampling techniques, all sampling studies help to increase our understanding of the extent and significance of bat rabies. In fact, if we are to fully assess their relationship to public health, it is imperative that we consider data from both randomly collected as well as laboratory-submitted specimens.

It is not uncommon that when spokesmen for bat rabies address the general public, only one or another type of study is emphasized. Conservationists, for example, may point to results generated by random collection techniques. They argue that the low incidence of naturally occurring infection and the small number of confirmed human deaths attributed to rabies of insectivorous-bat origin (19 in the United States, three in Canada, two in the former Soviet Union, and one each in Finland, India, and South Africa)[2] are indicative of its relative unimportance to public health. Furthermore, concern is sometimes voiced that many epidemiological investigations have little credibility (Taylor, Jr., 1987; Valega, 1992).

On the other hand, alarmists seeking to mount anti-bat campaigns may stress the higher prevalence of infection evident in laboratory-submitted specimens. Moreover, rather than consider bat-related human deaths from rabies on an absolute basis, they may emphasize the fact that a large percentage of all human deaths from rabies acquired in the United States in the last decade (75% between 1980 and 1990) has been bat related. These latter views have been alarmingly emphasized by tabloid journalism and other forms of irresponsible media sensationalism bent solely on eliciting fear and hysteria.

Be that as it may, each interpretation has merit, but each suffers from fallacies as well. While the true significance clearly lies somewhere between extremes of thought, it is not unusual that the full spectrum of data gets lost in a bid to propagate a singular point of view.

Species-Associated Geographic Distribution of Bat Rabies

Disease may be maintained enzootically only within certain species of bats, notably the red bat, hoary bat, big brown bat, Mexican free-tailed bat, and possibly the silver-haired bat and Florida yellow bat. Other species, such as members of the genus *Myotis* (which are reported rabid less frequently), may be infected by occasional spillover of virus from one of the major Chiropteran hosts (see page 192).

In the United States, confirmed reports of rabies in different bat species vary with geographic locale, although rabies-positive bats of migratory species are found throughout their range, which may extend for thousands of miles. The red bat is most commonly reported infected in southeastern and mid-Atlantic states. The silver-haired bat may be regionally important in the Pacific Northwest, the seminole bat in the Southeast, and the yellow bat in Florida. The hoary bat and big brown bat are most commonly reported rabid in Rocky Mountain, plains, and north-central states, and the Mexican free-tailed bat in the Southwest. In the Northeast, the big brown bat is the most commonly reported rabid bat species (Baer and Smith, 1991; Trimarchi, 1991, 1992, 1993, 1994).

[2]In using the number 19, this does not include one confirmed case of rabies in a six-year-old boy who was bitten on his thumb while asleep in bed by a bat subsequently confirmed to be rabid. He is one of the few human victims of rabies who have survived the disease (see page 35). It does include the case of a 37-year-old woman who died of rabies contracted through a corneal transplant from a donor who had died of rabies of bat origin (see page 234).

References

Baer, G. M. (1983). The Role of Wild Animals in Urban Rabies. *Animal Health in the Americas, 1983*. Proceedings of the III Inter-Agency Meeting, at the Ministerial Level, on Animal Health. Pan American Health Organization. Scientific Publication No. 476, p. 114. Washington, D. C. April 11-14, 1983

Baer, G. M. and D. B. Adams (1970). Rabies in insectivorous bats in the United States, 1953 - 1965. *Pub. Hlth. Repts.* 85(7): 637

Baer, G. M. and J. S. Smith (1991). Rabies in Nonhematophagous Bats. In G. M. Baer (ed.) *The Natural History of Rabies*. 2nd Edition. CRC Press, Inc. Boca Raton, Florida

Beauregard, M. (1969). Bat rabies in Canada 1963-1967. *Can. J. Comp. Med.* 33: 220

Bek, M. D., Smith, W. T., Levy, M. H., Sullivan, E., and G. L. Rubin (1992). Rabies case in New South Wales, 1990: Public health aspects. *Med. J. Australia.* 156(9): 596

Bigler, W. J., Hoff, G. L., and E. E. Buff (1975). Chiropteran rabies in Florida: A twenty-year analysis, 1954 to 1973. *Am. J. Trop. Med. Hyg.* 24(2): 347

Birney, E. C. and J. D. Rising (1967). Notes on distribution and reproduction of some bats from Kansas, with remarks on incidence of rabies. *Kansas Acad. Sci.* 70(4): 519

Brass, D. A. (1991). Some aspects of rabies surveillance in bats. *NSS (Natl. Speleol. Soc.) News.* 49(2): 53

Brosset, A. (1990). Les migrations de la pipistrelle de Nathusius, *Pipistrellus nathusii*, en France. Ses incidences possibles sur la propagation de la rage. *Mammalia.* 54(2): 207

Bucens, M. and L. O'Connor (1988). Rabies—It can happen here. *Med. J. Australia.* 149: 576

Burnett, C. D. (1989). Bat rabies in Illinois: 1965 to 1986. *J. Wildl. Dis.* 25(1): 10

Centers for Disease Control (1991). Human Rabies—Texas, Arkansas, and Georgia, 1991. *MMWR.* 40(44): 765

Constantine, D. G. (1967). Bat rabies in the southwestern United States. *Pub. Hlth. Repts.* 82(10): 867

Constantine, D. G. (1979). An updated list of rabies-infected bats in North America. *J. Wildl. Dis.* 15: 347

Constantine, D. G. (1988). Health Precautions for Bat Researchers. In T. H. Kunz (ed.) *Ecological and Behavioral Methods for the Study of Bats.* Smithsonian Institution Press. Washington, D. C.

Constantine, D. G. and D. F. Woodall (1966). Transmission experiments with bat rabies isolates: Reactions of certain carnivora, opossum, rodents, and bats to rabies virus of red bat origin when exposed by bat bite or by intramuscular inoculation. *Am. J. Vet. Res.* 27(116): 24

Constantine, D. G., Solomon, G. C., and D. F. Woodall (1968a). Transmission experiments with bat rabies isolates: Responses of certain carnivores and rodents to rabies viruses from four species of bats. *Am. J. Vet. Res.* 29(1): 181

Constantine, D. G., Tierkel, E. S., Kleckner, M. D., and D. M. Hawkins (1968b). Rabies in New Mexico cavern bats. *Pub. Hlth. Repts.* 83(4): 303

Constantine, D. G., Humphrey, G. L., and T. B. Herbenick (1979). Rabies in *Myotis thysanodes*, *Lasiurus ega*, *Euderma maculatum* and *Eumops perotis* in California. *J. Wildl. Dis.* 15: 343

Daniels, J. B., Stuart, G., Wheeler, R. E., Gifford, C., Ahearn, J. P., Philbrook, F. R., Hayes, R. O., and R. A. MacCready (1960). A search for encephalitis and rabies in bats of eastern Massachusetts. *New Engl. J. Med.* 263(10): 516

Dean, W. D., Maddy, K. T., Cockrum, E. L., and H. G. Crecelius (1960). Rabies in insectivorous bats of Arizona. *Arizona Med.* 17(2): 69

Dorward, W. J., Schowalter, D. B., and J. R. Gunson (1977). Preliminary studies of bat rabies in Alberta. *Can. Vet. J.* 18(12): 341

Dunn, K., Faoagali, J., DeBuse, P., Fraser, D., Stable, R., Patten, B., Martin, D., Laws, L. L., St. George, T., Ramm, R. A., Davison, R. P., and V. Kelk (1988). Imported human rabies—Australia. *MMWR.* 37(22): 351

Evans, C. S. (1987). Demographic Features of Rabid and Rabies Suspect Bats in Virginia. M. S. Thesis. College of Humanities and Sciences. Virginia Commonwealth University. Richmond, Virginia.

Faoagali, J. L., De Buse, P., Strutton, G. M., and H. Samaratunga (1988). A case of rabies. *Med. J. Australia.* 149: 702

Forman, A. J. (1993). The threat of rabies introduction and establishment in Australia. *Aust. Vet. J.* 70(3): 81

Frantz, S. C. (1989). Bat rabies management: New York State's holistic approach. *Fifth International Theriological Congress.* Rome, Italy. August 29, 1989

Girard, K. F. (1978). Letter to the editor. *New Engl. J. Med.* 288(16): 915

Girard, K. F., Hitchcock, H. B., Edsall, G., and R. A. MacCready (1965). Rabies in bats in southern New England. *New Engl. J. Med.* 272(2): 75

Glass, B. P. (1959). Recovery of rabies virus from the Mexican freetail bat in Oklahoma. *Proc. Oklahoma Acad. Sci.* 39: 83

Grattan-Smith, P. J., O'Regan, W. J., Ellis, P. S. J., O'Flaherty, S. J., McIntyre, P. B., and C. L. Barnes (1992). Rabies—A second Australian case, with a long incubation period. *Med. J. Australia.* 156: 651

Hill, Jr., R. E. and G. W. Beran (1992). Experimental inoculation of raccoons (*Procyon lotor*) with rabies virus of skunk origin. *J. Wildl. Dis.* 28(1): 51

Humphrey, G. L., Kemp, G. E., and E. G. Wood (1960). A fatal case of rabies in a woman bitten by an insectivorous bat. *Pub. Hlth. Repts.* 75(4): 317

Kough, R. H. (1954). Attack on a human being by a rabid insectivorous bat. *J. Am. Med. Assoc.* 155(5): 441

Krebs, J. W., Strine, T. W., and J. E. Childs (1993). Rabies surveillance in the United States during 1992. *J. Am. Vet. Med. Assoc.* 203(12): 1718

Kurta, A. (1979). Bat rabies in Michigan. *Michigan Academician.* XII(2): 221

Lennette, E. H., Soave, O. A., Kakamura, K., and G. H. Kellogg, Jr. (1960). A fatal human case of rabies following the bite of a rabid bat (*Lasionycteris noctivagans*). Isolation and identification of the virus from vector and victim. *J. Lab. Clin. Med.* 55(1): 89

Lewis, J. C. (1972). Factors influencing reports of rabid animals in Oklahoma. *J. Wildl. Dis.* 8: 245

Maddy, K. T., Cockrum, E. L., and H. G. Crecelius (1958). Bat rabies in Arizona. *Arizona Med.* 15(5): 344

Martin, R. L. (1959). A history of chiropteran rabies with special reference to occurrence and importance in the United States. *Wildl. Dis.* (No. 3): 1

Parker, R. L. (1969). Epidemiology of rabies. *Arch. Environ. Hlth.* 19: 857

Pool, G. E. and C. S. Hacker (1982). Geographic and seasonal distribution of rabies in skunks, foxes, and bats in Texas. *J. Wildl. Dis.* 18(4): 405

Pybus, M. J. (1986). Rabies in insectivorous bats of western Canada, 1979-1983. *J. Wildl. Dis.* 22(3): 307

Richardson, J. H., Ramsey, R. L., and L. E. Star (1966). Bat rabies in Georgia, 1956-1965. *Pub. Hlth. Repts.* 81: 1031

Rosatte, R. C. (1985). Bat rabies in Alberta 1979-1982. *Can. Vet. J.* 26: 81

Roueche, B. (1980). The Incurable Wound. In *The Medical Detectives.* Times Books. New York.

Rupprecht, C. E., Dietzschold, B., Wunner, W. H., and H. Koprowski (1991). Antigenic Relationships of Lyssavirus. In G. M. Baer (ed.) *The Natural History of Rabies.* 2nd Edition. CRC Press, Inc. Boca Raton, Florida.

Sasaki, D. M., Middleton, C. R., Sawa, T. R., Christensen, C. C., and G. Y. Kobayashi (1992). Rabid bat diagnosed in Hawaii. *Hawaii Med. J.* 51(7): 181

Scatterday, J. E. (1954). Bat rabies in Florida. *J. Am. Vet. Med. Assoc.* 12: 125

Scatterday, J. E. and M. M. Galton (1954). Bat rabies in Florida. *Vet. Med.* 49: 133

Schnurrenberger, P. R., Beck, J. R., and F. Burson (1964). Bat rabies. A discussion of problems existing in Ohio. *Ohio State Med. J.* 60(4): 361

Schowalter, D. B. (1980). Characteristics of bat rabies in Alberta. *Can. J. Comp. Med.* 44: 70

Sikes, R. K. (1962). Pathogenesis of rabies in wildlife. I. Comparative effect of varying doses of rabies virus inoculated into foxes and skunks. *Am. J. Vet. Res.* 23: 1041

Smith, J. S. (1989). Rabies Virus Epitopic Variation: Use in Ecologic Studies. In K. Maramorosch, F. A. Murphy, and A. J. Shatkin (eds.) *Advances in Virus Research.* Vol. 36. Academic Press, Inc. New York.

Smith, J. S. and G. M. Baer (1988). Epizootiology of Rabies: The Americas. In J. B. Campbell and K. M. Charlton (eds.) *Developments in Veterinary Virology—Rabies.* Kluwer Academic Publishers. Boston.

Smith, J. S. and H. D. Seidel (1993). Rabies: A new look at an old disease. *Prog. Med. Virol.* 40: 82

Smith, J. S., Yager, P. A., Bigler, W. J., and E. D. Hartwig, Jr. (1990). Surveillance and epidemiologic mapping of monoclonal antibody-defined rabies variants in Florida. *J. Wildl. Dis.* 26(4): 473

Smith, J. S., Orciari, L. A., Yager, P. A., Seidel, H. D., and C. K. Warner (1992). Epidemiologic and historical relationships among 87 rabies virus isolates as determined by limited sequence analysis. *J. Infect. Dis.* 166: 296

Steece, E. A., Erickson, T. J., Siem, R. A., and E. C. Birney (1982). Chiropteran rabies in Minnesota: 1976-1980. *J. Wildl. Dis.* 18(4): 487

Sulkin, S. E. and M. J. Greve (1954). Human rabies caused by bat bite. *Texas State J. Med.* 50: 620

Taylor, Jr., D. B. (1987). Bats take a bad rap. *The Potomac Caver* (newsletter of the Potomac Speleological Society). 30(3): 13. Reprinted from the newsletter of the Holston Valley Grotto, Tennessee.

Tinline, R. R. (1988). Persistence of Rabies in Wildlife. In J. B. Campbell and K. M. Charlton (eds.) *Rabies.* Kluwer Academic Publishers. Boston.

Trimarchi, C. V. (1978). Rabies in insectivorous temperate-zone bats. *Bat Res. News.* 19(1): 7

Trimarchi, C. V. (1980). Bat rabies in the United States. *Bull. Natl. Speleol. Soc.* 42: 64

Trimarchi, C. V. (1983). The Epidemiology and Control of Bat Rabies in New York State. *Proceedings of the North American Symposium on Wildlife Rabies.* Johns Hopkins University. Baltimore, Maryland. November 7-8, 1983.

Trimarchi, C. V. (1991). *Rabies Annual Summary, 1990.* Rabies Laboratory, Wadsworth Center for Laboratories and Research, New York State Department of Health. Albany, New York.

Trimarchi, C. V. (1992). *Rabies Annual Summary, 1991.* Rabies Laboratory, Wadsworth Center for Laboratories and Research, New York State Department of Health. Albany, New York.

Trimarchi, C. V. (1993). *Rabies Annual Summary, 1992*. Rabies Laboratory, Wadsworth Center for Laboratories and Research, New York State Department of Health. Albany, New York.

Trimarchi, C. V. (1994). *New York State Rabies Annual Summary, 1993*. Wadsworth Center for Laboratories and Research, New York State Department of Health. Albany, New York.

Trimarchi, C. V. and J. G. Debbie (1977). Naturally occurring rabies virus and neutralizing antibody in two species of insectivorous bats of New York State. *J. Wildl. Dis*. 13: 367

Trimarchi, C. V. and J. G. Debbie (1980). Report on the Northeastern Symposium on Bat Rabies Management. In D. E. Wilson and A. F. Gardner (eds.) *Proceedings of the Fifth International Bat Research Conference*. Texas Tech Press. Lubbock, Texas.

Tsiang, H. (1993). Pathophysiology of rabies virus infection of the nervous system. *Advances in Virus Research*. 42: 375

Valega, T. (1992). Caped crusaders. *NSS (Natl. Speleol. Soc.) News*. 50(8): 201

Venters, H. D., Hoffert, W. R., Scatterday, J. E., and A. V. Hardy (1954). Rabies in bats in Florida. *Am. J. Pub. Hlth*. 44: 182

Wampler, II, J. T. and G. L. Kirkland, Jr. (1981). Rabies in Pennsylvania. *Proc. Pennsylvania Acad. Sci*. 55: 47

Whitaker, Jr., J. O. and W. A. Miller (1974). Rabies in bats of Indiana. *Proc. Indiana Acad. Sci*. 83: 469

Witte, E. J. (1954). Bat rabies in Pennsylvania. *Am. J. Pub. Hlth*. 44: 186

World Health Organization (1992). *Expert Committee on Rabies. Eighth Report*. WHO Tech. Rpt. No. 824. Geneva.

Chapter 12: CLINICAL MANIFESTATIONS OF RABIES IN INSECTIVOROUS BATS

Incubation Period

As is true in other species, the incubation period of rabies virus in bats is highly variable. In experimental studies, incubation times between 2 and 25 weeks have been observed following intracerebral or intramuscular inoculation of virus. Moore and Raymond (1970) reported an incubation period of at least 209 days in a naturally infected big brown bat. The authors attributed the onset of viral activity to stress associated with captivity. Serial sampling of saliva for virus prior to onset of clinical signs had not been done. Rarely, incubation times of over one year have been reported (Kaplan, 1969; Trimarchi, 1978). Virus has been detected in saliva for varying periods of time (as much as 12 to 15 days) prior to the onset of clinical signs. Once clinical signs develop, a variety of manifestations may become apparent. No one sign is pathognomonic for rabies.

Lethal versus Nonlethal Cycles of Infection

In the highly gregarious Mexican free-tailed bat, Constantine (1971) described both a lethal and a nonlethal cycle of infection. In the nonlethal form, neither a clinically rabid state nor a salivary carrier state exists. Rather, the bat is believed to develop serum neutralizing antibodies to the rabies virus and survive infection, warding off development of disease. Thus, as is the case for other mammals, not all bats that are exposed to virus will succumb to its deadly effects. Bats may, for example, be exposed, but not infected, or they may become infected, but not ill. In exposed animals, the appearance of serum neutralizing antibodies, in the absence of clinical signs, may be suggestive of an incubating disease or exposure to rabies with subsequent development of immunity.

In the lethal rabies cycle of the Mexican free-tailed bat, clinical signs develop. Onset of disease is generally regarded as being fatal. Clinical signs are predominantly paralytic rather than furious in nature and include irritability or depression, weakness, anorexia, hypothermia, and paralysis (Constantine, 1967a). Although depression may be preceded by a period of belligerence, outright fury is rarely seen. Even though affected bats may attempt to bite nearby objects, they generally make no efforts to attack human observers. In general, they "seem concerned" mainly with their own debilitated state.

Constantine also noted that partially paralyzed and grounded bats may thrash about and squeak, especially when people approached. Squeaking and buzzing of rabid bats have been reported by others, healthy bats generally remaining quiet and motionless (Centers for Disease Control, 1954; Bell et al, 1955; Moore and Raymond, 1970; Schowalter, 1980; Haagsma, 1989). Clinically ill individuals may be thin, dehydrated, and hypothermic. They may often be found roosting alone (Sullivan et al, 1954; Constantine, 1988a).

Disorientation and Abnormalities of Flight

Bats are, by nature, creatures of the night. It is unusual to find them flying in broad daylight. Such activity frequently characterizes rabid individuals. Although all bats should be avoided and not molested, any bat seen active during daylight hours should be left strictly alone. In rabid individuals, flying during daylight may be part of a general disorientation complex. Disorientation of rabid bats may be further indicated by their repeatedly crashing into obstacles (Bell et al, 1957; Constantine, 1967a; Price and Everard, 1977). This may be recognized as a seeming purposelessness of flight and should not be confused with the momentary mid-flight collisions that cave explorers may be familiar with in narrow passageways (see page 311).

It should be noted, however, that a connection between rabies and daytime flying activity is somewhat of a generalization. Several species of bats can normally be found flying in the late afternoon, and many healthy bats will take to the wing during daylight hours if sufficiently disturbed. Speakman (1990) addressed the issue of daylight flying in British bats. Accordingly, he noted that insectivorous species sometimes emerged during daylight hours to both eat and drink, as well as at times when their survival was threatened, such as from overheating of the roost or the unexpected presence of a predator. Ollason et al (1992) observed a day-flying pipistrelle (*Pipistrellus pipistrellus*) in Scotland which they also believed to have been pursuing insects. Daylight flying may have energetic advantages for bats (see review by Speakman, 1991). However, they remain a principally nocturnal group. Speakman (1991) addressed several explanations for their infrequent daylight excursions, including:

1) Inability to dissipate the heat generated during flight in the heat of the afternoon.

2) Direct competition with aerial insectivorous birds.

3) Attack by diurnal avian predators of bats.

4) Attack by nonpredatory birds, including those which are not insectivorous.

Speakman's study suggested that the main reason for bats in Britain not feeding more frequently during the day was related to the increased risks of predation.

Furious versus Paralytic Disease and Provoked versus Unprovoked Attacks

In considering the public-health hazards associated with rabies in insectivorous bats, the nature of their interaction with man is of central importance. Bites from bats may follow from either "provoked" or "unprovoked" attacks. Since healthy bats generally avoid human contact, the impaired neurological status of rabid individuals (paresis or paralysis) or an aberrant behavior may lie at the heart of most bat/human encounters. Consideration of the clinically rabid bat, therefore, is essential to an understanding of their public-health significance.

Of particular interest, especially in regard to unprovoked bat attacks, is the development of a furious form of disease. Furious rabies has been reported in both solitary and colonial species of insectivorous bats that have been experimentally infected by intracerebral inoculation of virus. Ressang et al (1963) reported furious rabies in 4 of 67 fruit bats (flying foxes) in Indonesia that were intramuscularly or intracerebrally infected with virus. Intracerebral infection, however, is an unlikely route of natural infection and dosages received experimentally may be much higher than those obtained during natural infection.

Aggression has been observed in some species of solitary bats when rabid. It is believed that a furious form of rabies may typify infection in certain small, solitary species, such as the California myotis. In this species, the lethal, clinically rabid state may be similar to the furious form of rabies in dogs. According to Constantine (1971), they become furious, attack without provocation, and die with encephalitis. Intraspecific transmission of virus among solitary species may be dependent upon attacks by clinically rabid individuals on others of their kind.

A predominantly paralytic form of rabies, typically lacking in a significant furious phase, is frequently reported as characterizing rabies in colonial species. Furious rabies in various species of colonial bats has occasionally been claimed although, in many instances, reports of furious rabies may reflect excitement of observers (Constantine, 1988b). However, reports of furious rabies in naturally infected big brown bats have been confirmed and unprovoked attacks on humans have been documented (Trimarchi et al, 1979; Schowalter, 1980). Of course, carelessly handling any sick bat (solitary or colonial) is always hazardous. All wild animals, rabid or not, may be expected to bite in self-defense.

Burnett (1989) commented on the possibility that differences in major clinical manifestations of rabies between migratory and nonmigratory species of bats might be related, in part, to the stresses imposed by migration. However, aggressive behavior has been observed in the nonmigratory, colonial big brown bat and the migratory Mexican free-tailed bat is rarely reported to become aggressive when rabid.

The literature on animal rabies is replete with discussion of provoked versus unprovoked attacks. An historical account of provoked or unprovoked bite is often of great epidemiologic significance in medical decision making with respect to the need for administration of post-exposure rabies prophylaxis. Unfortunately, distinction between provoked and unprovoked attacks, particularly in instances of bat exposure, may be difficult to make. Provoked and unprovoked attacks are epidemiologic circumstances without adequate definition. Even in dogs, criteria distinguishing between the two have been considered highly subjective.[1]

Consider, for example, the case of a rabid bat that lands upon the shoulder of a hiker during a midday excursion. Frightened by the sudden appearance of the animal, the hiker attempts to brush the bat off and is bitten in the process. One may argue that the bat landed on the hiker's shoulder because of an increasing disorientation or failing flight capability related to a progressive neurological impairment. It was induced to inflict a bite only after being struck by the hiker's open hand. Thus, it is arguably an example of a provoked bite.

In keeping with the suggestion of disorientation or failing flight ability, however, one may also argue that the nature of the disease was responsible for placing the bat on the hiker's shoulder in the first place. From this perspective, the incident cannot be regarded as a provoked attack. Rather, the ill bat set off a train of events (culminating in a bite) by landing where it did. From this point of view, the bite may be considered to be unprovoked in nature (although not a manifestation of a furious form of disease per se). Similarly, the person who awakens to find a bat in bed may evoke a bite by accidentally rolling over onto the animal. Is such an attack provoked? Or, was it unprovoked and related to the aberrant behavior that placed the bat at the scene in the first place? The arguments lead us nowhere.

The distinction between these perspectives is, perhaps, academic, serving only to help clarify the nature of this disease in the Chiroptera. The fact that bat/human interactions do occur is significant, regardless of whether or not they are a manifestation of a truly furious form of disease. Suffice it to say that bats, like other rabid animals, suffer neurologic impairment and may behave in an aberrant fashion compared to nonrabid individuals. Motor deficits as well as behavioral alterations in infected individuals may both serve to increase the probability of bat/human interactions taking place. Regardless of the circumstances surrounding human exposure, any person who sustains a bite or scratch from a bat should seek medical attention. Unless proven not to be rabid, post-exposure rabies prophylaxis is recommended in all cases of bat bite.

---

[1] Although not necessarily applicable to instances of bat bite, the following activities defining dog attacks as provoked or unprovoked have been suggested by Siwasontiwat et al (1992).

Provoked Bite:

1) entering a strange compound with a guard dog.
2) walking past a dog.
3) stepping on or bumping into a dog.
4) interfering in a dog fight.
5) taking puppies from their mother.
6) taking food from a dog.
7) feeding a dog.
8) playing in an area where a dog is located.
9) beating a dog.
10) petting or playing with a strange dog.

Unprovoked Bite:

1) attack by a dog for an unknown reason and from an unknown site.
2) being bitten by the victim's own dog.

Salivary Carrier State and the Rio Bravo Virus

In the early history of paralytic rabies in South America, it was reported that vampire bats frequently recovered from a clinically rabid state. In this alleged state of recovery, however, they were believed to still be capable of transmitting rabies to livestock for several months because the virus survived in their salivary glands and was, therefore, present in saliva.[2]

In the years following discovery of bat rabies in the United States, two investigators reported that subclinical carrier states could be demonstrated in insectivorous bats. These bats were characterized as having rabies virus present in their saliva, but not in their brains, suggesting that they might have acted as symptomless carriers (Tierkel, 1958, 1959; Sulkin et al, 1959, 1960). Such observations are at odds with more recent work, in which virus was never found in salivary glands of bats in the absence of concomitant brain infection (Bell et al, 1962; Girard et al, 1965; Baer and Bales, 1967; Constantine, 1971; Johnson, 1971; Baer, 1975; Bell, 1975; Constantine, 1975; Moreno and Baer, 1980; Acha, 1981).

Bats may harbor a wide variety of bacterial and viral agents, the public-health significance of which may vary greatly. Dozens of different kinds of viruses and antibodies to dozens of others have been identified in bats (Constantine, 1971; Price, 1978a, 1978b). Like the rabies virus itself, many of these viruses have been isolated from salivary glands and may produce rabies-like signs in laboratory rodents. Some examples include: *Tamana bat virus* from Trinidad (Price, 1978a); *Tacaribe virus* from Trinidad (Downs et al, 1963; Price, 1978b); *Bukalosa bat virus* from Uganda (Williams et al, 1964; Simpson et al, 1968); *Entebbe bat salivary gland virus* from Uganda (Lumsden et al, 1961); *Bangui-M7 bat virus* from the Central African Republic (Chippaux and Chippaux-Hyppolite, 1965 [cited by Constantine, 1970]); *Mount Elgon bat virus* from Kenya (Metselaar et al, 1969 [cited by Constantine, 1970]; Murphy et al, 1970); and *Montana Myotis leukoencephalitis (MML) virus* from the United States (Bell and Thomas, 1964).

One such agent, the Rio Bravo virus (also known as the bat salivary gland virus), may be related to early reports of an asymptomatic salivary carrier state in insectivorous bats. This virus is antigenically related to the virus of St. Louis encephalitis (Burns and Farinacci, 1956; Sulkin et al, 1966a; Hendricks et al, 1983). The Mexican free-tailed bat is believed to be the natural reservoir of the Rio Bravo virus (Constantine, 1970). It has also been isolated from the house bat (*Molossus ater*) in Trinidad (Price, 1978a).

Depending on time of year and roost conditions (especially ventilation, crowding, and the presence of migrant populations), prevalence of infection with the Rio Bravo virus in apparently healthy Mexican free-tailed bats has been found to vary up to about 3.4% (Constantine, 1967a). Infection is not generally observed in suckling bats, virus appearing in salivary glands between 2 and 8 weeks of age. Baer and Woodall (1966) reported a prevalence of 8.7% (4 of 46) in weak and nonflying individuals, suggesting that infection with Rio Bravo virus may be more common in sick bats. The Mexican free-tailed bat may carry the virus in its salivary glands for two years. Other bats are believed to clear the virus from their glands (Constantine and Woodall, 1964).

Proposed mechanisms of transmission of the Rio Bravo virus from bat to bat include aerosol and bite. Infection is not known to produce clinical signs in bats (Constantine, 1970); however, it is pathogenic in humans and some animals (Sulkin et al, 1962; Constantine and Woodall, 1964; Constantine, 1970). The virus is known to cause fever, drowsiness, temporary weakness of the extremities, and nervousness in monkeys; and systemic or CNS illness (possibly aseptic meningitis), orchitis, or oophoritis in humans. Rio Bravo virus is lethal for mice. Signs of infection in these animals include a roughened hair coat, dehydration, decreased activity, a "humped" spine, and progressive paralysis (Constantine and Woodall, 1964).

The significance of Rio Bravo virus to the

[2]In rare instances, recovery from rabies infection, with prolonged shedding of virus, has been reported in dogs in Africa (Fedaku et al, 1981; Aghomo and Rupprecht, 1990a; Fedaku, 1991).

alleged salivary carrier state is twofold:

1) The similarity of clinical infection in mice to that of rabies.

2) The fact that the Rio Bravo virus is isolated from bat salivary glands.

If mouse inoculation tests (using salivary-gland extracts alone) are used to identify the presence of rabies virus, the Rio Bravo virus, in producing signs somewhat similar to those of rabies, may be mistakenly identified as rabies in a rabies-negative, Rio Bravo-positive bat. Microscopic examination of the bat's brain will reveal no evidence of rabies infection. In not succumbing to the Rio Bravo virus, the bat may then be regarded as an asymptomatic carrier of rabies and an interpretation of an asymptomatic bat, with rabies virus in its salivary glands but not brain, may be made. In actuality, however, the animal is a rabies-negative bat with Rio Bravo virus in its salivary glands.

Constantine (1975) suggested that a misinterpretation of this nature may have occurred in some of the earlier investigations, leading to erroneous reports of a salivary carrier state. Confusion may have been compounded by the pooling tissue techniques used by some investigators.

In the past, the existence of an asymptomatic salivary carrier state was a point of controversy (see Baier, 1973; Girard, 1973). Two criteria of an asymptomatic salivary carrier state have not been met by insectivorous bats:

1) Long-term presence of virus in saliva in the absence of clinical signs and brain infection.

2) Regular recovery of bats from a clinically rabid state.

The major body of modern evidence is consistent with the fact that clinically rabid bats succumb to the disease and die, just like other victims, and that an asymptomatic salivary carrier state does not exist. If the brain of a suspect bat tests negative for rabies with the fluorescent antibody test, medical authorities do not recommend antirabies treatment in a person who has sustained a bite.[3]

The Role of Hibernation in Rabies Pathogenesis

Work in the late 1950's and early 1960's pointed to the possibility of dormant viral infections in bats. In this instance, virus was sequestered in the body in a quiescent state. Under appropriate stimulation, the virus could be reactivated. Latency is a well-known feature of herpes infection, in which virus remains dormant for long periods of time in neuronal ganglia. Regarding such a "reservoiring mechanism" for the rabies virus, evidence has implicated brown adipose tissue (brown fat) deposits as possible depot sites during such a dormant state. Probably, the presence of virus in brown fat depots is related more to the centrifugal migration of virus than to any particular tissue tropism.

Although the precise function of brown fat was not known in the early 1960's, it was known to be intimately related, in some manner, to the process of hibernation.[4] Hence, it was often re-

[3]Despite the very high sensitivity and specificity of the fluorescent antibody test (FAT) on brain tissue from a rabies suspect, in cases where the FAT is negative and a human exposure is involved (particularly if rabies is still suspected on either clinical or epidemiological grounds), a backup test is usually performed. This may be a tissue-culture procedure (Rudd and Trimarchi, 1989), or a mouse inoculation test (Koprowski, 1973) which uses suspensions of brain tissue (not salivary gland) from the suspect animal. Recently, it has been suggested that a polymerase-chain-reaction protocol may be of enormous value in the diagnosis of rabies or as a backup test to confirm results of a negative FAT examination in cases involving human exposure (Kamolvarin et al, 1993; McColl et al, 1993).

[4]All animals must find external environments or maintain internal environments within which their many chemical processes can function efficiently. Migration to an area with a more hospitable climate represents behavioral defiance of local conditions whereas hibernation, torpidity, or an energetic regulatory response represent physiological acceptance. Hibernation is, essentially, a condition wherein an animal assumes a state of reduced body temperature, but still retains the capacity of rewarming itself back to normal levels. It is a basic solution to the problem of food shortage during the winter months, since the depression in metabolic rate enables the animal to get along on reserves of fuel stored within its body. Bats display a daily torpor, allowing their body temperature to drop when inactive during the day. The dormant

ferred to as the hibernating gland in earlier literature. Recognizing its role in this phenomenon, Sulkin et al (1957, 1959, 1960, 1966b) reasoned that temperature might be a significant factor in the pathogenesis of rabies infection in bats. These investigators studied the role of ambient temperature in the pathogenesis of rabies infection in two species of bats, Mexican free-tailed bats and little brown bats (*Myotis lucifugus*). The free-tailed bat is a quasi-hibernator, but the little brown bat is a true hibernating species, with well-developed deposits of brown fat.[5] Accordingly, they inoculated Mexican free-tailed and little brown bats intramuscularly with a canine strain (Thompson) of rabies virus (isolated from the brain of a human patient) and maintained some animals at an ambient temperature of 5° C (41° F) or 10° C (50° F) and some at 29° C (84° F). After a variable period of time, some of the animals maintained at 5° C and 10° C were transferred to the 29° C environment (Sulkin et al 1960).

In the 29° C group, 36.1% (35 of 97) of the little brown bats were shown to be rabies positive, compared to 7.5% (3 of 40) of those held at 5° C for 40 days. Of 47 animals held at 5° C for 14 days and then transferred to 29° C, 48.9% (23 of 47) were shown to be rabies positive by the 26th day following transfer to the warm environment.

Similar, but less marked, results were obtained with the Mexican free-tailed bats. In the 29° C group, 23.4% (32 of 137) of the bats were shown to be rabies positive, compared to 5.2% (4 of 77) of those held at 10° C. Of 26 animals held at 10° C for 70 to 106 days and then transferred to 29° C, 15.4% (4 of 26) were shown to be rabies positive by the 72nd day following transfer to the warm environment (Sulkin et al, 1960).

Bell and Moore (1960) reported isolation of rabies virus from the brown fat of naturally infected little brown bats. Using isolates from the pooled brown fat of two of these bats, Sulkin et al (1960) repeated the experiments described above using little brown bats. In the 29° C group, 50% (14 of 28) of the bats were shown to be rabies positive, compared to 4.3% (2 of 47) of those held at 5° C. Of 26 animals held at 5° C for 17 days and then transferred to 29° C, 42% (21 of 50) were shown to be rabies positive between 8 and 31 days following transfer to the warm environment (Sulkin et al, 1960).

The results of these studies suggested that ambient temperature can affect the progression of rabies infection in bats. "Cold storage" appeared to inhibit the progression of rabies infection in the cold-adapted bats. When these bats were transferred to the warmer environs, virus began to multiply in approximately the same time frame as in the initially warm-adapted group.

That the cold-induced torpid state shifts the time frame of disease onset was strikingly demonstrated by Sadler and Enright (1959). They inoculated groups of pallid bats (*Antrozous pallidus*) intracranially with virus isolated from a Mexican free-tailed bat. Respective groups were then maintained at a temperature of 4° C (39.2° F) for 9, 19, 29, 39, 44, and 90 days. Following this time, bats were transferred to 22° C (71.6° F) until onset of clinical signs. Respective incubation times at 22° C until manifestation of disease were 8, 13, 8, 9, 5, and 5 days. These are remarkably close, despite the marked difference in times bats were held at 4° C.

Virus was more frequently identified in salivary tissue following a cold-induced dormancy than in initially warm-adapted animals (Sulkin et al, 1960). This suggested an increased potential for bat-to-bat transmission of virus following hi-

state is associated with a decrease in activity, and a drop in heart rate, respiration, body temperature, and total metabolism. Hibernation is not to be looked upon as a deficient ability to maintain body temperature in the face of a cold stress. Rather, it is a carefully controlled physiologic function. If, when in the torpid state, the ambient temperature drops below freezing, internal heat production within the animal will carefully maintain body temperature at the preferred hibernating level.

[5] The two types of fatty tissues found in animals include brown and white adipose tissue, and they have markedly different functions. White adipose tissue serves principally as a storage form of energy. Brown adipose tissue, on the other hand, burns metabolic fuel for the express purpose of generating heat. This may play a role in both heat production (thermogenesis) as well as in the regulation of energy balance. Deposits of brown fat play a crucial role in the rewarming process during arousal from a state of hibernation.

bernation.

Bats undergo a daily torpor, in which their body temperature approaches ambient. In nonmigratory species a similar but more prolonged phenomenon occurs during winter hibernation. In both instances, as body temperature drops, metabolic activity falls in a commensurate fashion. The possibility that a temperature-dependent drop in metabolic activity was related to the observed effects of temperature on rabies pathogenesis was investigated by Sadler and Enright (1959).

Pallid bats were inoculated intracerebrally with rabies virus of Mexican free-tailed bat origin and held at an ambient temperature of 22° C (71.6° F) for 72 hours. Two control groups were held at 22° C or 30° C (86° F), respectively. Four remaining groups were held at 30° C for 48 hours and then transferred to a 4° C (39.2° F) environment and maintained for 48, 72, 96, or 120 hours, respectively. Because no clinical signs of disease were apparent in most of the animals, incubation time was defined as the total number of days from inoculation until death. The mean incubation time was greater for the group held at 22° C (18.7 days) compared to that held at 30° C (12.3 days). Salivary glands of all bats held at 22° C, but none of those held at 30° C, were positive for virus. Mean incubation times of groups held at 4° C for 48, 72, or 96 hours were twice as long (25.7, 26.2, and 25.5 days, respectively) as that of the control group held at 30° C (12.3 days). The mean incubation time of the group held at 4° C for 120 hours was approximately 40% greater (35.8 days) than that of the other three cold-maintained groups. Virus was isolated from salivary glands of 50% of the bats alternated between the two temperatures and from brains of all but one bat (held at 4° C for 48 hours). The authors believed that these results did not suggest any relationship between daily hibernation and survival of rabies-infected bats. However, there may be a correlation with prolonged hibernation (Sadler and Enright, 1959).

In their work with pallid bats, Sadler and Enright (1959) found that experimentally inoculated animals held at 4° C (39.2° F) for between 9 and 72 days had no detectable virus in either their brains or salivary glands. In contrast, 82% of brains and 47% of salivary glands of animals held at 22° C (71.6° F) for between 11 and 90 days and 79% of brains and 9% of salivary glands of animals held at 37° C (98.6° F) for between 8 and 88 days were virus positive. The authors interpreted this as being indicative of diminished viral replication in slowly metabolizing (i.e., cold) tissues.

They also postulated that despite the lack of viral replication in the cold, an immune response may still have been possible. If true, this is significant in that it could account for the survival of infected bats in nature and may be related to the finding of rabies-neutralizing antibodies in apparently healthy wild-caught bats. Alternatively, the cold-induced dormancy of rabies infections in bats may be a survival mechanism for the virus in nature and may, therefore, contribute to a viral reservoiring mechanism (Sulkin et al, 1959). Studies assessing the relationship between ambient temperature and the progression of rabies infection in bats should be repeated using modern laboratory technology.

Significance of Naturally Occurring Rabies-Neutralizing Antibodies

In an early study of bite-inflicted rabies, Constantine and Woodall (1966) subjected one skunk to 476 red bat bites (336 of which were from bats which had rabies-positive salivary glands at death) and a second skunk to 532 red bat bites (376 of which were from bats which had rabies-positive salivary glands at death). Neither of the skunks contracted rabies, but both developed serum neutralizing antibodies against the rabies virus. Development of antibodies has been reported in suckling mice, wood rats, deer mice, and raccoons following bite of rabid red bats (Constantine and Woodall, 1966); in skunks and raccoons following bite of rabid Mexican free-tailed bats (Constantine et al, 1968); in foxes and coyotes following intramuscular injection of red-bat virus (Constantine and Woodall, 1966); and in rabbits following intramuscular, intracerebral, or subcutaneous inoculation of virus of pallid-bat origin (Burns et al, 1958).

Raccoons naturally exposed to virus and with antibodies present in their blood, have been found in the vicinity of Texas bat caves (Quist et al, 1957; Irons, 1969 [cited by Baer, 1975]). During massive die-offs of bats at Carlsbad Caverns, New Mexico in 1955 and 1956, many thousands of Mexican free-tailed bats perished.[6] Deaths occurred at the onset of their fall migration and were characterized by convulsive seizures and pulmonary hemorrhage. Rabies could not be implicated as a cause (Constantine, 1967b; Constantine et al, 1968). Of 33 carnivores collected near the cave entrance (including foxes, ringtails, raccoons, and skunks), two skunks had rabies-neutralizing antibodies and the rest had neither antibody nor virus demonstrable (Constantine et al, 1968). Carey and McLean (1983) collected carnivores in the region of Bracken Cave (a Mexican free-tailed bat nursery cave in Texas) and found that 3.3% (4 of 120) of trapped raccoons and 7.4% (2 of 27) of trapped skunks had serum neutralizing antibodies against rabies virus.

It has been suggested that ingestion of low doses of virus contained in the carcasses of rabid animals may lead to the development of serum neutralizing antibodies. In studying bovine paralytic rabies in Argentina, Lord et al (1975a) suggested that consumption of rabid vampire bats may have contributed to the observed occurrence of antibody to rabies virus in foxes and skunks. Lawson et al (1987) reported that foxes consuming rabid mice developed protective levels of rabies-neutralizing antibody. Delpietro et al (1990) reported the development of rabies-neutralizing antibodies in rodents consuming brains of cattle that had died of vampire-induced rabies. Rosatte and Gunson (1984) reported the occurrence of rabies antibody in 9% (18 of 198) of skunks in an area of Alberta, Canada known to be free of skunk rabies. The authors suggested that consumption of rabid bats in the area may have been responsible for transmission of virus. However, monoclonal analyses by Webster et al (1986) do not support this hypothesis.

Although the significance of naturally occurring antibody titers against the rabies virus is not yet fully understood (incubation of disease versus development of immunity), there is a growing belief among epidemiologists that natural immunization, following exposure to virus in the wild, may occur frequently (Beran, 1992). By extension, one may consider that environments such as Frio Cave, rather than serving as aerosol infection centers, may play a role in immunizing wildlife. The extent to which this actually occurs and its epidemiologic significance is unknown.

Naturally occurring serum neutralizing antibodies to rabies have been detected in varying amounts in clinically normal specimens of several species of insectivorous bats (Burns and Farinacci, 1955; Burns et al, 1956a, 1956b; Constantine et al, 1968; Baer, 1975; Trimarchi and Debbie, 1977; Steece and Altenbach, 1989). A high rate of antibody development may exist in a population, despite a low incidence of clinical disease. In survey studies of Mexican free-tailed bats, as much as 65% to 80% of clinically normal specimens have had detectable antibody titers. Antibodies to the rabies virus have also been reported in up to 58% of clinically normal vampire bats in Latin America (Ryan, 1963; Villa-R. and Alvarez, 1963; Lord et al, 1975b; Ortega et al, 1985; Delpietro and Konolsaisen, 1991), and in 4% of straw-colored fruit bats (*Eidolon helvum*) in Nigeria (Aghomo et al, 1990). Detection of antibody or rabies virus in vampire bats is highly cyclic in nature (see page 95).

Maternally derived rabies antibodies may pass through the placenta to fetal bats. Antibodies acquired in utero may protect newborn bats against disease for a limited period of time. When antibody levels wane, animals may become vulnerable to infection. The loss of protective antibody in August or September may play a role in the increased incidence of disease at this time (Constantine, 1967a; Constantine et al, 1968).

Steece and Altenbach (1989) examined serum neutralizing antibodies to rabies virus in wild-caught Mexican free-tailed bats obtained in New Mexico from May through September. They found a high prevalence of IgG-class antibody and a low prevalence of IgM-class antibody in adult female bats. Kwiecinski et al (1993) reported that the primary immune response to inac-

[6]Several other major bat die-offs (unrelated to rabies) have been reported. These have been summarized by Clark, Jr. (1981).

tivated rabies virus in big brown bats and in the tropical fruit-eating species, *Artibeus jamaicensis* (the Jamaican fruit bat), resulted in the production of IgM-class antibody, whereas secondary responses to antigenic challenge resulted in production of IgG-class antibody. In the mammalian immune system, IgM-class antibodies are typically short-lived and their presence is generally representative of current or recent infection. The presence of IgG-class antibodies, on the other hand, indicates probable recovery from infection and development of immunity (Steece and Altenbach, 1989).

In view of the ease with which intraspecific transmission of virus may occur among colonial bats, the lack of reports of periodic rabies outbreaks among colonies and the relatively low incidence of naturally occurring disease is striking. The development of serum neutralizing antibodies following nonfatal exposure may account for the apparent lack of widespread disease in populations of colonial bats. Constantine (1988a) suggested that rabies may manifest itself predominantly in immunodeficient individuals, the rarity of disease in immunocompetent bats being reflective of a long-established, balanced relationship between the normally fatal virus and its reservoir host.

References

Acha, P. N. (1981). *A Review of Rabies Prevention and Control in the Americas 1970 to 1980—Overall status of Rabies.* Joint C.N.E.R. - WHO Scientific Meeting on Animal Rabies. Nancy and Malzeville, France. June 3-5, 1981

Aghomo, H. O. and C. E. Rupprecht (1990a). Further studies on rabies virus isolated from healthy dogs in Nigeria. *Vet. Microbiol.* 22: 17

Aghomo, H. O., Ako-Nai, A. K., Oduye, O. O., Tomori, O., and C. E. Rupprecht (1990b). Detection of rabies virus antibodies in fruit bats (*Eidolon helvum*) from Nigeria. *J. Wildl. Dis.* 26(2): 258

Baer, G. M. (1975). Rabies In Nonhematophagous Bats. In G. M. Baer (ed.) *The Natural History of Rabies.* Vol. I. Academic Press. New York.

Baer, G. M. and D. F. Woodall (1966). Bat salivary gland virus carrier state in a naturally infected Mexican freetail bat. *Am. J. Trop. Med. Hyg.* 15(5): 769

Baer, G. M. and G. L. Bales (1967). Experimental rabies infection in the Mexican freetail bat. *J. Infect. Dis.* 117: 82

Baier, J. H. (1973). Management of bat bites. Letter to the Editor. *New Engl. J. Med.* 288(19): 1027

Bell, J. F. (1975). Latency and Abortive Rabies. In G. M. Baer (ed.) *The Natural History of Rabies.* Vol. I. Academic Press. New York.

Bell, J. F. and G. J. Moore (1960). Rabies virus isolated from brown fat of naturally infected bats. *Proc. Soc. Exp. Biol. Med.* 103: 140

Bell, J. F. and L. A. Thomas (1964). A new virus, "MML," enzootic in bats (*Myotis lucifugus*) of Montana. *Am. J. Trop. Med. Hyg.* 13(4): 607

Bell, J. F., Hadlow, W. J., and W. L. Jellison (1955). Chiropteran rabies in Montana. *Pub. Hlth. Repts.* 70(10): 991

Bell, J. F., Hadlow, W. J., and W. L. Jellison (1957). A survey of chiropteran rabies in western Montana. *Pub. Hlth. Repts.* 72(1): 16

Bell, J. F., Moore, G. J., Raymond, G. H., and C. E. Tibbs (1962). Characteristics of rabies in bats in Montana. *Am. J. Pub. Hlth.* 52(8): 1293

Beran, G. W. (1992). Professor of Veterinary Epidemiology and Preventive Medicine. College of Veterinary Medicine, Iowa State University. Ames, Iowa. Personal communication.

Burnett, C. D. (1989). Bat rabies in Illinois: 1965 to 1986. *J. Wildl. Dis.* 25(1): 10

Burns, K. F. and C. J. Farinacci (1955). Rabies in nonsanguivorous bats of Texas. *J. Infect. Dis.* 97: 211

Burns, K. F. and C. J. Farinacci (1956). Virus of bats antigenically related to St. Louis encephalitis. *Science.* 123: 227

Burns, K. F., Farinacci, C. J., Murnane, T. G., and D. F. Shelton (1956a). Insectivorous bats naturally infected with rabies in the southwestern United States. *Am. J. Pub. Hlth.* 46: 1089

Burns, K. F., Farinacci, C. J., and T. G. Murnane (1956b). Rabies in insectivorous bats of Texas. *J. Am. Vet. Med. Assoc.* 128(1): 27

Burns, K. F., Shelton, D. F., and E. W. Grogan (1958). Bat rabies: Experimental host transmission studies. *Ann. N. Y. Acad. Sci.* 70: 452

Carey, A. B. and R. G. McClean (1983). The ecology of rabies: Evidence of co-adaptation. *J. Appl. Ecol.* 20: 777

Centers for Disease Control (1954). Midwestern CDC Services. *Report from the Rocky Mountain Laboratory.* Hamilton, Montana.

Chippaux, A. and C. Chippaux-Hyppolite (1965). Une souche d'arbovirus isolee a Bangui a partir de glandes salivaires de chauves-souris. *Bull. Soc. Pathol. Exot.* 58: 164

Clark, Jr., D. R. (1981). Bats and Environmental Contaminants—A Review. U. S. Fish and Wildlife Service. U. S. Department of the Interior. Special Scientific Report - Wildlife No. 235.

Constantine, D. G. (1967a). Bat rabies in the southwestern United States. *Pub. Hlth. Repts.* 82(10): 867

Constantine, D. G. (1967b). Activity patterns of the Mexican free-tailed bat. *University of New Mexico Publications in Biology.* 7: 8

Constantine, D. G. (1970). Bats in Relation to Health, Welfare, and Economy of Man. In W. A. Wimsatt (ed.) *Biology of Bats.* Vol. II. Academic Press. New York.

Constantine, D. G. (1971). Bat Rabies: Current Knowledge and Future Research. In Y. Nagano and F. M. Davenport (eds.) *Rabies.* University Park Press. Baltimore.

Constantine, D. G. (1975). Rabies virus in bats' brain and salivary glands. *New Engl. J. Med.* 292(1): 51

Constantine, D. G. (1988a). Health Precautions for Bat Researchers. In T. H. Kunz (ed.) *Ecological and Behavioral Methods for the Study of Bats.* Smithsonian Institution Press. Washington, D. C.

Constantine, D. G. (1988b). Public Health Veterinarian. Department of Health Services, State of California - Health and Welfare Agency, Veterinary Public Health Unit. Berkeley, California. Personal communication.

Constantine, D. G. and D. F. Woodall (1964). Latent infection of Rio Bravo virus in salivary glands of bats. *Pub. Hlth. Repts.* 79(12): 1033

Constantine, D. G. and D. F. Woodall (1966). Transmission experiments with bat rabies isolates: Reactions of certain carnivora, opossum, rodents, and bats to rabies virus of red bat origin when exposed by bat bite or by intramuscular inoculation. *Am. J. Vet. Res.* 27(116): 24

Constantine, D. G., Tierkel, E. S., Kleckner, M. D., and D. M. Hawkins (1968). Rabies in New Mexico cavern bats. *Pub. Hlth. Repts.* 83(4): 303

Delpietro, H. A. and J. F. Konolsaisen (1991). Dinamica da raiva em uma populacao de morcegos hematofagos (*Desmodus rotundus*) no nordeste Argentino, e sua relacao com a raiva paralitica dos herbivoros. *Arq. Biol. Tecnol.* 34(3/4): 381

Delpietro, H., Segre, L., Marchevsky, N., and M. Berisso (1990). Rabies transmission to rodents after ingestion of naturally infected tissues (English abstract). *Medicina - Buenos Aires.* 50(4): 356

Downs, W. G., Anderson, C. R., Spence, L., Aitken, T. H. G., and A. Greenhall (1963). Tacaribe virus, a new agent isolated from *Artibeus* bats and mosquitos in Trinidad, West Indies. *Am. J. Trop. Med. Hyg.* 12(4): 640

Fedaku, M. (1991). Latency and Aborted Rabies. In G. M. Baer (ed.) *The Natural History of Rabies.* 2nd Edition. CRC Press, Inc. Boca Raton, Florida.

Fedaku, M., Shaddock, J. H., and G. M. Baer (1981). Intermittent excretion of rabies virus in the saliva of a dog two and six months after it had recovered from experimental rabies. *Am. J. Trop. Med. Hyg.* 30: 1113

Girard, K. (1973). Management of bat bites. Letter to the Editor. *New Engl. J. Med.* 288(19): 1027

Girard, K. F., Hitchcock, H. B., Edsall, G., and R. A. MacCready (1965). Rabies in bats in southern New England. *New Engl. J. Med.* 272(2): 75

Haagsma, J. (1989). Rabies en vleermuizen: hoe te handelen? *Ned. Tijdschr. Geneeskd.* 133(11): 550. (Rabies in Bats: How should it be treated?) English translation courtesy of Dr. Nathan M. Appel.

Hemachudha, T., Chutivongse, S., Wilde, H., and P. Phanuphak (1991). Latent rabies. *New Engl. J. Med.* 324(26): 1890

Hendricks, D. A., Hardy, J. L., and W. C. Reeves (1983). Comparison of biological properties of St. Louis encephalitis and Rio Bravo viruses. *Am. J. Trop. Med. Hyg.* 32(3): 602

Johnson, H. N. (1971). General Epizootiology of Rabies. In Y. Nagano and F. M. Davenport (eds.) *Proceedings of Working Conference on Rabies.* Sponsored by the Japan-United States Cooperative Medical Science Program. University Park Press. Baltimore.

Kamolvarin, N., Tirawatnpong, T., Rattanasiwamoke, R., Tirawatnpong, S., Panpanich, T., and T. Hemachudha (1993). Diagnosis of rabies by polymerase chain reaction with nested primers. *J. Infect. Dis.* 167: 297

Kaplan, M. M. (1969). Epidemiology of rabies. *Nature.* 221 (5179): 421

Koprowski, H. (1973). The Mouse Inoculation Test. In M. M. Kaplan and H. Koprowski (eds.) *Laboratory Techniques in Rabies.* 3rd Edition. World Health Organization. Geneva.

Kwiecinski, G. C., Murphy, D. J., and C. E. Rupprecht (1993). An enzyme linked immunosorbant assay for detection of rabies specific IgG in bats. *23rd Annual North American Symposium on Bat Research.* Gainesville, Florida. October, 1993

Lawson, K. F., Black, J. G., Charlton, K. M., Johnston, D. H., and A. J. Rhodes (1987). Safety and immunogenicity of a vaccine bait containing ERA strain of attenuated rabies vaccine. *Can. J. Vet. Res.* 51: 460

Lord, R. D., Delpietro, H., Fuenzalida, E., de Diaz, A. M. O., and L. Lazaro (1975a). Presence of rabies neutralizing antibodies in wild carnivores following an outbreak of bovine rabies. *J. Wildl. Dis.* 11: 210

Lord, R. D., Fuenzalida, E., Delpietro, H., Larghi, O. P., de Diaz, A. M., and L. Lazaro (1975b). Observations on the epizootiology of vampire bat rabies. *Bull. Pan Am. Hlth. Org. 9: 189*

Lumsden, W. H. R., Williams, M. C., and P. J. Mason (1961). A virus from insectivorous bats in Uganda. *Ann. Trop. Med. Parasitol.* 55(4): 389

McColl, K. A., Gould, P. W., Hooper, P. T., Westbury, H. A., and J. S. Smith (1993). Polymerase chain reaction and other laboratory techniques in the diagnosis of long incubation rabies in Australia. *Aust. Vet. J.* 70(3): 84

Metselaar, D., Williams, M. C., Simpson, D. I. H., West, R., and F. A. Mutere (1969). Mount Elgon bat virus: A hitherto undescribed virus from *Rhinolophus hildebrandtii eloquens* K. Anderson. *Arch. Gesamte. Virusforsch.* 26: 183

Moore, G. J. and G. H. Raymond (1970). Prolonged incubation period of rabies in a naturally infected insectivorous bat, *Eptesicus fuscus* (Beavois). *J. Wildl. Dis.* 6: 167

Moreno, J. A. and G. M. Baer (1980). Experimental rabies in the vampire bat. *Am. J. Trop. Med. Hyg.* 29(2): 254

Murphy, F. A., Shope, R. E., Metselaar, D., and D. I. H. Simpson (1970). Characterization of Mount Elgon virus, a new member of the Rhabdovirus group. *Virology.* 40: 288

Ollason, J. G., Keller, V. E., and S. L. Frears (1992). Day-flying bat attacked by house martins. *J. Zool. (Lond.).* 227: 322

Ortega, J. R. V., Delgado, M. A. M., Campero, D. B., and D. O. Cordova (1985). Presencia de anticuerpos y virus rabico en *Desmodus rotundus* y otros murcielagos en una region de la zona humeda del Istmo de Tehuantepec. (Presence of rabies antibodies and virus in *Desmodus rotundus* and other bats in a region of the humid zone of the Tehuantepec Isthmus, Mexico.) *Tecnica Pecuaria en Mexico*. No. 49: 9 (English abstract) in *Vet. Bull.* (1987). 57(4): 283

Price, J. L. (1978a). Isolation of Rio Bravo and a hitherto undescribed agent, Tamana bat virus, from insectivorous bats in Trinidad, with serological evidence of infection in bats and man. *Am. J. Trop. Med. Hyg.* 27(1): 153

Price, J. L. (1978b). Serological evidence of infection of Tacaribe virus and arboviruses in Trinidadian bats. *Am. J. Trop. Med. Hyg.* 27(1): 162

Price, J. L. and C. O. R. Everard (1977). Rabies virus and antibody in bats in Grenada and Trinidad. *J. Wildl. Dis.* 13: 131

Quist, K. D., Eads, R. B., and A. Conklin (1957). Studies on bat rabies in Texas. *J. Am. Vet. Med. Assoc.* 130: 66

Ressang, A. A., Gwan, S. I., and S. Hardjosworo (1963). Bats, rodents and rabies in Indonesia. *Communications Veterinaire.* 7: 33

Rosatte, R. C. and J. R. Gunson (1984). Presence of neutralizing antibodies to rabies virus in striped skunks from areas free of skunk rabies in Alberta. *J. Wildl. Dis.* 20(3): 171

Rudd, R. J. and C. V. Trimarchi (1989). Development and evaluation of an in vitro virus isolation procedure as a replacement for the mouse inoculation test in rabies diagnosis. *J. Clin. Microbiol.* 27(11): 2522

Ryan, R. M. (1963). Rabies virus in the kidney and other tissues of vampire bats in western Mexico. *Zoonoses Res.* 2(2): 77

Sadler, W. W. and J. B. Enright (1959). Effect of metabolic level of the host upon the pathogenesis of rabies in the bat. *J. Infect. Dis.* 105: 267

Schowalter, D. B. (1980). Characteristics of bat rabies in Alberta. *Can. J. Comp. Med.* 44: 70

Simpson, D. I. H., Williams, M. C., O'Sullivan, J. P., Cunningham, J. C., and F. A. Mutere (1968). Studies on arboviruses and bats (Chiroptera) in East Africa. II. Isolation and haemagglutination-inhibition studies on bats collected in Kenya and throughout Uganda. *Am. Trop. Med. Parasit.* 62(4): 432

Siwasontiwat, D., Lumlertdacha, B., Polsuwan, G., Hemachudha, T., Chutivongse, S., and H. Wilde (1992). Rabies: Is provocation of the biting dog relevant for risk assessment? *Trans. Roy. Soc. Trop. Med.* 86: 443

Speakman, J. R. (1990). The function of daylight flying in British bats. *J. Zool. (Lond.).* 220: 101

Speakman, J. R. (1991). Why do insectivorous bats in Britain not fly more frequently? *Funct. Ecol.* 5(4): 518

Steece, R. and J. S. Altenbach (1989). Prevalence of rabies specific antibodies in the Mexican free-tailed bat (*Tadarida brasiliensis mexicana*) at Lava Cave, New Mexico. *J. Wildl. Dis.* 24(4): 490

Sulkin, S. E., Krutzsch, P. H., Wallis, C., and R. Allen (1957). Role of brown fat in pathogenesis of rabies in insectivorous bats. *Proc. Soc. Exp. Biol. Med.* 96: 461

Sulkin, S. E., Krutzsch, P. H., Allen, R., and C. Wallis (1959). Studies on the pathogenesis of rabies in insectivorous bats. I. Role of brown adipose tissue. *J. Exp. Med.* 110: 369

Sulkin, S. E., Allen, R., Sims, P., Krutzsch, P. H., and C. Kim (1960). Studies on the pathogenesis of rabies in insectivorous bats. II. Influence of environmental temperature. *J. Exp. Med.* 112: 595

Sulkin, S. E., Burns, K. F., Shelton, D. F., and C. Wallis (1962). Bat salivary gland virus: Infection of man and monkey. *Texas Repts. Biol. Med.* 20: 113

Sulkin, S. E., Sims, R. A., and R. Allen (1966a). Isolation of St. Louis encephalitis virus from bats (*Tadarida b. mexicana*) in Texas. *Science.* 152: 223

Sulkin, S. E., Allen, R., and R. Sims (1966b). Growth of Rabies Virus in Brown Adipose Tissue in Vivo and in Vitro. *International Symposium on Rabies*. Symp. Series Immunobiol. Standard. Vol. I. Karger, Basel. New York. Talloires, 1965

Sullivan, T. D., Grimes, J. E., Eads, R. B., Menzies, G. C., and J. V. Irons (1954). Recovery of rabies virus from colonial bats in Texas. *Pub. Hlth. Repts.* 69(8): 766

Tierkel, E. S. (1958). Recent developments in the epidemiology of rabies. *Ann. N. Y. Acad. Sci.* 70: 445

Tierkel, E. S. (1959). Rabies. In C. A. Brandy and E. L. Jungherr (eds.) *Advances in Veterinary Science.* Vol. 5: 183

Trimarchi, C. V. (1978). Rabies in insectivorous temperate-zone bats. *Bat Res. News.* 19(1): 7

Trimarchi, C. V. and J. G. Debbie (1977). Naturally occurring rabies virus and neutralizing antibody in two species of insectivorous bats of New York State. *J. Wildl. Dis.* 13: 367

Trimarchi, C. V., Abelseth, M. K., and R. J. Rudd (1979). Aggressive behavior in rabid big brown bats (*Eptesicus fuscus*). Report from the Division of Laboratories and Research, New York State Dept. Health. Albany, New York. *Rabies Information Exchange:* 34

Villa-Ramirez, B. and B. Alvarez L. (1963). Rabies virus in the kidney and other tissues of vampire bats in western Mexico. *Zoonoses Res.* 2(2): 77

Webster, W. A., Casey, G. A., and K. M. Charlton (1986). Major antigenic groups of rabies virus in Canada determined by anti-nucleocapsid monoclonal antibodies. *Comp. Immun. Microbiol. Infect. Dis.* 9(1): 59

Williams, M. C., Simpson, D. I. H., and R. C. Shepherd (1964). Studies on viruses in East African bats (Chiroptera). *Zoonoses Res.* 3(3): 141

Chapter 13:
MAINTENANCE OF ENZOOTIC RABIES IN INSECTIVOROUS BATS

Potential Sources of Virus

With regard to the source of virus in North American insectivorous bats, two possibilities have been suggested. The virus may have long been enzootic in various bat populations, but gone unnoticed by man until its initial discovery in 1953; or, the virus may have originated from an outside source in recent history, entering North American bat populations through one of two sylvatic routes (via predators or interspecific bat transmission).

Many species of carnivores are known to prey upon bats. A rabid fox, skunk, or raccoon may attack a bat, but fail to kill it. This type of exposure may be one way in which rabies may have originally entered this country's bat populations. Once within a local population, the virus may have established itself, leading to rabies in enzootic form. Although such a mechanism seems straightforward, serological evidence does not support it. Several variants of rabies virus are known to exist and can be differentiated from each other on both a geographic and species-specific basis. The different reservoirs of rabies harbor characteristic viral variants. Bats are known to carry multiple variants of virus that are markedly distinct both antigenically and genetically from those of terrestrial species (Smith et al, 1985).

After countless passages of virus through bat populations, however, viruses may have changed from an ancestral infecting form. This might account for the currently observed serologic and genetic differences and could be consistent with infection of bats by local wildlife at some time in the distant past, however unlikely. Isolation of a terrestrial variant of virus from any species of bat has not been confirmed.

A more commonly believed theory, at one time, was that vampire bats served as the source of virus for North American species. Presumably, this could have occurred either as a result of infected vampire bats migrating (or being passively transported) into the United States or of northern bat species migrating in a southerly direction.

It had been suggested that rabid vampire bats may have been introduced into Tampa, Florida as stowaways on banana boats (Scatterday and Galton, 1954). According to banana importing companies, however, commonly seen stowaways included the tree mouse, mouse opossum, snakes, and spiders. Stowaway bats had reportedly never been observed. Habitual migration of modern vampires into temperate climes is also unlikely.

However, many migrating bats (particularly Mexican free-tails) overwinter in Mexico, where they may share roosts with vampire bats (Figure 13-1). Prior to monoclonal antibody analyses, it had been suggested frequently that cohabitation of these bats with vampires could have led to rabies infection from bite or aerosol exposure (Courter, 1954; Burns and Farinacci, 1955; Burns et al, 1956; Enright et al, 1955; Grimes et al, 1955; Quist et al, 1957; Arnstein, 1958; Maddy et al, 1958; Kent and Finegold, 1960; Verts and Barr, 1961; Davis et al, 1962; Constantine et al, 1968; Smith, 1971; Greenhall, 1972). When housed in captivity with Mexican free-tails, vampire bats have been observed to attack and feed upon them (Constantine et al, 1968), which could lead to transmission of virus. Infected Mexican free-tailed bats, in turn, may have infected others during the course of their northerly migration back to the United States. This may have resulted in the eventual spread of rabies virus into bat populations (via both intra- and interspecific transmis-

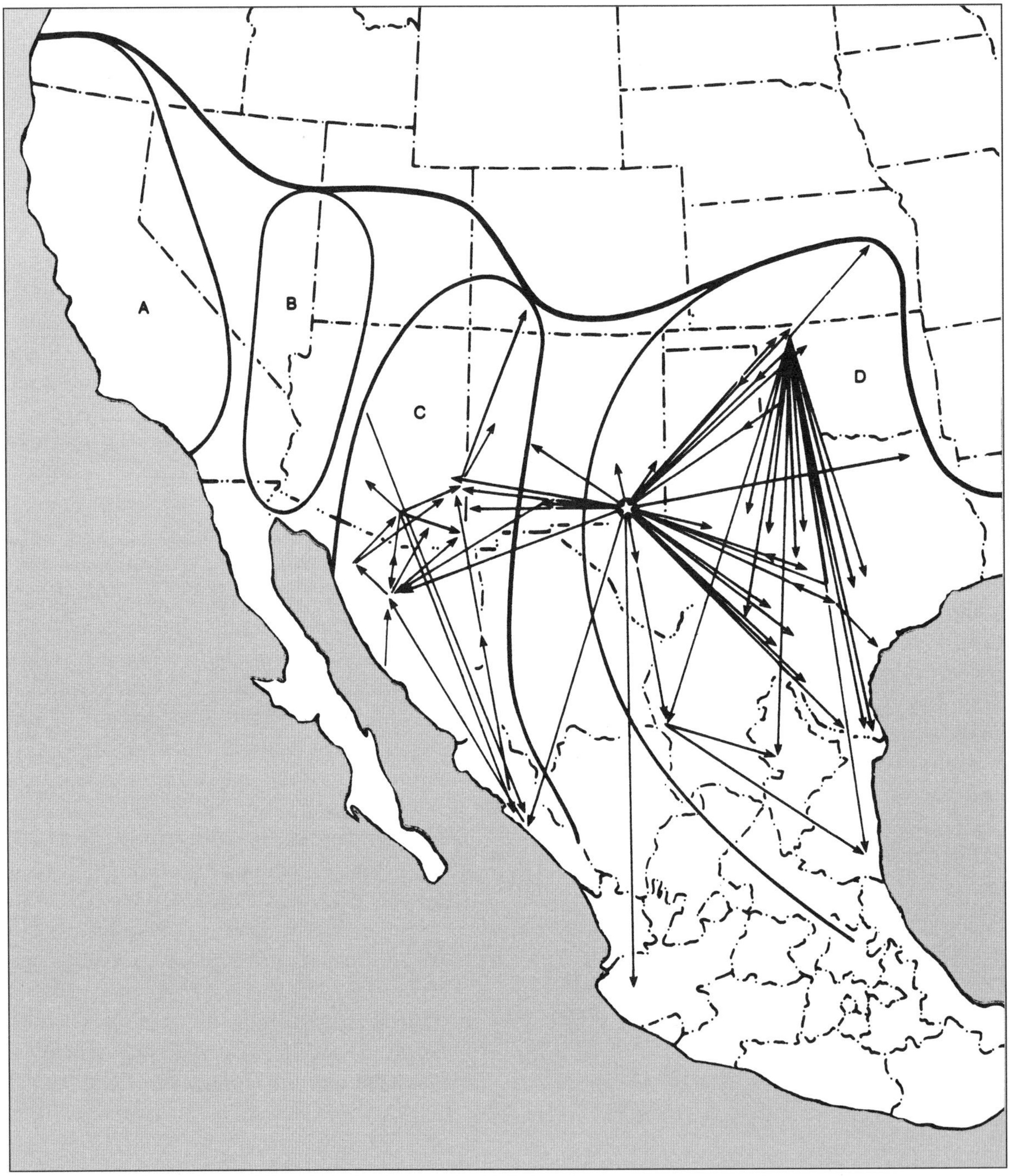

Figure 13-1. Population movement of the Mexican free-tailed bat based on banding studies. Although some populations are believed to be relatively non-migratory (regions A and B), others (regions C and D) make extensive seasonal migrations. Arrows represent movement from the banding site to a point of recovery. The star represents Carlsbad Caverns, New Mexico. (From Hill, J. E. and J. D. Smith. *Bats—A Natural History.* British Museum of Natural History. London, 1984. Reproduced with permission.)

sion) throughout the Southwest and, ultimately, across the United States and Canada.

Malaga-Alba (1957) did not believe the Mexican free-tailed bats to be infected by vampires because of no observed coexistence in Mexican caves. However, Constantine's field observations in Mexico revealed that such cohabitation does occur (Constantine, 1967 [cited by Constantine et al, 1968]). According to Arellano (1986), although vampires share roosts with other species of bats, mixing never occurs. Such behavior patterns, however, may only be a feature of healthy bats and not rabid ones. Because of the alterations in behavior that often typify rabies infection in animals, behavioral observations of healthy individuals have only limited value in predicting the actions of rabid ones. Observations of segregated populations of healthy bats do not necessarily form a valid foundation for speculation about their interactions with rabid individuals.

Differences in pathogenic properties of rabies isolates collected from naturally infected Mexican free-tailed bats and those from vampires suggest separate origins. Rabies isolates from Mexican free-tailed bats have been shown to produce death in mice after an incubation period of 4 to 5 days, with marked neuronal destruction. Vampire isolates, in contrast, do not kill mice before 11 to 17 days (depending on dosage), causing considerably less neuronal pathology (Johnson, 1966; Baer et al 1980). The relatively long incubation period of vampire isolates is typical of street virus isolated from naturally infected animals. The shorter incubation period of free-tailed bat isolates is more characteristic of fixed virus. In their resemblance to fixed virus, isolates of rabies from Mexican free-tailed bats are apparently unique (Baer et al, 1980), consistent with the premise that they are probably not of vampire origin. Johnson (1960 [cited by Kent and Finegold, 1960]) commented on differences in virulence between vampire and Mexican free-tailed isolates and expressed the opinion, at that time, that this source of transmission was unlikely.

Based on monoclonal antibody studies (Rupprecht, 1986; Dietzschold et al, 1988), the viral isolates from vampire bats of Latin America are now known to be distinct from those of North American insectivorous species (Figure 13-2),

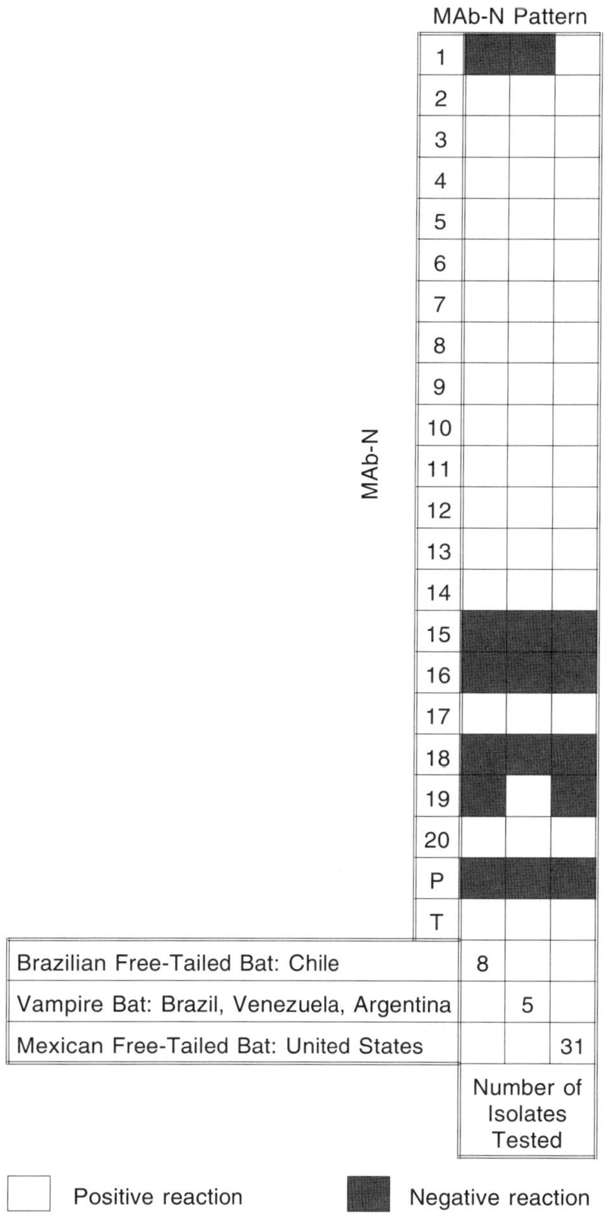

Figure 13-2. MAb-N variants of rabies virus associated with Mexican free-tailed and vampire bats. Viral isolates collected from each species were reacted with a panel of monoclonal antibodies (MAb-N) to the rabies N protein. (From Baer, G. M. and J. S. Smith. Rabies in Nonhematophagous Bats. In G. M. Baer (ed.) *The Natural History of Rabies.* 2nd Edition. © CRC Press, Inc. Boca Raton, Florida, 1991. Reproduced with permission.)

suggesting that regular transmission of virus between hematophagous and insectivorous bats does not occur. Rabies isolates from eight infected Brazilian free-tailed bats collected in Chile, as well as that isolated from a rabid cat in the same area, were also found to be antigenically distinct both from known vampire isolates as well as from those found in dogs in areas of enzootic canine rabies (Smith, 1989).

It cannot be excluded that such transmission may have occurred hundreds or even thousands of years ago, providing ample time for significant antigenic variation to have occurred (see page 265). After countless years of viral passage through successive generations of Mexican free-tailed bats, a vampire variant may have become "fixed" in the free-tail, with antigenic properties slightly different from an ancestral (i.e., vampire) form. The close genetic relatedness of the two isolates (Smith, 1994) also suggests the possibility of a common ancestry. In observing an isolated frame in a continuum of possible viral evolutionary change, it is difficult, if not impossible, to make definitive judgment regarding the original source of virus in North American bat populations. In the present state of knowledge, however, transmission of rabies from vampire bats to insectivorous species, in regions where their ranges overlap, does not appear to be of epidemiologic significance in the maintenance of infection in North American bats.

Horizontal Transmission of Virus Among Insectivorous Bats

Once rabies is introduced into an animal community, maintenance of virus in enzootic form requires continued transmission throughout a susceptible population. In the absence of intraspecific transmission, infected animals will die without the disease being propagated to others. Bat-to-bat transmission of rabies virus can occur through several possible avenues. Horizontal transmission occurs between contemporaries, or individuals of more or less the same generation.

Many species of bats are colonial, living in great numbers within caves, buildings, or similar habitats. Among some species, both inter- and intraspecific biting have been observed, providing at least one possible mechanism for the propagation of disease.

Populations of Mexican free-tailed bats may be extremely dense in southwestern bat caves. As many as 300 bats may occupy a square foot of ceiling. Davis et al (1962) defined a variety of behavioral patterns in the Mexican free-tailed bat related to the physical stresses imposed by their enormous colony structure. Crowding in maternity colonies is so extensive that freedom of movement may be severely curtailed. Pushing and shoving are often required if bats are to nudge themselves into an appropriate roosting location or free themselves from a tight cluster prior to flight. More aggressive action may sometimes be required. Davis (1959) reported that Mexican free-tailed bats fight amongst themselves and bite each other as they fly into the roost. Even juveniles bite one another, presumably in attempts to keep from falling. It is common in this species to find bleeding wounds on membranous areas of wings. Richly supplied with nerve endings, these sites may be favorable routes of viral infection.

The relatively high population densities characteristic of colonial species would seem to favor maintenance of a rabies enzootic in these species, without recourse to development of furious signs. If, on the other hand, disease is to be maintained in or spread among solitary species, a furious form of rabies may be necessary (although transmission from mother to offspring has been suspected in both colonial and solitary bats during the perinatal, and perhaps prenatal, period).

Interspecific aggression has been observed in hoary bats. In 1946, a hoary bat was seen in upstate New York with a small pipistrelle (*Pipistrellus subflavus obscurus*) in its jaws. The hoary bat reportedly maintained its death grip on the pipistrelle even when picked up by the nape of its neck (Bishop, 1947). In 1947, a hoary bat was observed chasing another bat along a cliff in California's San Joaquin Valley (Orr, 1950). A similar observation was made in 1978 by Bell in Arizona, where a hoary bat was reportedly seen attacking a silver-haired bat, a Mexican free-tailed bat, and a big brown bat. A captured bat, believed to be rabid, was thought to be the one under observation. Bell believed that such aggressive behavior was not normal, but a manifestation of furious rabies (Bell, 1980). Aggressive behavior, such as these cases illustrate, suggests another means of viral transmission between bats.

Engler (1943) reported several instances of carnivorous activity among captive insectivorous bats, including observation of a big brown bat devouring a long-eared myotis (*Myotis evotis chrysonotus*) and of a pallid bat partially eating a Mexican free-tailed bat. Although circumstances of their captivity may have been instrumental in inducing these behaviors, such feeding activity, if it occurs naturally, could be a potential source of viral transmission from bat to bat. Naturally occurring carnivorous behavior among typically insectivorous bats has been described by others (Norberg and Fenton, 1988).

Vertical Transmission of Virus Among Insectivorous Bats

Another route whereby community infection may be propagated is through vertical transmission, which refers to the transmission of an infectious agent from an individual of one generation to those of a succeeding generation (offspring). This might occur transovarially, in utero, or via ingestion of milk. Schneider et al (1957) reported infection in suckling bats, although they did not speculate on the mode of transmission.

Sims et al (1963) reported the presence of rabies virus in one (of 23) fetal and three newborn Mexican free-tailed bats whose mothers had been experimentally infected (intramuscular injection of a canine strain of rabies virus isolated from the brain of a human patient). Constantine (1986) suggested that the data presented by Sim's group were not entirely representative of infection in the wild, experimental bats having been inoculated with a relatively large volume of viral-laden fluid.

Of 28 fetuses collected from 22 naturally infected Mexican free-tailed bats, Constantine (1986) found none infected with virus by fluorescent antibody test. Of 284 suckling bats less than five days old, none were found to be infected. Infection among suckling bats was not apparent by fluorescent antibody test until they were between 5 and 11 days of age. Of the suckling Mexican free-tailed bats found to be naturally infected, 84% were between 7 and 11 days old. Constantine believed this to be indicative of infection at or shortly after the time of birth.

Steece and Calisher (1989) reported rabies infection in cultured fetal bat cells derived from fetuses harvested from wild-caught Mexican free-tailed bats. They concluded that these fetuses had been infected in utero, making this the first observation of prenatal transmission of rabies virus in naturally infected bats. The significance of such transmission to rabies epizootiology remains unknown.

References

Arellano, C. (1986). Vampire Bat Rabies in Cattle. *Rabies Control Symposium.* Washington, D. C. November 3-5, 1986

Arnstein, P. (1958). The Role of Bats as Rabies Vectors. *Symposium on Rabies.* University of Kansas Medical Society. Kansas City, Kansas. April 18, 1958

Baer, G. M. and J. S. Smith (1991). Rabies in Nonhematophagous Bats. In G. M. Baer (ed.) *The Natural History of Rabies.* 2nd Edition. CRC Press, Inc. Boca Raton, Florida.

Baer, G. M., Harrison, A. K., Bauer, S. P., Shaddock, J. H., and F. A. Murphy (1980). A bat rabies isolate with an unusually short incubation period. *Exp. Molec. Pathol.* 33: 211

Bell, G. P. (1980). A possible case of interspecific transmission of rabies in insectivorous bats. *J. Mammal.* 61(3): 528

Bishop, S. C. (1947). Curious behavior of a hoary bat. *J. Mammal.* 28(3): 293

Burns, K. F. and C. J. Farinacci (1955). Rabies in nonsanguivorous bats of Texas. *J. Infect. Dis.* 97: 211

Burns, K. F., Farinacci, C. F., Murnane, T. G., and D. F. Shelton (1956). Insectivorous bats naturally infected with rabies in the southwestern United States. *Am. J. Pub. Hlth.* 46: 1089

Constantine, D. G. (1967). Activity patterns of the Mexican free-tailed bat. *University of New Mexico Publications in Biology.* No. 7. University of New Mexico Press. Albuquerque, New Mexico.

Constantine, D. G. (1986). Absence of prenatal infection of bats with rabies virus. *J. Wildl. Dis.* 22(2): 249

Constantine, D. G., Tierkel, E. S., Kleckner, M. D., and D. M. Hawkins (1968). Rabies in New Mexico cavern bats. *Pub. Hlth. Repts.* 83(4): 303

Courter, R. D. (1954). Bat rabies. *Pub. Hlth. Repts.* 69(1): 9

Davis, D. E. (1959). *Proceedings of Conference on Research in Bat Rabies.* National Institutes of Health. Bethesda. P. 49. July 10-11, 1959

Davis, R. B., Herreid, C. F., and H. L. Short (1962). Mexican free-tailed bats in Texas. *Ecol. Monogr.* 32(4): 311

Dietzschold, B., Rupprecht, C. E., Tollis, M., Lafon, M., Mattei, J., Wiktor, T. J., and H. Koprowski (1988). Antigenic diversity of the glycoprotein and nucleocapsid proteins of rabies and rabies-related viruses: Implications for epidemiology and control of rabies. *Rev. Infect. Dis.* 10(Suppl. 4): S785

Engler, C. H. (1943). Carnivorous activities of big brown and pallid bats. *J. Mammal.* 24: 96

Enright, J. B., Sadler, W. W., Moulton, J. E., and D. Constantine (1955). Isolation of rabies virus from an insectivorous bat (*Tadarida mexicana*) in California. *Proc. Soc. Exp. Biol. Med.* 89: 94

Greenhall, A. M. (1972). The problem of bat rabies, migratory bats, livestock and wildlife. *Transactions of the North American Wildlife and Natural Resources Conference*—No. 37. Mexico City, Mexico. March 12-15, 1972

Grimes, J. E., Eads, R. B., and J. V. Irons (1955). An additional species of insectivorous bat naturally infected with rabies. *Am. J. Trop. Med. Hyg.* 4(3): 554

Hill, J. E. and J. D. Smith (1984). *Bats—A Natural History*. British Museum of Natural History. London.

Johnson, H. N. (1966). Sporadic Cases of Rabies in Wildlife: Relation to Rabies in Domestic Animals and Character of Virus. *Proceedings of the National Rabies Symposium*. National Communicable Disease Center. U. S. Dept. of Health, Education, and Welfare. Public Health Service. Atlanta, Georgia. May 5-6, 1966

Kent, J. R. and M. F. Finegold (1960). Human rabies transmitted by the bite of a bat. *New Engl. J. Med.* 263(21): 1058

Maddy, K. T., Cockrum, E. L., and H. G. Crecelius (1958). Bat rabies in Arizona. *Arizona Med.* 15(5): 344

Malaga-Alba, A. (1957). Rabies in wildlife in middle America. *J. Am. Vet. Med. Assoc.* 130: 386

Norberg, U. M. and M. Brock Fenton (1988). Carnivorous bats? *Biol. J. Linn. Soc.* 33: 383

Orr, R. T. (1950). Unusual behavior and occurrence of a hoary bat. *J. Mammal.* 31: 456

Quist, K. D., Eads, R. B., and A. Conklin (1957). Studies on bat rabies in Texas. *J. Am. Vet. Med. Assoc.* 130: 66

Rupprecht, C. E. (1986). *The Epidemiology of Wildlife Rabies Within North America: Characterization Via Monoclonal Antibodies*. Ph.D. Thesis. The University of Wisconsin. Milwaukee, Wisconsin.

Scatterday, J. E. and M. M. Galton (1954). Bat rabies in Florida. *Vet. Med.* 49: 133

Schneider, N. J., Scatterday, J. E., Lewis, A. L., Jennings, W. L., Venters, H. D., and A. V. Hardy (1957). Rabies in bats in Florida. *Am. J. Pub. Hlth.* 47(8): 983

Sims, R. A., Allen, R., and S. E. Sulkin (1963). Studies on the pathogenesis of rabies in insectivorous bats. III. Influence of the gravid state. *J. Infect. Dis.* 112: 17

Smith, C. W. (1971). Rabies and the caver. A review of the pertinent literature. *NSS (Natl. Speleol. Soc.) News*. 29: 60

Smith, J. S. (1989). Rabies Virus Epitopic Variation: Use in Ecologic Studies. In K. Maramorosch, F. A. Murphy, and A. J. Shatkin (eds.) *Advances in Virus Research*. Vol. 36. Academic Press, Inc. New York.

Smith, J. S. (1994). Research Microbiologist. Rabies Laboratory, Centers for Disease Control. Atlanta, Georgia. Personal communication.

Smith, J. S., Sumner, J., Roumillot, F., Baer, G. M., and W. Winkler (1985). Epidemiological Analysis of Street Rabies Viruses From Enzootic Areas of the United States. In E. Kuwert, C. Merieux, H. Koprowski, and K. Bogel (eds.) *Rabies in the Tropics*. Springer-Verlag. New York.

Steece, R. S. and C. H. Calisher (1989). Evidence for prenatal transfer of rabies virus in the Mexican free-tailed bat (*Tadarida brasiliensis mexicana*). *J. Wildl. Dis.* 25(3): 329

Verts, B. J. and T. R. B. Barr (1961). An effort to identify rabies in bats from northwestern Illinois. *Cornell Vet.* 51: 384

Chapter 14:
AIRBORNE TRANSMISSION OF RABIES VIRUS

Human Case Studies

On January 1, 1956, an entomologist with the Texas State Health Department, was stricken with impaired vision and fitful sleep. The following day, he suffered through two convulsive seizures. In the hospital, he volunteered the information that he was suffering from rabies, but maintained that he had been subjected to no animal bite, bat or otherwise. He died on January 4 and rabies was confirmed as the cause of death (Irons et al, 1957).

The patient had been part of the state's rabies investigative team. In the course of his job, he handled thousands of bats. In particular, he worked extensively with Mexican free-tailed bats in Texas bat caves. Several months prior to his death, he had spent time working with bats in Wilson Cave, Kerr County; Bracken Cave, Comal County; and Frio Cave, Uvalde County. Bracken and Frio Caves harbored two of the largest maternity colonies of Mexican free-tailed bats in the country (Irons et al, 1954; Eads et al, 1957).

On June 1, 1959, a consultant mining engineer was admitted to a hospital in Los Angeles, California. His chief complaints were shortness of breath and retching. He died on June 3 and rabies was confirmed as the cause of death. The patient had spent time investigating Mexican and Texas caves for their guano-mining potential.[1] Two months prior to his death, he had explored several caves in Mexico. A little over a month prior to his death, he had been working in various Texas caves, including Hawkey Cave, Pecos County; Fern Cave, Valverde County; Dunbar Cave, Edwards County; and Frio Cave, Uvalde County. In the course of his explorations, he noted the extraordinary number of bats in Frio Cave. As in the case of the entomologist, he denied having been bitten by any animal (Humphrey et al, 1960; Kent and Finegold, 1960). Additional medical details of these two cases can be found on pages 236-237.

In the alleged absence of animal bites, these two cases of rabies were somewhat reminiscent of circumstances surrounding the early human deaths in Trinidad. However, investigations would ultimately point to a quite different mechanism of viral transmission. In a series of experiments conducted in Frio Cave, Uvalde County, Texas and Lava Cave, Socorro County, New Mexico between 1960 and 1966, Constantine (1962, 1967) demonstrated the possibility that rabies could, under certain conditions, be transmitted by aerosolization of virus.

Bat Populations of Frio Cave

Frio Cave (also sometimes known as Annandale Ranch Cave, Florea Cave, Uvalde Cave, and Verdi Cave) is the roosting site for a remarkably large number of bats. According to Constantine (1967), it is home to three species. During the spring, summer, and autumn months, between 10,000 to 20,000 cave myotis bats (*Myotis velifer*) can be found in various chambers. Predomi-

[1]In supporting prodigious colonies of Mexican free-tailed bats, the various nursery caves of the Southwest are living factories of guano production. Guano, the accumulated excrement of the colony, has been mined extensively in caves throughout Texas and New Mexico. Early settlers retrieved guano from Frio Cave to use as fertilizer, driving wagons directly into the cave for loading. The nitrate-rich excrement was also used to make saltpeter for gunpowder during the Civil War (Reddell, 1961).

nantly in the winter months, but sometimes in summer, several thousand leaf-chinned bats (*Mormoops megalophylla*) are present. By far, the most numerous of the three Chiropteran inhabitants is the Mexican free-tailed (or Mexican guano) bat. In summer months, they use the cave as a nursery and an estimated 20 to 30 million free-tails could be found. The highly gregarious Mexican free-tailed bats form the largest colonies of any mammal (Greenhall, 1982).

Rabies among the Mexican free-tails is most commonly reported between April and November, particularly when young begin to fly from August through October. Two distinct peaks in occurrence of disease correspond to the seasonal migratory patterns of the bat and to increased submission of specimens at these times. The first peak occurs in June and corresponds to their migration north to the United States from Mexico and Central America. The second peak occurs in September on their flight south (Constantine, 1967; Constantine et al, 1968; Baer and Adams, 1970).

Experimental Studies Within Frio Cave

In a series of increasingly refined experiments, sentinel animals were exposed to the atmosphere of Frio Cave in different locations for varying periods of time. A diversity of animals were held in the cave for times ranging from a week to a month. Animals were selected with regard to their possible role in sylvatic rabies cycles (predators or native cave inhabitants) or their potential usefulness as future indicators of aerosol transmission of virus (rodents). The animals were carefully housed so as to allow exposure to the atmosphere of the cave while excluding cave-dwelling arthropods.

Among animals that developed rabies, foxes and coyotes proved highly susceptible. Several opossums developed rabies as well. The opossum has generally been considered to be less susceptible to rabies infection than many other mammals. However, susceptibility, as measured by parenteral inoculation, may differ from susceptibility to aerosolized virus (Constantine, 1967). Susceptibility may also vary with the variant of virus used in experimental studies.

Two general elements in the study believed to be critical to viral transmission were the presence of large numbers of bats combined with poor ventilation. Specific factors of concern were those related to dose/time interactions, including turbinate anatomy and physiology, mucociliary pattern, breathing habits, and atmospheric conditions within the cave. The portals of viral entry might have been skin wounds, the alimentary tract, or respiratory mucosa. Possible sources of exposure that were considered included:

1) Virus from urine or saliva of infected bats.
2) Contamination of environment by infective droplets.
3) Inhalation of viral-laden air.
4) Mechanical transmission by arthropods.

Constantine believed that the primary source of virus was droplets in the air. These were thought to have emanated from the vocalizations of the bats. Although larger droplets would have been filtered out by the upper respiratory system and removed by the mucociliary escalator after inhalation, a droplet nucleus might have invaded to the alveolar level. During the course of their residence within the cave, animals might have sustained minute trauma to the respiratory mucosa, caused by cave gases and guano dust. These traumatic lesions may have enhanced the uptake of virus. Stress might also have played a role in increasing the susceptibility of test animals to disease.

Rabies virus has been found in olfactory mucosa of infected Mexican free-tailed bats collected from Frio Cave (Constantine et al, 1972) and it is known that olfactory neuroepithelial cells are readily infected with rabies virus. Murphy et al (1973) demonstrated widespread oronasal distribution of rabies virus following centrifugal migration from the brain and several investigators have demonstrated that laboratory rodents can be infected with rabies virus following experimental intranasal instillation (Selimov et al, 1969; Hronovsky and Benda, 1969a, 1969b; Murphy, 1986; Lafay et al, 1991). These facts are consistent with the possibility that the respiratory system, under certain circumstances, may be a significant portal of entry for aerosolized virus.

Constantine et al (1972) suggested that the constant vocalizations of the free-tailed bats may have contributed to the presence of airborne virus within Frio Cave. Results obtained in Frio Cave were consistent with those of experimental studies, in which various animals could be infected by exposure to aerosolized rabies virus (Constantine et al, 1972; Winkler, 1975).

Constantine (1966) produced rabies in dogs, cats, coyotes, raccoons, striped skunks, and spotted skunks by intramuscular inoculation of a salivary gland suspension obtained from a rabid coyote. This coyote had been infected by injection of a salivary gland suspension obtained from another coyote which had previously been infected by aerosol exposure in a bat cave. These results were consistent with the possibility that animals infected by aerosol exposure might subsequently transmit disease to others.

In 1966, rabies virus was isolated from the atmosphere of Frio Cave using a mechanical air-sampling device (Winkler, 1968). Although exact quantities of virus in the air were not evaluated, the demonstration of air-borne virus was significant. The isolates recovered by Winkler were lethal only to foxes, which may have been highly susceptible.

The finding that many of the sentinel animals exposed to the atmosphere of Frio Cave developed rabies, and the subsequent isolation of virus from the atmosphere, suggested a mechanism whereby the two human deaths might have occurred. It has generally been accepted that the deaths of the entomologist and the mining engineer were due to rabies infection secondary to inhalation of aerosolized virus within Frio Cave or a similar free-tailed bat nursery site (Constantine et al, 1972).

Historical accounts of human illness associated with working in Frio Cave have been reported frequently, although their etiology remains unknown. Christensen (1946) wrote,

> *Guano has been mined from the tremendous, multi-apertured Rio Frio Cave for more than a century. Nitrates extracted from guano at this cave are said to have supplied much of the gunpowder for the Confederate armies during the War Between the States. Huge quantities of guano still remain, for miners in this cave seem to contract a violent disease and mining operations have not been completed.*

Constantine (1967) suggested that these early records may reflect historical evidence of aerosol-induced human rabies infection. Sulkin et al (1962), on the other hand, postulated that the neurologic disease observed in Latin American guano miners may have been due to infection with the Rio Bravo virus (see page 154). Systemic fungal infection due to histoplasmosis (Sulkin and Allen, 1971) and ammonia-induced pneumonia (Knutson, 1984) may also cause debilitating disease and have been reported in persons exploring densely populated nursery caves of the southwestern United States.

Evidence in Support of Inhalation Exposure

In support of an inhalation mechanism of transmission, Winkler (1975) cited Baer as communicating to him that a red fox, exposed deep within Frio cave for less than 12 hours, had become infected with rabies. It has generally been considered that foxes are among the most susceptible of animals to rabies infection. Our perceptions of species susceptibility, however, must change with respect to the route of exposure and the nature of the infecting isolate. Baer (1988) believes that humans, in general, are quite resistant to aerosolized rabies virus.

In further support of inhalation as a mechanism of exposure, it should be noted that experimental transmission of aerosolized rabies virus has been documented in laboratory rodents. There have also been two subsequent cases of human rabies believed to have been due to aerosol transmission of virus.

A somewhat different perspective can be gleaned from an unusual occurrence at the Public Health Service's Southwest Rabies Investigation Station in Las Cruces, New Mexico. This laboratory was established primarily to investigate the role of bats in rabies epidemiology in the southwestern United States. In the latter half of 1967, an unexplained rabies outbreak ravaged the unit's animal colony, killing 39 animals with no known history of exposure to rabies (Winkler et al, 1972;

HUMAN RABIES FOLLOWING EXPOSURE TO AEROSOLIZED VIRUS

At the turn of the century, two persons were reported to have developed rabies following exposure to "the hot breath of the [rabid] wolf" (Babes, 1912 [cited by Fishbein, 1991]). In recent years, two other cases of human rabies following inhalation of viral aerosols have been documented.

One involved a 56-year-old veterinarian working in a commercial laboratory producing rabies vaccine (Winkler et al, 1973). On March 1, 1972, he began suffering from headaches, vomiting, diarrhea, abdominal cramps, and generalized weakness. On admission to the hospital, physical examination was within normal limits, but his temperature increased to 102.9° F and confusion developed within several hours. By 36 hours after the onset of clinical signs, his temperature had increased to 104.9° F. His confusion worsened and he passed into a stuporous and then comatose state. On the second day of illness, he was transferred to Scott and White Memorial Hospital, still in deep coma, with irregular respiration. Pupils were pinpoint and his left arm and leg were hyperreflexic. He remained in a decerebrate posture. He died eight days after the onset of symptoms.

On February 17, the patient had participated for an hour in the preparation of a batch of experimental rabies vaccine. In the course of this procedure, it is believed that he had spent time breathing above a kitchen-type blender, which was being used to homogenize the brains of 11 rabid goats. The blender had been covered with a loose-fitting lid and it was subsequently found that its use resulted in the production of visible aerosols. Infection was believed to have been due to inhalation of substantial amounts of aerosolized virus during the course of vaccine production. Although unlikely, the possibility that other mechanisms of transmission may have been responsible could not be completely ruled out. These included oral inoculation and entry through skin lesions. The patient had received four doses of an experimental rabies vaccine in 1958, but did not have a positive serum antibody titer when tested the following year (Winkler et al, 1973).

Another case involved a 32-year-old laboratory technician at the New York State Department of Health in 1977. He was part of a research effort endeavoring to produce an orally effective wildlife rabies vaccine. This involved coating small pellets with aerosolized virus. During the course of the work, he was accidentally exposed to a heavy dose of aerosolized virus. On February 14, he developed malaise and a headache and left work early. Over the next several days, he experienced nausea and chills in the afternoon. On April 18, he felt weak and feverish.

He was admitted to the Albany Medical Center on April 20, where he was observed to be lethargic, with expressive aphasia. The following day, he passed into a comatose state, which remained unchanged through May 3. After this time, his condition began to slowly improve. Although this technician suffered from a confirmed case of paralytic rabies, he survived. With time, he recovered use of his arms and legs, and partial recovery of speech (Tillotson et al, 1977a, 1977b), although considerable neurologic impairment remains to date.

Winkler, 1975). Animals that died included 10 coyotes, 12 gray foxes, 14 red foxes, 2 kit foxes, and 1 raccoon.

By May of 1968, measurable titers (1:5) of serum neutralizing antibodies against the rabies virus were found in four animals which had survived the outbreak. These animals had been serologically negative on arrival at the facility and had never been knowingly exposed to rabies while there. An interesting feature of this laboratory outbreak was the rabies attack rate (number of new cases in a given time interval per population at risk initially exposed) for certain species. These were comparable to those measured in sentinel animals by Constantine at Frio Cave (Table 14-1).

The epidemiological evidence, although admittedly circumstantial, pointed to aerosol dissemination of virus as the cause of the SWRIS epizootic. It was believed that the virus was of

Table 14-1

Rabies Attack Rates Measured During the SWRIS Epizootic Compared With Attack Rates for Sentinel Animals Exposed to Aerosolized Virus in Frio Cave

Animal	Laboratory Outbreak	Frio Cave Exposures
Coyote	92%	100%
Gray Fox	71%	94%
Kit Fox	48%	73%
Red Fox	34%	56%
Opossum	18%	37%
Raccoon	5%	-
Skunk	-	-

From Winkler, W. G., Baker, Jr., E. R., and C. C. Hopkins. An outbreak of non-bite transmitted rabies in a laboratory animal colony. *Am. J. Epidemiol.* 95(3): 267, 1972. Reproduced with permission.

bat origin and shed by several animals intentionally infected sometime previously. In using bat variants of virus in their experiments, Winkler (1975) suggested that the investigators may have "selected for a strain of virus well adapted for airborne dissemination." The water sprayer used to clean cages was suspected of aerosolizing virus shed in secretions of infected animals and contaminating the cages. The problem may have been compounded by a malfunctioning air-exchange system.

In the course of five months, in the midst of the rabies epizootic at the Southwest Rabies Investigation Station, repeated air samples were negative for rabies virus (Winkler, 1975). However, these air samples were necessarily obtained after the exposures occurred, rather than 1 to 2 months prior to the onset of clinical signs, when the exposures most likely occurred.

Inhalation Exposure in Frio Cave?

While inhalation of a viral aerosol was certainly a possible mode of disease transmission, it was, by no means, the only one. Constantine's suggestion that human intruders into Frio Cave easily suffer bumps and bruises, scratches from flying bats, and bites from arthropods points to possible modes of transmission other than inhalation. The key to belief in an inhalation exposure lies in the alleged absence of any other likely means of transmission, particularly animal bites or scratches. According to Constantine (1962), both individuals were reliable observers who, while still conscious and alert, denied being bitten.

In describing the account of the mining engineer, Humphrey et al (1960) reported that he had been emphatic in his denial of having sustained an animal bite. However, he had emerged from Frio Cave with a small bleeding wound on his face. In the medical case history, Kent and Finegold (1960) reported that his denials of bat bite had been made in a state of progressively worsening confusion and conflicted with the story he had earlier told his friend. There is no substantial evidence to indicate how this wound was incurred. Humphrey et al (1960) and Kent and Finegold (1960) reported that he had been "nicked" in the face by a bat.

In reality, the possibilities are numerous and include, among others, bat bite, bat scratch, or a scrape due to falling or stumbling within the cave. Although bats tend to hang on tenaciously when biting, it remains a possibility that he had been bitten without his realizing it. Kent and Finegold (1960) believed that the patient had been bitten by a bat in Frio Cave.

In their studies of Mexican free-tail maternity caves in Texas, Davis et al (1962) found that swarms of bats would often crawl over investigators. On exposed skin surfaces, the bats would scratch enough to cause reddening of the skin. Whether or not a scratch by a rabid bat constitutes an exposure to rabies is not known. In an environment such as Frio Cave, where virus appears able to exist in the atmosphere, it seems possible that virulent virus may linger on the claws of a bat (perhaps even a noninfected one). This remains unsubstantiated. It is also possible that virus may persist for a short period of time on the claws of a rabid bat following contamination with saliva during grooming (Constantine, 1988). With thousands of bats flying around him, as the patient reported, an infectious scratch may have occurred.

Other nonbite sources of exposure may have included contact with fomites or exposure of open wounds (such as the one on his face) to an infectious aerosol.[2] The patient reported "wading" through knee-deep guano. In the context of the unique environment of Frio Cave, or other similar environments, surface contamination of guano by aerosolized droplets might also have been a possible (although unsubstantiated) source of infection.

In the case of the entomologist, Irons et al (1957) reported that he had a chronic skin eruption on his neck. A site of dermatitis might also have been a point of viral infection. Irons et al (1957) were of the opinion that the source of exposure was rubbing his neck with contaminated gloves. Such a source of exposure can be entertained on a theoretical basis only in context of the unique environment of a Frio Cave-like ecosystem.

Final consideration must be given to the time frame involved. In the experiments reported from Frio Cave, animals were exposed to the cave's atmosphere for extended periods of time. Human exposure, however, would have been measured in hours at most. The lesions in the respiratory tract that Constantine spoke of might not have occurred in so short a time. But it is impossible to say how much of the time spent in the cave by sentinel animals was actually pre-exposure.

Although Constantine commented briefly on the possibility of other routes of exposure in his 1967 report, inhalation has generally been emphasized as the probable mechanism involved. Inhalation of aerosolized virus certainly may have occurred, but it is not the only possible route of infection in these cases. Despite the widespread acceptance of inhalation as the source of human exposure in the Frio Cave system, the evidence of an inhalation mechanism is not at all conclusive (Constantine, 1986).

References

Babes, V. (1912). *Traite de la Rage*. Librarie J. B. Balliere et Fils, Paris.

Baer, G. M. (1988). Chief, Rabies Laboratory. Centers for Disease Control. Atlanta, Georgia. Personal communication.

Baer, G. M. and D. B. Adams (1970). Rabies in insectivorous bats in the United States, 1953-1965. *Pub. Hlth. Repts.* 85(7): 637

Bell, J. F., Hadlow, W. J., and W. L. Jellison (1957). A survey of chiropteran rabies in western Montana. *Pub. Hlth. Repts.* 72(1): 16

Bell, J. F., Moore, G. J., and G. H. Raymond (1969). Protracted survival of a rabies-infected insectivorous bat after infective bite. *Am. J. Trop. Med. Hyg.* 18(1): 61

Bisseru, B. (1972). *Rabies*. Woolnough Ltd. Wellingborough, Great Britain.

Christensen, E. (1946). The bats of Carlsbad Caverns. *Animal Kingdom*. XLIX(3): 98

Constantine, D. G. (1962). Rabies transmission by nonbite route. *Pub. Hlth. Repts.* 77(4): 287

Constantine, D. G. (1966). Transmission experiments with bat rabies isolates: Responses of certain carnivora to rabies virus isolated from animals infected by nonbite route. *Am. J. Vet. Res.* 27(116): 13

Constantine, D. G. (1967). *Rabies Transmission by Air in Bat Caves*. Public Health Service Publication No. 1617. National Communicable Disease Center. Atlanta, Georgia.

Constantine, D. G. (1986). Public Health Veterinarian. Department of Health Services, State of California - Health and Welfare Agency, Veterinary Public Health Unit. Berkeley, California. Personal communication.

Constantine, D. G. (1988). Health Precautions for Bat Researchers. In T. H. Kunz (ed.) *Ecological and Behavioral Methods for the Study of Bats*. Smithsonian Institution Press. Washington, D. C.

Constantine, D. G., Tierkel, E. S., Kleckner, M. D., and D. M. Hawkins (1968). Rabies in New Mexico cavern bats. *Pub. Hlth. Repts.* 83(4): 303

Constantine, D. G., Emmons, R. E., and J. D. Woodie (1972). Rabies virus in nasal mucosa of naturally infected bats. *Science*. 175: 1255

Davis, R. B., Herreid, C. F., and H. L. Short (1962). Mexican free-tailed bats in Texas. *Ecol. Monogr.* 32(4): 311

[2]Although the virus is present in saliva and, to a limited extent, other secretions, a marked viremia is not normally a feature of clinical rabies. Thus, despite some earlier reports to the contrary, vectors of blood-borne diseases, such as biting flies, mites, ticks, etc., which abound in free-tailed bat nurseries, have not been considered significant in rabies transmission (Remlinger and Bailly, 1939; Reagan et al, 1956; Bell et al, 1957, 1969; Nicolitsch, 1959 [cited by Bisseru, 1972]). Similarly, nonrabid vampire bats have not been shown to become infected from feeding on rabid cattle.

Eads, R. B., Wiseman, J. S., and G. C. Menzies (1957). Observations concerning the Mexican free-tailed bat, *Tadarida mexicana*, in Texas. *Texas J. Sci.* 9(2): 227

Fishbein, D. (1991). Rabies in Humans. In G. M. Baer (ed.) *The Natural History of Rabies*. 2nd Edition. CRC Press, Inc. Boca Raton, Florida.

Greenhall, A. M. (1982). *House Bat Management*. Resource Publication No. 143. United States Fish and Wildlife Service. Washington, D. C.

Hronovsky, V. and R. Benda (1969a). Experimental inhalation infection of laboratory rodents with rabies virus. *Acta Virol.* 13: 193

Hronovsky, V. and R. Benda (1969b). Development of inhalation rabies infection in suckling guinea pigs. *Acta Virol.* 13: 198

Humphrey, G. L., Kemp, G. E., and E. G. Wood (1960). A fatal case of rabies in a woman bitten by an insectivorous bat. *Pub. Hlth. Repts.* 75(4): 317

Irons, J. V., Eads, R. B., Sullivan, T., and J. E. Grimes (1954). The current status of rabies in Texas. *Texas Repts. Biol. Med.* 12: 489

Irons, J. V., Eads, R. B., Grimes, J. E., and A. Conklin (1957). The public health importance of bats. *Texas. Repts. Biol. Med.* 15: 292

Kent, J. R. and M. F. Finegold (1960). Human rabies transmitted by the bite of a bat. *New Engl. J. Med.* 263(21): 1058

Knutson, S. (1984). American Caving Accidents, 1983. *NSS (Natl. Speleol. Soc.) News*. 42(11): 353

Lafay, F., Coulon, P., Astic, L., Saucier, D., Riche, D., Holley, A., and A. Flamand (1991). Spread of the CVS strain of rabies virus and of the avirulent mutant AvO1 along the olfactory pathways of the mouse after intranasal inoculation. *Virology*. 183: 320

Murphy, F. A. (1986). *Pathogenesis of Rabies Infection—Rabies Control Symposium*. Washington, D. C. November 3-5, 1986

Murphy, F. A., Harrison, A. K., Washington, B. S., Winn, C., and S. P. Bauer (1973). Comparative pathogenesis of rabies and rabies-related viruses: Infection of the central nervous system and centrifugal spread of virus to peripheral tissues. *Lab. Invest.* 29(1): 1

Reagan, R. L., Tromba, F. G., Geumlek, M., and A. L. Brueckner (1956). Transmission of a street rabies virus strain (R-174) from the cave bat (*Myotis lucifugus*) to the tick (*Ornithodoros*) by blood feeding: A preliminary report. *Cornell Vet.* 46: 3

Reddell, J. R. (1961). The caves of Uvalde County. Part I. Texas Speleological Survey. *Texas Speleol. Assoc.* 1(3): 10

Remlinger, P. and J. Bailly (1939). *Ann. Inst. Pasteur.* 62: 463

Selimov, M. A., Marinina, V. P., Nikitina, L. F., and R. Sh. Ilyasova (1969). Experimental respiratory infection induced by rabies virus variants adapted to tissue culture. *Acta Virol.* 13: 135

Sulkin, S. E. and R. Allen (1971). Potential hazards to investigators of bat inhabited caves. In E. L. Lundelius, Jr. and B. H. Slaughter (eds.) *Natural History of Texas Caves*. Gulf Natural History. Dallas, Texas.

Sulkin, S. E., Burns, K. F., Shelton, D. F., and C. Wallis (1962). Bat salivary gland virus: Infection of man and monkey. *Texas Repts. Biol. Med.* 20: 113

Tillotson, J. R., Axelrod, D., and D. O. Lyman (1977a). Rabies in a laboratory worker—New York. *MMWR*. 26(22): 183

Tillotson, J. R., Axelrod, D., and D. O. Lyman (1977b). Follow-up on rabies—New York. *MMWR*. 26(31): 249

Winkler, W. G. (1968). Airborne rabies virus isolation. *Bull. Wildl. Dis. Assoc.* 4: 37

Winkler, W. G. (1975). Airborne Rabies. In G. M. Baer (ed.) *The Natural History of Rabies*. Vol. II. Academic Press. New York.

Winkler, W. G., Baker, Jr., E. R., and C. C. Hopkins (1972). An outbreak of non-bite transmitted rabies in a laboratory animal colony. *Am. J. Epidemiol.* 95(3): 267

Winkler, W. G., Fashinell, T. R., Leffingwell, L., Howard, P., and J. P. Conomy (1973). Airborne rabies transmission in a laboratory worker. *J. Am. Med. Assoc.* 226(10): 1219

Chapter 15:

VIRAL TRANSMISSION STUDIES AND RETROSPECTIVE ANALYSES

Are Insectivorous Bats a Special Link in the Spread of Disease?

The discovery of a previously unknown reservoir of rabies virus in the early 1950's certainly had far-ranging public-health implications, demanding the attention of medical authorities (Tjalma and Wentworth, 1957; Tierkel, 1958). The finding of rabies virus in insectivorous bats prompted early concern that these animals might be of special significance in sylvatic rabies cycles (Figure 15-1). Favoring such an association, early investigators pointed to the possibility that the migrations of rabid bats could explain the occurrence of enzootic rabies in geographically widely separated wildlife populations.

Based only on highly speculative evidence, proposals had been advanced, time and time again, that bats were important links in maintaining an ongoing infection of wildlife (Venters et al, 1954; Burns and Farinacci, 1955; Irons et al, 1957; Schneider et al, 1957). An editorial in the *New England Journal of Medicine* (1957), for example, suggested that "the dog, wolf and the fox, like man, are merely incidental sparks from a smoldering fire of chiropterous [bat] rabies." Early suggestions were made that serious consideration be given to population-reduction programs (Burns and Farinacci, 1955). Within two years of their discovery, rabid bats (and by extension, all bats) in the United States had been labeled a menace to public health.[1]

Wildlife populations believed to be directly at risk from this newly uncovered source of virus were those which preyed upon bats or other cave-dwelling species, and those which utilized bat caves as shelters. Skunks and raccoons, the predominant wildlife reservoirs of rabies in the United States, as well as foxes, are all known to feed to a varying extent upon bats and are among the most common terrestrial mammals visiting caves (Constantine, 1948; Stamm et al, 1956; Eads et al, 1955, 1957; Irons et al, 1957; Reddell, 1961; Davis et al, 1962; Constantine et al, 1968a; Harris, 1971; Winkler and Adams, 1972). Results of fecal analysis have shown that, in some areas, over 90% of a raccoon's diet may consist of bats (Winkler and Adams, 1972). Skunks and raccoons have also been observed using southwestern bat caves as dens (Davis et al, 1962; Winkler and Adams, 1972).

The suggestion that bats might serve as important reservoirs of wildlife rabies marked the advent of studies seeking to elucidate the relationships, if any, among bats, caves, and rabies in terrestrial wildlife. These have generally taken one of three basic forms: viral transmission studies (inoculation, forced bite, and ingestion), consideration of epidemiologic associations and retrospective analyses, and monoclonal antibody surveys.

[1]At present, an analogous situation is emerging in this country with regard to the American pit bull terrier. Real or imagined, deserved or not, this dog is quickly gaining a reputation as a vicious, unpredictable killer. In the face of expanded, and generally highly biased, media coverage, the breed has been swept into a growing arena of public controversy. In fact, in England, the *Dangerous Dogs Act* of 1991 has been enacted with the express intent of eliminating the breed from the country (Comment, 1993). As the saga of the pit bull evolves, it provides valuable insight into the shaping of public sentiment towards animals like bats. Time, publicity, fear, fact, and fancy will continue to intertwine in complex fashion to either exonerate or condemn creatures who do not conveniently fit into the mainstream of human affection.

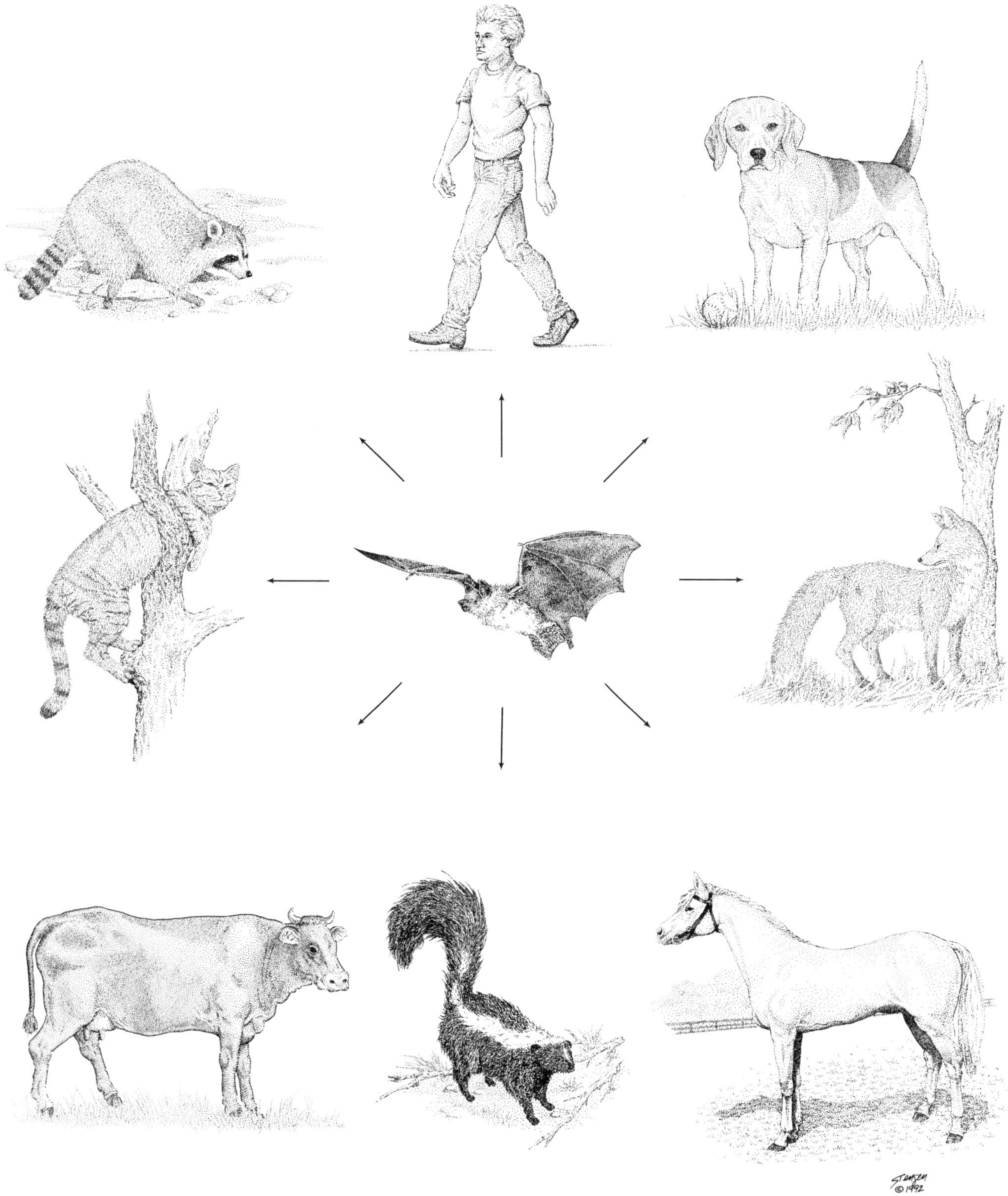

Figure 15-1. The discovery of rabies in North American bat populations led to the belief among some early investigators that bats played a pivotal role in the initiation and maintenance of infection in terrestrial species. Today, this is known not to be the case. Although sporadic transmission of rabies from bats to other animals (including humans) has been documented, modern epidemiologic evidence is consistent with the fact that nonterrestrial and terrestrial rabies cycles are largely independent of each other.

Limitations of Inoculation and Forced-Bite Studies

Viral-transmission studies were designed to test the validity of interspecies transmission of rabies from bats to other animals. These early investigations primarily included inoculation and forced-bite studies, in which test animals were either inoculated with virus isolated from infected bats or made to suffer repeated bites from experimentally infected bats. Inoculation studies attest to the susceptibility of test mammals to infection with nonterrestrial viral isolates. Susceptibility to parenteral challenge with bat isolates suggests that a test animal might be infected if bitten by a rabid bat. These approaches, while certainly shedding some light on the question of wildlife viral transmission, both suffered from certain inherent limitations.

With regard to viral inoculations, these do not precisely simulate natural bat bites. Injection, as a means of depositing virus within a test subject's body, is extremely efficacious. It allows for clean transmission of virus, with complete assuredness of delivery. It also permits the investigator to select the most appropriate injection site, as well as dose and variant of virus. No margin is allowed for natural variables, which might affect transmission during a natural encounter. These would include considerations such as propensity to bite; capacity to bite; location, number, and effectiveness of bites; amount of saliva discharged with bite; and viral titer in that saliva.

While bite studies more nearly approximate natural conditions, these have often involved repeated bites on mucous membranes, or in thin-skinned suckling animals, conditions that may not be entirely representative of circumstances in the wild. The potential for experimental viral transmission is optimized and the extent to which such an experimental protocol mimics natural encounters may be suspect. Failure to establish viral transmission by forced biting may reflect a time when virus is not present in the saliva of an infected bat, a relative lack of susceptibility of test animals to the particular variant of virus being used, or an inadequate vector competence (perhaps related to a bat's inability to bite deeply enough to pierce the skin of a test subject).

Although confirmation that the biting bat is infected with rabies is made, saliva has not always been tested for the presence of virus at the time of the forced bite. This may be significant because a bat may have virus in its brain, but not in its salivary glands (Constantine, 1966a; Bell et al, 1969). Virus may be present in salivary glands of an individual bat at one particular time, but not at another (Constantine and Woodall, 1966; Baer and Bales, 1967; Bell et al, 1969). A cycle of salivary infection may exist.[2] In rabid dogs, salivary secretion of virus prior to death may be of an intermittent or steady nature (King, 1991a). King (1991b) reported the isolation of rabies virus from 6 of 7 samples of saliva obtained daily from a woman in Zambia until three days prior to her death, at which time virus could no longer be isolated in salivary samples.

Experimental Parenteral Transmission of Rabies Virus

Burns et al (1958) found that isolates of virus from naturally infected Mexican free-tailed bats could produce rabies when injected intramuscularly, subcutaneously, or intracerebrally into guinea pigs, hamsters, rabbits, and goats. Pooled salivary glands from Mexican free-tailed bats experimentally infected with homologous rabies virus (virus isolated from a naturally infected member of the same species), when injected intramuscularly, were shown to produce rabies in dogs, foxes, coyotes, raccoons, skunks, ringtail cats, and other Mexican free-tailed bats. Domestic cats and opossums were unaffected (Constantine, 1966a). Intramuscular inoculation of pooled salivary glands from red bats experimentally infected with homologous virus produced rabies in skunks and ringtail cats, but not dogs, cats, foxes, coyotes, opossums, deer mice, or wood rats (Constantine and Woodall, 1966). Trimarchi et al (1986) demonstrated development of rabies in cats following intramuscular inoculation of virus obtained from the salivary glands of a naturally infected big brown bat.

[2]This does not imply the presence of an asymptomatic salivary carrier state (see page 154).

Experimental Transmission of Rabies Virus by Forced Biting

Bite-induced transmission of rabies virus from rabid bats has been studied in several species of laboratory animals. Rabies was produced in suckling mice following bites on the thigh by naturally infected California myotis (*Myotis californicus californicus*) and silver-haired bats (Bell, 1959; Bell et al, 1962). Suckling mice were also infected by bites from red bats experimentally infected with homologous virus (Constantine and Woodall, 1966). Naturally infected silver-haired and big brown bats could transmit rabies to older mice in some instances (Bell et al, 1962). Burns et al (1958) were unable to demonstrate infection of mice or guinea pigs following multiple bites on the ears and abdomen by pallid bats experimentally infected with rabies virus of Mexican free-tailed bat origin. The authors believed these bats to be incapable of inflicting a wound of sufficient depth to vector the rabies virus.

Constantine et al (1968b) demonstrated transmission of virus to a hamster, but not to suckling mice, by the bite of a leaf-nosed bat (*Macrotus waterhouseii*) experimentally infected with homologous rabies virus. They were unable to produce infection in suckling mice, hamsters, or various carnivores by bites from hoary, silver-haired, or big brown bats experimentally infected with homologous virus. In their inoculation studies, varying dosages of rabies virus from hoary and big brown bats experimentally infected with homologous virus, failed to produce infection in hamsters. The authors concluded that these species of bats do not readily transmit virus to other animals in nature. Recent evidence attests to the fact that big brown bats, both experimentally and naturally infected, can transmit virus to terrestrial species (Trimarchi, 1984, 1986a, 1986b; Centers for Disease Control, 1985; Smith et al, 1986).

Burns et al (1958) enclosed individual monkeys in cages with between 50 and 100 rabid Mexican free-tailed bats. Bats were either naturally infected or experimentally infected with homologous virus. The monkeys and bats had many vicious encounters, with bats often being dismembered or devoured. The monkeys sustained multiple bite wounds on the hands and digits, as well as stab wounds to the throat and gums. In no instance did monkeys become rabid or develop measurable titers of rabies-neutralizing antibody. That they were susceptible to the viral isolates used was demonstrated by infection following intracerebral inoculation. However, this does not mimic naturally occurring bites.

Constantine (1966b) subjected foxes and coyotes to bites by Mexican free-tailed bats experimentally infected with homologous virus. Each test animal was subjected to bites on the labial mucosa, free edge of lip, area between lip and nose, and on the nose. It seems justifiable that a bat predator would incur bites about the face. Deaths from rabies were subsequently observed in both species.

In the course of experimental infection, however, each coyote was subjected to 724 bat bites and each fox to 660 bat bites. Constantine said, "...one might wonder if a comparable occurrence would be found in nature." The likelihood of such an occurrence being real seems remote and the significance of these findings, therefore, remains equivocal. Constantine could come to no firm conclusion regarding the number of bites required to produce infection, although he considered it possible that successful transmission had occurred early in the sequence.

Based only on these preliminary transmission studies, the role of bats in sylvatic rabies cycles remained obscure (Anonymous, 1973; National Research Council Subcommittee on Rabies, 1973). Transmission of virus from bats to other animals had been accomplished, but only with difficulty. However, even rabid dogs do not transmit virus to bite victims consistently. Probability of disease among untreated persons bitten by confirmed rabid dogs varies between 15% and 60%, depending on numerous factors.

Experimental Transmission of Rabies Virus by Ingestion

Carnivores frequently consume fallen bats at the entrance to bat caves, or capture bats emerging from low-level cave entrances. Davis et al (1962) reported that raccoons in residence in Texas bat caves consumed grounded bats, but did not hunt bats roosting on accessible walls or ceilings. Bats on cave floors are more readily consumed and more likely to be ill (perhaps rabid) than individuals roosting high on walls or ceilings. A great many bats, sick or injured, frequently collapse during emergence flights. Some of these bats may also be rabid and the potential exists for viral transmission to predators by bite or ingestion (Stamm et al, 1956; Lord et al, 1975). Moreover, animals that have already died of rabies may also serve as potential sources of virus for scavengers which devour the body.

Experiments with mice have shown that these animals can become infected by consuming tissues of mice infected with rabies virus of canine, insectivorous-bat, and vampire-bat origin, as well as those infected with the CVS strain of virus (Soave, 1966; Correa-Giron et al, 1970; Delpietro et al, 1990). Shen and Shumeikina (1958) reported that rats could become infected following oral administration of rabies virus in either solution or brain tissue. The degree of oral infectivity varied with the particular variant. Fischman and Ward, III (1968) reported that oral administration of rabies virus produced rabies in neonatal mice, rabbits, guinea pigs, and hamsters. They also reported oral transmission to mother mice following cannibalism of experimentally infected infants. Fedaku et al (1988) found that oral inoculation (cannibalization of infected sucklings) of a viral isolate from a big brown bat, as well as a Danish bat isolate, was lethal to female breeder mice. Delpietro et al (1990) reported the transmission of rabies to rodents following ingestion of brain tissue from cattle that had died of vampire-induced rabies.

Bell and Moore (1971) were unable to document oral infection of ferrets or cats, even after consumption of as many as 25 rabid mouse carcasses infected with virus of skunk, hoary bat, silver-haired bat, or little brown bat origin. Antibody titers were not demonstrable in these animals. However, skunks did become infected after consumption of a single carcass. Ramsden and Johnston (1975) observed development of rabies in foxes and skunks fed varying numbers of rabid mice infected with virus of skunk or red-fox origin.

Two human deaths in China due to rabies following the preparation and consumption of rabid dogs have been reported by Kureishi et al (1992), although handling and skinning of these animals, rather than ingestion, may have been the source of infection (see page 107).

The significance of oral transmission of virus to sylvatic rabies cycles is not readily apparent. Bell and Moore (1971) postulated that ingestion of rabid bats may be an important feature of transmission of virus to local predators. To date, there is no evidence to support an important contribution to maintenance of wildlife infection. However, Delpietro et al (1990) suggested that the consumption of rabid carcasses may increase the potential risks to humans from rodent bites.

Retrospective Analyses: Associations on a Local Level

Fischman and Young (1976) studied associations[3] among caves, bats, and the presence of rabies in fox populations. Prior to monoclonal and genetic analyses of viral isolates, a great number of observational and experimental difficulties existed in testing the hypothesis of causal relation between rabies in bats and that in wildlife (e.g., foxes). With respect to these difficulties, Fischman and Young (1976) wrote,

> *The direct natural observation of appropriate contact of a fox with a bat, followed by development of disease in the fox and the subsequent spreading of the disease to other members of the species is not going to be made. Testing of a bat-fox hypothesis would have to include observational studies, such as an examination of the strength of the association found with fox rabies and caves,*

[3]An association refers to the nature of relationships between two variables. If two variables occur together more often than can be accounted for by chance alone, the association is positive in nature. If they occur together less often than would be expected by chance alone, the association is negative. An association between a disease and a potential causative agent can be considered nonstatistical if it arises by chance alone and statistical if variables are positively related. In establishing a causal relationship between variables, consideration must be given to: 1) the time sequence of events, 2) the strength of the association, 3) the biological gradient, 4) consistency, and 5) compatibility with existing knowledge (Thrusfield, 1986).

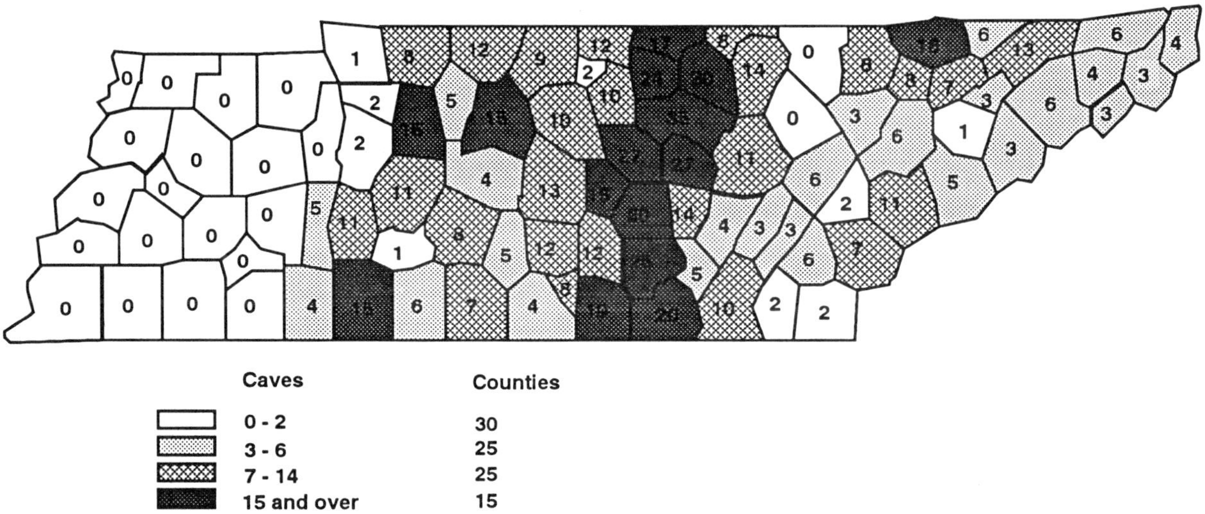

Figure 15-2. Number of caves in Tennessee, by county. (From Fredrickson, L. E. and L. Thomas. Relationship of fox rabies to caves. *Pub. Hlth. Repts.* 80(6): 495, 1965. Redrawn with permission.)

retrospective studies of the occurrence of fox rabies from a time and place point of view and prospective population and disease studies of foxes and bats in cave and non-cave areas accompanied by antibody and virus isolation studies. Evidence incriminating the bat as a basic reservoir animal, if forthcoming, will have to be based on epidemiologic proof and data demonstrating convincing biologic plausibility.

Such an observational analysis was first made in Tennessee by Fredrickson and Thomas in 1965, a time which predated development of the monoclonal antibody technology that now allows researchers to antigenically characterize rabies viruses. They proposed a close association between the reported incidence of fox rabies and the location of caves in the state. Accordingly, a retrospective study of fox rabies in the years between 1946 and 1961 indicated that 1.3% of the caves and 0.1% of the cases of fox rabies had been in the western part of the state, 74% of the caves and 70.1% of the cases of fox rabies had been in the central part of the state, and 24.8% of the caves and 29.8% of the cases of fox rabies had been in the eastern part of the state. The authors considered that the caves served as a "catalyst in bringing the rabid bat and the susceptible fox together in a manner that permits the fox to become infected."

While these data are suggestive of a close relationship between caves and fox rabies, certain aspects of the analysis are questionable. In particular, if each of the state's counties is considered individually, the observed correlation between the number of caves and rabid foxes breaks down. The authors reported counties as having 0 to 2, 3 to 6, 7 to 14, or greater than 15 caves; and 0, 1 to 9, 10 to 19, or greater than 20 reported cases of fox rabies over the 15-year period. Of 15 counties with more than 15 caves, only 3 (20%) reported more than 20 cases of fox rabies, whereas 28% (7 out of 25) of those counties with 7 to 14 caves reported more than 20 cases of fox rabies. Twenty-nine percent (4 of 14) of the counties reporting more than 20 cases of fox rabies had less than 6 caves (Figures 15-2 and 15-3).

When considered from this perspective, a less significant correlation is suggested, instead of the directly positive one reported in the study. In reexamining the data, Hayne and Neeley (1967 [cited by Editorial, 1967]) concluded that there is "no important relationship between the number of caves per county and any of the factors they

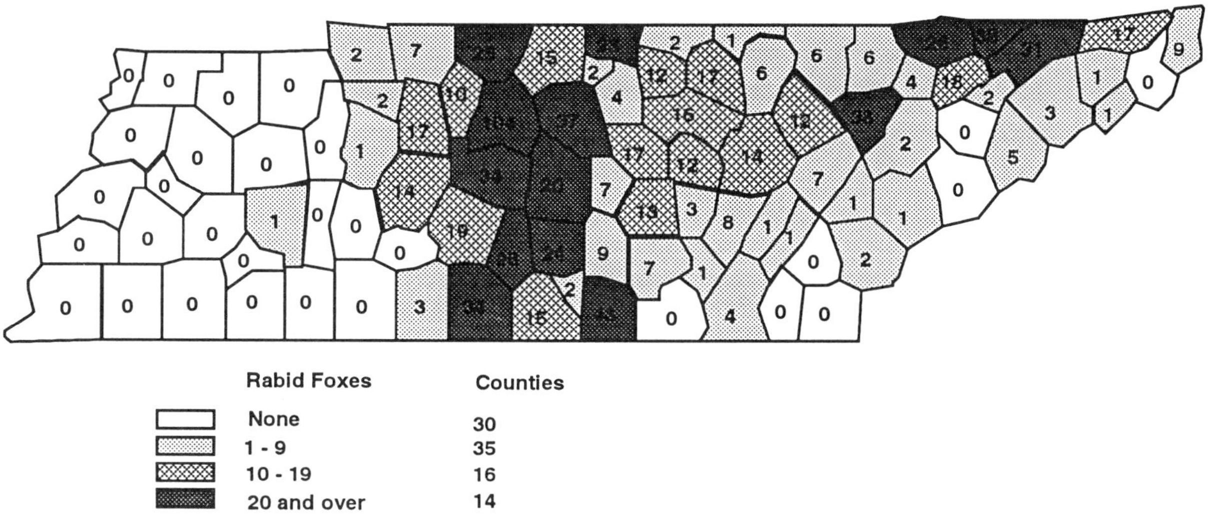

Figure 15-3. Number of rabid foxes in Tennessee, by county, 1946-1961. (From Fredrickson, L. E. and L. Thomas. Relationship of fox rabies to caves. *Pub. Hlth. Repts.* 80(6): 495, 1965. Redrawn with permission.)

examined." Rather, the findings may have been an artifact of their method of pooling data (Hayne, 1993).

Mahan (1973) examined the relationship between bats, caves, and fox rabies in Tennessee. No significant differences in fox utilization of caves were observed between caves with or without bats and no correlations were found between the incidence of rabies in bats and that in foxes. In Georgia, no evidence could be found for a role of bats in the transmission of rabies virus to foxes (Carey, 1974).

More recently, Smith et al (1990) studied the antigenic relationship between rabies in bats and other wildlife, particularly raccoons, in Florida (see page 199). In this state, the raccoon is the major reservoir of terrestrial rabies. Based on results of monoclonal antibody studies, the authors found no evidence of any relationship.

Retrospective Analyses: Associations on a National Level

A similar association was made on a national level by Fischman and Young (1976). These authors noted the overlap between regions of enzootic fox rabies and karst areas in the United States. In considering the relationship between caves and fox rabies, Fischman (1976) discussed several reasons that would explain apparently positive associations, including:

1) **Direct Association** - There is a real association between caves and fox rabies, and the bats are directly or indirectly responsible for infecting foxes.

2) **Indirect Association** - There is a real association between caves and fox rabies, but neither the bats nor the caves are causal agents. An unknown factor or factors are involved. For example, cave areas may be superior fox habitats, supporting vastly greater fox populations.

3) **Artifactual, Spurious, or Biased Association** - The reporting of cases is biased because of predominant fox or human population densities.

While a number of remarkably positive associations existed, many unexplained negative ones did also. Thus, while fox rabies appeared to be enzootic in major karst regions, this was evidently true in many nonkarst regions, as well. Regarding final proof, Fischman (1976) considered that the strength of the statistical association of caves and fox rabies would necessarily be based upon retrospective analysis (in which past epidemiologic patterns are studied) and prospective analysis (in which continuous surveillance programs and experimental studies provide up-to-date information on various aspects of the disease). Biologic plausibility seemed to dominate as a mechanism for establishing the strength of the association. Several questions posed by Fischman (1976) are pertinent in this regard, including:

1) Do bats inhabit the caves in fox-rabies areas?
2) To what extent are these bats infected with virus?
3) Do foxes visit these caves?
4) What is the route whereby a fox may become infected?
5) To what extent are these foxes infected with virus?

Central to these types of population studies is an evenly distributed population of foxes in karst and nonkarst areas. In Texas, for example, Irons et al (1957) found that the population of raccoons, skunks, and foxes is considerably higher near caves. However, Carey (1982) reported that even in the high-population-density bat caves of the Southwest, foxes were not observed to concentrate at entrances to feed on bats as other predators do. In the absence of adequate population surveys, studies trying to correlate wildlife rabies with the presence of caves lack plausibility. Limited availability of information compounded the difficulties in developing final satisfactory proof of bats as reservoirs of sylvatic rabies.

It is interesting to note that reported cases of bat rabies are not well correlated with cave locations. This may be a reflection of migratory habit, habitat preference, or biased reporting due to geographic differences in human population density.

Insectivorous Bats and Sylvatic Rabies Cycles

Arguments have been advanced to suggest an association between bats, caves, and rabies in wildlife. The authors of these discussions have looked upon bats as providing the material upon which a long-sought "unifying hypothesis" of rabies transmission could be based and which would presumably be of value in developing plans to eradicate the disease (Fischman, 1976). There is no doubt that the potential for viral transmission from bats to terrestrial wildlife exists. Limited numbers of such instances (including 19 cases in foxes) have already been documented (see Table 16-1). The degree to which this potential is realized, however, while not fully known, does not appear to be extensive. In fact, it is believed to be relatively uncommon. Studies seeking to relate fox rabies with the presence of caves (and by association, bats) have simply not stood the test of time.

If bats were important agents in transmitting virus to local wildlife, terrestrial rabies would be more extensive in regions of enzootic bat rabies. Such a relationship, however, has not been found (Richardson et al, 1966 and Whitaker, Jr. et al, 1969 [cited by Kurta, 1979]; Friend, 1968; Whitaker, Jr. and Douglas, 1986). Although certainly a reflection of the extent of study and the method of statistics employed, it seems highly improbable that positive correlations, if they exist, should be so limited in geographic distribution.

Of significance, in this respect, is the fact that in the years between 1961 and 1992, there have been 294 recorded instances of states annually reporting cases of bat rabies alone (see Table 11-2). Nineteen states have reported rabies in bats, but not terrestrial animals, for at least two consecutive years and many for considerably longer. Similar associations are also known on local levels, bat rabies being exclusively present in particular locales (Carey, 1974). In British Columbia, rabies in insectivorous bats has been known since 1954 and has been reported continually in the virtual absence of known rabies in other species. Similar observations have been reported in Europe as well, where several countries have reported rabies in insectivorous bats in the absence of known infection in terrestrial species. In fact, bat rabies in Europe is often reported from areas without disease in foxes (Muller, 1992). In Europe, rabies in foxes has also been reported from areas in which bat rabies is reportedly absent. In Romania, for example, no rabies-positive specimens have been found among more than 900 insectivorous bats collected from an area of enzootic fox rabies (Stirbu et al, 1973).

These facts speak against an important role of bats in infecting terrestrial species of wildlife. Commenting on sylvatic cycles, Steele (1973) wrote, "...if the native bats of Canada and the United States were a reservoir of virus for wildlife or domestic farm animals and pets, the evidence would have been forthcoming by now." Twenty years later, the validity of this statement is supported by widespread surveillance studies (see Chapter 16). Baer (1985), on the other hand, in considering the future directions of rabies research, asked the question, "When rabies is controlled in wild animals will bats serve as a continuing source of reintroduction of the virus?" As we begin to make inroads in the elimination of wildlife rabies (see Chapter 21), time alone will provide the answer to this question, although current epidemiologic concepts do not support the likelihood of significant overlap of terrestrial and nonterrestrial rabies cycles.

The oral vaccination programs targeting red foxes in Europe have been highly successful in eliminating fox rabies from large portions of Europe. Eradication of fox rabies has been followed by the simultaneous disappearance of rabies in other terrestrial species living in the same regions (Wandeler, 1991). Bat rabies in these areas has remained essentially unchanged. These findings validate the premise that terrestrial and nonterrestrial rabies exist in largely independent cycles.

In the United States, infection in terrestrial animals may still be sporadically reported from states in which rabies is generally known to occur only in bats. In assessing the potential sources of exposure in these instances, Smith (1988) considered the following possibilities:

1) Exposure by contact with an infected bat.

2) Vaccination with live, attenuated rabies vaccine, followed by reversion of the vaccine strain to a virulent form.

3) Infection in an area in which rabies is enzootic in terrestrial species, followed by transport or migration to an area known to be free of terrestrial rabies.

The decline in canine rabies in the United States in recent decades has increased the relative importance of wildlife reservoirs of disease. Understanding the importance of wildlife reservoirs and the interactions among them is critical to our understanding of the epidemiology and epizootiology of this dreaded disease. Only an accurate perception of pertinent epidemiologic associations will provide a solid basis for intelligent disease control. In this respect, monoclonal antibodies have proven to be an exceptional tool in the evaluation of possible roles that bats may play in initiating and/or maintaining enzootic rabies in terrestrial species.

References

Anonymous (1973). Animal reservoirs of rabies. *The Lancet*. 1(7794): 89

Baer, G. M. (1985). Research Directions in Rabies. In W. G. Winkler (ed.) *Rabies Concepts for Medical Professionals*. Merieux Institute. Miami, Florida.

Baer, G. M. and G. L. Bales (1967). Experimental rabies infection in the Mexican freetail bat. *J. Infect. Dis*. 117: 82

Bell, J. F. (1959). Transmission of rabies to laboratory animals by bite of a naturally infected bat. *Science*. 129: 1490

Bell, J. F. and G. J. Moore (1971). Susceptibility of carnivora to rabies virus administered orally. *Am. J. Epidemiol*. 93(8): 176

Bell, J. F., Moore, G. J., Raymond, G. H., and C. E. Tibbs (1962). Characteristics of rabies in bats in Montana. *Am. J. Pub. Hlth*. 52(8): 1293

Bell, J. F., Moore, G. J., and G. H. Raymond (1969). Protracted survival of a rabies-infected insectivorous bat after infective bite. *Am. J. Trop. Med. Hyg*. 18(1): 61

Burns, K. F. and C. J. Farinacci (1955). Rabies in nonsanguivorous bats of Texas. *J. Infect. Dis*. 97: 211

Burns, K. F., Shelton, D. F., and E. W. Grogan (1958). Bat rabies: Experimental host transmission studies. *Ann. N. Y. Acad. Sci*. 70: 452

Carey, A. B. (1974). *An Analysis of an Apparent Rabies Epizootic in Rockbridge County, Virginia*. M.S. Thesis. Virginia Polytechnic Institute and State University. Blacksburg, Virginia.

Carey, A. B. (1982). The ecology of red foxes, gray foxes, and rabies in the eastern United States. *Wildl. Soc. Bull*. 10(1): 18

Centers for Disease Control (1985). An epidemiologic study of sylvatic rabies in Texas and New York using monoclonal antibodies. *CDC Rabies Surveillance Report.* U. S. Department of Health and Human Services, Public Health Service.

Comment (1993). Dangerous dogs and the law. *Vet. Rec.* 132(3): 49

Constantine, D. G. (1948). Great bat colonies attract predators. *Bull. Natl. Speleol. Soc.* 10: 100

Constantine, D. G. (1966a). Transmission experiments with bat rabies isolates: Reaction of certain carnivora, opossum, and bats to intramuscular inoculations of rabies virus isolated from free-tailed bats. *Am. J. Vet. Res.* 27(116): 16

Constantine, D. G. (1966b). Transmission experiments with bat rabies isolates: Bite transmission of rabies to foxes and coyotes by free-tailed bats. *Am. J. Vet. Res.* 27(116): 20

Constantine, D. G. and D. F. Woodall (1966). Transmission experiments with bat rabies isolates: Reactions of certain carnivora, opossum, rodents, and bats to rabies virus of red bat origin when exposed by bat bite or by intramuscular inoculation. *Am. J. Vet. Res.* 27(116): 24

Constantine, D. G., Tierkel, E. S., Kleckner, M. D., and D. M. Hawkins (1968a). Rabies in New Mexico cavern bats. *Pub. Hlth. Repts.* 83(4): 303

Constantine, D. G., Solomon, G. C., and D. F. Woodall (1968b). Transmission experiments with bat rabies isolates: Responses of certain carnivores and rodents to rabies viruses from four species of bats. *Am. J. Vet. Res.* 29(1): 181

Correa-Giron, E. P., Allen, R., and E. Sulkin (1970). The infectivity and pathogenesis of rabies virus administered orally. *Am. J. Epidemiol.* 91(2): 203

Davis, R. B., Herreid, C. F., and H. L. Short (1962). Mexican free-tailed bats in Texas. *Ecol. Monogr.* 32(4): 311

Delpietro, H., Segre, L., Marchevsky, N., and M. Berisso (1990). Transmision de rabia a roedores por la ingestion de tejidos extraidos de animales naturalmente infectados (Rabies transmission to rodents after ingestion of naturally infected tissues). *Medicina (Buenos Aires).* 50(4): 356 (English abstract) in *Vet. Bull.* (1991). 61(10): 1037

Eads, R. B., Wiseman, J. S., Grimes, J. E., and G. C. Menzies (1955). Wildlife rabies in Texas. *Pub. Hlth. Repts.* 70: 995

Eads, R. B., Wiseman, J. S., and G. C. Menzies (1957). Observations concerning the Mexican free-tailed bat, *Tadarida mexicana,* in Texas. *Texas J. Sci.* 9(2): 227

Editorial (1957). The rabid bat. *New Engl. J. Med.* 256(25): 1203

Editorial (1967). On caves and bats and rabies. *Bat Res. News.* 8(3): 20

Fedaku, M., Shaddock, J. H., Chandler, F. W., and D. W. Sanderlin (1988). Pathogenesis of rabies virus from a Danish bat (*Eptesicus serotinus*): Neuronal changes suggestive of spongiosis. *Arch. Virol.* 99: 187

Fischman, H. R. (1976). Consideration of an association between geographic distribution of caves and occurrence of rabies in foxes. *J. Am. Vet. Med. Assoc.* 169(11): 1207

Fischman, H. R. and F. E. Ward, III (1968). Oral transmission of rabies virus in experimental animals. *Am. J. Epidemiol.* 88: 132

Fischman, H. R. and G. S. Young (1976). An association between the occurrence of fox rabies and the presence of caves—Geographic relationships. *Am. J. Epidemiol.* 104(6): 593

Fredrickson, L. E. and L. Thomas (1965). Relationship of fox rabies to caves. *Pub. Hlth. Repts.* 80(6): 495

Friend, M. (1968). History and epidemiology of rabies in wildlife in New York. *New York Fish Game J.* 15: 71

Harris, A. H. (1971). Use of Texas Caves by Terrestrial Mammals. In E. L. Lundelius, Jr. and B. H. Slaughter (eds.) *Natural History of Texas Caves.* Gulf Natural History. Dallas, Texas.

Hayne, D. W. (1993). Institute of Statistics (retired). North Carolina State University. Raleigh, North Carolina. Personal communication.

Hayne, D. W. and D. L. R. Neeley (1967). Re-examination of reported relationships between caves and fox rabies in Tennessee. *Pres. 47th Annual Meeting of the American Society of Mammalogy.* Nags Head, North Carolina. June 18-22, 1967

Irons, J. V., Eads, R. B., Grimes, J. E., and A. Conklin (1957). The public health importance of bats. *Texas. Repts. Biol. Med.* 15: 292

King, A. A. (1991a). Rabies: A review. *J. Comp. Path.* 108: 1

King, A. A. (1991b). *Studies of the Antigenic Relationships of Rabies and Rabies-Related Viruses Using Anti-Nucleoprotein Monoclonal Antibodies.* Ph.D. Thesis. School of Biological Sciences, University of Surrey. Guildford, United Kingdom. Courtesy of Dr. Arthur A. King.

Kureishi, A., Xu, L. Z., Wu, H., and H. G. Stiver (1992). Rabies in China: Recommendations for control. *Bull. Wld. Hlth. Org.* 70(4): 443

Kurta, A. (1979). Bat rabies in Michigan. *Michigan Academician.* XII(2): 221

Lord, R. D., Delpietro, H., Fuenzalida, E., de Diaz, A. M. O., and L. Lazaro (1975). Presence of rabies neutralizing antibodies in wild carnivores following an outbreak of bovine rabies. *J. Wildl. Dis.* 11: 210

Mahan, W. E. (1973). *An Evaluation of the Relationship Between Cave-Dwelling Bats and Fox Rabies in Appalachia.* M.S. Thesis. University of Georgia.

Athens, Georgia.

Muller, W. W. (1992). 4.3 Review of reported rabies case data in Europe to the WHO Collaborating Centre Tubingen from 1977 to 1992. 4.3.3 Bat rabies cases. *Rabies Bulletin Europe*, 4th quarter. Information Surveillance Research. WHO Collaborating Centre for Rabies Surveillance and Research. Tubingen, Federal Republic of Germany. 4/92: 18

National Research Council Subcommittee on Rabies (1973). *Control of Rabies*. National Academy of Sciences. Washington, D. C.

Ramsden, R. O. and D. H. Johnston (1975). Studies on the oral infectivity of rabies virus in carnivora. *J. Wildl. Dis.* 11: 318

Reddell, J. R. (1961). The caves of Uvalde County. Part I. Texas Speleological Survey. *Texas Speleol. Assoc.* 1(3): 10

Richardson, J. H., Ramsey, R. L., and L. E. Star (1966). Bat rabies in Georgia, 1956-1965. *Pub. Hlth. Repts.* 81: 1031

Schneider, N. J., Scatterday, J. E., Lewis, A. L., Jennings, W. L., Venters, H. D., and A. V. Hardy (1957). Rabies in bats in Florida. *Am. J. Pub. Hlth.* 47(8): 983

Shen, N. J. and I. A. Shumeikina (1958). Susceptibility of white rats to oral infection with rabies strain of street virus (In Russian). Cited in *Biol. Abstr.* 44: 6 (October - December, 1963), Entry # 24515

Sikes, R. K. (1962). Pathogenesis of rabies in wildlife. I. Comparative effect of varying doses of rabies virus inoculated into foxes and skunks. *Am. J. Vet. Res.* 23: 1041

Smith, J. S. (1988). Monoclonal antibody study of bat rabies. *Rev. Infect. Dis.* 10(Suppl. 4): S637

Smith, J. S., Reid-Sanden, F. L., Roumillat, L. F., Trimarchi, C., Clark, K., Baer, G. M., and W. G. Winkler (1986). Demonstration of antigenic variation among rabies virus isolates by using monoclonal antibodies to nucleocapsid proteins. *J. Clin. Microbiol.* 4: 573

Smith, J. S., Yager, P. A., Bigler, W. J., and E. D. Hartwig, Jr. (1990). Surveillance and epidemiologic mapping of monoclonal antibody-defined rabies variants in Florida. *J. Wildl. Dis.* 26(4): 473

Soave, O. A. (1966). Transmission of rabies to mice by ingestion of infected tissue. *Am. J. Vet. Res.* 27(116): 44

Stamm, D. D., Kissling, R. E., and M. E. Eidson (1956). Experimental rabies infection in insectivorous bats. *J. Infect. Dis.* 98: 10

Steele, J. H. (1973). The epidemiology and control of rabies. *Scand. J. Infect. Dis.* 5: 299

Stirbu, A., Filotti, A., and E. Toacsen (1973). Epidemo-epizootia de turbare in Romania si rolul liliecilor in transmiterea acestei boli (The rabies epidemic in Roumania and the role of bats in transmission). *Studii si Cercetari de Virusologie*. 24(2): 95 (English abstract) in *Vet. Bull.* (1973). 43(10): 551

Thrusfield, M. (1986). *Veterinary Epidemiology*. Butterworths. Boston.

Tierkel, E. S. (1958). Recent developments in the epidemiology of rabies. *Ann. N. Y. Acad. Sci.* 70: 445

Tjalma, R. A. and B. B. Wentworth (1957). Bat rabies —Report of an isolation of rabies virus from native Ohio bats. *J. Am. Vet. Med. Assoc.* 130: 68

Trimarchi, C. V. (1984). *Rabies Annual Summary, 1984*. Rabies Laboratory, Wadsworth Center for Laboratories and Research, New York State Department of Health. Albany, New York.

Trimarchi, C. V. (1986a). *Rabies Laboratory Monthly Report. November, 1986*. Rabies Laboratory, Wadsworth Center for Laboratories and Research, New York State Department of Health. Albany, New York.

Trimarchi, C. V. (1986b). *Rabies Annual Summary, 1986*. Rabies Laboratory, Wadsworth Center for Laboratories and Research, New York State Department of Health. Albany, New York.

Trimarchi, C. V., Rudd, R. J., and M. K. Abelseth (1986). Experimentally induced rabies in four cats inoculated with a rabies virus isolated from a bat. *Am. J. Vet. Res.* 47(4): 777

Venters, H. D., Hoffert, W. R., Scatterday, J. E., and A. V. Hardy (1954). Rabies in bats in Florida. *Am. J. Pub. Hlth.* 44: 182

Wandeler, A. I. (1991). Oral Immunization of Wildlife. In G. M. Baer (ed.) *The Natural History of Rabies*. 2nd Edition. CRC Press, Inc. Boca Raton, Florida.

Whitaker, Jr., J. O. and L. R. Douglas (1986). *Bat Rabies in Indiana, 1965-1984*. Indiana State University, Terre Haute and Indiana State Board of Health, Indianapolis.

Whitaker, Jr., J. O., Miller, W. A., and W. L. Boyko (1969). Rabies in Indiana bats. *Proc. Indiana Acad. Sci.* 82: 469

Winkler, W. G. and D. B. Adams (1972). Utilization of southwestern bat caves by terrestrial carnivores. *Am. Midl. Nat.* 87(1): 191

Chapter 16: MONOCLONAL ANTIBODY CHARACTERIZATION OF BAT-RABIES ISOLATES

Value in Epidemiologic Investigation

In recent years, monoclonal antibodies have been used with increasing frequency to characterize the many viruses isolated from various species infected with rabies. Five protein components of the rabies virus have been identified: L (large viral polymerase), N (nucleocapsid protein), G (glycoprotein), and M_1 and M_2 (matrix proteins). Highly specific monoclonal antibodies have been developed to both nucleocapsid and glycoprotein components of a great many viral variants.

Probing viral isolates with monoclonal panels has allowed investigators to detect minor antigenic differences among various rabies isolates. Characterization of selected antigenic features of individual variants permits distinction among the viruses present in different reservoir hosts, in different geographic regions, and among those with different passage histories. This has proven to be a powerful tool in the study of epidemiologic associations, allowing researchers to identify the probable source of exposure in a rabid animal or person. Monoclonal antibody analyses have provided an enormous amount of information, revolutionizing our understanding of rabies epidemiology.

Rupprecht (unpublished observations [cited by Rupprecht et al, 1991]) studied the phenotypic variation in viruses over time. Accordingly, the antigenic stability of street viruses was studied following serial passage through several species of animal hosts and continuous cultivation in cell culture. Isolates recovered after apparent vaccine failures and from naturally infected animals were also examined. The data do not support a high likelihood of significant change (antigenic shift) in the makeup of viral antigens. Minor variation was observed to be restricted to the G antigen, the N protein being highly conserved. The N protein is a major internal structural protein, bound to the viral RNA and required for its replication and transcription. The G antigen, on the other hand, is an external protein associated with the viral envelope. The G antigen is probably under considerable selection pressure and, therefore, more likely to undergo limited change. These changes may be reflected in minor variations in reactivity with select monoclonal antibody panels.

The characteristic virus isolated from members of a reservoir species is referred to as an ecotype. The term encompasses a variety of factors, including those related to the antigenic makeup of the specific variant as well as ecological data pertaining to the host species. Aspects of the virus relating to its antigenic makeup alone define a variant. A single viral variant may comprise more than one ecotype if it is found, to a significant extent, in more than one host species (Smith, 1993).

Compartmentalization of Rabies Variants

Investigators have studied reactivity patterns of viral isolates from both reservoir species and sporadically infected individuals of other species in areas of enzootic terrestrial rabies throughout the United States, as well as from adjacent areas of both Canada and Mexico. Among terrestrial reservoirs in the United States, five distinct antigenic reactivity patterns (Figure 16-1) charac-

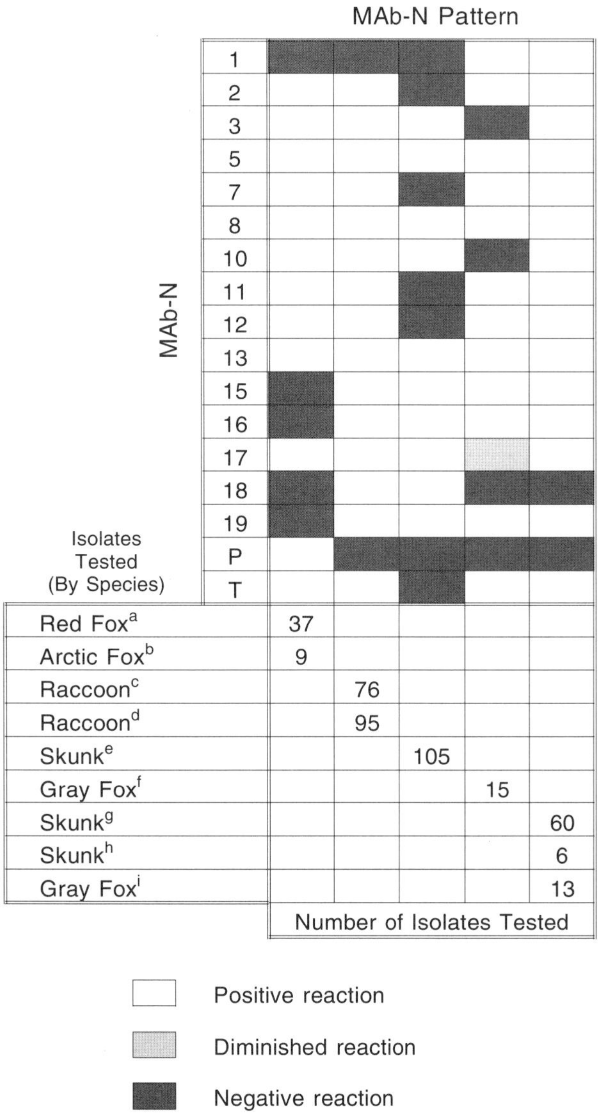

[a]Collected from Ontario, Quebec, and New York; [b]Collected from Alaska and the Northwest Territories; [c]Collected from mid-Atlantic USA; [d]Collected from southeastern USA; [e]Collected from south-central USA; [f]Collected from Arizona; [g]Collected from Manitoba, Saskatchewan, and the north-central USA; [h]Collected from California; [i]Collected from central Texas.

Figure 16-1. MAb-N variants found in terrestrial mammals in the United States. Viral isolates were collected from each of the major terrestrial reservoir species from defined major areas of enzootic terrestrial rabies and reacted with a panel of monoclonal antibodies (MAb-N) to the rabies N protein. (From Smith, J. S. and G. M. Baer. Epizootiology of Rabies: The Americas. In J. B. Campbell and K. M. Charlton (eds.) *Developments in Veterinary Virology—Rabies.* Kluwer Academic Publishers. Boston, 1988. Redrawn with permission.)

terize viral isolates in regions of enzootic rabies (Smith, 1988; Smith and Baer, 1988). These include the following:

1) Isolates from the area of enzootic red-fox rabies in the northeastern United States (identical reactivity pattern to isolates found in Ontario and Quebec).

2) Isolates from an expanding region of enzootic raccoon rabies in the Southeast, Northeast, and mid-Atlantic states.

3) Isolates from an area of enzootic skunk rabies in south-central states.

4) Isolates from an area of enzootic gray-fox rabies in Arizona.

5) Isolates from separated areas and hosts, including areas of enzootic skunk rabies in north-central states, Appalachian states, and California; and areas of rabies in dogs and gray foxes in California, Arizona, and Texas that border Mexico (identical reactivity pattern characterizes isolates from rabid dogs in Mexico).

Furthermore, six major and four minor areas of enzootic sylvatic terrestrial rabies have been defined (see Figure 11-1). The major areas include: 1) the north-central focus of skunk rabies, 2) the south-central focus of skunk rabies, 3) the northern California focus of skunk rabies, 4) the southeastern focus of raccoon rabies, 5) the mid-Atlantic focus of raccoon rabies, and 6) the northeastern focus of raccoon rabies. The minor areas include: 1) a region of red-fox rabies in New York, 2) regions reporting a few cases of rabies in arctic and red foxes in Alaska, 3) a small region of gray-fox rabies in Arizona, and 4) a small focus of rabies among gray foxes and coyotes in Texas.

Antigenic Characterization of Bat-Rabies Isolates

Rabies variants isolated from bats have been shown to be antigenically different from those found in terrestrial reservoirs (compare Figures 16-1, 16-2, and 16-3). Monoclonal analyses of rabies viruses have shown that there is a lack of distinct homogeneity of bat-rabies isolates, both within a species and within a particular geo-

MONOCLONAL ANTIBODIES

Although antibodies are generally considered to be specific with respect to the antigens against which they are directed, their specificity is not absolute. With the advent of a technology for fusing cells together, a means was devised for producing immortal clones of cells secreting large quantities of identical antibody with a single specificity.

Monoclonal antibodies are produced by first immunizing a mouse against a particular antigen. Antibody-secreting white blood cells (plasma cells) from the mouse's spleen are then fused with special cancerous cells (mouse myeloma cells). The hybrid cells (hybridomas) made from fusion of the cancerous myeloma cells and the plasma cells are then isolated and clones of hybrid cells that produce the specific antibody required can be selected and grown in cell culture. The hybridoma cells will secrete large quantities of antibody, the specificity of which will be determined by the original plasma cell used in the fusion.

Because the specificity of monoclonal antibodies is determined by the researcher, they will be standard from laboratory to laboratory worldwide. The very high specificity of monoclonal antibodies and the fact that they can be produced in virtually unending supply make them powerful tools, with almost limitless biomedical use. They have proven value both in the research and diagnostic laboratory as well as in the setting of clinical practice.

graphic zone (Smith et al, 1984, 1985; Rupprecht, 1986).

This is in contrast to isolates from terrestrial reservoirs in a given area of enzootic rabies. Isolates from the mid-Atlantic raccoon epizootic have been shown to remain temporally stable for as long as 6 to 7 years (Smith et al, 1984, 1985). Isolates from rabid foxes in France, the former Federal Republic of Germany (West Germany), and Italy have remained stable for as long as 20 years (Dietzschold et al, 1988). Rupprecht (unpublished observations [cited by Dietzschold et al, 1988]) demonstrated antigenic stability of field strains of virus after more than 40 passages in cell culture or heterologous hosts. Results of genetic analyses of defined genomic regions of rabies isolates from the same geographic area have shown stability of nucleotide sequences over 30 years (Smith et al, 1992; Smith and Seidel, 1993).

The existence of species-associated antigenic variants of bat virus may reflect the cycling of an array of stable, but distinct, isolates. Smith and Baer (1988) reported separate antigenic reactivity patterns of isolates collected from Mexican free-tailed bats, red bats, hoary bats, and big brown bats in the United States (Figure 16-2). These ecotypes typically characterize isolates from infected bats of that particular species throughout its range (Figures 16-4, 16-5, and 16-6) and are only sporadically found in other species. Thirteen separate variants have been identified in big brown bats: 2 from the Northeast, and 11 from western states (Baer and Smith, 1991). These variants appear to be restricted in distribution to this species and its subspecies (Figures 16-2, 16-7, and 16-8). Further studies of rabies variants isolated from big brown bats may provide evidence for colonial or territorial boundaries, accounting for this geographic compartmentalization (Smith, 1989).

Isolates from yellow bats in Florida exhibit an antigenic reactivity pattern similar to pattern 3 (Figure 16-2), suggesting a variant distinct from the four important Chiropteran reservoirs in the United States (Smith et al, 1990). An immunologically indistinguishable variant characterizes isolates from silver-haired bats. At present, the antigenic variant, common to both species, cannot be easily differentiated by monoclonal analysis (CDC monoclonal panel). Distinction between them has been based on the known ranges of these two bat species. In areas where their ranges overlap, discrimination between the two isolates using monoclonal antibodies has not been readily possible. However, newly applied techniques of modern genetic analysis have revealed that isolates from silver-haired and Florida yellow bats are, in fact, distinct and can be distinguished from each other (Smith, 1993).

Isolates from species of *Myotis* reveal no con-

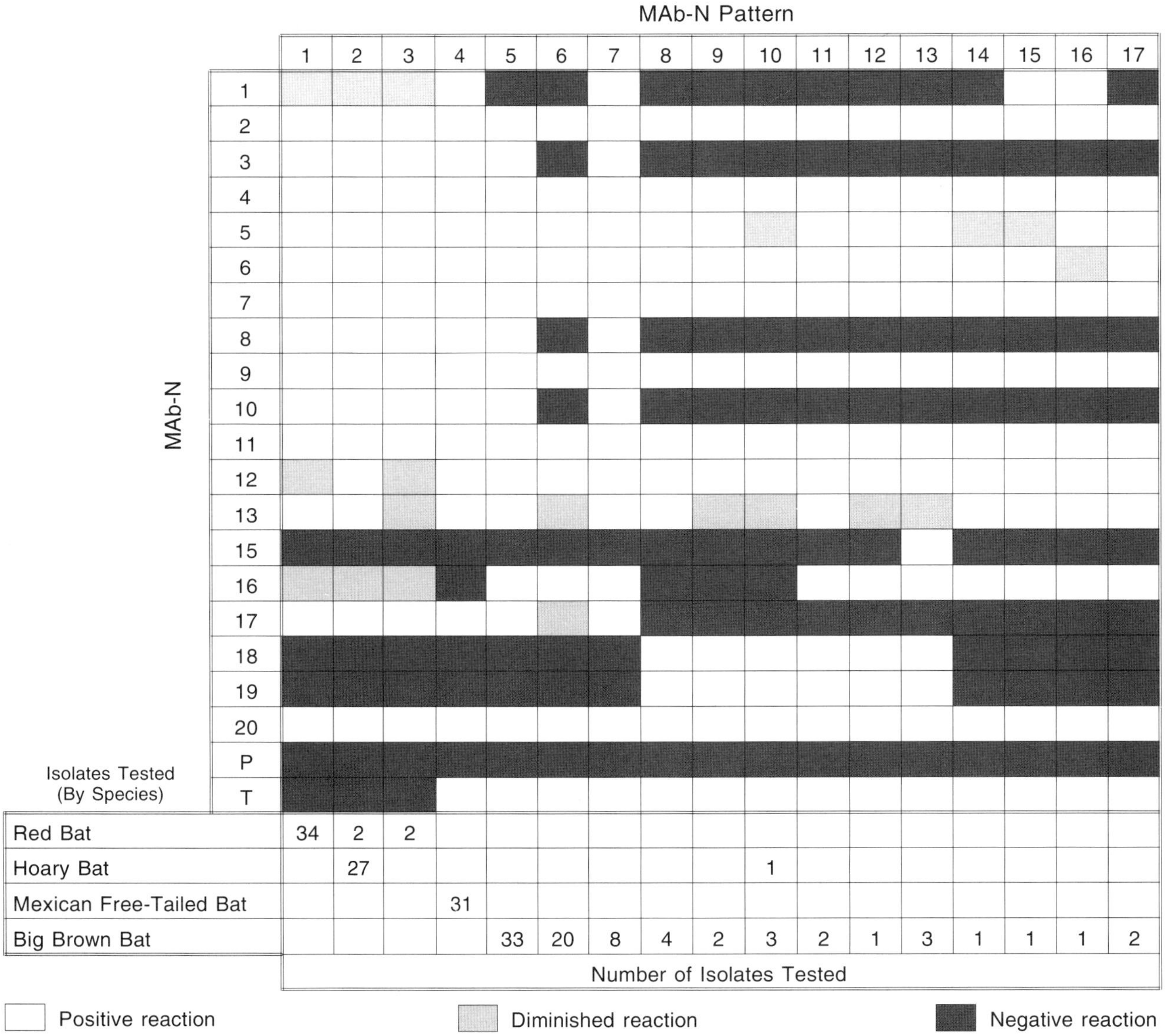

Figure 16-2. MAb-N variants found in insectivorous bats in the United States. Viral isolates were collected from each of the four major nonterrestrial host species and reacted with a panel of monoclonal antibodies (MAb-N) to the rabies N protein. (From Baer, G. M. and J. S. Smith. Rabies in Nonhematophagous Bats. In G. M. Baer (ed.) *The Natural History of Rabies*. 2nd Edition. © CRC Press, Inc. Boca Raton, Florida, 1991. Redrawn with permission.)

sistent antigenic reactivity pattern (Smith and Baer, 1988). Rather, the observed variants are generally characteristic of the major nonterrestrial reservoir of the area. This suggests that there is no independent rabies cycle in *Myotis* species, but that they are infected by spillover of virus from other bat species following sporadic contact (compare Figures 16-2 and 16-3).

Some monoclonal reactivity patterns cannot be associated with any of the major Chiropteran reservoirs; however, too few samples are available to define the host species that maintain these variants in the wild.

The finding of separate reactivity patterns in various bat species may be a reflection of viral compartmentalization, similar to that known to occur in terrestrial animals (Smith, 1989). Although certain species of bats may be more commonly reported rabid in a particular geographic locale (see page 147), no discrete geographic

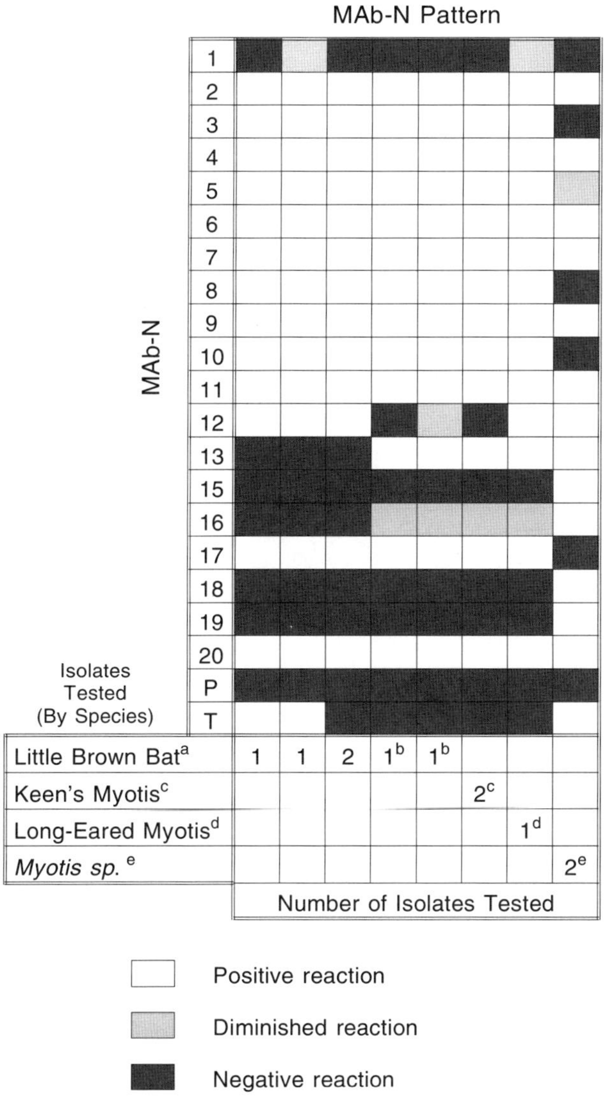

[a] Collected from New York.

[b] Identical reactivity pattern to that found in rabid red bats in the area.

[c] Collected from New York and Maryland. Identical reactivity pattern to that found in rabid red bats in the area.

[d] Collected from Colorado. Identical reactivity pattern to that found in rabid hoary bats in the area.

[e] Collected from Arizona and Nevada. Identical reactivity pattern to that found in rabid big brown bats in the area.

Figure 16-3. MAb-N variants found in insectivorous bats of the genus *Myotis* in the United States. Viral isolates were collected from various species of *Myotis* and reacted with a panel of monoclonal antibodies (MAb-N) to the rabies N protein. (From Smith, J. S. and G. M. Baer. Epizootiology of Rabies: The Americas. In J. B. Campbell and K. M. Charlton (eds.) *Developments in Veterinary Virology—Rabies.* Kluwer Academic Publishers. Boston, 1988. Redrawn with permission.)

boundaries of enzootic disease in bats are known. Rabies-positive specimens of migratory species, for example, are reported throughout their geographic range, which may extend for thousands of miles.

The specific viral ecotype associated with each of the major Chiropteran reservoirs is associated with that species throughout its geographic range and is only rarely reported from other bat species (Smith and Baer, 1988; Baer and Smith, 1991). This suggests that rabies in these bats exists as separate, independent enzootics, maintained principally by intraspecies transmission (Baer and Smith, 1991). The presence of rabies infection in nonreservoir species, such as members of the genus *Myotis*, reflects natural interspecific transmission of virus among bats. None of the reactivity patterns identified in bat isolates are known from major terrestrial rabies enzootics (Smith and Baer, 1988).

Transmission of Nonterrestrial Virus to Terrestrial Species

In studying viral isolates from rabid specimens across the country, important information has been gathered regarding the role of bats in rabies epidemiology and epizootiology. In particular, comparison of isolates from infected animals with species-associated reference variants has provided valuable information about the likely source of the original exposure. Based on these studies, it is believed that only sporadic (but definite and measurable) transfer of virus occurs from bats to terrestrial mammals, including both wild and domestic species (Tables 16-1 and 16-2).

The finding of a particular viral isolate in an animal does not absolutely define the source of viral exposure. It only indicates the reference group of the infecting variant (Rupprecht et al, 1987). The finding of a characteristic nonterrestrial isolate in an infected cow does not, as a matter of course, mean that a bat bit the cow. It may be that the cow was exposed by another species, itself previously infected by a bat. While the possibility of such secondary transmission does exist, it is not likely.

In many instances, known epidemiologic circumstances surrounding the exposure of domestic animals help to corroborate the probability of bat

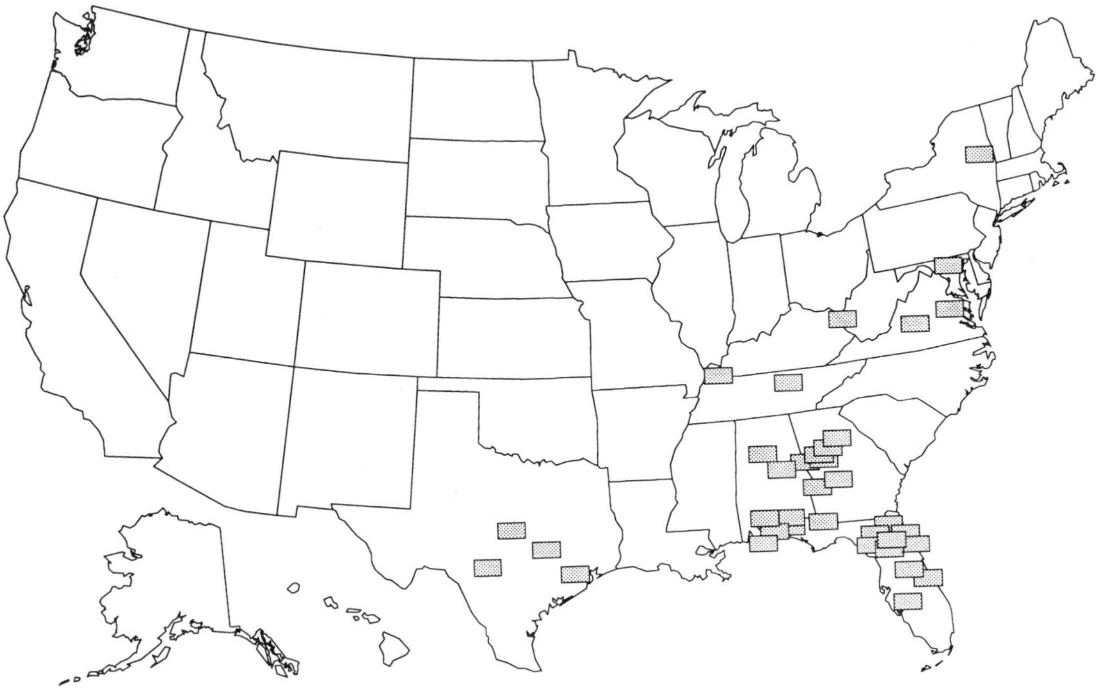

Figure 16-4. Distribution of rabies variants associated with infected red bats in the United States. Hatched boxes represent collection sites of isolates from red bats displaying MAb-N reactivity pattern 1, as indicated in Figure 16-2. (From Baer, G. M. and J. S. Smith. Rabies in Nonhematophagous Bats. In G. M. Baer (ed.) *The Natural History of Rabies*. 2nd Edition. © CRC Press, Inc. Boca Raton, Florida, 1991. Redrawn with permission.)

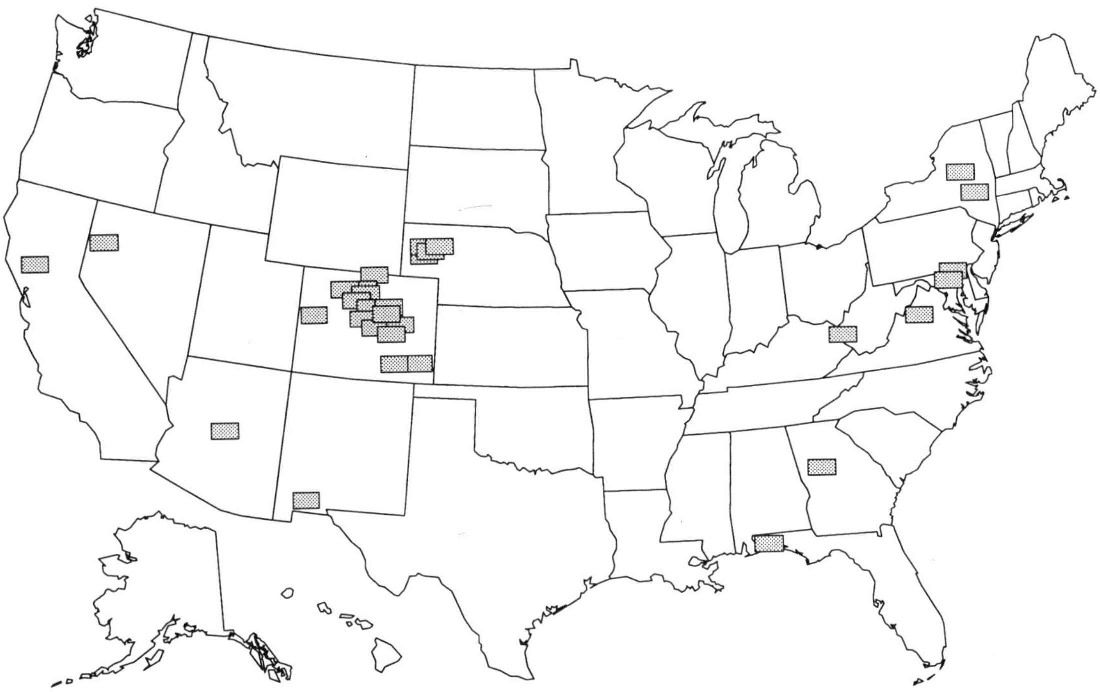

Figure 16-5. Distribution of rabies variants associated with infected hoary bats in the United States. Hatched boxes represent collection sites of isolates from hoary bats displaying MAb-N reactivity pattern 2, as indicated in Figure 16-2. (From Baer, G. M. and J. S. Smith. Rabies in Nonhematophagous Bats. In G. M. Baer (ed.) *The Natural History of Rabies*. 2nd Edition. © CRC Press, Inc. Boca Raton, Florida, 1991. Redrawn with permission.)

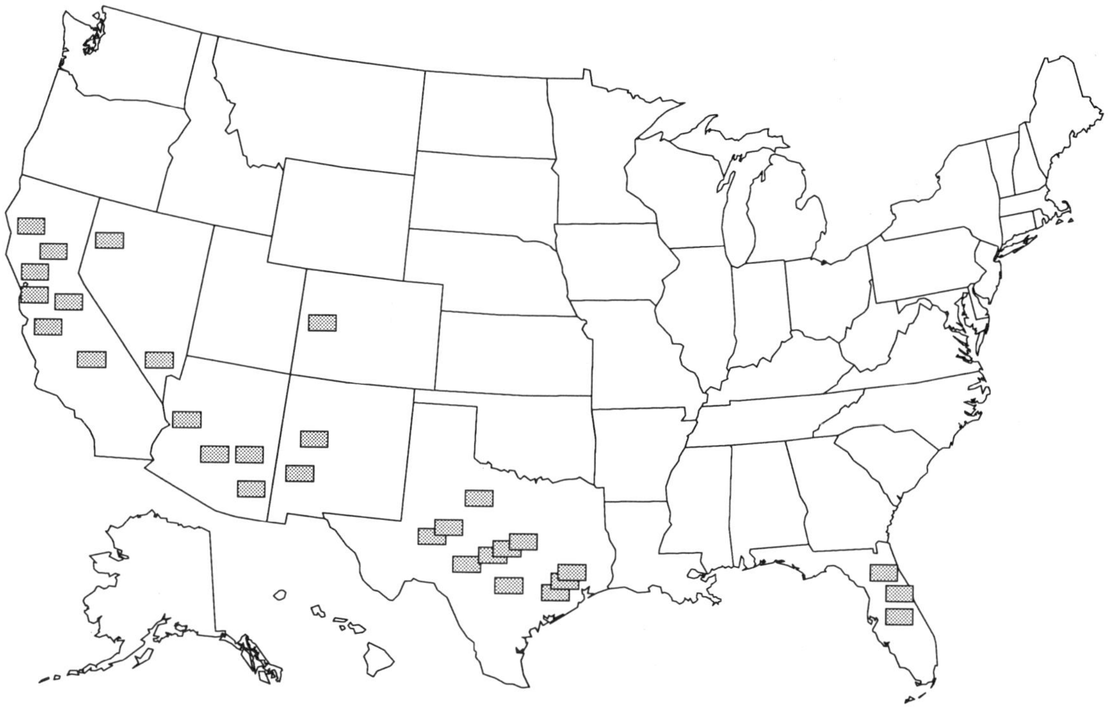

Figure 16-6. Distribution of rabies variants associated with infected Mexican free-tailed bats in the United States. Hatched boxes represent collection sites of isolates from Mexican free-tailed bats displaying MAb-N reactivity pattern 4, as indicated in Figure 16-2. (From Baer, G. M. and J. S. Smith. Rabies in Nonhematophagous Bats. In G. M. Baer (ed.) *The Natural History of Rabies*. 2nd Edition. © CRC Press, Inc. Boca Raton, Florida, 1991. Redrawn with permission.)

bite as the original source of infection. In the case of the rabid cow from Pennsylvania (Table 16-2), there was evidence highly suggestive of a bat bite. Two months prior to the onset of clinical signs, the farmer removed a bat which had apparently been clinging to the cow's chest (Glickman et al, 1983). The bat, however, was not tested for rabies.

Trimarchi (1983, 1986) reported the isolation of a nonterrestrial variant of virus from two unvaccinated cats in New York that had histories of catching bats, and Rupprecht et al (1987) reported the isolation of a nonterrestrial variant from a cat in Massachusetts, also with a history of catching bats.

Fuller (1984) reported that the horse from New Hampshire had been stabled in a barn occupied by bats. However, he also noted that an unusual amount of daytime fox activity had been observed on the premises for two months prior to the onset of signs in the horse. It was not possible in this instance to distinguish between primary bat-to-horse or secondary bat-to-fox-to-horse transmission of virus. With respect to the horse in New York (1986),[1] a rabid big brown bat had been found in a shed near the stable a few years prior to the onset of clinical signs. The antigenic reactivity pattern of the the bat isolate was identical to that isolated from the horse (Trimarchi, 1986; Smith, 1988). In the experience of researchers at the New York State Department of Health, if rabies is found in a colony of big brown

[1]This particular horse had been admitted to the Teaching Hospital of the New York State College of Veterinary Medicine, Cornell University. It was hospitalized for three days prior to euthanasia. Thirty-nine persons, including 30 veterinary students and hospital staff, required post-exposure rabies prophylaxis. Such widespread exposure is not an altogether unusual condition when rabid animals are admitted to university veterinary hospitals.

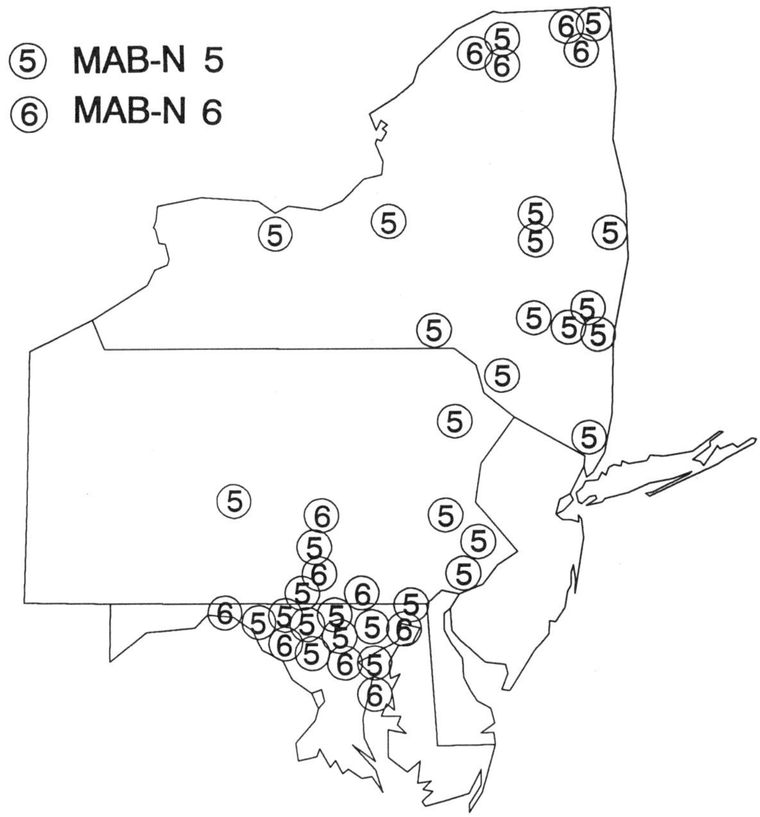

Figure 16-7. Distribution of rabies variants associated with infected big brown bats in New York, Pennsylvania, and Maryland. Numbers represent collection sites of isolates from big brown bats displaying MAb-N reactivity patterns 5 and 6, as indicated in Figure 16-2. (From Baer, G. M. and J. S. Smith. Rabies in Nonhematophagous Bats. In G. M. Baer (ed.) *The Natural History of Rabies*. 2nd Edition. © CRC Press, Inc. Boca Raton, Florida, 1991. Redrawn with permission.)

bats, another rabid individual is likely to occur every few years (Trimarchi, 1989).

Whetstone et al (1984) reported that a rabid dog from California had been infected by a bat. Epidemiologic circumstances included the finding of a dried bat carcass in the dog's pen and a report by the dog's owner that it had been playing with a bat about one week prior to the onset of clinical signs. Monoclonal antibody analysis of the viral isolate obtained from this animal revealed a nonterrestrial variant of virus. However, an abbreviated monoclonal panel was used and the validity of this work has been criticized (Constantine, 1988).[2] More recently, Neill (1993) re-

[2]Two European variants of rabies virus (one isolated from a sheep in the former Socialist Federal Republic of Yugoslavia and the other from a fox in France), when tested with a reduced panel of monoclonal antibodies, were mistakenly identified as European bat lyssaviruses (rabies-related virus of bat origin). However, when these isolates were tested with a larger panel of monoclonal antibodies, they were classified as being terrestrial in nature, belonging to serotype 1 (Montano Hirose et al, 1990; Lafon, 1993). Abbreviated monoclonal antibody panels must be rigorously tested before being relied upon to provide useful epidemiological data. They suffer the limitation of reduced capacity to recognize a new reactivity pattern which may characterize a previously unidentified viral isolate. Moreover, the possibility exists that a new isolate may react with a variable portion of an abbreviated panel, leading to classification in a known reactivity group. Subsequent testing with a wider battery of monoclonals may reveal a distinctive reactivity pattern.

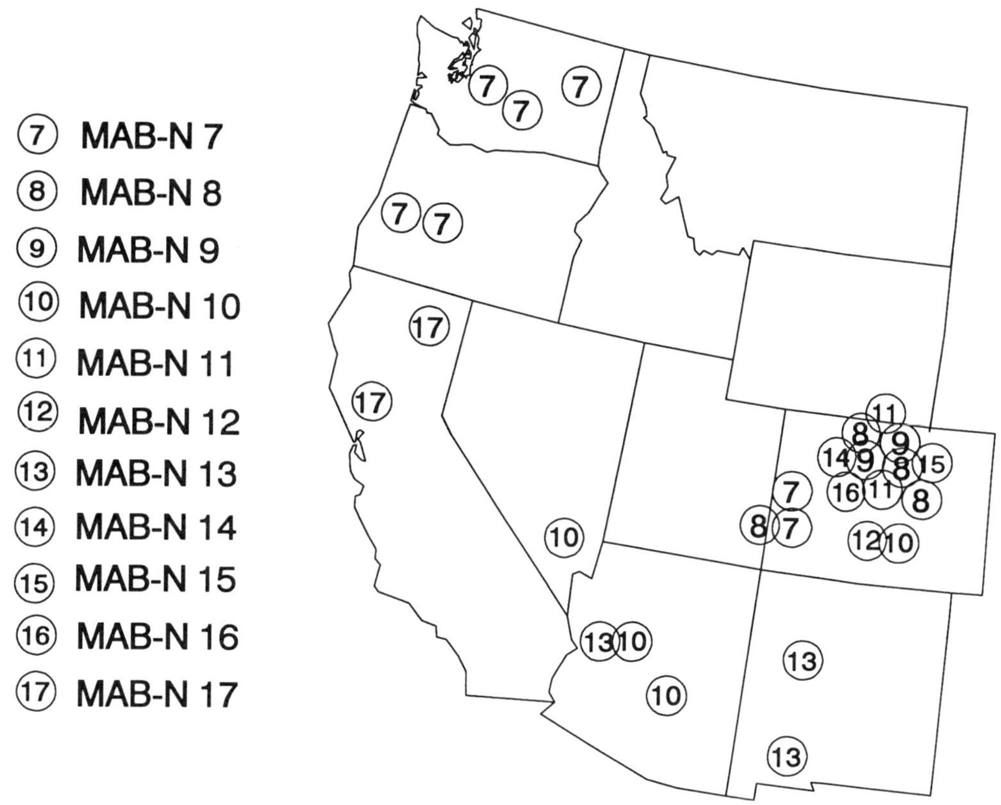

Figure 16-8. Distribution of rabies variants associated with infected big brown bats in the western United States. Numbers represent collection sites of isolates from big brown bats displaying MAb-N reactivity patterns 7 to 17, as indicated in Figure 16-2. (From Baer, G. M. and J. S. Smith. Rabies in Nonhematophagous Bats. In G. M. Baer (ed.) *The Natural History of Rabies*. 2nd Edition. © CRC Press, Inc. Boca Raton, Florida, 1991. Redrawn with permission.)

ported the isolation of a nonterrestrial viral variant (characteristic of Mexican free-tailed bats) from a dog in Texas. These results have been confirmed by the Centers for Disease Control (Smith, 1994). Isolates obtained in 1977 from a rabid dog in California, also suspected of having been infected by a bat (Emmons, 1994), were recently shown to be characteristic of those found in Mexican free-tailed bats (Smith, 1994).

In 1992, a previously unknown variant of rabies virus was isolated from a ringtailed cat in Nevada. Although suggestive of a nonterrestrial variant of virus, this remains unsubstantiated. Until more isolates are found and the variant better characterized, it remains unknown if the source of virus in this animal was terrestrial or nonterrestrial in nature (Smith, 1993).

In 1983, rabies virus was isolated from a gray fox in Dutchess County, New York, an area far from the region of enzootic red-fox rabies in the northeastern part of the state along its border with Canada (Figure 16-9). Gray foxes are rarely reported rabid in the Northeast and rabies in terrestrial species had been unknown in this county for 25 years (Centers for Disease Control, 1985). In the following year, three additional isolates (one from Rensselaer County and two from Ulster County) were identified in gray foxes (Trimarchi, 1984). In 1987, three more rabid gray foxes were identified in the state. They were found in close proximity to each other in Putnam County (Trimarchi, 1987). In 1988, a case of rabies was identified in a gray fox from Saratoga County (Trimarchi, 1988).

Concern was voiced that these findings represented an expansion of the red-fox rabies enzo-

Table 16-1

Isolation of Nonterrestrial Variants of Rabies Virus From Terrestrial Wildlife in the United States, by Species and Year

Source of Isolate	Place/Year	Reference Strain	Reference
Fox	NY/1978	Nonterrestrial	Trimarchi, 1989
Fox	OR/1982	Nonterrestrial	Smith, 1988
Fox	NY/1983	Big Brown Bat	CDC, 1985
Fox	NY/1984	Big Brown Bat	Trimarchi, 1984
Fox	NY/1984	Big Brown Bat	Trimarchi, 1984
Fox	NY/1984	Red Bat	Trimarchi, 1984
Fox	RI/1986	Big Brown Bat	Smith et al, 1986
Fox	AZ/1986	Big Brown Bat	Smith, 1988
Fox	MI/1986	Big Brown Bat	Smith, 1988
Fox	NY/1987	Red Bat	Trimarchi, 1987
Fox	NY/1987	Red Bat	Trimarchi, 1987
Fox	NY/1987	Red Bat	Trimarchi, 1987
Fox	NY/1988	Big Brown Bat	Trimarchi, 1989
Fox	IN/1989	Silver-Haired Bat	Smith, 1992
Fox	CA/1989	Mexican Free-Tail	Smith, 1992
Fox	MA/1991	Nonterrestrial	Smith, 1992
Fox	MA/1991	Nonterrestrial	Smith, 1992
Fox	VA/1992	Silver-Haired Bat	Smith, 1992
Fox	TX/1992	Silver-Haired Bat	Smith, 1992
Skunk	NY/1978	Nonterrestrial	Smith, 1992
Skunk	CO/1987	Big Brown Bat	Smith, 1988
Skunk	CA/1987	Nonterrestrial	Smith, 1992
Skunk	CA/1987	Nonterrestrial	Smith, 1992
Skunk	CO/1992	Nonterrestrial	Smith, 1992
Skunk	WY/1991	Silver-Haired Bat	Smith, 1992
Skunk	WY/1991	Silver-Haired Bat	Smith, 1992
Raccoon	DE/1983	Nonterrestrial	Smith, 1992

otic into both a new region and a new species. Monoclonal antibody analysis of these viral isolates from gray foxes, however, revealed that they were distinct from that found in red foxes. Rather, the antigenic reactivity patterns were nonterrestrial in nature, four being identical to isolates found in big brown bats and four to isolates found in red bats.

These findings were consistent with the fact that no expansion of the area of enzootic red-fox rabies had occurred (gray foxes found infected within the region of enzootic red-fox rabies being infected with the red-fox variant of virus). The data were consistent with transmission of virus from bats to terrestrial carnivores.

This small cluster of cases of gray-fox rabies of bat origin in New York State was important because it hinted at the possibility that bats may initiate epizootics of rabies among terrestrial animals (reiterating concerns voiced by investigators in the 1950's). However, the small number of cases and the fact that two separate nonterrestrial variants were involved suggested that such was not the case. Nevertheless, New York State remains an important site for continued surveillance. Monoclonal antibody analysis of a further case of rabies in a gray fox (Sullivan County, New York) in 1990 indicated viral spillover from the advancing raccoon epizootic (Trimarchi, 1990). To date, no additional cases of bat-to-fox transmission of rabies virus have been documented in New York State.

Smith et al (1990) studied the relationship between rabies in bats and raccoons in Florida, com-

Table 16-2

Isolation of Nonterrestrial Variants of Rabies Virus From Domestic Animals in the United States, by Species and Year

Source of Isolate	Place/Year	Reference Strain	Reference
Cat	CA/1976	Big Brown Bat	Smith, 1988
Cat	MA/1980	Nonterrestrial	Rupprecht et al, 1987
Cat	NY/1981	Big Brown Bat	Smith, 1992
Cat	CA/1983	Big Brown Bat	Smith, 1988
Cat	NY/1983	Nonterrestrial	Trimarchi, 1983
Cat	OR/1984	Big Brown Bat	Smith, 1988
Cat	NM/1985	Mexican Free-Tail	Smith, 1992
Cat	GA/1985	Red Bat	Smith, 1988
Cat	CO/1985	Nonterrestrial	Smith, 1988
Cat	UT/1986	Nonterrestrial	Smith, 1988
Cat	TX/1986	Mexican Free-Tail	Smith, 1988
Cat	NY/1986	Big Brown Bat	Trimarchi, 1986
Cat	TX/1988	Mexican Free-Tail	Neill, 1992
Cat	TX/1988	Mexican Free-Tail	Neill, 1992
Cat	TX/1989	Mexican Free-Tail	Neill, 1992
Cat	TX/1990	Mexican Free-Tail	Neill, 1992
Cat	TX/1991	Mexican Free-Tail	Neill, 1992
Cat	ID/1991	Silver-Haired Bat	Smith, 1992
Cat	ME/1991	Lasiurine?	Smith, 1992
Cat	ID/1992	Silver-Haired Bat	Smith, 1992
Cat	TX/1993	Mexican Free-Tail	Neill, 1993
Cow	PA/1982	Big Brown Bat	Smith et al, 1986
Cow	VA/1983	Nonterrestrial	Smith et al, 1988
Dog	CA/1977	Mexican Free-Tail	Smith, 1994
Dog	TX/1993	Mexican Free-Tail	Neill, 1993
Horse	NH/1983	Big Brown Bat	Smith et al, 1986
Horse	NY/1986	Big Brown Bat	Trimarchi, 1986
Horse	NV/1986	Big Brown Bat	Smith, 1988
Horse	CA/1988	Silver-Haired Bat	Smith, 1992
Horse	VA/1988	Red Bat	Smith, 1992
Horse	TX/1991	Mexican Free-tail	Neill, 1992
Horse	NY/1991	Big Brown Bat	Trimarchi, 1991
Sheep	IL/1986	Big Brown Bat	Smith, 1992

paring viral isolates from rabid bats and terrestrial carnivores found within the state during 1987 and 1988. Figure 16-10 shows a comparison of the prevalence of rabies in bats, foxes, and raccoons in Florida from 1951 to 1988, broken down into four districts (Figures 16-11 and 16-12). As shown, an increase in reported cases of raccoon rabies was, on occasion, accompanied or preceded by an increase in reported cases of bat rabies.

Results of monoclonal antibody analyses of viral isolates obtained from rabies cases between 1987 and 1988 indicated that terrestrial and nonterrestrial isolates could be easily distinguished (Figure 16-13). Isolates from terrestrial species (including raccoons and a limited number of others) were identical to those infecting raccoons throughout Florida and the southeastern United States. In no case was a nonterrestrial variant of virus isolated from a terrestrial species, despite the geographic and temporal overlap of disease in bats and raccoons. Thus, the authors found no

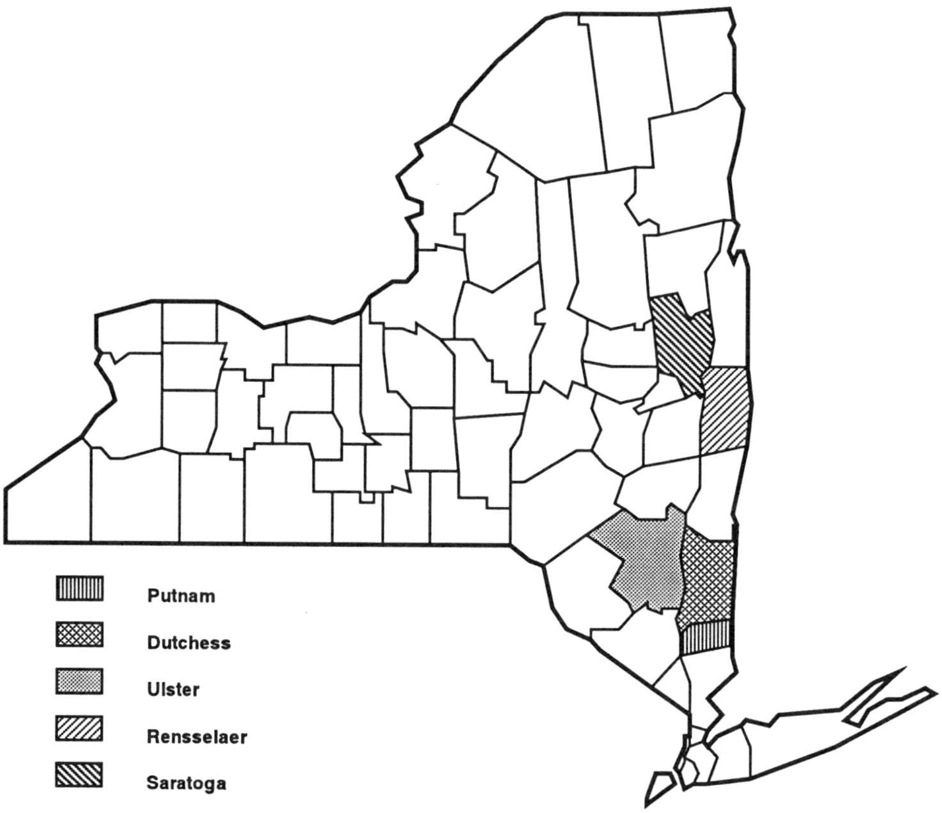

Figure 16-9. Nonterrestrial variants of rabies virus isolated from gray foxes in New York State. (Data from Trimarchi, C. V. *Rabies Annual Summaries, 1985-1991.* Rabies Laboratory, Wadsworth Center for Laboratories and Research, New York State Department of Health. Albany, New York.)

evidence to support the occurrence of viral transmission from rabid bats to terrestrial animals in the state. These results were consistent with findings of earlier studies comparing rabies isolates from the mid-Atlantic raccoon epizootic to those known to be present in bats in the same geographic area (Smith et al, 1984).

In Canada, there have been only eight documented cases of rabies transmission from bats to terrestrial animals and only three to humans (Webster et al, 1985, 1988, 1989; Casey et al, 1989; Whitney, 1989; Wandeler and Casey, 1993; Wandeler, 1992; Loewen, 1993). Animal cases included a horse from British Columbia; a cow, squirrel, and skunk from Ontario; a fox from Newfoundland; a skunk from Alberta; and a fox and cow from Nova Scotia. With respect to the squirrel, this remains the only documented case of rabies transmission from a bat (big brown) to a rodent in North America.

Insectivorous Bats and Sylvatic Rabies Cycles

As monoclonal antibody technology became more widely applied to the characterization of rabies viruses, the respective roles of various wildlife species in the maintenance of sylvatic rabies cycles and the mechanisms whereby various viral isolates cycle within and among different bat populations became more clearly defined.

The presence of nonterrestrial variants of rabies virus in infected terrestrial species is most often identified in areas that are free of enzootic terrestrial disease. This is primarily because isolates from infected animals found in areas of enzootic terrestrial rabies are usually not tested. Infection in these animals is generally secondary to spillover of virus from the major terrestrial reser-

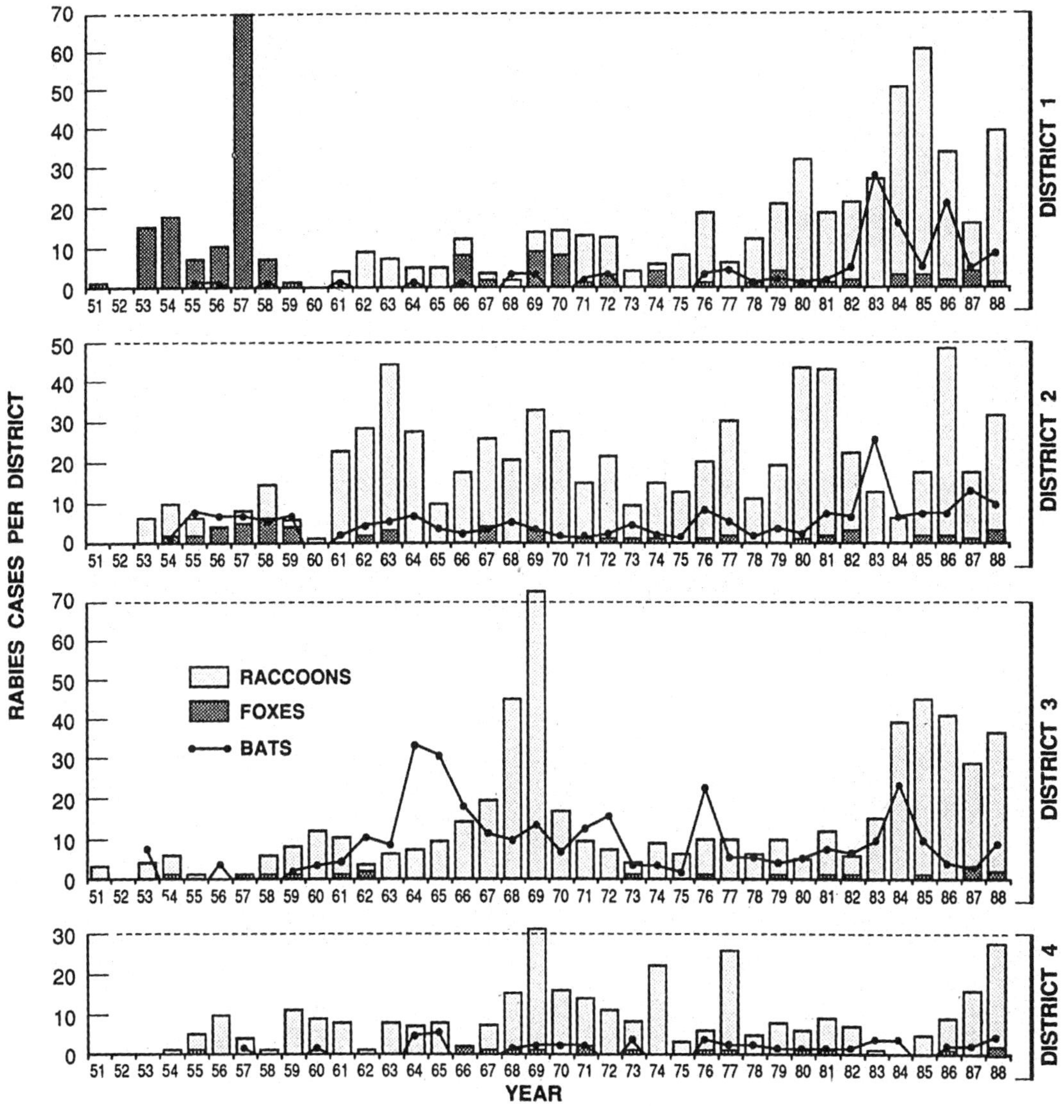

Figure 16-10. Numbers of cases of rabies in raccoons, foxes, and bats in Florida, by district, 1951-1988. (From Smith, J. S., Yager, P. A., Bigler, W. J., and E. C. Hartwig, Jr. Surveillance and epidemiologic mapping of monoclonal antibody-defined rabies variants in Florida. *J. Wildl. Dis.* 26(4): 473, 1990. Reproduced with permission.)

voir of the area.

Although the potential for transmission of virus from insectivorous bats to other wildlife exists, monoclonal antibody surveys have documented the fact that such transmission occurs relatively infrequently (although it undoubtedly occurs more frequently than is reported). To date, results of monoclonal antibody surveys across the United States (as well as Canada and Europe) support the epidemiologic concept that enzootic rabies in insectivorous bats cycles largely independently of that in terrestrial mammals.

Sporadic transmission of nonterrestrial virus to a terrestrial species has not been shown to result in the establishment of enzootic disease in that species (World Health Organization, 1992). The accumulated evidence documents the fact that insectivorous bats are not an important maintenance source of virus for other wildlife populations.

There is no evidence to support the long-held belief that the presence of enzootic rabies in some

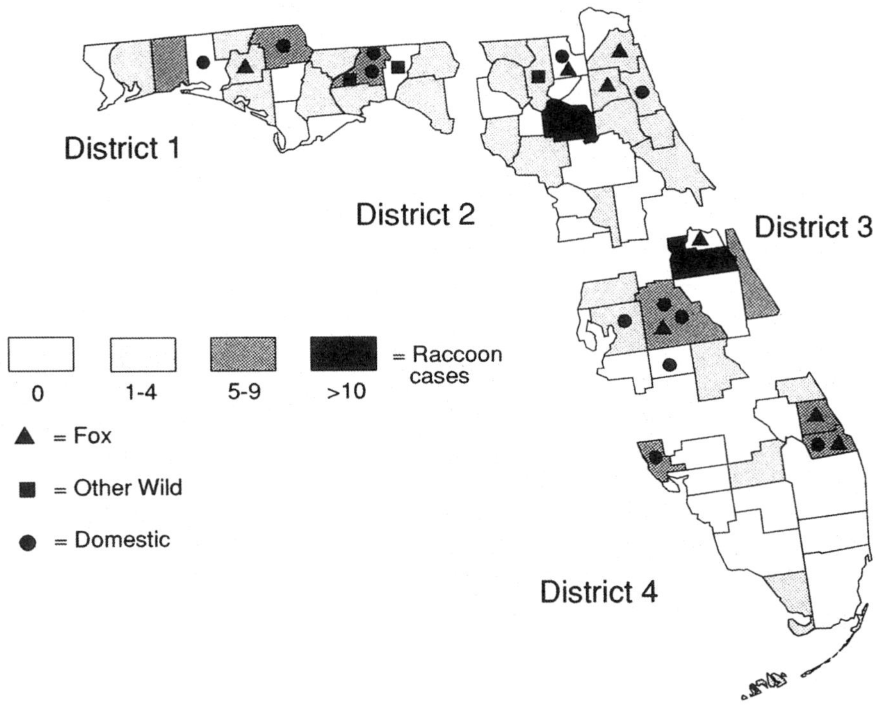

Figure 16-11. Prevalence and distribution of terrestrial rabies cases, by county, in Florida, 1988. (From Smith, J. S., Yager, P. A., Bigler, W. J., and E. C. Hartwig, Jr. Surveillance and epidemiologic mapping of monoclonal antibody-defined rabies variants in Florida. *J. Wildl. Dis.* 26(4): 473, 1990. Reproduced with permission.)

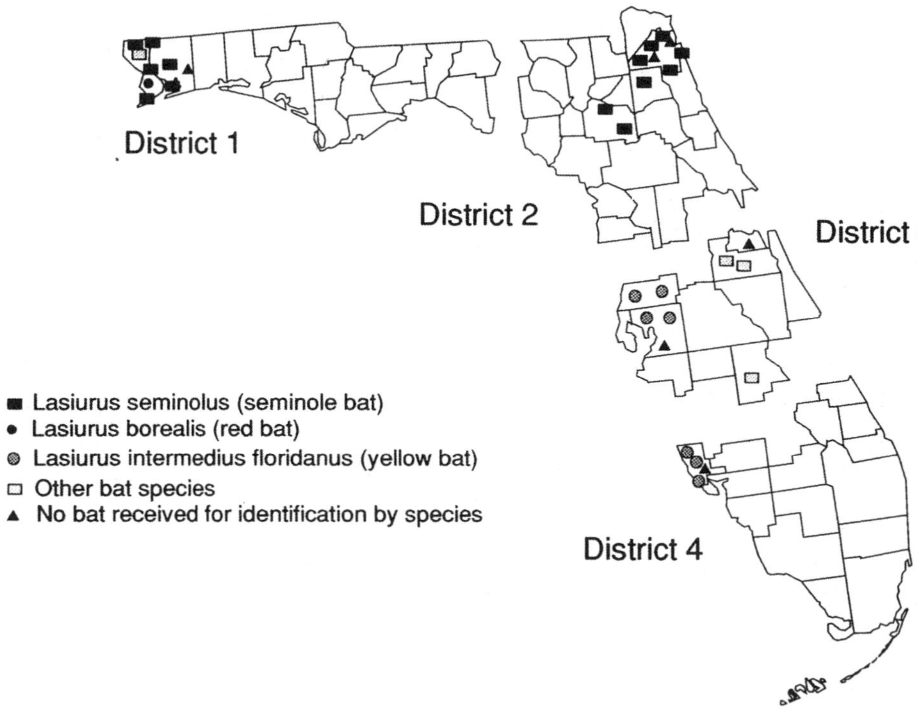

Figure 16-12. Distribution of bat rabies cases, by species, in Florida, 1988. (From Smith, J. S., Yager, P. A., Bigler, W. J., and E. C. Hartwig, Jr. Surveillance and epidemiologic mapping of monoclonal antibody-defined rabies variants in Florida. *J. Wildl. Dis.* 26(4): 473, 1990. Reproduced with permission.)

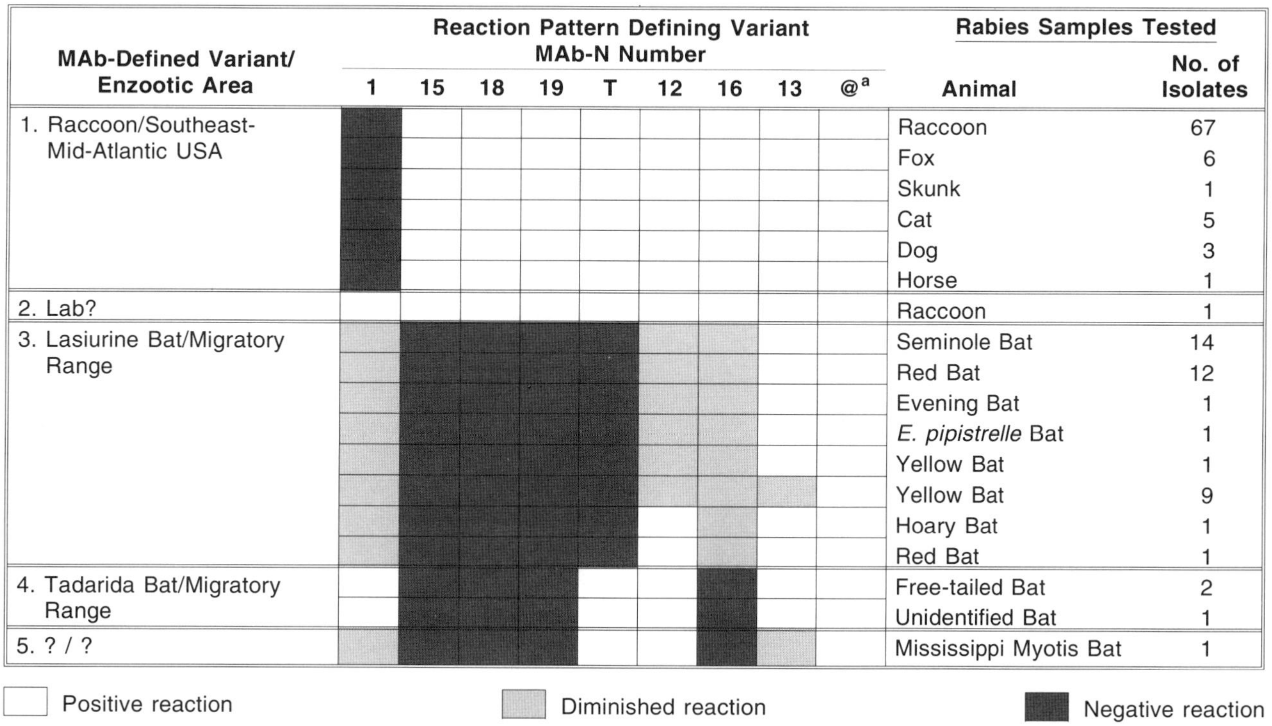

[a]@ 12 MAbs which react with all rabies isolates from the southeastern United States.

Figure 16-13. Antigenic analysis of 128 rabies samples from Florida, 1986-1987. (From Smith, J. S., Yager, P. A., Bigler, W. J., and E. D. Hartwig, Jr. Surveillance and epidemiologic mapping of monoclonal antibody-defined rabies variants in Florida. *J. Wildl. Dis.* 26(4): 473, 1990. Redrawn with permission.)

species of insectivorous bats has had any significant influence on the prevalence or distribution of rabies in the predominant terrestrial reservoirs of disease (see page 265). Transmission of virus from nonterrestrial to terrestrial species is a relatively infrequent occurrence. Rather, the presence of rabies in both domestic animals and nonreservoiring species of wildlife is typically the result of spillover of virus from the major terrestrial reservoir of the region.

Genetic Analysis of Rabies Isolates

The widespread availability of monoclonal antibodies has allowed investigators to define precise antigenic parameters for identifying (and then subclassifying) the serotypes of rabies and rabies-related viruses. The yield from monoclonal analyses in epidemiologic investigations has been substantial. Despite extensive application of monoclonal technology, however, it is not without limitations. In particular, monoclonal analysis is limited in its capacity to differentiate between antigenically closely related viral variants.

A more definitive examination of the relatedness of different viral variants is provided by newly applied techniques of genetic analysis. Amplification of viral genetic material using a polymerase chain reaction (PCR) has enabled researchers to directly sequence the nucleotide substitutions of portions of the viral genome (Ermine et al, 1990; Bourhy et al, 1992, 1993; Sacramento et al, 1992; Smith et al, 1992; Kulonen and Boldina, 1993; McColl et al, 1993; Nadin-Davis et al, 1993; Smith and Seidel, 1993). The degree of similarity among sequences from different viral isolates (from related and unrelated hosts and from local and distant geographic regions) can then be defined by computer algorithms (Figures 16-14 and 23-4).

Application of modern genetic analysis to studies of the molecular epidemiology of rabies is currently in its infancy. To date, molecular

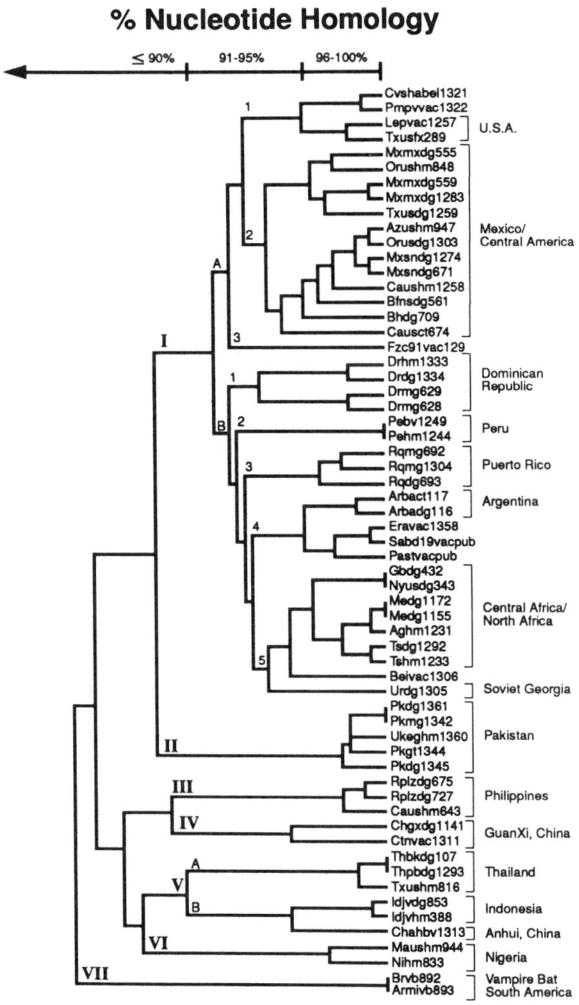

Figure 16-14. Dendrogram showing the percentage of genetic relatedness (% nucleotide homology) among globally dispersed terrestrial rabies isolates of serotype 1, several vaccine strains, and isolates from vampire bats in Latin America. The numerical values for sequence divergence between pairs of samples were used to arbitrarily divide the sample clusters in the dendrogram into three categories. Pairwise comparisons between nucleotide sequences were made using computer algorithms. The first category includes clusters of the most closely related samples (differing by <5%). These consisted of field samples collected from the same outbreak area. The second category (differing from each other by <10%) included clusters that were related by historical, political, and cultural connections, as well as geographic proximity. The third category (differing from each other by ≥10%) consisted of clusters that were only distantly related. Horizontal branch lengths indicate the percent relatedness of pairs, measured at the level of the vertically oriented lines (the latter included for clarity). As can be seen, samples from rabid vampire bats (group VII) were only distantly related to viral isolates from terrestrial species, even those from the same relative geographical region. Sequence analysis is a relatively new application in rabies epidemiology. Analysis of isolates from defined genomic areas and populations will greatly improve our understanding of rabies epidemiology worldwide. (From Smith, J. S. and H. D. Seidel. Rabies: A new look at an old disease. *Prog. Med. Virol.* 40: 82, 1993. Reproduced with permission.)

analyses have substantiated the fact that nonterrestrial and terrestrial rabies cycles are largely independent of each other.

Direct sequencing of amplified viral genomic material has proven valuable in both public-health investigations (Ou et al, 1992) and biomedical research. Continued genetic analysis will ultimately lead to a broader understanding of the historical spread and global epidemiology of the disease, providing more definitive information than monoclonal studies alone. This will better enable researchers to speculate on the global evolution of the rabies and rabies-related viruses. PCR technology will probably also be incorporated into sophisticated rabies diagnostic applications as well (Sacramento et al, 1991; Kamolvarin et al, 1993).

References

Baer, G. M. and J. S. Smith (1991). Rabies in Nonhematophagous Bats. In G. M. Baer (ed.) *The Natural History of Rabies*. 2nd Edition. CRC Press, Inc. Boca Raton, Florida.

Bourhy, H., Kissi, B., Lafon, M., Sacramento, D., and N. Tordo (1992). Antigenic and molecular characterization of bat rabies virus in Europe. *J. Clin. Microbiol.* 30(9): 2419

Casey, A., Webster, A., and K. Charlton (1989). Cross-Canada Disease Report—Eastern Canada. *Can. Vet. J.* 30: 522

Centers for Disease Control (1985). An epidemiologic study of sylvatic rabies in Texas and New York using monoclonal antibodies. *CDC Rabies Surveillance Report*. U. S. Department of Health and Human Services, Public Health Service.

Constantine, D. G. (1988). Health Precautions for Bat

Researchers. In T. H. Kunz (ed.) *Ecological and Behavioral Methods for the Study of Bats*. Smithsonian Institution Press. Washington, D. C.

Dietzschold, B., Rupprecht, C. E., Tollis, M., Lafon, M., Mattei, J., Wiktor, T. J., and H. Koprowski (1988). Antigenic diversity of the glycoprotein and nucleocapsid proteins of rabies and rabies-related viruses: Implications for epidemiology and control of rabies. *Rev. Infect. Dis.* 10(Suppl. 4): S785

Emmons, R. W. (1994). Chief, Viral and Rickettsial Disease Laboratory, Department of Health Services, State of California. Berkeley, California. Personal communication.

Ermine, A., Larzul, D., Ceccaldi, P. E., Guesdon, J. L., and H. Tsiang (1990). Polymerase chain reaction amplification of rabies virus nucleic acids from total mouse brain RNA. *Mol. Cell. Probes.* 4(3): 189

Fuller, Jr., J. E. (1984). A case of equine rabies. *New Engl. J. Med.* 310(8): 525

Glickman, L., Russell, H., Maher, J., McCarthy, M., White, E. J., Hays, C.W., and G. Landis (1983). Exposure to a rabid cow—Pennsylvania. *MMWR.* 32(9): 128

Kamolvarin, N., Tirawatnpong, T., Rattanasiwamoke, R., Tirawatnpong, S., Panpanich, T., and T. Hemachudha (1993). Diagnosis of rabies by polymerase chain reaction with nested primers. *J. Infect. Dis.* 167: 297

King, A. A. (1991). *Studies of the Antigenic Relationships of Rabies and Rabies-Related Viruses Using Anti-Nucleoprotein Monoclonal Antibodies. Ph.D. Thesis.* School of Biological Sciences, University of Surrey. Guildford, United Kingdom. Courtesy of Dr. Arthur A. King.

Kulonen, K. and I. Boldina (1993). Differentiation of two rabies strains in Estonia with reference to recent Finnish isolates. *J. Wildl. Dis.* 29(2): 209

Lafon, M. (1993). Rabies Unit. World Health Organization Collaborating Center for Rabies, Pasteur Institute. Paris, France. Personal communication.

Loewen, K. (1993). Animal Diseases Research Institute. Lethbridge, Alberta. Personal communication.

McColl, K. A., Gould, P. W., Hooper, P. T., Westbury, H. A., and J. S. Smith (1993). Polymerase chain reaction and other laboratory techniques in the diagnosis of long incubation rabies in Australia. *Aust. Vet. J.* 70(3): 84

Montano Hirose, J. A., Bourhy, H., and M. Lafon (1990). A reduced panel of anti-nucleocapsid monoclonal antibodies for bat rabies virus identification in Europe. *Res. Virol.* 141: 571

Nadin-Davis, S. A., Casey, G. A., and A. Wandeler (1993). Identification of regional variants of the rabies virus within the Canadian province of Ontario. *J. Gen. Virol.* 74: 829

Neill, S. U. (1992/1993). Supervisor, Medical Virology. Texas Department of Health. Austin, Texas. Personal communication.

Ou, C.-Y., Ciesielski, C. A., Myers, G., Bandea, C. I., Luo, C.-G., Korber, B. T. M., Mullins, J. L., Schochetman, G., Berkelman, R. L., Economou, N., Witte, J. J., Furman, L. J., Satten, G. A., Macinnes, K. A., Curran, J. W., and H. W. Jaffe (1992). Laboratory Investigation Group, Epidemiologic Investigation Group: Molecular epidemiology of HIV transmission in a dental practice. *Science.* 256: 1165

Rupprecht, C. E. (1986). *The Epidemiology of Wildlife Rabies Within North America: Characterization Via Monoclonal Antibodies.* Ph.D. Thesis. The University of Wisconsin. Milwaukee, Wisconsin.

Rupprecht, C. E., Glickman, L. T., Spencer, P. A., and T. J. Wiktor (1987). Epidemiology of rabies virus variants: Differentiation using monoclonal antibodies and discriminant analysis. *Am. J. Epidemiol.* 126(2): 298

Sacramento, D., Bourhy, H., and N. Tordo (1991). PCR technique as an alternative method for diagnosis and molecular epidemiology of rabies virus. *Mol. Cell. Probes.* 5: 229

Sacramento, D., Badrane, H., Bourhy, H., and N. Tordo (1992). Molecular epidemiology of rabies virus in France: Comparison with vaccine strains. *J. Gen. Virol.* 73: 1149

Smith, J. S. (1988). Monoclonal antibody study of bat rabies. *Rev. Infect. Dis.* 10(Suppl. 4): S637

Smith, J. S. (1989). Rabies Virus Epitopic Variation: Use in Ecologic Studies. In K. Maramorosch, F. A. Murphy, and A. J. Shatkin (eds.) *Advances in Virus Research.* Vol. 36. Academic Press, Inc. New York.

Smith, J. S. (1992/1993/1994). Research Microbiologist. Rabies Laboratory, Centers for Disease Control. Atlanta, Georgia. Personal communication.

Smith, J. S. and G. M. Baer (1988). Epizootiology of Rabies: The Americas. In J. B. Campbell and K. M. Charlton (eds.) *Developments in Veterinary Virology—Rabies.* Kluwer Academic Publishers. Boston.

Smith, J. S. and H. D. Seidel (1993). Rabies: A new look at an old disease. *Prog. Med. Virol.* 40: 82

Smith, J. S., Sumner, J. W., Roumillat, L. F., Baer, G. M., and W. G. Winkler (1984). Antigenic characteristics of isolates associated with a new epizootic of raccoon rabies in the United States. *J. Infect. Dis.* 149(5): 769

Smith, J. S., Sumner, J., Roumillot, F., Baer, G. M., and W. Winkler (1985). Epidemiological Analysis of Street Rabies Viruses From Enzootic Areas of the United States. In E. Kuwert, C. Merieux, H. Koprowski, and K. Bogel (eds.) *Rabies in the Tropics.*

Springer-Verlag. New York.

Smith, J. S., Yager, P. A., Bigler, W. J., and E. D. Hartwig, Jr. (1990). Surveillance and epidemiologic mapping of monoclonal antibody-defined rabies variants in Florida. *J. Wildl. Dis.* 26(4): 473

Smith, J. S., Orciari, L. A., Yager, P. A., Seidel, H. D., and C. K. Warner (1992). Epidemiologic and historical relationships among 87 rabies virus isolates as determined by limited sequence analysis. *J. Infect. Dis.* 166: 296

Trimarchi, C. V. (1983). The Epidemiology and Control of Bat Rabies in New York State. *Proceedings of the North American Symposium on Wildlife Rabies.* Johns Hopkins University. Baltimore. November 7-8, 1983.

Trimarchi, C. V. (1984). *Rabies Annual Summary, 1984.* Rabies Laboratory, Wadsworth Center for Laboratories and Research, New York State Department of Health. Albany, New York.

Trimarchi, C. V. (1986). *Rabies Annual Summary, 1986.* Rabies Laboratory, Wadsworth Center for Laboratories and Research, New York State Department of Health. Albany, New York.

Trimarchi, C. V. (1987). *Rabies Annual Summary, 1987.* Rabies Laboratory, Wadsworth Center for Laboratories and Research, New York State Department of Health. Albany, New York.

Trimarchi, C. V. (1988). *Rabies Laboratory Monthly Report. May, 1988.* Rabies Laboratory, Wadsworth Center for Laboratories and Research, New York State Department of Health. Albany, New York.

Trimarchi, C. V. (1989). Director, Rabies Laboratory. Wadsworth Center for Laboratories and Research, New York State Department of Health. Albany, New York. Personal communication.

Trimarchi, C. V. (1990). *Rabies Annual Summary, 1990.* Rabies Laboratory, Wadsworth Center for Laboratories and Research, New York State Department of Health. Albany, New York.

Wandeler, A. I. (1992). Head, Rabies Unit. Animal Diseases Research Institute. Nepean, Ontario. Personal communication.

Wandeler, A. I. and G. A. Casey (1993). Rabies diagnoses in eastern Canada, January 1, 1992 - June 30, 1992. Cross-Canada Disease Report. *Can. Vet. J.* 34: 123

Webster, W. A., Casey, G. A., Charlton, K. M., and T. J. Wiktor (1985). Antigenic variants of rabies virus isolates from eastern, central and northern Canada. *Can. J. Comp. Med.* 49: 186

Webster, W. A., Casey, G. A., and K. M. Charlton (1988). Rabies in a squirrel. *Can. Vet. J.* 29(12): 1015

Webster, W. A., Casey, G. A., and K. M. Charlton (1989). Bat-induced rabies in terrestrial mammals in Nova Scotia and Newfoundland. *Can. Vet. J.* 30: 679

Whetstone, C. A., Bunn, T. O., Emmons, R. W., and T. J. Wiktor (1984). Use of monoclonal antibodies to confirm vaccine-induced rabies in ten dogs, two cats, and one fox. *J. Am. Vet. Med. Assoc.* 185(3): 285

Whitney, H. G. (1989). Update on rabies—Newfoundland. Cross-Canada Disease Report. *Can. Vet. J.* 30: 522

World Health Organization (1992). *Expert Committee on Rabies. Eighth Report.* WHO Tech. Rpt. No. 824. Geneva.

Chapter 17:
INSECTIVOROUS BATS AND RABIES IN CANADA

Reservoirs of Disease

In Canada, rabies is enzootic in skunks, foxes, and insectivorous bats. Foxes and striped skunks are the primary wildlife reservoirs (Gregory, 1985). Predominant geographic reservoir associations include the skunk in Manitoba and Saskatchewan; the red fox and skunk in Ontario and Quebec; the Arctic fox in Northwest Territories; and bats throughout Canada (Prins and Yates, 1986; Dolman and Charlton, 1987; Prins and Loewen, 1988). As is the case in the United States, rabid bats are widely dispersed throughout Canada.

Rabies in insectivorous bats has been reported from all provinces of Canada, except Newfoundland and Prince Edward Island (Beauregard and Stewart, 1964; Tabel et al, 1974; Prins and Yates, 1986). The majority of rabid bats have been reported from Ontario and Alberta (Table 17-1). Rabid bats are not commonly reported from Canada's Atlantic provinces, only four cases having been reported between 1972 and 1989 (Webster et al, 1989). However, rabid bats have been reported throughout western Canada (including the western Northwest Territories, the Yukon Territory, and the provinces of Manitoba, Saskatchewan, Alberta, and British Columbia). Bats are the only known reservoirs of rabies virus in British Columbia. As was the case in the United States, the early recognition of rabies in insectivorous bats in Canada was followed by heightened media publicity and survey studies of bat populations.

Epidemiology and Epizootiology

As reported in the United States and Europe, the majority of bat submissions (and the majority of rabies-positive findings) have been during the summer months (Figure 17-1). Similarly, the greatest number of submissions are from regions with a dense human populace. Species identified as rabid from western provinces include the little brown bat (*Myotis lucifugus*), big brown bat, long-eared bat (*Myotis evotis*), California bat, Yuma bat (*Myotis yumanensis*), hoary bat, and silver-haired bat.

The most common bat in western Canada, and therefore the one most likely to be encountered by man, is the little brown bat. It is the species of bat most commonly submitted to diagnostic laboratories. However, suspect specimens are not commonly reported to be infected (Pybus, 1986). Between 1977 and 1985, 2.7% (8 of 300) of suspect little brown bats in British Columbia were found to be infected (Prins and Loewen, 1988). The species of bat most commonly reported to be infected in Canada is the big brown bat, although the reported prevalence of infection may vary from province to province. Due to its habit of roosting in buildings, the big brown bat lives in close association with humans.

Beauregard (1969) suggested that migratory species, in moving south into the United States, may become infected by mingling with rabid resident American bats. A similar concern was voiced anonymously in 1954. Schowalter (1980) observed that migratory silver-haired bats could occasionally be found in the midst of colonies of both little and big brown bats. The author cited these findings as evidence that infected migratory bats may play a role in carrying virus into north temperate-zone bat communities. By the same reasoning, infected Canadian bats may also carry virus south into the United States (Figure 17-2).

Schowalter (1980) believed that rabies among bats in Alberta occurred as a series of local outbreaks, rather than existing at a constant low level

Table 17-1

Rabies-Positive Bats Identified in Canada, by Province and Year, 1976-1986

Province	1976	1977	1978	1979	1980	1981	1982	1983	1984	1985	1986	Total
Ontario	9	17	14	22	32	19	22	47	51	35	45	313
Alberta	28	9	5	12	11	9	7	5	5	4	6	101
British Columbia	8	8	1	5	10	8	7	9	5	11	9	81
Saskatchewan	6	9	5	4	3	3	2	2	3	7	5	49
Manitoba	1	-	-	-	-	-	-	-	1	-	-	2
Quebec	-	2	-	-	1	-	2	-	2	1	1	9
Nova Scotia	-	-	-	-	-	-	-	-	-	-	1	1
New Brunswick	-	-	-	-	-	-	-	-	1	-	-	1
Total	52	45	25	43	57	39	40	63	68	58	67	557

From Rosatte, R. C. Bat rabies in Canada: History, epidemiology and prevention. *Can. Vet. J.* 28(12): 754, 1987. Reproduced with permission.

(enzootic), as reported elsewhere. The local outbreaks were considered to be short-lived and follow-up survey studies were characterized by a diminished prevalence. Such outbreaks are not known to characterize rabies in insectivorous bats in the United States or elsewhere and there is no good evidence to suggest that they occur (see pages 139 and 265).

Bats are the only known reservoirs of rabies virus in British Columbia. Since the fluorescent antibody test became the standard for rabies diagnosis in 1968, four cats (one in 1968, two in 1992, and one in 1993), one horse (1984), and one beaver (1985) are the only animals, other than bats, that have been confirmed as rabies positive in British Columbia (Copeland et al, 1985; Prins and Yates, 1986; Prins and Loewen, 1988, 1991; Wandeler, 1992; Loewen, 1993). A nonterrestrial variant of virus was isolated only from the horse. The finding of the first rabid cat predated availability of monoclonal antibody testing and viral isolates from this cat are no longer available for testing (Wandeler, 1992). The horse had been stabled in an area in which bat rabies was enzootic. Virus isolated from the horse was identical to that found in bats of British Columbia, Alberta, Saskatchewan, and Ontario. Although indicative of the fact that transmission of virus from bats to other animals can occur, it has been reported only rarely in Canada.

There have been only eight documented cases of rabies transmission from bats to terrestrial animals in Canada (Webster et al, 1985, 1988, 1989; Casey et al, 1989; Whitney, 1989; Wandeler, 1992; Loewen, 1993; Wandeler and Casey, 1993). These include a red fox and a cow from Cape Breton Island, Nova Scotia; a silver fox from the southern coast of Newfoundland; a cow, squirrel, and skunk from Ontario; a skunk from Alberta; and a horse from British Columbia.

The rabid squirrel identified in Ottawa was submitted for testing after it had bitten a person (Webster et al, 1988). This finding remains the only documented case of a rodent (squirrel) being infected with a bat variant of rabies virus. The squirrel had been infected with a variant of virus identical to that found in big brown bats in Ontario. Virus had been found in the salivary glands of this animal. Canadian public-health policy insures that all specimens (including rodents) submitted for rabies evaluation are tested, regardless of whether or not a human exposure is involved (Webster et al, 1988; Prins, 1991).

These findings are consistent with those of large-scale serological surveys conducted in the United States and Europe. The results do not sup-

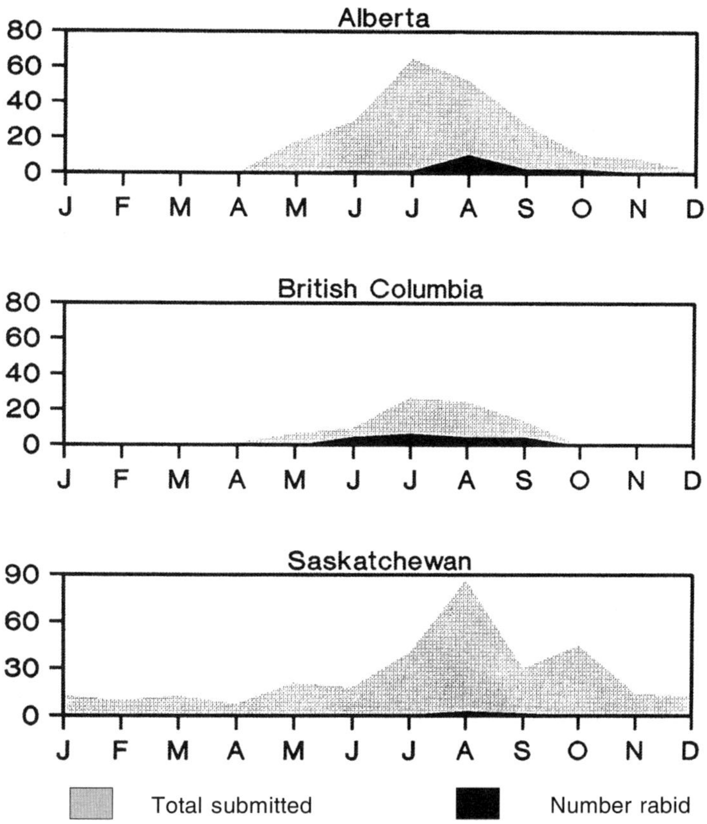

Figure 17-1. Big brown bats submitted and those found rabid in Alberta, British Columbia, and Saskatchewan, by month, 1979-1983. This species, the most commonly reported rabid bat in Canada, is nonmigratory in habit and hibernates from November through March. Hence, both submissions and positive findings are most common in the summer months. (From Baer, G. M. and J. S. Smith. Rabies in Nonhematophagous Bats. In G. M. Baer (ed.) *The Natural History of Rabies*. 2nd Edition. © CRC Press, Inc. Boca Raton, Florida, 1991. Reproduced with permission.) Original data from Pybus, M. J. Rabies in insectivorous bats of western Canada, 1979-1983. *J. Wildl. Dis.* 22(3):307, 1986

port a significant role of bats in the initiation or maintenance of rabies infection in terrestrial species. Investigations have consistently documented the fact that rabies cycles in insectivorous bats are largely independent of those in terrestrial wildlife.

Antigenic Characterization of Rabies Isolates from Canadian Bats

Rabies isolates from bats in Canada have been divided into four major groups (Figures 17-3 and 17-4). The B-1 group consists of isolates obtained from big brown bats in Ontario plus one isolate from Nanaimo, British Columbia (Webster et al, 1986). The antigenic reactivity of isolates from big brown bats in Ontario is generally uniform, although minor variations in reactivity patterns were noted from isolates in different regions of the province. Big brown bats are the most commonly submitted Chiropteran species in Ontario. They are also the species of bat most commonly reported rabies positive. Other bat species (including various species of *Myotis, Lasionycteris*, and *Lasiurus*) are submitted to diagnostic laboratories less frequently and are not commonly diagnosed rabid. The authors found no evidence to support the occurrence of interspecific transmission of virus between big brown bats in Ontario and other Chiropteran species.

Isolates from various species and geographical regions make up the B-2 group. These include isolates from long-eared bats and hoary bats in British Columbia; little brown bats, big brown

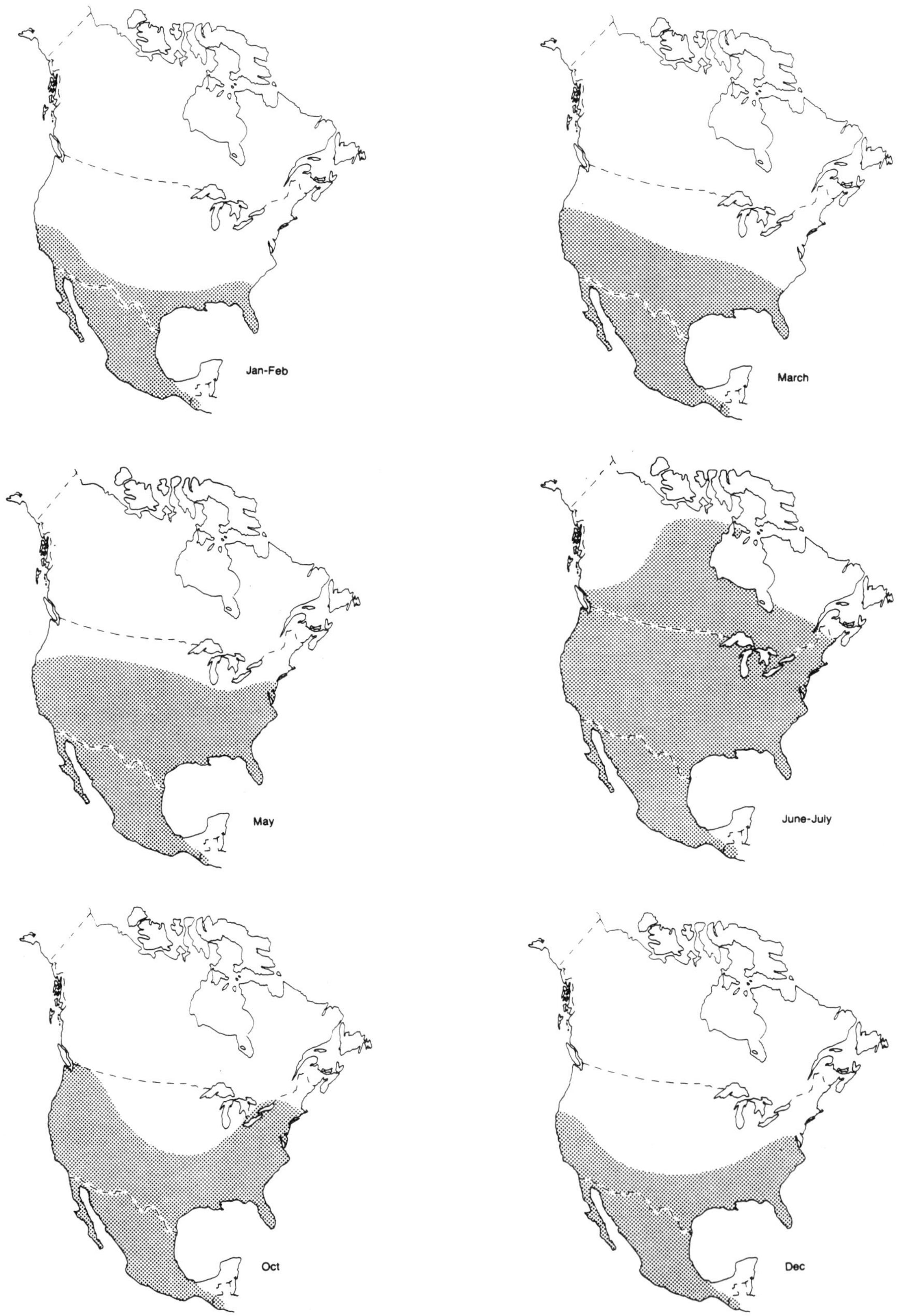

Figure 17-2. Migratory pattern of the hoary bat. (From Hill, J. E. and J. D. Smith. *Bats—A Natural History*. British Museum of Natural History. London, 1984. Reproduced with permission.)

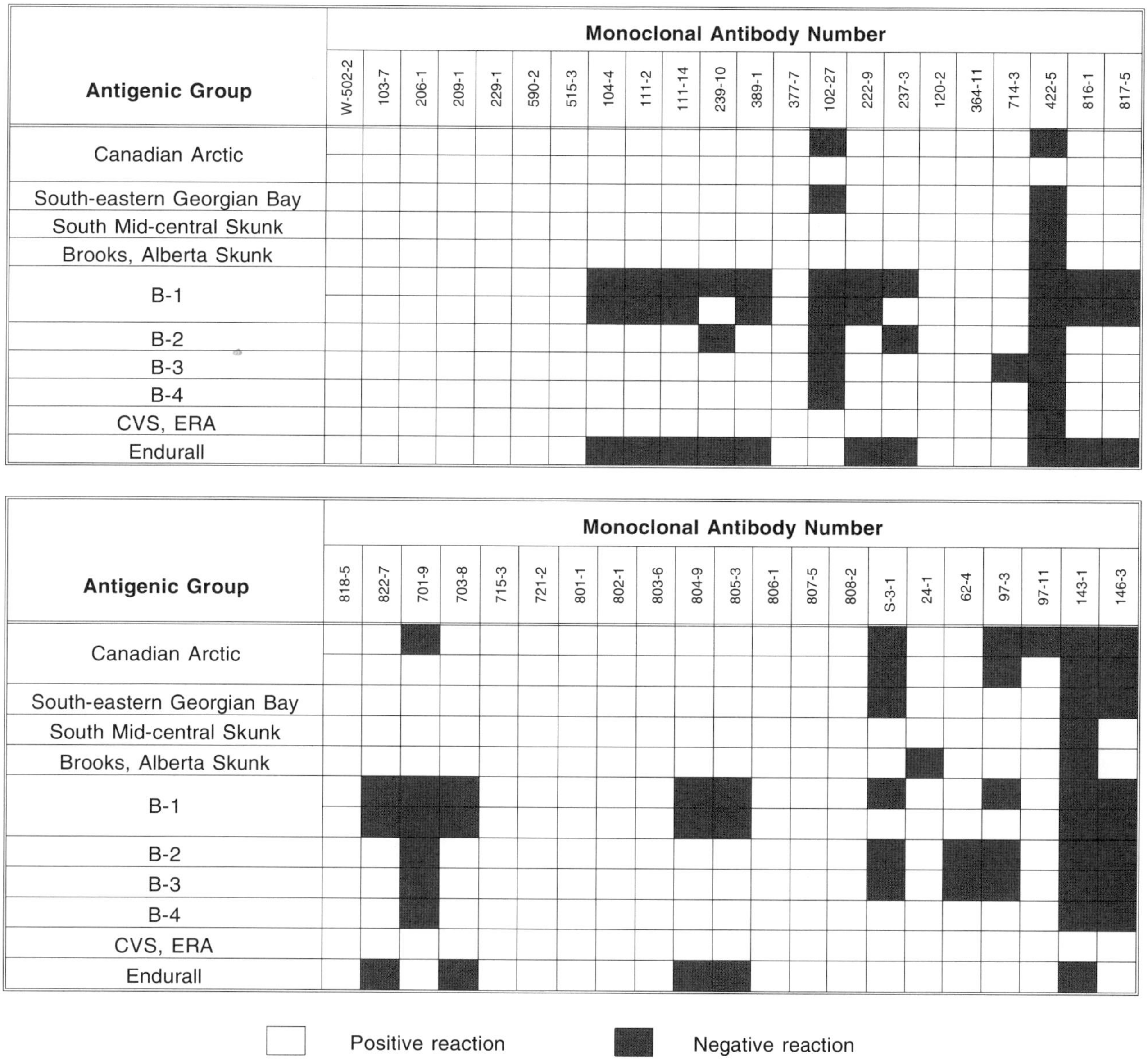

Figure 17-3. Reactivity of anti-nucleocapsid monoclonal antibodies with viral isolates from Canada and from fixed viruses. (From Webster, W. A., Casey, G. A., and K. M. Charlton. Major antigenic groups of rabies virus in Canada determined by anti-nucleocapsid monoclonal antibodies. *Comp. Immun. Microbiol. Infect. Dis.* 9(1): 59, 1986. © Pergamon Press Ltd, Headington Hill Hall, Oxford OX3 OBW, UK. Reproduced with permission.)

bats, silver-haired bats, and hoary bats from Alberta; hoary bats from Saskatchewan; plus a single isolate from a silver-haired bat in Ontario. The antigenic profiles of these isolates were identical. Webster et al (1986) suggested that the widely dispersed range and host distribution of isolates characterized by this reactivity pattern may be related to migratory behavior (*Lasionycteris* and *Lasiurus*) and interactions with resident bat populations.

Two isolates from a little brown bat in Ontario plus one from *Myotis keenii* (Keen's myotis) in New Brunswick constitute the B-3 group.

The B-4 group comprises isolates of big brown bats from Saskatoon, Saskatchewan and from the mid-southern portion of Alberta.

Single isolates from several regions which differ from the four major groupings by their re-

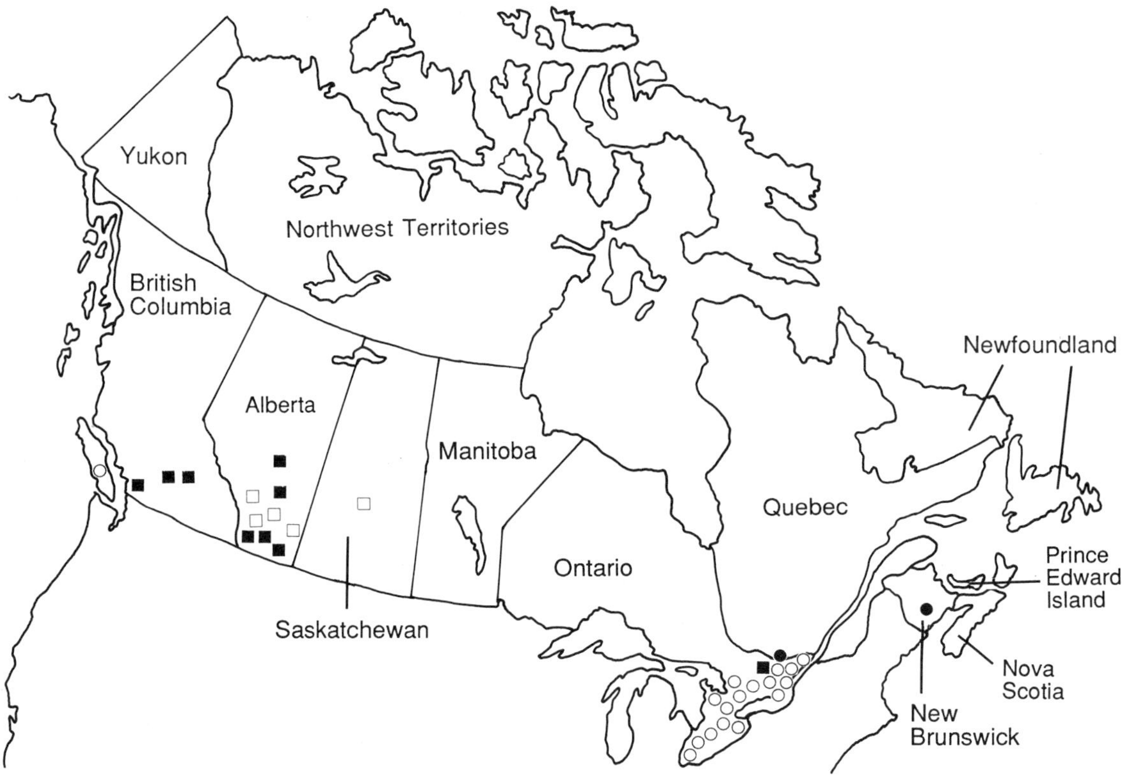

Figure 17-4. Distribution of major antigenic groups of rabies virus in bats from Canada. B-1○ ; B-2■ ; B-3●; B-4□. (From Webster, W. A., Casey, G. A., and K. M. Charlton. Major antigenic groups of rabies virus in Canada determined by anti-nucleocapsid monoclonal antibodies. *Comp. Immun. Microbiol. Infect. Dis.* 9(1): 59, 1986. © Pergamon Press Ltd, Headington Hill Hall, Oxford OX3 OBW, UK. Redrawn with permission.)

activity patterns to one or more monoclonal antibodies have not been grouped.

The relationship between reactivity profiles of nonterrestrial isolates from geographically separated regions of Canada (e.g., B-1 and B-4 variants of big brown bat isolates) and those from the United States (e.g., 13 reactivity patterns identified in big brown bats across the country) have not been fully investigated. There is also little available information on which species of bats in Canada represent important reservoirs of virus and which, if any, are infected primarily by spillover from the major Chiropteran host in the area.

British Columbia

Between 1979 and 1983, only 0.1% (1 of 769) of survey bats, randomly collected from buildings in western Canada, was found to be infected. This is in contrast to 5.1% (95 of 1,874) of clinically ill, suspect specimens submitted for testing (Pybus, 1986). As discussed earlier (see page 140), however, disease prevalence among randomly collected bats and suspect submissions may differ markedly and results should be interpreted accordingly. In British Columbia alone (Table 17-2), 8.4% (152 of 1,810) of suspect submissions were found to be rabid between 1971 and 1989 (Prins and Loewen, 1988, 1991). Bat species which are migratory in Alberta and Saskatchewan may be year-round residents in British Columbia.

Alberta

Bat rabies in Alberta was first detected in 1971. Between 1971 and 1975, 1.8% (23 of 1,252) of randomly collected survey specimens were found to be rabid. Of the infected bats included in this sampling, 1.9% (21 of 1,107) were little brown bats and 1.4% (2 of 145) were big brown bats. Fifty-nine of 1,249 (4.7%) suspect submission bats were confirmed rabid (Dorward et al, 1977).

Between 1973 and 1975, the most commonly infected submission suspect in Alberta was the silver-haired bat, with a disease prevalence of 9.9% (22 of 222), followed by the big brown bat with a disease prevalence of 7.0% (19 of 272). Nine of 464 (1.9%) little brown bats were infected (Dorward et al, 1977). The relatively high prevalence of infection in silver-haired bats between 1973 and 1975 was an unusual occurrence. In previous and subsequent years, the big brown bat was the most commonly reported rabid Chiropteran species.

Between 1979 and 1982, the overall prevalence of infection among eight species of bats submitted to diagnostic laboratories was found to be 4.6% (Rosatte, 1985). Of 39 bats reported to be rabid during this time, 22 were big brown bats, 10 were silver-haired bats, 5 were hoary bats, and 2 were little brown bats. Respective species-specific prevalence was 9.7%, 6.3%, 24%, and 0.5% Although big brown bats were the most commonly infected species, the prevalence was highest among hoary bats. As discussed previously (see page 142), this is not an unusual finding for solitary-bat submissions. Rabies prevalence in little brown bats was considerably lower than the 1.9% reported between 1973 and 1975.

Gunson and Schowalter (1974) suggested an association between rabid bats and rabid coyotes in Alberta, similar to the one suggested by Fredrickson and Thomas (1965) for bats and foxes in Tennessee. Both associations, however, remain unsubstantiated by monoclonal antibody analyses.

Table 17-2

Prevalence of Rabies Among Specimens of Bats Submitted for Testing in British Columbia, 1971-1985[a]

Year	Number Positive/Tested	Percent Positive
1971	0/0	0
1972	1/4	25.8
1973	4/35	11.4
1974	3/28	10.7
1975	17/146	11.6
1976	9/110	8.2
1977	9/115	7.8
1978	1/58	1.7
1979	5/41	12.2
1980	10/65	15.4
1981	8/59	13.6
1982	7/104	6.7
1983	9/101	8.9
1984	5/128	3.9
1985	11/160	6.9
Total	99/1,154	8.6

[a] Between 1986 and 1989, 53 of 656 suspect submissions were found to be rabies positive, leading to an overall prevalence of 8.4% (152 of 1,810) between 1971-1989.

From Prins, B. and K. Loewen. Bat rabies in British Columbia 1971 to 1985. *Can. Vet. J.* 29: 41, 1988. Reproduced with permission.

Early Reports of Human Exposure

In Greater Vancouver, on June 3, 1957, a 13-year-old boy found a big brown bat in some stones in a schoolyard. He picked the bat up and was bitten on his index finger. The bat clung tenaciously and was removed only after the boy's teacher killed it with ether. It was subsequently confirmed rabies positive. Post-exposure rabies prophylaxis was administered. This was the first reported case of bat rabies in Canada, although disease among bats was likely present prior to this discovery (Avery and Tailyour, 1960; Tabel et al, 1974).

On July 16, 1958, an obviously ill big brown bat was found by a boy along a beach in the Okanagan Region of British Columbia. When he picked the bat up, it bit him on the hand and he dropped it back onto the beach. After hearing the story, the boy's mother retrieved the bat (which by then was dead). The bat was found to be rabid

Table 17-3

Symptoms and Contacts Reported in Rabid Bats in Ontario, 1963-1967

	Symptoms				Contacts				
					Persons		Pets		
Species	Flying Abnormally	Partially Paralyzed	Not Reported	Total Bats	Bite	Handling	Cats	Dogs	Total Contacts
Big Brown bat	5	7	20	32	20	2	1	1	24
Hoary Bat		1	2	3		2	1		3
Silver-Haired Bat		1	2	3		1			1
Little Brown Bat		1	1	2	1	1			2
Eastern Pipistrelle		1		1					
Keen's Myotis			1	1	1				1
Red Bat		1		1					
Not Identified			1	1					
Total	5	12	27	44	22	6	2	1	31

From Beauregard, M. Bat rabies in Canada 1963-1967. *Can. J. Comp. Med.* 33: 220, 1969. Reproduced with permission.

and post-exposure rabies prophylaxis was administered.

A month later (August 21, 1958), the caretaker of the Community Hall at Osoyoos, British Columbia found a silver-haired bat in an old shoe. As it crawled out, the caretaker picked it up and was bitten on the thumb and index finger. The bat was diagnosed as rabid and post-exposure rabies prophylaxis administered.

Human Rabies of Bat Origin in Canada

Hundreds of people in Canada have received post-exposure rabies prophylaxis following alleged contact with a bat (Tables 17-3, 17-4, and 17-5). Many of these contacts involved confirmed rabid animals, and many culminated in a bite. Most of the reported cases of human exposure involved the careless handling of sick bats, a repeating theme in circumstances of bat/human interaction.

Since 1925, 21 human deaths due to rabies have been documented in Canada (Rosatte, 1987). Epidemiologic data are available for the six cases occurring after 1960. Three of the five (60%) indigenously acquired cases (Saskatchewan, 1970; Nova Scotia, 1977; and Alberta, 1985) are known to have been bat related.

1) In September of 1970, a 15-year-old boy from Meadow Lake, Saskatchewan came downstairs from his bedroom with a dead bat in his hand. He told his parents that he had smothered

Table 17-4

Bat/Human Contacts Requiring Post-Exposure Rabies Prophylaxis in Ontario, 1980-1986

Year	Number of Humans Treated	Percent of Total Human Exposure
1980	45	2.5
1981	41	2.6
1982	61	2.5
1983	108	4.4
1984	78	3.8
1985	71	3.3
1986	88	2.1
Total	492	2.9

From Rosatte, R. C. Bat rabies in Canada: History, epidemiology and prevention. *Can. Vet. J.* 28(12): 754, 1987. Reproduced with permission.

Table 17-5

Human Contact With Bats Submitted for Rabies Testing in Western Canada, 1968-1989

Province	Human Contact Reported		No Human Contact Reported		Total
	Neg	Pos	Neg	Pos	
Alberta	310	16	3,785	154	4,265
Saskatchewan	200	15	1,555	72	1,842
British Columbia	211	27	1,288	114	1,640
Northwest Territories	0	0	6	0	6

From Bradley, J. A. Laboratory diagnosis of rabies in western Canada (1968-1977). *Can. Vet. J.* 20: 186, 1979; Prins, L. and W. D. G. Yates. Rabies in western Canada, 1978-1984. *Can. Vet. J.* 27: 164, 1986; and Prins, B., and K. Loewen. Rabies diagnosis in western Canada, 1985-1989. *Can. Vet. J.* 32: 487, 1991. Adapted with permission.

it in his bed clothes after it had flown into his face and bitten him.

On September 22, the boy was admitted to the University Hospital in Saskatoon with fever; pain in his head, neck, and shoulder; and dysphagia. Symptoms quickly worsened until his death on September 29. This was the first reported human death from rabies of bat origin in Canada (Dempster et al, 1972). Additional medical details can be found on page 238.

2) While trying to remove a bat from his home, a 62-year-old man from Parrsboro, Nova Scotia was bitten on his left hand. Approximately one year later, the man was admitted to the Victoria General Hospital with an undiagnosed neurological illness. Within 40 hours of his admission, he lapsed into a coma and died. Autopsy confirmed rabies as the cause of death (King et al, 1978). Additional medical details can be found on page 238.

3) In July of 1985, a 25-year-old man was scratched or bitten on the left cheek by a bat in northern Alberta. The bat had fallen from the top of his tent. The man threw the bat outside and it was gone the following morning. No post-exposure rabies prophylaxis was administered, local antiseptic being the only treatment received. On October 24, he developed a "kink" in his neck, chest discomfort, and a general state of malaise. Rabies immune globulin was administered, but he became comatose. He died on November 26, when artificial life support was discontinued. Virus isolated from a brain biopsy prior to death was identical to that commonly found in bats of western Canada (McLean et al, 1985; Dolman and Charlton, 1987; Varughese, 1987; Webster et al, 1987). Additional medical details can be found on page 237.

References

Anonymous (1954). Possibility of bats carrying rabies virus into Canada. *Can. J. Comp. Med.* XVIII(9): 313

Avery, R. J. and J. M. Tailyour (1960). The isolation of the rabies virus from insectivorous bats in British Columbia. *Can. J. Comp. Med. Vet. Sci.* 24: 145

Baer, G. M. and J. S. Smith (1991). Rabies in Nonhematophagous Bats. In G. M. Baer (ed.) *The Natural History of Rabies.* 2nd Edition. CRC Press, Inc. Boca Raton, Florida.

Beauregard, M. (1969). Bat rabies in Canada 1963-1967. *Can. J. Comp. Med.* 33: 220

Beauregard, M. and R. C. Stewart (1964). Bat rabies in Ontario. *Can. J. Comp. Med. Vet. Sci.* 28: 43

Bradley, J. A. (1979) Laboratory diagnosis of rabies in western Canada (1968-1977). *Can. Vet. J.* 20: 186

Casey, A., Webster, A., and K. Charlton (1989). Cross-Canada Disease Report—Eastern Canada. *Can. Vet. J.* 30: 522

Copeland, L., Gregory, D., and A. Webster (1985). Rabid beaver incident—British Columbia. *Can. Dis. Wkly. Rept.* 11(51): 214

Dempster, G., Grodums, E. I., Bayatpour, M., and A. Zbitnew (1972). A human case of unsuspected rabies in Saskatchewan diagnosed by virus isolation. *Can. J. Pub. Hlth.* 63: 215

Dolman, C. L. and K. M. Charlton (1987). Massive necrosis of the brain in rabies. *Can. J. Neurol. Sci.* 14: 162

Dorward, W. J., Schowalter, D. B., and J. R. Gunson (1977). Preliminary studies of bat rabies in Alberta. *Can. Vet. J.* 18(12): 341

Fredrickson, L. E. and L. Thomas (1965). Relationship of fox rabies to caves. *Pub. Hlth Repts.* 80(6): 495

Gregory, D. J. (1985). Rabies in Canada, 1984. *Rabies Bulletin Europe.* Information Surveillance Research. WHO Collaborating Centre for Rabies Surveillance and Research, Tubingen, Federal Republic of Germany. 1: 10

Gunson, J. R. and D. B. Schowalter (1974). Rabies-Related Studies of Wildlife in Alberta. *Regional Sylvatic Rabies Conference.* Billings, Montana. September 17, 1974

Hill, J. E. and J. D. Smith (1984). *Bats—A Natural History.* British Museum of Natural History. London.

King, D. B., Sangalang, V. E., Manuel, R., and T. Marrie (1978). A suspected case of human rabies—Nova Scotia. *Can. Dis. Wkly. Rept.* 4(13): 49

Loewen, K. (1993). Animal Diseases Research Institute. Lethbridge, Alberta. Personal communication.

Loewen, K. and B. Prins (1988). Rabies diagnoses January 1 - June 30, 1987. Western Canada. *Can. Vet. J.* 29: 173

McLean, R. G. (1970). Wildlife rabies in the United States: Recent history and current concepts. *J. Wildl. Dis.* 6: 229

McLean, A. E., Noble, M. A., Black, W. A., and W. A. Kettyls (1985). A human case of rabies—British Columbia. *Can. Dis. Wkly. Rept.* 11(51): 213

Prins, B. (1991). Animal Diseases Research Institute. Lethbridge, Alberta. Personal communication.

Prins, B. and K. Loewen (1988). Bat rabies in British Columbia 1971-1985. *Can. Vet. J.* 29: 41

Prins, B. and K. Loewen (1991). Rabies diagnosis in western Canada, 1985-1989. *Can. Vet. J.* 32: 487

Prins, L. and W. D. G. Yates (1986). Rabies in western Canada, 1978-1984. *Can. Vet. J.* 27: 164

Pybus, M. J. (1986). Rabies in insectivorous bats of western Canada, 1979-1983. *J. Wildl. Dis.* 22(3): 307

Rosatte, R. C. (1985). Bat rabies in Alberta 1979-1982. *Can. Vet. J.* 26: 81

Rosatte, R. C. (1987). Bat rabies in Canada: History, epidemiology and prevention. *Can. Vet. J.* 28(12): 754

Rosatte, R. C. and J. R. Gunson (1984). Presence of neutralizing antibodies to rabies virus in striped skunks from areas free of skunk rabies in Alberta. *J. Wildl. Dis.* 20(3): 171

Schowalter, D. B. (1980). Characteristics of bat rabies in Alberta. *Can. J. Comp. Med.* 44: 70

Tabel, H., Corner, A. H., Webster, W. A., and C. A. Casey (1974). History and epizootiology of rabies in Canada. *Can. Vet. J.* 15(10): 271

Varughese, P. V. (1987). Rabies and post-exposure treatment in Canada, 1985. *Can. Dis. Wkly. Rept.* 13(5): 17

Wandeler, A. I. (1992). Head, Rabies Unit. Animal Diseases Research Institute. Nepean, Ontario. Personal communication.

Wandeler, A. I. and G. A. Casey (1993). Rabies diagnosis in eastern Canada, January 1, 1992 - June 30, 1992. Cross-Canada Disease Report. *Can. Vet. J.* 34: 123

Webster, W. A., Casey, G. A., Charlton, K. M., and T. J. Wiktor (1985). Antigenic variants of rabies virus isolates from eastern, central and northern Canada. *Can. J. Comp. Med.* 49: 186

Webster, W. A., Casey, G. A., and K. M. Charlton (1986). Major antigenic groups of rabies virus in Canada determined by anti-nucleocapsid monoclonal antibodies. *Comp. Immun. Microbiol. Infect. Dis.* 9(1): 59

Webster, W. A., Casey, G. A., Charlton, K. M., Sayson, R. C., McLaughlin, B., and M. A. Noble (1987). A case of human rabies in western Canada. *Can. J. Pub. Hlth.* 78: 412

Webster, W. A., Casey, G. A., and K. M. Charlton (1988). Rabies in a squirrel. *Can. Vet. J.* 29(12): 1015

Webster, W. A., Casey, G. A., and K. M. Charlton (1989). Bat-induced rabies in terrestrial mammals in Nova Scotia and Newfoundland. *Can. Vet. J.* 30: 679

Whitney, H. G. (1989). Cross-Canada Disease Report. Update on rabies—Newfoundland. *Can. Vet. J.* 30: 522

Chapter 18:
HUMAN EXPOSURE TO RABIES VIRUS OF INSECTIVOROUS-BAT ORIGIN

Limitations in the Collection of Human Exposure Data

When reported, it is not always easy for public-health authorities to unravel the circumstances surrounding an alleged bat attack. People have, for example, mistaken night-flying birds and even large moths for bats. Bats that pass in close proximity to a person while chasing down insect prey have been mistakenly thought of as attacking without provocation. Subjective fear may cloud an individual's impression of a bat "attack" and subsequent reflection may appreciably alter perception of the incident. Although most confirmed bites from insectivorous bats have been provoked in some manner, outright aggression and unprovoked attacks by rabid bats on humans have been documented. Most incidents of apparently unprovoked attacks have involved solitary species.

In the absence of substantiating physical evidence (e.g., a bite wound, a captured bat, or a witness to an alleged exposure), it is impossible for medical authorities to authenticate the account of an individual claiming to have been bitten by a bat. Tuttle and Kern (1981) have voiced concern regarding the validity of many such reports.

Even in cases in which human interaction with a bat can be documented, establishing the fact that a significant exposure (requiring post-exposure rabies prophylaxis) occurred may still remain difficult. As such, post-exposure rabies prophylaxis may or may not be recommended and the incident may or may not be recorded as a bat attack. Bat-inflicted attacks on humans (with corroborative evidence) do occur. But, the percentage of all such reports that are genuine attacks/encounters is not really known (Brass, 1993).

On December 15, 1987 a 13-year-old boy died of rabies in California. It was widely reported in the news media that the boy had been bitten by a rabid bat. In fact, there was no history of any animal bite and reports by the news media were completely unfounded. Monoclonal antibody analysis of the viral isolate obtained from the child revealed a reactivity pattern identical to that of rabid terrestrial animals in the area, indicating that a bite by a rabid bat was not responsible (Centers for Disease Control, 1988). Sadly, exaggerated and sometimes highly biased media coverage has heightened public fear of bats (Acha, 1981). Furthermore, irresponsible tabloid journalism continues to elicit strong fear of bats.

Some of the difficulties involved in establishing the incidence of naturally occurring infection in wild bat populations have been discussed (see pages 139). Assorted problems also hamper the collection of human exposure data. It is, therefore, virtually impossible to determine the number of bat/human encounters that occur annually or to precisely clarify their nature (real or imagined, provoked or unprovoked). Some of the difficulties involved include the following:

1) In most states, multiple facilities exist for distribution of the biologicals required for post-exposure rabies prophylaxis. Thus, no centralized source of distribution or record keeping exists. In many of these states, it is not required for physicians or health-care facilities to report either animal bites or administration of post-exposure rabies prophylaxis to the state health department. Therefore, no readily accessible record exists and a substantial amount of pertinent epidemiologic data is lost.

2) Computerized records of whatever information is on file are not always available, making retrieval of pertinent data virtually impossible.

Table 18-1

Human Contact With Bats Submitted for Rabies Testing in New York State, 1985-1991

	1985	1986	1987	1988	1989	1990	1991
Total Number of Bats Submitted	1,184	953	1,312	1,177	1,271	1,782	1,663
Number (%) of Submitted Bats Having Human Contact	125 (10.5)	98 (10.3)	75 (5.7)	95 (8.1)	114 (8.9)	176 (9.9)	216 (12.9)
Number (%) of Rabies-Positive Submissions	43 (3.6)	46 (4.8)	48 (3.7)	38 (3.2)	4 (4.2)	584 (4.7)	79 (4.8)
Number (%) of Rabies-Positive Bats Having Human Contact	8 (18.6)	3 (6.5)	3 (6.3)	8 (21.1)	6 (11.1)	8 (9.5)	12 (15.2)

Data from Trimarchi, C. V. *Rabies Annual Summaries, 1985-1991.* Rabies Laboratory, Wadsworth Center for Laboratories and Research, New York State Department of Health. Albany, New York.

3) Some health departments file case reports only if the animal involved is proven to be rabid by state laboratories. Histories involving nonrabid animals are often discarded.

4) Case histories are often vague and unsubstantiated. The victim's subjective impression of the animal involved and the nature of the encounter are often all that exist. They are of limited value.

5) Many times the animal involved is not recovered or is in a condition that is unsuitable for rabies testing. Thus, there is no laboratory documentation of infection.

Limited Survey Information

Both the New York and Colorado State Departments of Health keep very complete records of animal rabies in their respective states. Emerson (1986) and Pape (1992) reported that between 1983 and 1991, 74 persons received post-exposure rabies prophylaxis in Colorado following contact with a bat. In 34 of these cases, the bat was unavailable for testing; in 30 cases, the captured bat was positive for rabies; in four cases, the test results were equivocal or the specimen not testable; in two cases, the person was bitten by a cat that had bitten a bat (in one case, the bat escaped and, in the other, it was found to be positive for rabies); and in four cases, a report of the incident was not available. In 1981 and 1982, 32 persons in Colorado received post-exposure rabies prophylaxis following alleged bat exposure. Information surrounding the circumstances of these exposures was not available.

Between 1985 and 1991, 9.6% of all bats submitted to the New York State Department of Health and 12% of those confirmed rabies positive had reportedly interacted with a human (Table 18-1). In Arizona, 5.6% of 480 suspect submissions and 22.3% of 121 confirmed rabid bats between January, 1988 and September, 1993 reportedly interacted with a human (Levy, 1993). Two (of 27) of these human exposures were unconfirmed.

In a 20-state survey conducted between 1980 and 1981, Helmick (1983) reported that 9.8% (555 of 5,654) of persons who received post-exposure rabies prophylaxis sought treatment because of exposure to a bat (see Table 3-1). Of states reporting human post-exposure rabies prophylaxis following alleged encounters with bats alone, Idaho reported 37 cases; New Hampshire, 40; New Jersey, 57; Oregon, 38; Rhode Island, 13; Utah, 45; and Washington, 104.

In Georgia, Montana, and New Jersey, the state health departments, rather than local health-care facilities, had distributed needed rabies vaccine and immunoglobulin for a time (Centers for Disease Control, 1985, 1986). For a short period of time these states maintained excellent records of post-exposure rabies prophylaxis. Accordingly, the number of persons treated for an alleged exposure to a bat in 1985 were 16, 9, and 35 in Georgia, Montana, and New Jersey, respectively. Beyond an actual count of the number of cases of post-exposure rabies prophylaxis, however, these numbers have only limited meaning, since additional information concerning the epidemiologic circumstances surrounding these and many other such encounters are not readily available.

In western Canada, human involvement was reported in 12% of rabies-positive and 9% of rabies-negative bats submitted for testing between 1968 and 1989.

Common Circumstances of Human Exposure

The highest incidence of bat bites occurs in persons who pick up sick or injured animals. While usually not actively aggressive (and often too weak to even be capable of aggression), these animals may bite in self-defense when handled. Both the curious passerby and the Good Samaritan risk exposure to bite when handling grounded animals (Girard et al, 1965; Baer and Adams, 1970; Bigler et al, 1975; Prather et al, 1975; Constantine, 1966, 1967; Trimarchi and Debbie, 1980; Haagsma, 1989). Fallen and partially paralyzed bats found by people or easily captured by cats, dogs, or other animals, may bite in self-defense and transmit virus as readily as might an overtly aggressive individual. All persons, children in particular, should be warned against handling such bats. Even toddlers have been bitten by grounded rabies-positive bats when parental attention has momentarily lapsed. According to Tuttle (1988), hoary bats are the most likely of American species to bite when grounded. Rabies infection may significantly alter the disposition of any grounded individual.

Human exposure may also follow from occasional encounters with bats that have found their way into homes. Constantine (1988) suggested that bats brought home by cats and released in the home may subsequently wander onto beds, biting persons who roll onto them at night.[1] Least common are reports of unprovoked aggression in rabid bats.

Bat/Human Exposure Histories

Despite the generalized lack of human exposure statistics, many exposure profiles have been recorded nationwide. Some typical examples, culled from the literature and from state health department records, follow. Please note the difficulties that medical authorities would have in substantiating some of these accounts or in determining their exact nature. Medical histories of confirmed human deaths due to rabies of bat origin are reported in Chapter 19.

The Colorado State Health Department (Emerson, 1986; Pape, 1992) reported the following case histories (summarized with permission). The large number of case reports from Colorado is not reflective of a hazardous environment. Rather, it reflects the excellent record keeping of the Colorado State Health Department.

1) On September 9, 1990, an 11-year-old girl noticed the family cat carrying what she believed was a bird in its mouth. She tried to "rescue" the bird, which was actually a bat. She was bitten on the finger. The bat was captured and found to be positive for rabies. Post-exposure rabies prophylaxis was administered.

2) At around 8:00 p.m on the evening of September 2, 1990, a man was barbecuing at his home when a bat flew out of the bushes and landed on his left arm. It bit him several times, leaving multiple puncture wounds. He shook the bat off, but it flew at him again. It then flew away. It was not recovered. Post-exposure rabies prophylaxis was administered.

3) A 41-year-old man, vacationing at a mountain resort, was cycling at about 1:30 p.m. on August 19, 1990. During a rest, a bat flew out of some bushes and landed on him. He knocked the bat to the ground, but it flew up at him again. He brushed it off again and began riding away.

---

[1]If not previously vaccinated, pets believed to have been bitten by any rabid animal must be either destroyed or held in extensive quarantine. Adequately immunized animals should receive a booster immunization and may require a period of quarantine as well (National Association of State Public Health Veterinarians, 1992, 1993, 1994).

The bat flew after him, landing on him yet again. The man grabbed the bat and killed it. It was subsequently confirmed as rabid. He did not recall being bitten and no lacerations or puncture wounds could be found. Post-exposure rabies prophylaxis was, nonetheless, recommended.

4) On the afternoon of August 5, 1990, a seven-year-old girl was playing in her backyard when a bat apparently became entangled in her hair.[2] She brushed it off, throwing it to the ground. It flew back onto her head. Her mother killed the bat and discarded it. It was subsequently retrieved and refrigerated. The bat was found to be positive for rabies. No evidence of a bite wound could be found and the girl did not report feeling a bite at the time. The physical examination, however occurred four days after the encounter and so post-exposure rabies prophylaxis was initiated.

5) At around 11:00 a.m. on July 11, 1989, a four-year-old boy was playing outside with friends when they heard a hissing and squeaking sound from a nearby tree. A bat was found in the tree. The children were told to back away by one of the adults present, but before they did, the bat flew out of the tree and landed on the boy. It bit him several times on the neck and flew away. The following day, the groundskeeper found a bat about 100 feet from the tree. The bat was squeaking loudly, but unable to fly. It was found to be rabies positive and post-exposure rabies prophylaxis was administered.

6) On May 15, 1989, a three-year-old girl found a bat flopping around on the ground. While she and other family members were watching the animal, it suddenly flew up and "struck" the girl in the face. It then flew away. The girl was bleeding from a small cut at the corner of her mouth. The risk of rabies transmission was considered small, but post-exposure rabies prophylaxis was administered.

7) On August 25, 1988, a 68-year-old man observed a bat flying around the porch of his home in the afternoon. When he stepped outside, the bat alighted on his shirt. He was unable to get the bat off and eventually took his shirt off. The bat was stepped on and killed. The man's wife noted some blood on his chin and four small puncture wounds were observed when the blood cleaned away. The bat was positive for rabies and post-exposure rabies prophylaxis was administered.

8) In mid-August, 1987, a woman reported that her 22-year-old boyfriend had fallen asleep on the porch of her home. Later in the evening, he awoke screaming and exclaimed that something had bitten him on the inner thigh. The blanket was tossed aside. In the morning, they found a bat in the blanket. It was alive and hissing, but apparently unable to fly. The bat was found to be rabies positive and post-exposure rabies prophylaxis was begun.

9) On July 7, 1987, a five-year-old boy told his mother that he had located a dead bird in the back yard. The mother picked the animal up and realized it was a bat. The boy indicated that he had handled the bat and, although reportedly not bitten, he did have a two-day-old cut on one hand. The bat was found to be positive for rabies and, despite a low probability of infection, post-exposure rabies prophylaxis was administered.

10) On the morning of June 3, 1987, a 47-year-old woman reported that an animal, which she thought was a bird, flew into her home through the open front door. It landed behind a curtain. She captured the animal in both hands and was bitten on her left hand. She then realized it was a bat and dropped it. The animal flew out the door. Post-exposure rabies prophylaxis was administered.

11) In August of 1986, a 24-year-old woman on a camping trip stepped out of her cabin and instantly felt a furry object on her face. She realized it was a bat and brushed it off, but it flew

[2]The threat of bats becoming entangled in one's hair is a common myth, but one with little basis in fact. It probably arose from the occasional reports of interactions with rabid bats as indicated above, and from periodic situations in which bats may fly very close to a person's head. One of these occasions occurs when a bat is flying indoors. As it approaches a wall, it slows down and turns to avoid a collision. As it does so, it will stall in flight and gain airspeed by diving towards the center of the room (where a frightened person is often standing). The second situation in which bats appear to fly at a person's hair is when they are chasing insects that happen to be very close to an individual, such as a swarm of mosquitos. There is no evidence to support the belief that healthy bats will deliberately seek out a person's hair.

directly towards her again. It landed on her coat. She brushed it off again, whereupon it flew into the cabin and crashed into a wall. It was captured and sent to the state health department for testing. The woman had lacerations on her lower lip and chin. The wound on her lip bled very slightly. The bat was found to be positive for rabies and post-exposure rabies prophylaxis was begun.

12) On the evening of June 3, 1986, a 35-year-old woman was awakened when her cat jumped up onto the bed. She apparently attempted to push the cat off the bed and felt a sharp pain in her left arm. When she got up, she found a bat on the floor, which the cat grabbed and ran away with. Two small puncture wounds were present on her forearm. The bat was not recovered. Post-exposure rabies prophylaxis was administered.

13) On a Friday evening in October of 1985, a young man was fishing at a local reservoir. A bat apparently alighted and clung to his shoulder and when he reached to brush it away, it may have bitten his right index finger. He suffered a small bleeding laceration. The bat escaped. Post-exposure rabies prophylaxis was administered.

14) A young woman was bitten in the perineal region by a bat on the evening of September 12, 1985. She discovered the bat wrapped in a blanket on her bed. The bat was recovered and found to be rabid. Post-exposure rabies prophylaxis was administered.

15) In August of 1985, a woman reported that her cat had brought a live bat home. Her husband separated the bat from the cat but, in the process, the cat turned and bit her on the back of the hand, causing at least one puncture wound. At that time, the patient did not seek medical treatment nor did she adequately clean the wound. The bat was thrown into the alley and disappeared. The secondary transmission of rabies virus by the bite of an animal which had mouth contact with a potentially rabid animal was considered a possibility. Post-exposure rabies prophylaxis was administered. The cat, which had been adequately immunized against rabies, was revaccinated and retained by the owner.

16) On August 8, 1985, a 25-year-old man caught a bat and, in the process of handling it, was bitten several times on the finger and thumb. The bat was subsequently recovered and found to be rabid. Post-exposure rabies prophylaxis was administered.

17) On July 18, 1985, an Animal Control Officer was exterminating bats at the town's City Hall. He had already shot five bats with a .38 caliber pistol loaded with rubber bullets when a bat he had not seen flew down from its roost. He threw up his arms in defense and was struck by the bat, resulting in a 4 cm scratch on his left forearm. Although the wound did break the skin, it was superficial and bled sparingly. The attacking bat was dispatched with a rubber bullet. The examining physician recommended post-exposure rabies prophylaxis, but delayed treatment until the bat was tested. Although the probability of viral transmission was thought to be low, the possibility could not be ruled out. Post-exposure rabies prophylaxis was administered.

18) A nine-year-old boy awoke screaming early on the morning of June 7, 1985 with a bat attached to his right thumb. His mother took him into the bathroom and shook the bat off into the sink. A physician observed two puncture wounds, one of which was slightly lacerated, and which reportedly bled sparingly. The bat was recovered and found to be rabid. Post-exposure rabies prophylaxis was administered.

19) Early Sunday morning, May 26, 1985, a woman was awakened by a very sharp pain in her right hand. She saw what she believed to be a bat flying in the room. The woman captured the animal in a towel and, believing it to be smothered, placed the towel outside. Nothing was found in the towel when it was examined later. A relative took her to the local emergency room, where she was treated for superficial puncture wounds and scratches to her middle finger. Post-exposure rabies prophylaxis was administered.

20) A 44-year-old man was camping on Saturday, May 4, 1985 at an altitude of about 9,000 feet. He heard something falling through a tree above him and felt a "fluttering" on his face. When he brushed at it, he discovered that his cheek was bleeding. This occurred in darkness and he had not been able to identify the source, although he claimed he heard a squeaking sound at the time. He did not report feeling pain. He

did note numerous bats flying in the area during the evening. A physician found several superficial scratches on the patient's face. The health department considered the possibility of a bat encounter to be remote. Nevertheless, the patient was apprehensive and believed that he had encountered a bat. Because this possibility could not be completely ruled out, the decision was made to administer post-exposure rabies prophylaxis.[3]

21) On October 11, 1984, a 13-year-old girl was bitten by the family cat. Apparently, the cat had captured a bat and bitten the girl on the arm when she tried to take it away. The bat was found to be rabid. Because of the possibility of mechanical transfer of virus, post-exposure rabies prophylaxis was administered.

22) A 30-year-old woman reported that during the course of a drive, a bat flew into the window of her rental truck. It went down the back of her shirt and inflicted several scratches on her back before she got her shirt off. The bat was taken, confined in her shirt, to a local veterinarian, who put it in a plastic bag with chloroform. The bat was found to be rabid by the health department and post-exposure rabies prophylaxis was administered.

23) An eight-year-old girl was bitten by something, possibly a bat, on the evening of August 25, 1984. As she emerged from the family car, a small living creature reportedly dropped on her head and fell down the back of her shirt, inflicting minor scratches and possible puncture wounds on her neck and back. The creature dropped out of her shirt and disappeared. Neither she nor her parents saw it. They had observed bats flying in the area and believed that the animal in question was a bat. Her parents observed no blood from the scratches or punctures. The examining physician reported two small papules about half an inch apart on the child's back, which could have been puncture wounds. Based on the report and physical examination, the health department could not rule out the possibility that a bat had been involved, even though they thought it unlikely. Post-exposure rabies prophylaxis was administered.

24) While making deliveries, a 17-year-old girl found a bat. She stepped on it to kill it and then proceeded to remove its viscera in the hope of keeping the dried bat in her room. It was assumed that she had considerable contact with liquid secretions from the bat in the process. A break in the skin was noted on one hand. No brain tissue was available for rabies testing. Post-exposure rabies prophylaxis was administered.

25) On Tuesday, July 3, 1984, an 18-year-old girl, asleep in her bed, felt a fluttering on her leg and a sensation of localized pain. She struck at the cause. Upon entering the room, her father observed a bat on the curtain. Both assumed that the bat was associated with the leg wound. The animal was thrown outside and it disappeared. The physician who examined the girl reported a small healed puncture wound that could have been a bat bite. Post-exposure rabies prophylaxis was administered.

26) At 3:00 a.m., on Friday, June 22, 1984, a 40-year-old man was bitten on the back of his neck by a bat. The bat was apparently in the patient's bed. The man felt a pain in his neck when he rolled over onto the bat. He struck at the animal, which was clinging momentarily, and apparently killed it. The dead bat was brought in for testing by his sister, who said she had noted minor bleeding from the wound. The patient apparently refused to consult with a physician until the rabies status of the bat was ascertained. The bat was found to be rabid and post-exposure rabies prophylaxis was administered.

27) At 4:00 p.m. on June 14, 1984, a young man fishing on a river noted a bat flying around. The bat settled on the end of his fishing pole and he struck it with his hand to knock it off. When he did, he felt a sharp pain near his right thumb. He apparently killed the bat with the blow and, after washing his hand in the river, noted that a small amount of blood was seeping from a slight puncture. The bat was recovered and found to be rabid. Post-exposure rabies prophylaxis was ad-

[3]Tuttle (unpublished observations reported by Tuttle and Kern, 1981) reported "several instances in which bats were blamed for attacks by resting screech owls. Many reported attacks [also] resulted from panicked people scratching themselves while attempting to 'escape' a bat that merely flew past."

ministered.

28) On June 8, 1984, a man observed a bat in a hardware store and caught it in his bare hands. He was bitten on the right thumb. He took the bat home and left it in a tree in his backyard. On June 12, his wife noted that it had fallen to the ground, dead. Local animal control officials retrieved it and submitted it to the local health department. The bat was identified as a big brown bat and was found to be rabid. Post-exposure rabies prophylaxis was administered.

29) On June 2, 1984, a woman reportedly found her cat playing with a bat. She picked up the bat from the cat and put it in the trash can. In the process, the bat bit her on the ring finger of her right hand, causing a puncture wound. She later opened the trash can lid and the bat flew away. Because of the potential transmission of virus, post-exposure rabies prophylaxis was administered.

30) On May 24, 1984, a 50-year-old man was bitten on the finger by a bat which he observed floating on the surface of a lake where he was fishing. Thinking that the animal was a bird, he had apparently reached to pick it up, at which time he was bitten. Fortunately, he retained the incapacitated bat and placed it in a plastic bag. The specimen was subsequently identified as a red bat and was found to be rabid. Post-exposure rabies prophylaxis was administered.

31) A young married couple were awakened at about 2:00 a.m. while sleeping at a ranch. They found a bat on the sheet beneath which they were sleeping. After the bat had been killed, the couple went to the emergency room of the local hospital. They reported no bites, but this was not verified by physical examination. The bat was submitted for testing and the people left the state to return to their home in Texas. The bat was found to be rabid and the people contacted. Post-exposure rabies prophylaxis was administered.

32) A 17-year-old boy claimed that a bat swooped down on him at about 11:30 p.m. on Thursday, October, 27. When he raised his arms to fend it off, he was bitten on the left index finger. He shook the bat off and it disappeared. The examining physician reported four puncture wounds on the boy's fingertip. Post-exposure rabies prophylaxis was administered.

33) A young woman was apparently bitten near her right thumb by a big brown bat as she reached into an old paint can. The bat was recovered and found to be rabid. Post-exposure rabies prophylaxis was administered.

34) On July 29, 1983, a young woman was bitten on the index finger of her right hand by a bat she was trying to separate from her cat. The cat may also have been bitten. The bat was found to be rabid and post-exposure rabies prophylaxis was administered.

35) Around dusk on May 10, 1983, an 11-year-old girl was walking in an alley near her home. She reported that a bat flew down and bit her on the left upper arm and then flew off. The examining physician reported a puncture wound with a V-shaped flap of torn skin. Post-exposure rabies prophylaxis was administered.

36) On Monday afternoon, May 9, 1983, a woman was working in her yard when a bat alighted on her gloved hand. She was wearing heavy cotton gloves at the time. It apparently bit through an index finger of the glove, causing an imprint on her finger, but no visible break in the skin. The bat was killed in the yard and subsequently identified as a big brown bat. It was found to be rabid. Since the possibility of exposure to virus could not be ruled out with certainty, post-exposure rabies prophylaxis was administered.

Chabala et al (1991) reported the first case of a pregnant woman who received post-exposure rabies prophylaxis with HRIG and human diploid rabies vaccine.

37) A 27-year-old woman, in her 14th week of pregnancy, was bitten by a bat that she had found in a tree and prodded into a cage using a stick. She was bitten on the tip of her left index finger while attempting to feed the animal. Physical examination by the emergency-room physician revealed three small puncture wounds on the tip of her finger. The wound was cleaned and post-exposure rabies prophylaxis begun. Three days after initiation of treatment, the Lansing (Michigan) Department of Health reported that the bat was rabies positive. Although the child was born with a transposition of the great

vessels, the infant did well and the mother remained in good health after 11 months of follow-up (Chabala et al, 1991).

Several studies have documented the value of post-exposure rabies prophylaxis in pregnant women (Cates, Jr., 1974; Spence et al, 1975; Varner et al, 1982; Chutivongse and Wilde, 1989; Chabala et al, 1991). If exposed to a rabid animal, pregnancy should not be a contraindication to treatment.

The Arizona Department of Health Services reported the following incidents:

38) On September 7, 1991, a pet cat captured and played with a grounded bat. The cat brought the chewed-up bat home. It was found in the hands of the family's ten-month-old baby. It may have been in the child's mouth. The bat was confirmed rabies positive and post-exposure rabies prophylaxis recommended. The cat had not been immunized against rabies and was euthanatized at the owner's request (Levy, 1991).

39) On October 8, 1991, a bat flew into a boarding-school dormitory through an open door. A boy was bitten when he attempted to pick the bat up. The bat was confirmed as rabid and post-exposure rabies prophylaxis was initiated (Levy, 1991).

40) Two people were bitten by a bat that flew into their hotel room. The guests were bitten as they attempted to swat and/or capture the bat. The State Health Laboratory determined that the bat was not rabid (Levy, 1991).

41) A man was bitten when he poked at a sick bat with a stick. The bat reportedly flew up at the man, who lost his balance and fell on top of the bat. The man was bitten on the arm (Doll et al, 1989).

Hoff et al (1993) reported the following incidence in Kansas City, Missouri:

42) In September of 1990, a woman was awakened by a bat landing on her chest. She sustained a wound when she swatted the bat, caused either by a bite or by the bat's teeth being driven into her skin when it was hit. Post-exposure rabies prophylaxis was administered. The bat was found to be rabid. The residence had numerous openings through which bats could gain access and bat-related problems had been reported previously by tenants in the apartment directly above. The health department ordered the building's owner to bat-proof the premises.

43) In May of 1989, a bat that apparently flew into a darkened home through an open door was swatted by a man as it flew past him. The bat returned and bit him on the face. Post-exposure rabies prophylaxis was administered. The bat was found to be rabid.

Schnurrenberger et al (1964) reported the following incidents recorded by the Ohio State Department of Health:

44) At 4:00 p.m. on July 2, 1957, an 11-year-old girl found her cat playing with a bat. She tried to pick the bat up and was bitten. The bite broke the skin, but the wound did not bleed. The bat died two days later and was found to be negative for rabies. It was not identified.

45) On July 7, 1957, a bat was noted to be flying repeatedly over a crowded swimming pool at around 1:00 p.m. It was knocked into the water and then bit a 42-year-old man, causing a bleeding wound. He had to shake his hand to dislodge the bat. The bat was destroyed. It was neither identified nor tested for rabies. Post-exposure rabies prophylaxis was administered.

46) At 4:00 p.m. on July 10, 1957, a four-year-old boy and his slightly younger sister were playing in their backyard when a "red baby bird" flew down, bit the girl once on the arm, and then flew away. Two bleeding wounds, slightly smaller than a pinhead, were observed. Post-exposure rabies prophylaxis was administered.

McChesney et al (1983) described the following typical histories reported to the Arkansas Health Department:

47) A bat landed on my shoulder and bit me when I tried to brush it off.

48) I didn't see the bat roosting in the tree. It bit me as I reached up to pick an apple.

49) The family cat brought a live bat home, which bit my son as he tried to take it away.

50) A neighbor's child captured a bat and

brought it to school. It may have bitten my daughter.

---

51) *Bat Research News* (1982) quotes *The Louisville Times* of January, 1982 as reporting that rock n' roll singer Ozzy Osbourne had been treated for a possible case of rabies after biting the head off a bat during a concert in Des Moines, Iowa. Osbourne has a reputation for sticking birds and other things into his mouth during performances.

52) On December 28, 1983, 11 children in Corpus Christi, Texas found 29 dead Mexican free-tailed bats beneath a bridge. The bats had succumbed to very cold weather and fallen from their roosts. The children, aged 4 to 14 years, found the bats partially thawed. Many bats had blood oozing from their mouths. Some of the children placed the bats in their own mouths, in imitation of a popular singer (see case #51) and in a free-for-all, they threw the carcasses at one another. Due to the possibility of mucous-membrane exposure to infectious secretions, the children were treated with post-exposure rabies prophylaxis. The incident was reported in the news media and another group of children that had played with dead bats was identified. These children were also treated for possible rabies exposure (Buttery et al, 1984).

53) According to Allanach (1981), a 41-year-old telephone-company repairman was attacked by a bat in New Brunswick, Canada, while opening the door of a telephone tower. He was bitten on the right hand, drawing blood. The bat attacked twice and was killed the second time. The Department of Agriculture confirmed that the bat was rabid and post-exposure rabies prophylaxis was initiated.

54) Near midnight on October 4, 1976, a fringed myotis (*Myotis thysanodes*) landed on a man's face just outside his home in California. The bat hung from the man's upper lip. He brushed it off and killed it. The bat was found to be rabid (Constantine et al, 1979).

55) A rabid yellow bat was picked up off the ground by a man in California on the morning of July 27, 1976. The bat bit him (Constantine et al, 1979).

56) On March 7, 1973, at 10:00 a.m., a rabid yellow bat (*Lasiurus ega*) landed on the bare foot of a woman hiking in California. The bat punctured her big toe. Authorities were not certain if this was due to a bite wound or to a claw puncture (Constantine et al, 1979).

57) While a young boy was running alongside some shrubbery in California, a rabid yellow bat "fell" onto his back. No bites or scratches were noted (Constantine et al, 1979).

58) Baer (1975) reported the case of a man asleep on an outside hammock in Ohio during the afternoon of August 2, 1965. He was awakened by the sudden appearance of a big brown bat clinging to his face. The bat was diagnosed as rabid.

59) On October 19, 1963, in Ohio, a lethargic big brown bat was found on a boy's pillow. His window had been left open during the evening. The child had scratches on his face. The bat was recovered and diagnosed as rabid (Baer, 1975).

60) A rabid hoary bat circled playing children at midday in New Mexico (Constantine 1967). It landed on a girl's back and bit her clothing.

61) A rabid hoary bat in California swooped down from a tree, bit a child on the back, fell to the ground and died (Constantine, 1967). Constantine also reported a similar incident that involved a big brown bat.

62) Wiseman et al (1962) reported that a rabid red bat had either fallen or been thrown into a swimming pool in Austin, Texas. A girl was bitten by the bat as she attempted to push it aside.

63) On August 27, 1961, a man was sitting on the patio of his home in Texas watching a red bat flying overhead. The animal suddenly swooped down and bit him on the forearm. The bat was recovered and found to be rabid (Wiseman et al, 1962)

64) Lou and Wenner (1962) reported the case of a five-year-old boy who, early in the afternoon of September 23, 1960, was playing in front of his home in Kansas. He hit a ball into a tree and knocked a bat to the ground. The boy kicked the bat, which then bit him on the right ankle. Post-exposure rabies prophylaxis was administered. The bat was subsequently found to be rabid.

65) Dean et al (1960) reported that a fisherman in Arizona was being bothered by a hoary bat that was flying near him during broad daylight. It bit him and was subsequently diagnosed as rabid.

66) On September 7, 1957, a child in Arizona was bitten by a rabid cat. The cat would not release its jaws from the child and was shot by the child's father. Prior to the incident, the cat had been seen daily for several weeks trying to capture a bat roosting on the ceiling of a fruit storage cave. Following the cat bite, the bat could not be found (Maddy et al, 1958; Dean et al, 1960).

67) On November 28, 1953, a man was bitten by a bat in a tavern in Pennsylvania. The bat had been flying around the bar and was repeatedly swatted at by patrons until it was knocked to the ground. The man was bitten on the hand as he investigated the downed animal. The bat was mutilated by those in the bar, and possibly by animals after it was subsequently thrown outside. Sufficient brain material was not available for rabies testing (Martin, 1959).

68) Bell (1959) reported the case of a California myotis that attacked an elk hunter in the mountains of Montana on September 21, 1958. Around noon, on a sunny day, a bat suddenly alighted on the shirt of one of the hunters while he stood in camp. The bat bit at the shirt. The hunter, aware of the potential danger of bat rabies, did not touch the animal. The bat quickly flew away and the campers entered their cabin. Three or four minutes later, the hunters emerged from the cabin and the bat once again landed on the same hunter's shirt and bit at the fabric. The bat was recovered and found to be rabid. Prior to its death, the bat was used in several viral transmission studies. Its bite induced rabies in suckling mice.

In 1967, Bell commented further on this case. He found it interesting that the bat repeatedly landed on the heart region of the same individual, despite the fact that other people were present. Bell believed that some sort of sound was attracting the animal. A number of years after the incident, Bell sought out the victim and auscultated his chest. He found the individual to have an unusually loud heart murmur. Schowalter (1980) also believed that auditory stimuli could play a role in inciting rabid bats to attack. Constantine (1988) suggested that a hyperesthesia to sound may cause annoyance in infected bats, stimulating unprovoked attacks by certain solitary species. There is no evidence, however, to even remotely suggest that persons with heart disease are at increased risk of unprovoked bat attacks.

69) A big brown bat was found on the floor of an unoccupied house in Montana by a young boy. He took the bat home with him to keep as a pet. It died the following day. The bat was subsequently confirmed as rabies positive. He denied being bitten (Bell et al, 1957). This case points out the importance of educating children against handling wild animals. Some of the dangers in keeping wild animal "pets" have been emphasized by the World Health Organization (1978).

1) No rabies vaccine is licensed for use in wildlife.
2) Animals may have been infected with rabies prior to capture.
3) More persons contact an exotic "pet" in captivity than would in the wild.
4) When disease becomes manifest, many persons may be exposed and require post-exposure prophylaxis.
5) People handling "cute and helpless" animals often allow these animals to lick and "kiss" them. Thus, they may be exposed to infectious saliva and not know it.

"Because of the risk of rabies in wild animals (especially raccoons, skunks, coyotes, and foxes), the American Veterinary Medical Association, the National Association of State Public Health Veterinarians, and the Conference of State and Territorial Epidemiologists strongly recommend the enactment of state laws prohibiting the importation, distribution, relocation, or keeping of wild animals and wild animals crossbred to domestic dogs and cats as pets" (National Association of State Public Health Veterinarians, 1992, 1993, 1994). Human exposure to clinically normal, rabies-positive, wild-animal "pets" has occurred and will continue as long as such animals are extracted from the wild (Schneider and Bogel, 1983;

Woodruff et al, 1991; World Health Organization, 1992).

The period of rabies virus shedding in infected wild or exotic animals is unknown. As such, confinement and observation of those animals that bite humans are inappropriate (National Association of State Public Health Veterinarians, 1992, 1993, 1994).

References

Acha, P. N. (1981). *A Review of Rabies Prevention and Control in the Americas 1970 to 1980—Overall status of Rabies.* Joint C.N.E.R. - WHO Scientific Meeting on Animal Rabies. Nancy and Malzeville, France. June 3-5, 1981

Allanach, J. R. (1981). Treatment of rabid-bat bite. *Can. Med. Assoc. J.* 124: 1432

Baer, G. M. (1975). Rabies In Nonhematophagous Bats. In G. M. Baer (ed.) *The Natural History of Rabies.* Vol. II. Academic Press. New York.

Baer, G. M. and D. B. Adams (1970). Rabies in insectivorous bats in the United States, 1953 - 1965. *Pub. Hlth. Repts.* 85(7): 637

Bell, J. F. (1959). Transmission of rabies to laboratory animals by bite of a naturally infected bat. *Science.* 129: 1490

Bell, J. F. (1967) Notes of interest on bats. *Bat Res. News.* 8(2): 18

Bell, J. F., Hadlow, W. J., and W. L. Jellison (1957). A survey of chiropteran rabies in western Montana. *Pub. Hlth. Repts.* 72(1): 16

Bigler, W. J., Hoff, G. L., and E. E. Buff (1975). Chiropteran rabies in Florida: A twenty-year analysis, 1954 to 1973. *Am. J. Trop. Med. Hyg.* 24(2): 347

Brass, D. A. (1993). Insectivorous bats as reservoirs of rabies. *Compen. Cont. Educ. Pract. Vet.* 15(12): 33

Buttery, C. M. G., Rodriguez, R. M., McLerran, G., Villarreal, T., Green, J., Sieber, O., Gustafson, T. L., and C. E. Alexander (1984). Possible rabies exposure from bats—Texas. *MMWR.* 33(26): 375

Cates, W., Jr. (1974). Treatment of rabies exposure during pregnancy. *Obstet. Gynecol.* 44(6): 893

Centers for Disease Control (1985). An epidemiologic study of sylvatic rabies in Texas and New York using monoclonal antibodies. *CDC Rabies Surveillance Report.* U. S. Department of Health and Human Services, Public Health Service.

Centers for Disease Control (1986). Bat rabies—Europe. *MMWR.* 35(26): 430

Centers for Disease Control (1988). Human Rabies—California, 1987. *MMWR.* 37(19): 305

Chabala, S., Williams, M., Amenta, R., and A. F. Ognjan (1991). Confirmed rabies exposure during pregnancy: Treatment with human rabies immune globulin and human diploid cell vaccine. *Am. J. Med.* 91: 423

Chutivongse, S. and H. Wilde (1989). Postexposure rabies vaccination during pregnancy: Experience with 21 patients. *Vaccine.* 7: 546

Constantine, D. G. (1966). Recent Advances in Our Knowledge of Bat Rabies. *International Symposium on Rabies.* Symp. Series Immunobiol. Standard. Vol. I. Karger, Basel. New York. Talloires, 1965

Constantine, D. G. (1967). Bat rabies in the southwestern United States. *Pub. Hlth. Repts.* 82(10): 867

Constantine, D. G. (1988). Health Precautions for Bat Researchers. In T. H. Kunz (ed.) *Ecological and Behavioral Methods for the Study of Bats.* Smithsonian Institution Press. Washington, D. C.

Constantine, D. G., Humphrey, G. L., and T. B. Herbenick (1979). Rabies in *Myotis thysanodes, Lasiurus ega, Euderma maculatum* and *Eumops perotis* in California. *J. Wildl. Dis.* 15: 343

Dean, W. D., Maddy, K. T., Cockrum, E. L., and H. G. Crecelius (1960). Rabies in insectivorous bats of Arizona. *Arizona Med.* 17(2): 69

Doll, J. M., Wright, M. E., and C. Levy (1989). Rabies in Arizona, 1988. Division of Disease Prevention, Vector-Borne and Zoonotic Diseases, Arizona Department of Health Services.

Emerson, J. K. (1986). Chief, Environmental Epidemiology. Colorado Department of Health. Denver, Colorado. Personal communication.

Girard, K. F., Hitchcock, H. B., Edsall, G., and R. A. MacCready (1965). Rabies in bats in southern New England. *New Engl. J. Med.* 272(2): 75

Haagsma, J. (1989). Rabies en vleermuizen: hoe te handelen? *Ned. Tijdschr. Geneeskd.* 133(11): 550. (Rabies in Bats: How should it be treated?) English translation courtesy of Dr. Nathan M. Appel.

Helmick, C. G. (1983). The epidemiology of human rabies postexposure prophylaxis, 1980-1981. *J. Am. Med. Assoc.* 250(15): 1990

Hoff, G. L., Mellon, G. F., Thomas, M. C., and D. H. Giedinghagen (1993). Bats, cats, and rabies in an urban community. *South. Med. J.* 88(10): 1115

Levy, C. (1991). Bat rabies update: Two persons exposed in Yavapai County. Division of Disease Prevention, Vector-Borne and Zoonotic Diseases, Arizona Department of Health Services.

Levy, C. (1993). Epidemiology Specialist. Division of Disease Prevention, Vector-Borne and Zoonotic Diseases, Arizona Department of Health Services. Phoenix, Arizona. Personal communication.

Lou, T. Y. and H. A. Wenner (1962). Bats and rabies. *J. Kansas Med. Soc.* LXIII(VI): 217

The Louisville Times (1982). Rabid for rock 'n roll.

January, 1982. Reprinted in *Bat Res. News* (1982). 23(2): 21

Maddy, K. T., Cockrum, E. L., and H. G. Crecelius (1958). Bat rabies in Arizona. *Arizona Med.* 15(5): 344

Martin, R. L. (1959). A history of chiropteran rabies with special reference to occurrence and importance in the United States. *Wildl. Dis.* (No. 3): 1

McChesney, T. C., Spatz, H., and M. Edelman (1983). Bat rabies in Arkansas. *J. Arkansas Med. Soc.* 80(4): 181

National Association of State Public Health Veterinarians (1992). Compendium of Animal Rabies Control. *J. Am. Vet. Med. Assoc.* 200(2): 145

National Association of State Public Health Veterinarians (1993). Compendium of Animal Rabies Control. *J. Am. Vet. Med. Assoc.* 202(2): 199

National Association of State Public Health Veterinarians (1994). Compendium of Animal Rabies Control. *J. Am. Vet. Med. Assoc.* 204(2): 173

Pape, J. (1992). Colorado Department of Health. Denver, Colorado. Personal communication.

Prather, E. C., Bigler, W. J., Hoff, G. L., and J. A. Tomas (1975). *Rabies in Florida—History, Status, Trends.* Division of Health, Department of Health and Rehabilitative Services, State of Florida. Monograph Series #114. Jacksonville, Florida.

Schneider, L. G. and K. Bogel (1983). The Current Global Situation of Human and Canine Rabies and its Control. *Animal Health in the Americas, 1983.* Proceedings of the III Inter-Agency Meeting, at the Ministerial Level, on Animal Health. Pan American Health Organization. Scientific Publication No. 476, p. 97. Washington, D. C. April 11-14, 1983

Schnurrenberger, P. S., Beck, J. R., and F. Burson (1964). Bat rabies: A discussion of problems existing in Ohio. *Ohio State Med. J.* 60: 361

Schowalter, D. B. (1980). Characteristics of bat rabies in Alberta. *Can. J. Comp. Med.* 44: 70

Spence, M. R., Davidson, D. E., Dill, Jr., G. S., Boonthai, P., and J. W. Sagartz (1975). Rabies exposure during pregnancy. *Am. J. Obstet. Gynecol.* 123: 655

Trimarchi, C. V. and J. G. Debbie (1980). Report on the Northeastern Symposium on Bat Rabies Management. In D. E. Wilson and A. F. Gardner (eds.) *Proceedings of the Fifth International Bat Research Conference.* Texas Tech Press. Lubbock, Texas.

Tuttle, M. D. (1988). *America's Neighborhood Bats.* University of Texas Press. Austin, Texas.

Tuttle, M. D. and S. J. Kern (1981). Bats and Public Health. *Contributions in Biology and Geology.* No. 48. Milwaukee Public Museum.

Varner, M. W., McGuinness, G. A., and R. P. Galask (1982). Rabies vaccination in pregnancy. *Am. J. Obstet. Gynecol.* 143(6): 717

Wiseman, J. S., Davis, B. L., and J. E. Grimes (1962). Rabies infection in the red bat, *Lasiurus borealis borealis* (Muller), in Texas. *J. Mammal.* 43(2): 279

Woodruff, B. R., Jones, J. L., and T. R. Eng (1991). Human exposure to rabies from pet wild raccoons in South Carolina and West Virginia, 1987 through 1988. *Am. J. Pub. Hlth.* 81(10): 1328

World Health Organization (1978). "Pet" wild animals: A health hazard to man. *Rabies Bulletin Europe.* Information Surveillance Research. WHO Collaborating Centre for Rabies Surveillance and Research. Tubingen, Federal Republic of Germany. 4/78

World Health Organization (1991). *World Survey of Rabies 24 (for the year 1988).* World Health Organization, Veterinary Public Health Unit, Division of Communicable Diseases. Geneva, Switzerland. WHO/Rabies/91.202. Unpublished document (reviewed with permission).

World Health Organization (1992). 4.2 Extension of the raccoon rabies epizootic—United States, 1992. New Hampshire. *Rabies Bulletin Europe*, 4th quarter. Information Surveillance Research. WHO Collaborating Centre for Rabies Surveillance and Research. Tubingen, Federal Republic of Germany. 4/92: 15

Chapter 19:
HUMAN RABIES OF INSECTIVOROUS-BAT ORIGIN

Recognizing the Source of Exposure

The source of exposure has not been identified in 30% (41 of 136) of the cases of human rabies diagnosed in the United States between 1950 and 1993 (Fishbein, 1991; Centers for Disease Control, 1991, 1993). Explanations for this include difficulty in obtaining a history because of frequent occurrence of unrecognized exposures, language barriers, and speech impairment or memory loss due to encephalitis. Even without a history of exposure, rabies should be suspected in any patient with encephalitis who has lived in a country where rabies is enzootic in dogs. Eighteen of 55 (33%) cases of human rabies (not necessarily bat induced) reported in the United States between 1960 and 1993 were proven or believed to be acquired outside of the United States or its territories (see Figure 3-1).

In those cases of human rabies in which a characteristic nonterrestrial variant of virus has been isolated, but in which no bat bite has been substantiated, an exposure to a rabid bat is presumed. The possibility of secondary transmission, however unlikely, must always be borne in mind.

Globally, 28 cases of rabies in humans have been attributed to direct or indirect interaction with rabid insectivorous bats. These are shown in Table 19-1 and the medical case histories are discussed in the following section. Among the 20 cases reported from the United States, one involved a woman who developed rabies following a corneal transplant from a rabid donor. Although she died from rabies of nonterrestrial origin, an actual encounter with a bat played no role in the transmission. Her case history, nevertheless, is included and her death is considered to be due to bat rabies. Also included among these cases is that of a six-year-old boy who developed rabies after being bitten by a rabid bat. Despite confirmed clinical rabies, he survived.

Since 1980, 5 of the 7 cases of human rabies in the United States in which bats have been implicated have been attributed to silver-haired bats. These exposures have been very puzzling to researchers and characterization of viral isolates from this species continues.

Outside of the United States, there have been eight reports of human rabies following confirmed bat bite. It is likely, although unsubstantiated, that bat exposure has been responsible for, but unidentified in, other cases of human rabies. Countries that have reported human deaths due to bat rabies include Canada (3), South Africa (1), India (1), Finland (1), and the former Soviet Union (2).

The vast majority of human deaths from bat-induced rabies in Latin America have been due to bites from vampire bats; however, a limited number of cases of human rabies believed to have been due to interaction with nonhematophagous bats have been reported. Unfortunately, an accurate assessment of the number of such cases and information regarding the epidemiologic circumstances surrounding them is unavailable.

Clinical Case Histories: The United States

1) In mid-November, 1993, an 82-year-old man in New Boston, Texas died of an undiagnosed neurological illness. At postmortem, rabies was confirmed as the cause of death. Viral isolates from samples obtained at autopsy were characteristic of those found in silver-haired bats. The source of exposure remains unknown (Neill, 1993; Smith, 1993). Details of this case, as well

Table 19-1

Known Human Rabies Cases Following Exposure to Virus of Insectivorous-Bat Origin

Year	Location	Nature of Exposure	Reference
1951	Texas	Bite	Sulkin and Greve, 1954
1956	Texas	Unknown[1]	Irons et al, 1957
1958	California	Bite	Lennette et al, 1960
1959	Texas/Mexico	Unknown[2]	Irons et al, 1957
1959	Wisconsin	Bite	Centers for Disease Control, 1959
1970	Ohio	Bite[3]	Hattwick et al, 1972
1971	New Jersey	Bite	Goldfield et al, 1971
1973	Kentucky	Bite	Taormino et al, 1974
1976	Maryland	Bite	Centers for Disease Control, 1977
1978	Idaho	Corneal Transplant	Centers for Disease Control, 1981
1978	Oregon	Unknown[4]	Centers for Disease Control, 1981
1979	Oklahoma	Unknown[4]	Kerton et al, 1979
1979	Kentucky	Unknown[4]	Cowherd et al, 1979
1983	Michigan	Unknown[4]	Centers for Disease Control, 1985
1984	Pennsylvania	Unknown[4]	Zeidner et al, 1984
1990	Texas	Bite	Martin et al, 1991
1991	Arkansas	Bite	Gonzales et al, 1991
1991	Georgia	Unknown[4]	Gonzales et al, 1991
1993	New York	Unknown[4]	Smith, 1993
1993	Texas	Unknown[4]	Smith, 1993
1970	Saskatchewan	Bite	Dempster et al, 1972
1977	Nova Scotia	Bite	King et al, 1978
1985	Alberta	Bite or Scratch	McLean et al, 1985
1977	former U.S.S.R.	Bite	Selimov et al, 1986
1985	former U.S.S.R.	Bite	Selimov et al, 1986
1954	India	Bite	Veeraraghavan, 1955
1970	South Africa	Bite	Meredith et al, 1971
1985	Finland	Bite[1,4,5]	Berger, 1986

[1]Worked with bats; [2]Frequented bat caves; [3]Survived the disease; [4]Nonterrestrial (bat) variant of rabies virus isolated; [5]Multiple bat bites documented.

as a medical case history, are not yet available.

2) On July 5, 1993, an 11-year-old girl from Mamakating, New York complained to her parents of difficulty sleeping. The young girl was experiencing pain in her left hand and arm, which extended as far as her shoulder over the course of the next two days. A pediatrician believed the child to have been suffering the aftermath of exercise earlier in the week. A throat culture was taken and amoxicillin prescribed because of bilateral ear effusions. The family then left for a camping trip, but ended it abruptly when the girl became feverish and began hallucinating. She died on July 11 (Altman, 1993; Debbie et al, 1993; Linden, 1993).

On July 9, the girl developed fever and severe muscle spasms of her left arm. Walking was difficult and she was experiencing hallucinations. She was examined at an emergency room on July 10 and noted to have had a fever of 101.1° F, otitis media of the left ear, a nonexudative pharyngitis, and a maculopapular rash on her chest. Focal neurologic or meningeal signs were absent. The throat culture was positive for presumed group A Streptococcus. Recurrent streptococcal pharyngitis and otits media were diagnosed. She was treated with fluids and antibiotics and discharged (Debbie et al, 1993).

After discharge, she stopped drinking and had difficulty swallowing oral secretions. On July, 11, she was taken to an emergency room. At that time, her temperature was 105.3° F. Although no focal neurologic abnormalities were evident on physical examination, results of cerebrospinal fluid analysis led to a diagnosis of viral meningoencephalitis or meningococcal infection. She was treated with ceftriaxone and dexamethasone and admitted to the pediatric intensive care unit of a tertiary-care medical center.

On admission, she was alert and oriented. She was cooperative, but agitated. The patient soon developed respiratory distress, hypertension, and tachycardia. She was placed on a mechanical ventilator. Cardiac arrhythmias developed, leading to irreversible cardiac arrrest.

At autopsy, cerebral edema was observed. Histopathological studies revealed encephalitis and possible Negri bodies. A culture of cerebrospinal fluid obtained on July 11 for rabies virus and tests by the New York State Department of Health for the presence of rabies antibody in serum and cerebrospinal fluid were negative. The fluorescent antibody test for rabies virus was positive and confirmed by the Centers for Disease Control. Fifty-five people who may have had contact with infectious secretions of this patient required post-exposure rabies prophylaxis (Debbie et al, 1993; Trimarchi, 1994).

Genetic analysis of the viral isolate by researchers at the Centers for Disease Control has confirmed a nonterrestrial variant characteristic of that found in silver-haired bats, a solitary species that is not commonly submitted for rabies testing in New York State. A dead bat had been found in the child's home a short time prior to her illness; however, it had been discarded and no history of animal bite could be determined (Smith, 1993). The parents had been unable to make an identification of a silver-haired bat from study skins. The circumstances of the exposure remain unknown. Secondary exposure remains a possibility.

3) On October 2, 1991, a woman from Walker County, Georgia was treated with antibiotics at the local emergency room for symptoms of sore throat, headache, and fever. By October 4, swallowing was difficult and painful and she had a fever of 104° F. She was admitted to the hospital, but her condition progressively worsened until death from cardiac arrest on October 8. Rabies was confirmed as the cause of death. Monoclonal analysis of the viral isolate was consistent with a variant of virus characteristically identified in silver-haired bats. No history of animal exposure came to light, despite extensive questioning of friends and family (Gonzales et al, 1991).

4) On August 17, 1991, a 29-year-old man from Clark County, Arkansas complained of sore throat, headache, and difficulty swallowing. Two days later, his physician noted that he was agitated and tremulous. Pharyngitis was detected and antibiotics were prescribed. At home, he was observed to be fearful, anxious looking, and pacing. Later that evening he was taken to the emergency room, complaining of headache, generalized pruritus, dysphagia, a sensation of gagging, and frequent spitting. He remained agitated and was photophobic. Intubation was required by August 20 because of repeated vomiting. He was obtunded with an intermittently elevated body temperature, as high as 106° F. Three days later he suffered a cardiac arrest and, while attempts at resuscitation were successful, he died two days later.

Samples of brain tissue obtained at postmortem were positive for rabies. Monoclonal analysis of the viral isolate was consistent with a variant characteristic of that found in silver-haired bats. A friend of the victim indicated that she had witnessed a bat landing on the man's mouth early in the previous month. It had been killed and the remains discarded. No bites had been observed on the man's mouth or face, but others reported that he had, in fact, incurred either bites or scratches on both his thumb and chest. The patient had not notified the health department of the incident and the bat had not been made available for testing. Post-exposure rabies prophylaxis was administered to 99 persons (including family members, friends, coworkers, and health-care professionals) who may have had possible exposure to the victim's saliva from various sources, including shared utensils or beverage containers (Gonzales et al, 1991; Anonymous, 1992).

5) On May 30, 1990, a 22-year-old man in Hidalgo County, Texas complained of weakness in his right hand, which progressed to numbness of the entire arm by June 1. Hand pain and intermittent episodes of staring were followed by unresponsiveness on June 2.

He was prescribed for by a physician in Mexico, until his admission to an emergency room in a Texas hospital on the evening of June 2. At that time, he was treated with antibiotics and tetanus toxoid because of a history of puncture wound from a catfish fin sustained earlier in the week. On June 3, he again presented to the emergency room, with evidence of spasms and hyperventilation.

He was discharged after some improvement, but still continued to have episodes of muscle rigidity, breath holding, difficulty in swallowing, and hallucinations. He was admitted into the intensive care unit of a different hospital on the evening of June 3. A tentative diagnosis of either encephalitis or tetanus was made. Signs, at that time, included spasms of the face, mouth, and neck, stuttering of speech, hyperventilation, and a body temperature of 100.1° F. The following morning, he was confused and areflexic. His electroencephalogram (EEG) was abnormal and his body temperature had increased to 107° F.

On June 4, a history of bat bite came to light. He had been bitten on the right index finger in a tavern in Mercedes, Texas on April 13. No medical care had been obtained at that time.

On June 5, the patient became comatose and died. Rabies was confirmed as the cause of death. Monoclonal antibody analysis of virus obtained from postmortem brain tissue revealed a variant of virus characteristic of Mexican free-tailed bats.

On May 22, eight days prior to the development of clinical signs, this patient had donated blood. Although all blood was subsequently destroyed, one person did receive some of his blood products (platelet transfusion). This individual received post-exposure rabies prophylaxis (Martin et al, 1991).

6) On September 14, 1984, a 12-year-old boy from western Pennsylvania developed a runny nose and a sore throat. He became feverish, with chills and drenching sweats. He choked when he tried to eat. On September 17, he was having muscle spasms and difficulty breathing.

He was brought to the emergency room on September 17 in an agitated state and with a body temperature of 103° F. He was sweating profusely and was dehydrated. Generalized hyperreflexia and muscle fasciculations were evident. His pupils were dilated. By the next day, he was unable to swallow fluids and was having cardiac arrhythmias. He sometimes yelled inappropriately and violently, particularly when cool breezes crossed his face. Periods of lucidity alternated with hallucinations and disorientation. On September 20, a skin biopsy confirmed rabies.

By September 23, he was becoming less responsive to commands and was intubated because of profuse foamy salivation and periodic respiratory depression. His condition continued to worsen and he died on September 29. There was no known history of exposure to a rabid animal. Monoclonal antibody analysis of the viral isolate revealed a characteristic nonterrestrial variant of virus (Zeidner et al, 1984; Centers for Disease Control, 1985).

7) The Centers for Disease Control (1985) reported the case of a five-year-old Michigan girl who, on February 7, 1983, was experiencing pain and weakness in her right arm, malaise, anorexia, a sore throat, and pain in her left heel. She was alert and cooperative by February 11, but had tenderness in her right wrist, elbow, shoulder, and left heel. By February 13, she was becoming ir-

ritable and lethargic, had difficulty swallowing, developed progressive right arm weakness, urinary incontinence, hypertension, and a body temperature of 103.9° F. Her EEG was diffusely abnormal.

By February 14, she had become depressed, and required mechanical ventilation for respiratory distress. She was comatose by February 17. On February 23, 1983, the family remembered a possible bat bite in late August of 1982. The girl died on March 9, 1983, 32 days after the onset of clinical signs. Rabies was confirmed as the cause of death. Monoclonal analysis of the viral isolate revealed a characteristic nonterrestrial variant of virus.

8) On November 20, 1979, signs of dizziness, vomiting, profuse perspiration, and an incoordinated gait developed in a 45-year-old man from Frankfort, Kentucky. Over the course of the next two days, difficulty in swallowing, double vision, speech impediment, and spasms in the limbs were also noted. On admission to a local hospital, a diagnosis of tetanus was made. At that time he was alert, with a body temperature of 101.7° F, and having generalized muscle spasms in his extremities. He was treated for tetanus. On November 23, he was transferred to a hospital in Lexington with evidence of mild renal failure and hypotension. Three days later, he became comatose and remained that way until his death on November 30.

On December 6, rabies was confirmed as the cause of death. While still coherent, the patient reported that he was unaware of any exposure to a potentially rabid animal. Family and friends were also unaware of any such exposure (Cowherd et al, 1979). Recently, monoclonal antibody analysis of preserved viral isolates obtained from this patient revealed a reactivity pattern consistent with a nonterrestrial variant of virus (Smith, 1992). The circumstances of exposure remain unknown.

9) On September 15, 1979, a 24-year-old man from northeastern Oklahoma developed insomnia, headache, nausea and vomiting, malaise, myalgia, and a fever of 101° F. This progressed within two days to trembling and intermittent confusion. Hallucinations began to occur. He was then hospitalized and observed to be hyperactive. Impaired speech and facial nerve palsy developed. By the sixth day of illness, generalized seizures began. He became progressively more unresponsive, until death on October 4. Rabies was confirmed as the cause of death. The man worked as a woodcutter. No exposure to a potentially rabid animal was reported (Kerton et al, 1979). Recently, monoclonal antibody analysis of preserved isolates obtained from this patient revealed a reactivity pattern consistent with a nonterrestrial origin (Smith, 1992). The circumstances of exposure remain unknown.

10/11) On October 10, 1978, a 37-year-old woman from Boise, Idaho died of rabies, seven weeks after receiving a corneal transplant. The donor had been a 39-year-old man from Baker, Oregon, who had presumably died of Guillain-Barré syndrome. A virus of nonterrestrial origin was isolated from the donor subsequent to its isolation from the recipient at autopsy (Centers for Disease Control, 1981; Anderson et al, 1984).

On July 28, the donor developed pain in his back. This progressed to weakness in his arms and legs, diplopia, and ataxia. In the hospital, he suffered a cardiopulmonary arrest, became comatose and, on August 20, died. On the following day, one cornea was transplanted into the woman's eye.

Thirty days postoperatively, the recipient developed a progressively worsening retro-orbital headache, facial hyperesthesia, dysphagia, dysarthria, and difficulty walking. This progressed to flaccid paralysis and depression, ultimately culminating in death. Friends and family of both individuals could identify no source of exposure; however, the donor had been a professional lumberman and an avid trapper. Both cases were from areas where the only known reports of rabies since 1963 have been in bats. This was the first known case of rabies following a tissue transplant.

12) On May 10, 1976, a 55-year-old Maryland woman was bitten by a big brown bat on a finger of her left hand. She washed the wound with soap and water. The bat was recovered and

TRANSMISSION OF RABIES BY CORNEAL TRANSPLANT

Since 1978, there have been six fatal cases of human rabies transmitted by corneal transplant (World Health Organization, 1979, 1981, 1982; Gode and Bhide, 1988; O'Day, 1989; Sureau, 1990). The first case was reported from the United States in 1978. The second case to occur was in France (1979). The third and fourth cases (both from the same donor) occurred in Thailand (1981). The fifth and sixth cases (both from the same donor) occurred in India (1987).

In all but one case, rabies was diagnosed retrospectively in the donor only after the onset of clinical signs of rabies in respective recipients. In one case (India, 1987), rabies was diagnosed in the donor prior to the onset of clinical signs in one of two recipients. After rabies was diagnosed in one of the recipients, a course of post-exposure rabies prophylaxis was instituted in the second. However, a full course of post-exposure treatment was refused by the recipient because his transplant seemed to be functioning well. Perhaps if he had continued the treatment, he would have survived. In another case in France (1981), rabies was confirmed in the donor on the day following the corneal transplant. In this instance, post-exposure rabies prophylaxis was administered. The recipient has remained symptom free.

Human-to-human transmission of rabies is rare. These six cases of transmission by corneal transplant are the only well-documented instances known. Helmick et al (1987) reported six other cases between 1600 and 1934, but these were not well documented and occurred in areas in which animal rabies was enzootic. Thus, the possibility of animal bite could not be ruled out. Medical records reveal no instance of human-to-human transmission despite the hospitalization of thousands of rabies victims.

Helmick et al (1987) suggested that viral titers in human saliva may be too low to be effective in transmission. Nevertheless, viral transmission from patients to hospital staff remains a possibility and hospital personnel should take appropriate steps as needed to prevent exposure, including use of goggles, masks, and gloves (Dutta et al, 1992; World Health Organization, 1992). Additionally, it has been recommended that hospital personnel at permanent risk of infection, such as those staffing intensive care units in countries where human rabies cases are common, be pre-exposure immunized (Sureau, 1990).

The Expert Committee on Rabies (World Health Organization, 1992) has recently expressed the view that organs of patients who have died from any neurologic condition should not be used for transplantation. In its revised standards governing screening policy for transplant donors, the Eye Bank Association of America (1993) stated that death from viral encephalitis, from encephalitis of unknown origin, or from any central nervous system disease of unknown origin are absolute contraindications to organ donation.

found to be rabid. Forty-four hours after the bite, she was given human rabies immunoglobulin and started on a prescribed course of 21 doses of duck-embryo vaccine. This was completed on June 2.

Two days prior to completion of the series, the woman developed myoclonic twitching of both arms and of intercostal musculature. On June 4 (five days after development of the myoclonic twitching), she developed a painful paresthesia of her left hand and arm, abdominal pain, and vomiting. On June 7, she was admitted to the intensive care unit of The Medical Center of Delaware, Wilmington with a presumptive diagnosis of postvaccinal disease.

On admission, she was observed to be oriented and apprehensive. Vital signs were normal. Over the course of the next several days, she developed weakness and diminished sensation in her left hand and arm, and a left-sided Babinski sign (which eventually became bilateral). Visual hallucinations of kaleidoscopic designs (Pick's visions) were also noted by the patient. She eventually began talking of having distorted hallucinations, seeing hospital personnel walking through walls (peduncular hallucinosis). The patient carried on conversations with imaginary people and her attitude varied from polite and apologetic to profane, angry, and combative. She salivated profusely, but manifested no evidence of hydrophobia. She had an abnormal nystagmus, pinpoint pupils, anesthesia of the left side of her face, and a flaccid left arm devoid of sensation.

By June 10, she was agitated and felt tightness in her chest. A tracheostomy was performed and the patient was placed on a mechanical respirator, which she remained on until her death. She developed a fever of 101.6° F, with myoclonus in all extremities, and developed grand mal seizures. By June 14, the patient was comatose, demonstrating no response to painful stimuli, no reflexes, hypotension, and markedly abnormal cranial nerve function. By her 16th day in the hospital, a cardiac pacemaker was required to alleviate bradycardia (40 beats/min). Diabetes insipidus developed by the following day, which was unresponsive to pitressin. Four of 11 full-thickness skin biopsies were positive for rabies, five were suspicious, and two were negative. Corneal impression smears were also positive. Antibody titer (RFFIT) increased from 1:50 to 1:1100 during the course of her hospitalization. She died on June 27 from cardiac arrest, 23 days after the onset of signs (Centers for Disease Control, 1977; Nelson and Berry, 1993).

In those cases in which a definitive diagnosis of rabies by serological findings, skin biopsy, or corneal impression is not made, there may be difficulty in distinguishing the early onset of rabies from postvaccinal disease. Postmortem findings in this case (acute rabies encephalomyelitis and coexisting extensive perivenous demyelination) suggested the possibilities of a postvaccinal reaction, direct viral infection, or both. The combination of inflammatory and demyelinating disease is believed to have been responsible for the patient's rapidly changing neurological status (Nelson and Berry, 1993).

13) On September 7, 1973, a 26-year-old Kentucky man developed signs of paresthesia, pain in his ears, headache, sore throat, difficulty swallowing, anorexia, fever, intermittent confusion, and changes in behavior. He was admitted to the hospital drooling saliva, with pharyngeal spasms, spontaneous spasms in his legs and arms, stiffness in his neck, and a fever of 105° F. He developed respiratory arrest on September 14 and was resuscitated and placed on a respirator. By September 17, the patient's pupils were poorly responsive to light. He had intermittent facial paralysis, flaccid extremities, diminished response to pain, and decreased tendon reflexes. On September 22, he died from cardiac arrest (Taormino et al, 1974).

On September 15, his family said that he had been bitten on the right ear one month earlier by a bat while asleep. The bat was not recovered and the patient did not seek medical attention at the time.

14) On September 19, 1971, a 64-year-old man was bitten on the left side of his lower lip by a bat while on the porch of his rural home in Sussex County, New Jersey. The bat was not recovered. A course of duck-embryo vaccine was initiated.

By November 17, he was suffering from severe malaise. By November 19, he had a severe headache and paresthesia of the left face, neck, and shoulder. This progressed to dysphagia and hydrophobia. He was hospitalized on November 23, suffering from disorientation and hallucinations. He died on November 25 (Goldfield et al, 1971; Centers for Disease Control, 1972).

15) On October 10, 1970, a six-year-old boy in Lima, Ohio was bitten on his left thumb by a big brown bat, while asleep in his bed. The bat was believed to have entered the family's living quarters from the attic via an opening in the hall ceiling. The boy's father pulled the bat free and sent it to health-department officials. It was found to be rabid.

The wound was washed with soap and water and a 14-day course of duck-embryo vaccine started. Initial signs were pain in his neck, lethargy, malaise, and anorexia. He was admitted to the hospital on November 4, with a fever of 104° F. During the next ten days, his body temperature decreased, but he became increasingly lethargic.

By November 13, his neck was stiff and he had difficulty walking and writing. The following day he became incontinent, exhibited bizarre behavior, and responded only to repeated requests. He no longer spoke. His left leg, arm, and face became weaker. He was responsive only to deep pain. He developed signs of cardiac arrhythmias and spasms of the left side of his body. Throughout the course of his illness, the child was supported by continuous cardiopulmonary monitoring, prophylactic tracheostomy, and intense pulmonary assistance. He lapsed in and out of coma for a week, but then began to improve.

By November 30, he could sit up in bed and feed himself. He began to speak and walk and then to run by December 29. He was discharged from the hospital on January 27, exhibiting minimal neurological signs.

Although rabies virus was not isolated from the boy, the clinical, laboratory, and epidemiologic findings strongly supported a diagnosis of rabies. Problems in isolating virus after onset of clinical signs of rabies are not unusual. The demonstration of very high titers of rabies-neutralizing antibody was strong evidence of infection. The boy's recovery from the disease was remarkable (Centers for Disease Control, 1971; Hattwick et al, 1972; Carlson and Beran, 1986). Only two other well-documented cases of human recovery from clinical rabies have been reported (see page 35).

16) On August 8, 1959, a 44-year-old Wisconsin farmer was bitten on his right ear lobe by a bat while asleep in his home. The farmer caught the bat and squeezed it to death. The following morning, he threw the bat away. It was eaten by the family cat.

On August 29, symptoms of pain and tingling in his right ear were noted. These spread down his right arm. Subsequently, tremors began in this arm and gradually spread throughout his body. Pharyngeal spasms and delirium followed. He died on September 4. Rabies was confirmed as the cause of death. The cats and dogs on the farm were destroyed without examination (Centers for Disease Control, 1959).

17) On June 1, 1959, a 53-year-old consultant mining engineer was admitted to the Wadsworth Veterans Administration Hospital in Los Angeles, California. His chief complaints were shortness of breath and retching. Between April 9 and May 1, he had been engaged in investigations of Mexican and Texas caves for their guano-mining potential. Two months prior to his death, he had explored several caves in Mexico. A little over a month prior to his death, he had been working in various Texas caves, including Hawkey Cave, Pecos County; Fern Cave, Valverde County; Dunbar Cave, Edwards County; and Frio Cave, Uvalde County. In the course of his explorations, he noted the extraordinary number of bats in Frio Cave. He denied having been bitten by any animal, but a friend reported that he had blood on his face and had presumed this to have been due to a bat bite within Frio cave.

On May 22, nausea, vomiting, and diarrhea developed, lasting two days. While driving to California, he developed tenderness in his left arm and axilla. By May 25, he was short of breath and had retrosternal pain. On May 28, his left arm was tender and the hand numb. He had been admitted to the hospital on June 1 with a presumptive diagnosis of myocardial infarction by the referring physician.

On admission, he was apprehensive, restless, and confused. He retched violently and at frequent intervals, at which times he appeared to have difficulty breathing. His body temperature was 100.2° F. During his hospitalization, he became progressively more confused and disoriented, at times almost wild. Retching and labored breathing became more violent and frequent and could not be controlled. By June 2, his body temperature had increased to 101.6° F and his confusion had deepened. Reflexes were diminished and he began to spit up saliva.

On June 3, his body temperature had increased to 103° F and his blood pressure fell dramatically to 92/0. He died five hours later. Rabies was confirmed as the cause of death (Irons et al, 1957; Humphrey et al, 1960; Kent and Finegold, 1960). It has generally been accepted that this individual was infected by exposure to aerosolized rabies virus (see page 169).

18) On August 2, 1958, a 53-year-old

woman in Magalia Butte County, California was bitten on the middle finger of her left hand by a silver-haired bat. She believed the bat to have had a broken wing and was trying to place it in a tree, out of reach of her dogs. When she telephoned a veterinarian regarding treatment, she was advised to contact the local health department. Because of the Labor Day holiday, she contacted the Butte County Health Department on September 2. The health department confirmed that the bat was rabid.

Post-exposure rabies prophylaxis was administered from September 2 until September 26. On October 24, the woman visited a chiropractor with a complaint of numbness in her arms and fingers and pain in her back. The pain in her back progressed and abdominal pain developed as well. Concerned about the possibility of an intestinal obstruction, the chiropractor urged the woman to seek admission to a hospital, which she did on October 29.

During the course of her hospitalization, the woman experienced urinary incontinence and progressively worsening pain in many parts of her body, worse in her abdomen and down her legs. By the fifth day of her hospitalization, she was unable to feel hypodermic injections, but found wrinkles in the bed sheet discomforting. By the following day, she was unable to swallow mucus, which continuously ran from her mouth. On November 4, 66 days after exposure, the patient died.

The woman's husband knew of no animal exposure other than that of the bat. Two dogs and two cats belonging to the family remained well. This is considered by many to be the first fully documented human death due to bat-inflicted rabies in the United States (Humphrey et al, 1960; Lennette et al, 1960).

19) On January 1, 1956, an entomologist with the Texas State Health Department, was stricken with impaired vision and fitful sleep. The following day, he suffered through two convulsive seizures. In the hospital, he volunteered the information that he was suffering from rabies, but maintained that he had been subjected to no animal bite, bat or otherwise. He died on January 4 and rabies was confirmed as the cause of death (Irons et al, 1957). The patient had been part of the state's rabies investigative team. In the course of his job, he handled thousands of bats. In particular, he worked extensively with Mexican free-tailed bats in Texas caves. Several months prior to his death, he had spent time working with bats in Wilson Cave, Kerr County; Bracken Cave, Comal County; and Frio Cave, Uvalde County. Bracken and Frio Caves harbor two of the largest colonies of Mexican free-tailed bats in the country (Irons et al, 1954). It has generally been accepted that this individual was infected by exposure to aerosolized rabies virus (see page 169).

20) Although the presence of rabies in insectivorous bats was undiagnosed in the United States prior to 1953, the recognition of infection in bats prompted the belief that human exposure may have occurred previously. Sulkin and Greve (1954) reported the case of a 43-year-old woman who, on October 9, 1951, had been bitten on the left forearm arm by a sick bat she had picked up along a road in Parkland County, Texas.

Sixteen days later, she became ill and had pain in the bitten arm. Her body temperature was 103° F. By the following day, nausea, vomiting, and a generalized ache had developed. She was unable to move her left arm. She was treated for influenza, but her condition continued to deteriorate. On October 29, three weeks after the incident, she was admitted to a hospital in west Texas, where she was observed to have an inability to swallow. She was transferred to the Parkland City-County Hospital, Dallas in a comatose condition. A presumptive diagnosis of bulbar poliomyelitis was made. She remained in this condition until her death four days later. Negri bodies were demonstrated in her brain and, although the bat was never made available for examination, a retrospective diagnosis of bat-transmitted rabies was made.

Clinical Case Histories: Canada

1) During July of 1985, a 25-year-old man, working as a cook at a forest service camp in Smith, Alberta, was scratched or bitten on the left cheek by a bat in his tent. The bat had apparently fallen from the top of his tent. The man threw the bat outside and it was gone the following

morning. No post-exposure rabies prophylaxis was administered, local antiseptic being the only treatment received. The man remained at the camp in northern Alberta until the end of August.

After a five-day hiking trip near Nelson, British Columbia, he returned home to Vancouver, where he was a student at the University of British Columbia. On October 24, he began to experience pain in his neck, chest discomfort, profuse sweating, and a general state of malaise. Within a week, he had developed a fever of 104° F. The mere sight of water caused dry heaves and he began having convulsions, characterized by generalized body spasms. He was hospitalized on October 31, presenting with priapism and severe, but painless, muscle spasms in his neck and pharynx.

Fluorescent antibody examination of a brain biopsy was weakly positive for rabies. Rabies virus was isolated from both brain tissue and saliva. Monoclonal analysis of the isolate revealed a reactivity pattern identical to that seen in isolates obtained from insectivorous bats in Saskatchewan, Alberta, and British Columbia.

By November 1, the patient was incoordinated and had right-sided weakness. Rabies immune globulin was administered, but he became comatose. He died on November 26, when artificial life support was discontinued. All household contacts in Vancouver since October 18 and all hospital contacts since October 31 received post-exposure rabies prophylaxis. This was the first case of human rabies diagnosed in British Columbia, although it was actually imported from Alberta (McLean et al, 1985; Dolman and Charlton, 1987; Varughese, 1987; Webster et al, 1987).

2) While trying to remove a bat from his home, a 62-year-old man from Parrsboro, Nova Scotia was bitten on his left hand. Approximately one year later, on August 9, 1977, he was admitted to the Victoria General Hospital in Halifax, with an undiagnosed neurological illness. On admission, he was agitated and unable to perform fine movements with his left arm. Choreiform movements were present. Pain radiated from the fourth and fifth fingers and gradually spread up the arm, following the distribution of the ulnar nerve. Reflexes were not detectable in the affected arm and were exaggerated in the opposite one.

During 35 to 40 hours of hospitalization, the patient became progressively more agitated and disoriented. Violent agitation could not be controlled by sedation. On August 11, he lapsed into a coma and died. Postmortem examination confirmed rabies as the cause of death (King et al, 1978).

3) Early in September of 1970, a 15-year-old boy from Meadow Lake, Saskatchewan came downstairs from his bedroom with a dead bat in his hand. He told his parents that he had smothered it in his bed clothes after it had flown into his face and bitten him. The bat was displayed to friends and neighbors until it decomposed, at which time it was thrown away and the incident forgotten.

On September 22, the boy was admitted to the University Hospital in Saskatoon with fever, pain in his head, neck, and shoulder, and dysphagia. Symptoms quickly worsened until his death on September 29. Three weeks after death, a diagnosis of rabies was confirmed. It was, however, not until six weeks after the boy's death that the full account of the bat bite had been recalled by the boy's parents. This was the first reported human death from rabies of bat origin in Canada (Dempster et al, 1972).

Clinical Case Histories: Africa, Europe, and Asia

1) The only known case of bat-borne human rabies from the African continent was that of a 31-year-old man from Transvaal, South Africa. While asleep at the farm, Tooyskraal, he had been bitten on the lip by a bat, probably the insectivorous Natal clinging bat (*Miniopterus schreibersi natalensis*), one month prior to the onset of clinical signs (Meredith et al, 1971; Tignor et al, 1977; van der Merwe, 1982; World Health Organization, 1984a, 1984b).

The onset of illness commenced with headache, vertigo, and muscle aches in the neck and back. Continuous sweating and involuntary muscle spasms quickly developed, followed by progressive confusion, irritability, and aggressiveness. After three days, a physician was called to the farm. He observed the patient to be in a very agitated state, exhibiting muscle spasms of the neck and back. All reflexes were exaggerated. Mere touch provoked generalized convulsive spasms, most marked about the face, arms, and torso. The patient became wild and aggressive at these times. Attempts at drinking produced spasms of the throat muscles. He was admitted to the H. F. Verwoerd Hospital in Pretoria. The following day, he was reportedly "completely berserk," and forcible restraint was required. He died from respiratory arrest during a seizure less than 24 hours after admission (Meredith et al, 1971).

2) The only reported human death from bat-origin rabies in India occurred in 1954 in Srikakulam District, Andhra State. A 48-year-old railway pointsman was bitten near his wrist by an injured bat that he tried to place in a tree. The bat had been stoned by several boys. Clinical signs began three months later and consisted chiefly of malaise and difficulty in swallowing. His condition rapidly deteriorated and he died on May 24, within four days of the onset of symptoms. The species of bat was not determined, nor was it ever confirmed that the bat was rabid (Veeraraghavan, 1955; Humphrey et al, 1960).

3) On October 9, 1985, a 30-year-old Swiss biologist in Helsinki, Finland was admitted to the emergency ward of Meilahti Hospital in Helsinki with an ascending paralysis resembling the Guillain-Barré syndrome. Pain radiated to his right arm and neck. By the next day, he was having spasms, was hyperventilating, and had become hyperexcitable. Rabies was suspected because of the clinical signs and a history of multiple bat bites. The patient was a bat biologist and he had been bitten repeatedly by bats prior to the onset of clinical signs. He had been bitten 51 days earlier in Finland, one year earlier in Switzerland, and four and a half years earlier in Malaysia. The bat (*Myotis daubentoni*) from southern Finland had been behaving abnormally during a short observation period, but was released prior to onset of clinical signs in the patient. It may have bitten the patient several times. Apart from his trip to Malaysia, he had never been out of Europe, had never been in close contact with bats in other European countries, and had reportedly never sustained any other animal bites. He had never been immunized against rabies.

In late September of 1985, he developed persistent coryzal-like symptoms. Numbness in his right palm and pains in his neck were present by October 6, spreading to his right cheek within two days. By the following day he was unable to walk. On admission to the emergency ward, he was alert and oriented to his surroundings. He complained of generalized weakness, numbness of his right arm and neck, and retrosternal pain. Sensation was diminished in his upper limbs and neck.

Myoclonic twitching of his lower limbs, trismus, and marked agitation were present by October 10. He had inspiratory spasms and difficulty swallowing. He remained conscious and spoke of an overwhelming feeling of fear. Talking or being touched evoked laryngeal spasm. Rabies immunoglobulin and Acyclovir were administered, but his condition progressed to one of delirium, with shouting, muscle spasms, seizures, and respiratory insufficiency. Tracheal intubation was required and general anesthesia was necessary to relieve the muscle spasms. Diabetes insipidus, with associated polyuria, was present by October 12. Abrupt changes in blood pressure were recorded and the patient lapsed into unconsciousness. Neurological examination on October 22 revealed extremely diminished signs of brain stem function and the patient died in asystole on October 29, 1985.

Postmortem viral analysis confirmed the causative agent as being related to Duvenhage virus, but unique from other European bat lyssaviruses that have been found (Berger, 1986; Lumio et al, 1986; Roine et al, 1988; Bussereau et al, 1989; Haltia et al, 1989).

4) On May 8, 1985, an 11-year-old girl from Belgorod (in the former Russian Soviet Federative Socialist Republic) was bitten by a bat on her lower lip while standing on the balcony of an apartment house. The bat was pulled off of her and it escaped. No post-exposure rabies prophylaxis was administered. Evidence of illness developed 21 days later, manifesting as malaise, sleepiness, weakness of the legs, and pain in the

lower lip. During the course of her hospitalization, she developed a high fever, hyperesthesia, anxiety, excitation, ataxia, visual hallucinations, and convulsions. She eventually became comatose. She died six days after the onset of clinical signs and rabies was confirmed as the cause of death (Selimov et al, 1986 [cited by Selimov et al, 1989]; World Health Organization, 1987, 1989 [cited with permission]).

5) On August 16, 1977, a 15-year-old girl from Voroshilovgrad (in the former Ukrainian S.S.R.) was bitten on a finger by a bat. She died about five weeks later and rabies was confirmed as the cause of death (Shcherbak, 1984 [cited by World Health Organization, 1987]; Selimov et al, 1986 [cited by Selimov et al, 1989]).

Public-Health Implications of Rabies in Insectivorous Bats

The prevalence of rabies infection in insectivorous bats is low and investigations have not supported a role of infected bats in initiating wildlife epizootics. On rare occasions, however, they can vector virus to both domestic animals (see Table 16-2) and humans. They must, therefore, be considered of public-health significance, although relatively minor in nature.

The overall impact of bat rabies on human health depends, in large measure, on the general level of public awareness about the nature of the disease in bats. Education remains the single most effective means of minimizing the hazards of bat-induced disease. Although some human interactions with bats are quite unavoidable, simply leaving bats alone will eliminate the majority of potential exposures. The potential impact of bat rabies on public health is considerably lessened by the availability of efficacious treatments to prevent rabies following exposure to virus.

Regrettably, many of the public's perceptions of bats have been founded on sensationalized reporting by irresponsible newspapers and magazines. The relatively minor significance of insectivorous bats as vectors of rabies must always be weighed against their more important associations with human health. In keeping numbers of insect pests in check, bats may help to stem the tide of potentially dangerous arthropod-borne diseases. In the absence of bats, and other such natural checks and balances, these diseases might well engulf humanity in epidemic proportion.

References

Altman, L. K. (1993). A fatal case of rabies, and how it nearly went undetected. *The New York Times*. August 24: C3

Anderson, L. J., Williams, Jr., L. P., Layde, J. B., Dixon, F. R., and W. G. Winkler (1984). Nosocomial rabies: Investigation of contacts of human rabies cases associated with a corneal transplant. *Am. J. Pub. Hlth.* 74: 370

Anonymous (1992). Human rabies in Arkansas. *Vet. Hum. Toxicol.* 34(3): 260

Berger, R. (1986). A human rabies case in Finland possibly of bat origin. *Rabies Bulletin Europe*. Information Surveillance Research. WHO Collaborating Centre for Rabies Surveillance and Research. Tubingen, Federal Republic of Germany. 4: 12

Bussereau, F., Vincent, J., and P. Sureau (1989). Caractérisation d'une souche Finlandaise, d'origine humaine de virus rabique, par des anticorps monoclonaux: anti-virus Mokola. *Rec. Med. Vet.* 164(11): 895

Carlson, T. A. and G. W. Beran (1986). The first well documented case of recovery from clinical rabies in a human being. *Iowa State Univ. Vet.* 48(2): 107

Centers for Disease Control (1959). Human rabies. *MMWR.* 8(38): 2

Centers for Disease Control—Miscellaneous Pathogens Unit (1971). Followup on probable human rabies—Lima, Ohio. *MMWR.* 20(7): 54

Centers for Disease Control (1972). Rabies in the United States. *J. Infect. Dis.* 125(6): 674

Centers for Disease Control (1962-1988). *Rabies Surveillance Annual Summaries, 1961-1987.* U. S. Department of Health and Human Services, Public Health Service. Atlanta, Georgia.

Centers for Disease Control (1985). An epidemiologic study of sylvatic rabies in Texas and New York using monoclonal antibodies. *CDC Rabies Surveillance Report*. U. S. Dept. of Health and Human Services, Public Health Service. Atlanta, Georgia.

Centers for Disease Control (1991). Recommendations of the Immunization Practices Advisory Committee (ACIP). Vaccinia (Smallpox) Vaccine. *MMWR.* 40(No. RR-14): 1

Centers for Disease Control (1993). Editorial note. *MMWR.* 42(41): 805

Cowherd, H. J., Reeves, S., Riegler, S., Walzen, P. D., Hernandez, C., and J. W. Skaggs (1979). Human rabies—Kentucky. *MMWR.* 28: 590

Debbie, J. G., Frantz, S., Novick, L. F., Trimarchi, C. V., Birkhead, G. S., Baker, M., Hill, D., Fuchs, R., Valsamis, M., Vallejo, C., Roseman, B., and S. Schroeder (1993). Human rabies—New York. *MMWR.* 42(41): 799

Dempster, G., Grodums, E. I., Bayatpour, M., and A. Zbitnew (1972). A human case of unsuspected rabies in Saskatchewan diagnosed by virus isolation. *Can. J. Pub. Hlth.* 63: 215

Dolman, C. L. and K. M. Charlton (1987). Massive necrosis of the brain in rabies. *Can. J. Neurol. Sci.* 14: 162

Dutta, J. K., Dutta, T. K., and A. K. Das (1992). Human rabies: Modes of transmission. *J. Assoc. Physicians (India).* 40(5): 322

Eye Bank Association of America (1993). D1.000 Donor Screening. *Revised Medical Standards.* Eye Bank Association of America. Washington, D. C.

Fishbein, D. B. (1991). Rabies in Humans. In G. M. Baer (ed.) *The Natural History of Rabies.* 2nd Edition. CRC Press, Inc. Boca Raton, Florida.

Gode, G. R. and N. K. Bhide (1988). Two rabies deaths after corneal grafts from one donor. *The Lancet.* October 1 II(8614): 791

Goldfield, M., Altman, R., and O. Sussman (1971). Epidemiologic notes and reports. Human Rabies—New Jersey. *MMWR.* 25(51): 459

Gonzales, R., Ramirez, M., Jelinek, M., Milan, C., Kelley, M., Simpson, D. M., Brinkley, T., Taylor, G., Harris, A., Saugey, D., Edelmann, M., Lofgren, J. P., Berry, D., McChesney, T., Dean, D. L., Smith, J. D., Wilbur, J. A., Alexander, P., Kosanovich, M., Hawkins, S. S., Grant, J., Boaz, V. A., Roddy, H. W., Burke, T., Needham, D., Goforth, S., Jeradi, R. J., Allom, S., Waters, E., BeVille, J. M., and R. H. Hutcheson (1991). Human Rabies—Texas, Arkansas, and Georgia, 1991. *MMWR.* 40(44): 765

Haltia, M., Tarkkanen, A., and T. Kivela (1989). Rabies: Ocular pathology. *Br. J. Ophthalmol.* 73(1): 61

Hattwick, M. A., Weiss, T. T., Stechschulte, C. J., Baer, G. M., and M. B. Gregg (1972). Recovery from rabies. A case report. *Ann. Int. Med.* 76: 931

Helmick, C. G. (1983). The epidemiology of human rabies postexposure prophylaxis, 1980-1981. *J. Am. Med. Assoc.* 250: 1990

Helmick, C. G., Tauxe, R. V., and A. A. Vernon (1987). Is there a risk to contacts of patients with rabies? *Rev. Infect. Dis.* 9(3): 511

Humphrey, G. L., Kemp, G. E., and E. G. Wood (1960). A fatal case of rabies in a woman bitten by an insectivorous bat. *Pub. Hlth. Repts.* 75(4): 317

Irons, J. V., Eads, R. B., Sullivan, T., and J. E. Grimes (1954). The current status of rabies in Texas. *Texas Repts. Biol. Med.* 12: 489

Irons, J. V., Eads, R. B., Grimes, J. E., and A. Conklin (1957). The public health importance of bats. *Texas. Repts. Biol. Med.* 15: 292

Kent, J. R. and M. F. Finegold (1960). Human rabies transmitted by the bite of a bat. *New Engl. J. Med.* 263(21): 1058

Kerton, L., Schwartz, S., Cleaver, E. M., Reynolds, F. A., Grim, J., Roberts, M. A., and M. Ward (1979). Human rabies—Oklahoma. *MMWR.* 28: 476

King, D. B., Sangalang, V. E., Manuel, R., and T. Marrie (1978). A suspected case of human rabies—Nova Scotia. *Can. Dis. Wkly. Rept.* 4(13): 49

Lennette, E. H., Soave, O. A., Kakamura, K., and G. H. Kellogg, Jr. (1960). A fatal human case of rabies following the bite of a rabid bat (*Lasionycteris noctivagans*). Isolation and identification of the virus from vector and victim. *J. Lab. Clin. Med.* 55(1): 89

Linden, E. (1993). Beware of rabies. *Time.* August 23. 142(8): 58

Lumio, J., Hillbom, M., Roine, R., Ketonen, L., Haltia, M., Valle, M., Neuvonen, E., and J. Lahdevirta (1986). Human rabies of bat origin in Europe. *The Lancet.* I(8477): 378

Martin, J., Brattin, P., Acevedo, H., Kelly, M., and S. Neill (1991). Human rabies—Texas, 1990. *J. Am. Med. Assoc.* 265(11): 1365

McLean, A. E., Noble, M. A., Black, W. A., and W. A. Kettyls (1985). A human case of rabies—British Columbia. *Can. Dis. Wkly. Rept.* 11(51): 213

Meredith, C. D., Rossouw, A. P., and H. Van Praag Koch (1971). An unusual case of human rabies thought to be of chiropteran origin. *S. Afr. Med. J.* 45: 767

Nelson, D. A. and R. G. Berry (1993). Fatal rabies associated with extensive demyelination. *Arch. Neurol.* 50: 317

Neill, S. U. (1993). Supervisor, Medical Virology. Texas Department of Health. Austin, Texas. Personal communication.

O'Day, D. M. (1989). Diseases potentially transmitted through corneal transplantation. *Ophthalmol.* 96: 1133

Reddell, J. R. (1961). The caves of Uvalde County. Part I. Texas Speleological Survey. *Texas Speleol. Assoc.* 1(3): 10

Roine, R. O., Hillbom, M., Valle, M., Haltia, M., Ketonen, L., Neuvonen, E., Lumio, J., and J. Lahdevirta (1988). Fatal encephalitis caused by a bat-borne rabies-related virus. *Brain.* 111: 1505

Selimov, M. A., Tatarov, A. G., Antonova, L. A., Shcherbak, Y. N., Shablovskaya, E. A., Smekhov, A. M., and B. Y. Mogilevsky (1986). To the issue of chiropteric rabic infection. *Rabies Information Exchange.* June 14: 9

Selimov, M. A., Tatarov, A. G., Botvinkin, A. D.,

Klueva, E. V., Kulikova, L. G., and N. A. Khismatullina (1989). Rabies-related Yuli virus: Identification with a panel of monoclonal antibodies. *Acta Virol.* 33: 542

Selimov, M. A., Smekhov, A. M., Antonova, L. A., Shablovskaya, E. A., King, A. A., and L. G. Kulikova (1991). New strains of rabies-related viruses isolated from bats in the Ukraine. *Acta Virol.* 35: 226

Shcherbak, Yu. N. (1984). Virological Studies of Rabies in the Ukrainian Soviet Socialist Republic. In *Viruses and Viral Diseases.* 12: 11, Kiev (in Russian).

Smith, J. S. (1992/1993). Research Microbiologist. Rabies Laboratory, Centers for Disease Control. Atlanta, Georgia. Personal communication.

Sulkin, S. E. and M. J. Greve (1954). Human rabies caused by bat bite. *Texas State J. Med.* 50: 620

Sureau, P. (1990). Recent data on the epidemiology and prophylaxis of human rabies in France. *Comp. Immunol. Microbiol. Infect. Dis.* 13(2): 107

Taormino, V., Otero, R., Riley, K., Weiler, P., Skaggs, J., and C. Hernandez (1974). Rabies in humans. Centers for Disease Control. *Rabies Surveillance Annual Summary for the Year 1973.* U. S. Department of Health and Human Services, Public Health Service. Atlanta, Georgia.

Tignor, G. H., Murphy, F. A., Clark, H. F., Shope, R. E., Madore, P., Bauer, S. P., Buckley, S. M., and C. D. Meredith (1977). Duvenhage virus: Morphological, biochemical, histopathological and antigenic relationships to the rabies serogroup. *J. Gen. Virol.* 37: 595

Trimarchi, C. V. (1994). *New York State Rabies Annual Summary, 1993.* Wadsworth Center for Laboratories and Research, New York State Department of Health. Albany, New York.

van der Merwe, M. (1982). Bats as vectors of rabies. *S. Afr. J. Sci.* 78: 421

Varughese, P. V. (1987). Rabies and post-exposure treatment in Canada, 1985. *Can. Dis. Wkly. Rept.* 13(5): 17

Veeraraghavan, N. (1955). Scientific Report 1954. I. Rabies. E. A case of hydrophobia following a bat bite. *Trop. Dis. Bull.* 52(8): 764

Webster, W. A., Casey, G. A., Charlton, K. M., Sayson, R. C., McLaughlin, B., and M. A. Noble (1987). A case of human rabies in western Canada. *Can. J. Pub. Hlth.* 78: 412

World Health Organization (1984a). Hazard of importing rabies-like viruses from Africa. *Information Circular* #15. WHO Mediterranean Zoonoses Control Centre.

World Health Organization (1984b). *Expert Committee on Rabies. Seventh Report.* WHO Tech. Rpt. No. 709. Geneva.

World Health Organization (1987). Bat rabies in the Union of Soviet Socialist Republics. *Rabies Bulletin Europe.* Information Surveillance Research. WHO Collaborating Centre for Rabies Surveillance and Research. Tubingen, Federal Republic of Germany. 4/86: 12

World Health Organization/Veterinary Public Health (1989). *Report of the Fifth WHO Consultation on Monoclonal Antibodies in Rabies Diagnosis and Research.* Geneva, March 3, 1989. WHO/Rab. Res./ 89.33. Unpublished document (reviewed with permission).

World Health Organization (1991). *World Survey of Rabies 24 (for the year 1988).* World Health Organization, Veterinary Public Health Unit, Division of Communicable Diseases, Geneva. WHO/Rabies/ 91.202. Unpublished document (reviewed with permission).

World Health Organization (1992). *Expert Committee on Rabies. Eighth Report.* WHO Tech. Rpt. No. 824. Geneva.

Zeidner, D., Bowman, A., Dennehy, J., Hufnal-Miller, C., Leipold, R., Royer, T., Ryan, M., Toor, S., Martin, T., Maksimak, J., Kaiser, R. H., Lattimer, G., Hart, M., Sinner, C., Jones, B., Bowen, S., Witte, E., and C. Hays (1984). Human Rabies—Pennsylvania. *MMWR. 33(45): 633*

Chapter 20: MANAGEMENT OF UNWANTED BATS IN THE HOME

General Considerations

Of concern to homeowners is the problem of bats roosting in houses. This is not an uncommon problem and is one that occurs throughout the United States (Figure 20-1). Pest species living in and around human habitations (commensal or synanthropic pests) generally prefer inaccessible harborage. They can cause damage to property, may disperse a variety of microorganisms or allergens, and are generally difficult to eradicate once established (Frantz, 1988). Building roosts often show signs of having been used for several years (Davis et al, 1962).

Many species of colonial bats may form colonies of several hundred individuals within human dwellings (Frantz, 1988), roosting in buildings for various reasons (Wells, Jr. and Girard, 1977; Greenhall, 1982). Laidlaw and Fenton (1971) discussed four types of occurrences of bats in buildings:

1) Accidental forays during nocturnal activity.
2) Establishment of diurnal roosts or shelters.
3) Utilization as nursery colonies for parturition and rearing of young.
4) Utilization as hibernation sites.

In general, bats prefer houses near woods, wetlands, ponds, streams, and other bodies of water where insects are abundant. Considerations of temperature, humidity, vegetation, and physical characteristics are poorly understood. Older buildings may be more frequently colonized, perhaps because of a greater number of access openings. In Brigham and Fenton's (1987) study, 18 of 21 buildings housing big brown bat colonies had been constructed prior to 1940. No relationships between colonization and building material, height, style of architecture, location within town, or compass orientation were observed by Davis et al (1962). Sometimes bats are forced to roost in man-made structures when their natural habitats are destroyed. Others seem to prefer them to natural roosting sites (Greenhall, 1982) and man-made structures may even contribute to population expansions among some species in certain areas (Frantz, 1989).

The most commonly observed bats in buildings are the little brown bat, big brown bat, and Mexican free-tailed bat. These are colonial species that may form nursing colonies within buildings in summer months. Big brown bats are commonly year-round residents within buildings. Red bats, hoary bats, and silver-haired bats are solitary species which occasionally enter buildings during migration, but don't remain long. They may enter through open windows while hunting moths attracted to lights. A discussion of the roosting habits of those species most commonly encountered in human dwellings can be found in the review by Greenhall (1982).

In their investigations of home infestations by Mexican free-tailed bats in Texas, Davis et al (1962) found that as many as 25% of homeowners with bat infestations were not even aware of the presence of the bats. Brigham and Fenton (1987) reported that almost 50% (10 of 21) of residents in a Canadian village were unaware of the presence of bat colonies in their homes.

Although some homeowners may welcome bats because of their consumption of large quantities of pestiferous insects or a simple interest in watching them, others consider their presence to be a nuisance. Home infestations of bats may cause annoying noises, and their foul-smelling excrement and urine may stain walls and attract in-

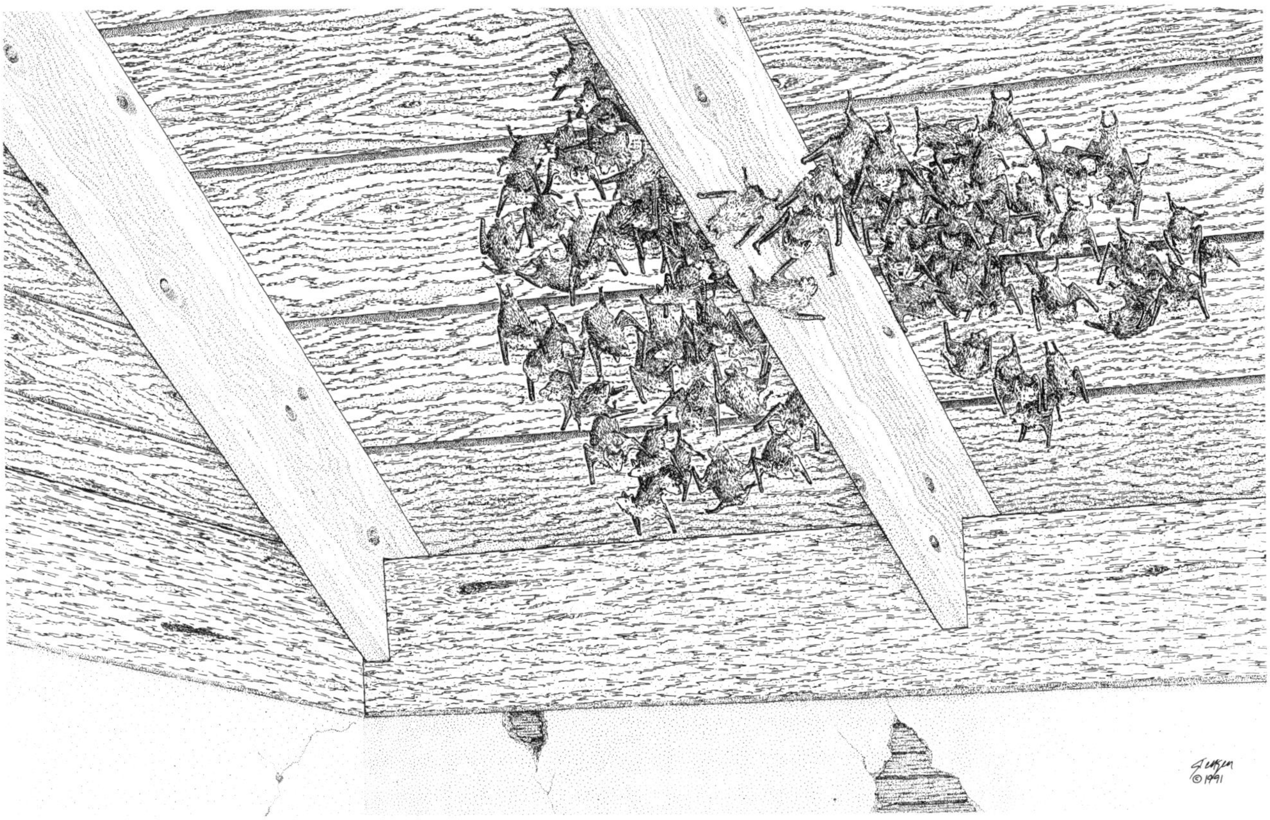

Figure 20-1. Bat infestation in the attic of a home. Even though some buildings may support large colonies of bats, the health hazards associated with bat infestations in homes remain very small.

sects (Barclay et al, 1980; Greenhall, 1982; Corrigan, 1983; Fenton, 1992; Ward, 1994). Extensive accumulations of guano may actually cause collapse of drop ceilings (Frantz, 1989). Over the course of several years, roosting bats may, on rare occasion, cause a mild deterioration in wood beams. Arthropods associated with indoor bat colonies may become household pests (Frantz and Trimarchi, 1984), although bat ectoparasites rarely bother humans.

Other homeowners seeking to rid their homes of a bat infestation may simply be responding to cultural phobias (Brigham and Fenton, 1987) or to the hysteria so commonly generated by tabloid journalism. The desire of many homeowners to eliminate house bats is, therefore, entirely understandable. School buildings, in particular, as well as other areas of high-risk human contact, such as hospitals, nursing homes, factories, and prisons, should be free of bat colonies (Cope, 1959; Constantine, 1970; Trimarchi, 1983).

Possible Health Hazards Associated with Bats in the Home

The presence of bats should be no reason for homeowners to give in to hysterical fears of mites, ticks, tuberculosis, histoplasmosis, rabies, or other diseases. Of all the bats infesting homes nationwide, there is no doubt that some of them are rabid. However, the chances of rabid bats roosting in any given home are small. If a rabid bat is present, the likelihood of its interacting with family members (let alone, transmitting disease) is not very high, but does remain a possibility.

Maddy et al (1958) reported the interesting case of a boy in Willcox, Arizona who, on May 14, 1957, had been bitten by a big brown bat he had taken to school. There had been a colony of big brown bats living in the attic of his home, with as many as five or six apparently sick bats falling to the floor and dying each day. It had been one of these fallen bats which the boy had taken to school. It was subsequently confirmed as rabid by the Arizona State Department of Health Laboratory. The cause of illness in the other bats of the colony remains unknown. According to Cockrum (1993), the other bats at the house had never been made available for examination. Rabies outbreaks have never been documented as a cause of mass bat illness.

Trimarchi (1986) reported that six rabid big brown bats were found in a colony roosting in a home in Clinton County, New York. So many infected bats in a home-dwelling colony had not been reported in New York before. Researchers in New York State have observed that if a rabid big brown bat is found in a home roost, there will probably be a rabid individual present at least every few years (Trimarchi, 1989).

Brigham and Fenton (1987) suggested that colony exclusion might not be an appropriate management stratagem if one or more rabies-positive big brown bats have been reported from a building colony. Accordingly, they recommended that it would be more appropriate to monitor an infected colony within a known site rather than evict bats and have them disappear into the neighborhood. In some buildings, this might be an appropriate means of management. However, in other instances, it may not be.

The health hazards associated with bats in the home are probably minimal, but they do exist. There may be an increase in human contact with bats in shared dwellings (Brigham and Fenton, 1987). Many instances of people finding bats in their blankets and being bitten while asleep have been reported (Emerson, 1986; Trimarchi, 1989; Pape, 1992), although these are not necessarily related to home infestations. Isolated intruders have caused similar problems.

With regard to the presence of a home-dwelling colony of bats, it remains difficult to precisely define the level of risk. Sick bats, for example, may fall to the ground and be handled by inquisitive children, who may then be bitten. Unexplained wounds may cause family members considerable anxiety over the thought of a possible bat bite and suspected animal contacts may lead to unnecessary destruction of pets. The probability of transmission of virus from rabid bats to humans is very small. Nevertheless, the possibility does influence management decisions regarding bat infestations of homes (Frantz and Trimarchi, 1984).

Health Concerns Related to the Chemical Extermination of Bats

In considering ways to eliminate house bats, homeowners should be wary of extermination companies offering bat-elimination services. In general, one would do well to contact the nongame branch of the local Fish and Game Department, or the U. S. Fish and Wildlife Service for recommendations. These agencies may be very helpful in recommending companies providing safe and reliable services. Homeowners who are hesitant about eliminating bats themselves should be on guard against exterminating companies offering chemical means of control, particularly any of the following services:

Rozol Tracking Powder - This is an anticoagulant (chlorophacinone) which, until recently, had been approved for bat-control use in 17 states. It was generally ineffective in controlling bats. Although it was approved for restricted use in controlling nuisance bats (Section 24[c] - "Special Local Needs" of the Federal Insecticide, Fungicide, and Rodenticide Act), the Environmental Protection Agency (EPA) considered it to be a public-health hazard. It can be highly hazardous if inhaled and may be absorbed through the skin (Strohm, 1982; Tuttle, undated manuscript). Its hazardous nature was decided in Minnesota court (EPA, 1980 [cited by Greenhall, 1982]). According to Constantine (1979 [cited by Greenhall, 1982]), "this method was similarly unproductive, accounting for the destruction of not more than ten percent (usually far less) of resident bats, despite applications of massive amounts of the material to attic ceilings and walls." Exposure to this material may endanger persons occupying treated homes.

In late 1990 and early 1991, LiphaTech, the manufacturer, voluntarily withdrew all of its 24(c) EPA registrations for bat extermination. According to the manufacturer, this was done "out of concern for the endangered species of bats" (S. Smith, 1992). It is now legally available as a rodenticide only. Its use in the control of bats is illegal in the United States. States which had been registered under the 24(c) label to use Rozol Tracking Powder and dates of registration withdrawal include: Colorado (1/91), Connecticut (1/91), Georgia (1/91), Idaho (1/91), Kentucky (1/91), Maine (1/91), Maryland (3/91), Massachusetts (1/91), Michigan (1/91), Montana (1/91), Ohio (3/91), Pennsylvania (3/91), South Carolina (1/91), Texas (1/91), Washington (1/91), West Virginia (11/90), and Wyoming (1/91). Lipha-Tech no longer holds registrations for any pesticides containing directions for use against bats (Thorne, 1987; S. Smith, 1992).

Methyl Bromide - Rarely effective as used and highly dangerous to human health. This substance may also dissolve insulation, adding to the possibility of electrical fire (Tuttle, undated manuscript). Greenhall (1982) suggested that its use be limited to times when a distinct public-health emergency exists, and then only after other methods have failed. Buildings must be tented during treatment to prevent escape of poisoned bats, which could present a community health hazard (Frantz, 1989).

Naphthalene - Generally ineffective and it may generate intolerable fumes throughout the house. Some people are particularly sensitive to these fumes. This is the only chemical registered with the EPA for indoor use as a bat repellant. It will repel bats if used in high enough concentration, but bats will return when the fumes dissipate (Cope, 1959; Greenhall, 1982).

DDT - Ineffective against bats and extremely hazardous to use (Kunz et al, 1977; Barclay et al, 1980). Although Greenhall (1982) reported it to be very toxic to bats, he cautioned against its use because of the potential hazard of spreading poisoned bats through the community. In the recent past, DDT had been the only toxicant registered for use by the EPA. Special permission was required for its use and there must have been a demonstrable public-health hazard before permission was given. In 1987, the EPA registration of DDT was withdrawn (Frantz, 1989).

Poisons are generally ineffective in controlling house bats. At best, they may drive bats away for a short period of time. Reinfestation may follow quickly. At worst, poisons can sift through a home, endangering the health of human occupants. In past years, repeated treatment had been almost standard protocol and a source of increased revenue for exterminating companies (Constantine, 1978). According to Tuttle and Kern (1981), "killing bats is lucrative in generating repeat business for the pest control industry."

Poison application may cause bats to sicken. These bats may become grounded locally and present a hazard to children, pets, or Good Samaritans who happen upon them. The majority of human exposures to bats, resulting in a bite, have come from handling ill and grounded animals. Bats disabled by chemical toxicants may, therefore, add a health burden to the local community (Kunz et al, 1977; Constantine, 1978, 1988; Trimarchi, 1978; Barclay et al, 1980; Clark, Jr., 1981; Greenhall, 1982; Debbie, 1983). Poisoned bats will continue to sicken, and an increased frequency of bat/human contact may continue for as long as two years following the initial poisoning (Kunz et al, 1977). Whenever bats are disabled and left to die, a serious human health hazard may ensue. According to Constantine (1978), "The mismanagement creates a self-perpetuating cycle of hysteria." The potential exposure to bats, and subsequent need for post-exposure rabies prophylaxis or destruction of unvaccinated pets, may increase by a factor of ten following widespread application of toxicants (Constantine, 1988).

In view of their general ineffectiveness and the potential dangers they pose, the use of chemical poisons in the management of house bats cannot be justified. In fact, the liberal use of deadly poisons will invariably create a far greater health hazard to the community than that originally posed by the bat colony itself (Kunz et al, 1977; Greenhall, 1982). Howard (1967 [cited by Greenhall, 1985]) wrote,

> *There is no question that some people who are responsible for vertebrate pest control programs are inclined to minimize the injurious effects of the methods they use, while some of those who are primarily interested in the conservation of wildlife are equally inclined to maximize the intrinsic value of any animals lost due to control operations. However, there is no rebuttal to the statement that the use of toxic chemicals must be kept to the*

absolute minimum in the control of vertebrate animals.

Exterminating companies that routinely manage bats chemically should be avoided. Fortunately, they are no longer common and the National Pest Control Association is educating member pest-control operators regarding ecologically sound methods of managing vertebrate pests, particularly bats (E. Smith, 1992a).

Batproofing Homes as an Effective Means of Controlling House Bats

Proper management of house bats should entail denial of reentry by batproofing of the premises (Silver and Jones, 1961; Constantine, 1966; Barclay et al, 1980; Greenhall, 1982; Tuttle and Smith, 1992; National Association of State Public Health Veterinarians, 1992, 1993, 1994). This is the only safe and effective means of solving the problem.

Bats can crawl through very small openings. Cope (1959) reported that small bats could pass through a wire mesh opening of 5/8" x 7/8" and openings of this size, and perhaps smaller, should be sealed. Useful sealing materials include sheet metal, plywood, aluminum flashing, weatherstripping, insulation, lathe, hardware cloth, window screen, caulking compounds (such as oakum, putty, and various elastomeric materials which expand and contract), and others. Constantine (1982) recommended initial use of porous materials or wire mesh to help prevent changes in roost ventilation, since increasing roost temperatures may drive bats into the living quarters of a home. After all bats have been excluded, more permanent building materials may be substituted.

Commonly used portals of entry include louvres, vents, broken windows, worn sidings, spaces around eaves and cornices, and various other cracks (Constantine, 1970). Clues to location of openings include pre-emergence noise, odors, smudge marks, and the presence of droppings on the ground. Droppings are very friable and crumble easily in the hand. Small bits of undigested insects can be seen in them. Rodent droppings, on the other hand, are firmer, more uniform in shape, and often pointed at one or both ends. Reptile and bird droppings can be distinguished by the white uric acid paste in them. Other ways to locate openings take advantage of detecting moving air currents (Corrigan, 1983; Greenhall, 1982, 1983). Smoke blowers will generate smoke and blow them out attic openings. Strips of tissue paper or candle flames will waver near building openings. Air flow indicators can also be used to detect leaks. Entrance holes can also be located by observing bats exiting in the evening.

Once located, these openings can be sealed when the bats are out for the evening or when they are away for extended periods during winter months (Strohm, 1982; Debbie, 1983; Frantz, 1986). Although roost fidelity after eviction is high, bats will eventually seek shelter elsewhere. They will not gnaw through building material in attempts to regain indoor roosts (Greenhall, 1982).

If all bats have not left the roost, plugged entrance holes can be opened at dusk on subsequent evenings until all have left. It may also be possible to govern bat movement by the installation of unidirectional portals, that serve as one-way access doors to the outside. Constantine (1982) devised a valve-like tube apparatus that acts in a one-way valve capacity. A collapsible tube is fitted over and taped to a rigid tube. Although collapsed, the flexible tube allows bats to exit easily, but prevents others from entering. Another apparatus, called the EX-100 Hanks Bat Excluder, consists of a one-way valve and a metal mesh cone, and works in a similar fashion (Anonymous, 1983; Greenhall, 1983). The presence of bats for extended periods of time after sealing entry holes indicates that previously unused openings still exist. These must be sealed as well.

Frantz (1986) described the successful use of inexpensive polypropylene birdnetting checkvalves for batproofing homes. Generally available at hardware or garden-supply stores, these can be customized for a particular architectural design. According to Frantz, they are effective exclusion devices because they take advantage of behavioral characteristics of the bat. When returning to an entry hole, bats will be guided by visual, auditory, and olfactory cues. Because the birdnetting checkvalves do not appreciably alter any of these characteristics, returning bats will persist for a time in regaining the roost through the original entry point, making no attempt to explore the perimeter of the checkvalve. They will ultimately seek an alternate roost. The National Pest Control Association recommends structural-grade rather than standard-grade material because of its greater strength and smaller mesh size (Tuttle and Smith, 1992).

Bats should not be built out of homes from May through August, when flightless young may be present. Videography has confirmed persistent attempts at reentry by excluded mothers (Frantz, 1989), roost fidelity being strongest during the maternity period (Frantz, 1986). The young, left behind by their mother, will die and decay. This will create a rank odor throughout the home (Corrigan, 1983). Constantine (1982) has recommended the following calendar guidelines for bat exclusion:

Winter: The best time to build bats out. If bats are known to be absent, all known entry holes should be closed. If hibernating individuals are known or suspected to be present, batproofing should not be absolute. A few one-way valves should be installed to allow bats to exit the roost in spring.

Early Spring: Batproofing should be carried out from onset of warm weather until just prior to new births (sometimes as early as the beginning of May). Most entry holes should be sealed, but a few one-way valves should be put in place to assist stragglers in leaving. These can then be removed and the openings sealed when all bats are known to have left the roost.

May through August: At this time, nonflying young are present. The roost should be left undisturbed. Batproofing should not be attempted.

September through Winter: Same recommendations as in early spring.

On occasion, bats may enter the living quarters of a home. Most commonly, this occurs during spring and fall migrations (Greenhall, 1982) and during hot periods in the summer, when they move out of walls and attics to prevent heat prostration (McChesney et al, 1983). Invasion of living quarters may also occur following changes in ventilation secondary to plugging of entry holes or following accidentally sealing bats inside (Constantine, 1982).

In managing these occasional intruders, it may prove difficult to locate access holes, but sealing off attic and basement areas from living quarters is usually possible. In particular, gaps should be sealed around attic and basement doors, wall and ceiling electrical fixtures, ceiling moldings, and baseboards (Frantz, 1986). Exclusion of bats from living quarters can also be accomplished by using half-inch hardware cloth atop fireplace chimneys and across ventilation ducts, and by weatherstripping attic doors (Strohm, 1982).

Bats that wander indoors will often quickly find their way out again by following air currents. This can be facilitated by isolating the bat in one room, if possible, followed by opening windows and doors to the outside. Frightened homeowners should do their best to keep the intruding bat in sight at all times, otherwise it might disappear into a multitude of small, dark hiding places and be almost impossible to find again. If the bat doesn't quickly find its own way out, it can be captured in a net, box, can, or in gloved hands and released at night in a secluded area. Even though they may bite when handled, such bats are rarely aggressive and do not normally attack people. Unless contact with a person or pet is suspected, killing the bat is unnecessary. If such contact is believed to have occurred, however, the bat should be retained and submitted for rabies testing.

Although there may be rare instances in which bat infestations cannot be built out (Girard, 1978), batproofing of homes is generally both effective and inexpensive. In fact, proper use of insulation and other building materials will not only batproof a home, but markedly increase its energy efficiency as well. Batproofing is, therefore, consistent with financial savings (Greenhall, 1982). It does less harm to the bat population than chemical management, and presents no chemical danger to family members and considerably less health hazard to the community. It is currently the only practical and effective means of controlling unwanted bats in the home.

Persons who regularly batproof homes should

seriously consider obtaining pre-exposure rabies immunization. Furthermore, the National Pest Control Association recommends that pest-control operators managing bat infestations wear leather gloves and take precautions (i.e., use of dust-proof respirators) against inhalation of guano dust (E. Smith, 1992b).

Displacement of bats from roost sites may result in a temporary increase in risk of human or animal exposure until alternate roosting areas are found (Frantz, 1989). Brigham and Fenton (1985, 1987) studied the movements of big brown bat colonies after exclusion from buildings in a Canadian village and found that displaced colonies within the village moved to a roosting site in a nearby building within an average distance of 55 meters from the original site. Those living in buildings outside the village moved an average of 160 meters to find a new roost. Big brown bats evicted from roosts before giving birth tended to be less successful in rearing young to flying age than those not so evicted.

References

Anonymous (1983). Wisconsin firm develops bat excluder. *Pest Contr. Technol.* 11(6): 74

Barclay, R. M. R., Thomas, D. W., and M. Brock Fenton (1980). Comparison of methods used for controlling bats in buildings. *J. Wildl. Manage.* 44(2): 502

Brigham, R. M. and M. Brock Fenton (1985). The influence of roost closure and foraging behaviour of *Eptesicus fuscus* (Chiroptera: Vespertilionidae). *Can. J. Zool.* 64: 1128

Brigham, R. M. and M. Brock Fenton (1987). The effect of roost sealing as a method to control maternity colonies of big brown bats. *Can. J. Pub. Hlth.* 78(1): 47

Clark, Jr., D. R. (1981). *Bats and Environmental Contaminants—A Review.* U. S. Fish and Wildlife Service, U. S. Department of the Interior, Special Scientific Report - Wildlife No. 235.

Cockrum, E. L. (1993). Department of Zoology, University of Arizona. Tucson, Arizona. Personal communication.

Constantine, D. G. (1966). Recent Advances in Our Knowledge of Bat Rabies. *International Symposium on Rabies.* Symp. Series Immunobiol. Standard Vol. I. Karger, Basel. New York. Talloires, 1965

Constantine, D. G. (1970). Bats in Relation to Health, Welfare, and Economy of Man. In W. A. Wimsatt (ed.) *Biology of Bats.* Vol. II. Academic Press. New York.

Constantine, D. G. (1978). Bats, rabies and DDT. *New Engl. J. Med.* 298(16): 915

Constantine, D. G. (1982). Batproofing of buildings by installation of valvelike devices in entryways. *J. Wildl. Manage.* 46(2): 507

Constantine, D. G. (1988). Health Precautions for Bat Researchers. In T. H. Kunz (ed.) *Ecological and Behavioral Methods for the Study of Bats.* Smithsonian Institution Press. Washington, D.C.

Cope, J. B. (1959). Build bats out. *Pest Control.* 27: 28

Corrigan, B. (1983). Misunderstood bats. *Pest Control.* August: 61

Davis, R. B., Herreid, C. F., and H. L. Short (1962). Mexican free-tailed bats in Texas. *Ecol. Monogr.* 32(4): 311

Debbie, J. G. (1983). Rabies Control in Wildlife. In *Reports on Rabies.* Veterinary Learning Systems, Inc. Princeton Junction, New Jersey.

Emerson, J. K. (1986). Chief, Environmental Epidemiology. Colorado Department of Health. Denver, Colorado. Personal communication.

Fenton, M. B. (1992). *Bats.* Facts on File, Inc. New York.

Frantz, S. C. (1986). Batproofing structures with birdnetting checkvalves. *Proceedings of the 12th Vertebrate Pest Conference*: 260

Frantz, S. C. (1988). Architecture and Commensal Vertebrate Pest Management. In R. B. Kundsin (ed.) *Architectural Design and Indoor Microbiol Pollution.* Oxford University Press. New York.

Frantz, S. C. (1989). Vertebrate Vector Specialist. Rabies Laboratory, Wadsworth Center for Laboratories and Research, New York State Department of Health. Albany, New York. Personal communication.

Frantz, S. C. and C. V. Trimarchi (1984). Bats in human dwellings: Health concerns and management. In D. J. Decker (ed.) *Proceedings of the First Eastern Wildlife Damage Control Conference.* Cornell University. Ithaca, New York. September 27-30, 1983.

Girard, K. F. (1978). Letter to the Editor. *New Engl. J. Med.* 298(16): 915

Greenhall, A. M. (1982). House Bat Management. *Resource Publication* No. 143. United States Fish and Wildlife Service. Washington, D.C.

Greenhall, A. M. (1983). *Bats—Damage Prevention and Control Methods.* Great Plains Agricultural Council. Wildlife Resources Committee, Cooperative Extension Service, Institute of Agriculture and Natural Resources, University of Nebraska. Lincoln, Nebraska.

Greenhall, A. M. (1985). Effects of Vampire Bats and Paralytic Rabies on Livestock Production. In S. M.

Gaafar, W. E. Howard, and R. E. Marsh (eds.) World Animal Science B2-Disciplinary Approach. *Parasites, Pests, and Predators.* Elsevior Science Publishing Co., Inc. New York.

Howard, W. E. (1967). Biocontrol and Chemosterilants. In E. W. Kilgore and R. L. Doutt (eds.) *Pest Control—Biological, Physical and Selected Chemical Methods.* Academic Press. New York.

Kunz, T. H., Anthony, E. L. P., and W. T. Rumage, III (1977). Mortality of little brown bats following multiple pesticide applications. *J. Wildl. Manage.* 41(3): 476

Laidlaw, G. W. J. and M. B. Fenton (1971). Control of nursery colony populations of bats by artificial light. *J. Wildl. Manage.* 35(4): 843

Maddy, K. T., Cockrum, E. L., and H. G. Crecelius (1958). Bat rabies in Arizona. *Arizona Med.* 15(5): 344

McChesney, T. C., Spatz, H., and M. Edelman (1983). Bat rabies in Arkansas. *J. Arkansas Med. Soc.* 80(4): 181

National Association of State Public Health Veterinarians (1992). Compendium of Animal Rabies Control. *J. Am. Vet. Med. Assoc.* 200(2): 145

National Association of State Public Health Veterinarians (1993). Compendium of Animal Rabies Control. *J. Am. Vet. Med. Assoc.* 202(2): 199

National Association of State Public Health Veterinarians (1994). Compendium of Animal Rabies Control. *J. Am. Vet. Med. Assoc.* 204(2): 173

Pape, J. (1992). Colorado Department of Health. Denver, Colorado. Personal communication.

Silver, J. and J. C. Jones (1961). *Control of Bats.* U.S. Fish and Wildlife Service, Wildlife Leaflet. 333: 1

Smith, E. C. (1992a). What do bats have to do with pest control month. In Tuttle, M. D. and E. C. Smith (1992). Bats: Nature's own PCO. *Pest Manage.* 11(5): 10

Smith, E. C. (1992b). Are bats a public health hazard? In Tuttle, M. D. and E. C. Smith (1992). Bats: Nature's own PCO. *Pest Manage.* 11(5): 10

Smith, S. (1992). Government Affairs Specialist. Lipha-Tech, Inc. Milwaukee, Wisconsin. Personal communication.

Strohm, B. (1982). Most "facts" about bats are myths. *Natl. Wildl.* 20(5): 35

Thorne, J. (1987). Conservation dispatches. *NSS (Natl. Speleol. Soc.) News.* 45(8) 302

Trimarchi, C. V. (1978). Rabies in insectivorous temperate-zone bats. *Bat Res. News.* 19(1): 7

Trimarchi, C. V. (1983). Bats in Human Dwellings: Health Concerns and Management. *Proceedings of the First Eastern Wildlife Damage Control Conference.* Cornell Cooperative Extension. Ithaca, New York. September 27-30, 1983.

Trimarchi, C. V. (1986). *Rabies Annual Summary, 1986.* Rabies Laboratory, Wadsworth Center for Laboratories and Research, New York State Department of Health. Albany, New York.

Trimarchi, C. V. (1989). Director, Rabies Laboratory. Wadsworth Center for Laboratories and Research, New York State Department of Health. Albany, New York. Personal communication.

Tuttle, M. D. (undated manuscript). Why rozol tracking powder never should be used against bats. Bat Conservation International. Austin, Texas. Courtesy of Dr. M. D. Tuttle.

Tuttle, M. D. (undated manuscript). The hazards of house bat management. Bat Conservation International. Austin, Texas. Courtesy of Dr. M. D. Tuttle.

Tuttle, M. D. and S. J. Kern (1981). Bats and Public Health. *Contributions in Biology and Geology.* No. 48. Milwaukee Public Museum.

Tuttle, M. D. and E. C. Smith (1992). Evicting unwanted tenants. *Pest Manage.* 11(5): 18

Ward, C. (1994). Bats in church. *The Lancet.* 343(8896): 552

Wells, Jr., L. F. and K. F. Girard (1977). Bats, rabies, and DDT. *New Engl. J. Med.* 297(7): 390

Chapter 21:
CONTROL OF RABIES IN WILD BAT POPULATIONS

Programs for Oral Vaccination of Wildlife

Controlling wildlife reservoirs of disease is extremely difficult. In the past, control programs often involved widespread destruction of wildlife populations. Such wholesale slaughter is often not completely successful (requiring as much as a 70% to 80% reduction in the reservoir population), frequently evokes strong public sentiment from a concerned populace, and may result in significant ecological disruption (Winkler and Bogel, 1992; World Health Organization, 1992).

Some countries (e.g., Canada) have made limited use of trap-vaccinate-release programs to build a barrier of immune individuals in attempts to control rabies in terrestrial carnivores (Rosatte et al, 1992, 1993). However, many investigators believe that oral vaccination programs, using potent, self-replicating, attenuated or recombinant vaccines, are the only practical and cost-effective strategy for long-term control of rabies in free-ranging terrestrial carnivores (Baer, 1988; Rosatte et al, 1990, 1992; Rupprecht et al, 1992a). Principal requirements for an orally administered bait and vaccine are outlined in Tables 21-1 and 21-2. Others have expressed the view that oral vaccination of wildlife for the purpose of rabies eradication is not realistic (Coyne et al, 1989; Bruggemann, 1992).

Many current rabies control programs are utilizing attempts at oral immunization (using vaccine products which are absorbed across the oropharyngeal mucosa), based on pilot studies carried out by the Centers for Disease Control (Baer et al, 1971, 1975) and the New York State Department of Health (Debbie et al, 1972). In particular, foxes across much of Europe have been successfully immunized against rabies by using orally effective attenuated vaccines (Flamand et al, 1992; Muller and Blancou, 1992; Winkler and Bogel, 1992; Petkevicius, 1993). Effective baiting systems and oral rabies vaccines have been developed for use against red-fox rabies in Switzerland (Steck et al 1982; Wandeler et al, 1988); the former Federal Republic of Germany/West Germany (Wilhelm and Schneider, 1990); Belgium, France, and Luxembourg (Artois et al, 1987; Pastoret et al, 1987; Pastoret and Brochier, 1992; Brochier et al, 1988, 1991); Czechoslovakia (World Health Organization, 1992); and Canada (Johnston and Voight, 1982; MacInness et al, 1988; Charlton, 1992; Wandeler and Casey, 1993). An oral vaccination field trial in southern Finland eliminated rabies in the raccoon dog within a year (World Health Organization, 1992). Similarly effective baiting systems are being developed to target other wildlife reservoirs, notably skunks and raccoons (Rupprecht et al, 1987; Hadidian et al, 1989; Bachmann et al, 1990; Linhart et al, 1991; Linhart, 1993).

Development of a safe and effective vaccine is the first step in a successful program to control wildlife disease (Anderson, 1986). Although feasibility studies of oral vaccination of wildlife have proven successful and experimental studies have documented successful immunization of various target species, no wildlife vaccine, to date, has been licensed for use in North America. Vaccines that might be utilized for wildlife immunization include products incorporating either live (attenuated) or inactivated virus. There are problems associated with both types. The inactivated vaccines may be more limited in their capacity to generate an adequate immune response. Attenuated (modified live) vaccines, on the other hand, while producing a more effective immunity, suffer from the possibility of viral reversion to a fully

Table 21-1

Requirements of Baits to be Used as Vehicles For a Live Attenuated Rabies Vaccine

- Should be attractive to the target species.
- Should be eaten without being stored.
- Should be rejected by other species (including humans).
- Should reach a large proportion of the target population.
- Should not inactivate the vaccine.
- Should deliver the vaccine into the oral cavity.
- Should be able to incorporate a biologic marker (e.g., tetracycline).
- Should be easily available and inexpensive.

From Wandeler, A. I., Capt, S., Kappeler, A., and R. Hauser. Oral immunization of wildlife against rabies: Concept and first field experiments. *Rev. Infect. Dis.* 10(Suppl. 4): S649, 1988.

virulent form (Rupprecht et al, 1990; le Blois et al, 1990). Limited studies have shown that orally administered attenuated vaccines may be pathogenic in skunks. Indeed, no modified live rabies vaccine should ever be used to vaccinate an animal for which it was not specifically intended. Newly pioneered vaccines may make use of either inhibition of binding of the rabies virus to target organs (Bracci et al, 1988) or the technology of genetic engineering.

Vaccinia Virus as a Recombinant Vaccine

Little is known about the early history of the vaccinia virus. Today, it is considered to be a virus of unknown origin that is not known to exist naturally. Until recently, it had been found only in vaccine institutions and research laboratories.

Although itself a minor human pathogen, the importance of vaccinia has been in its use as a vaccine against smallpox, a more serious human pathogen. The success of the vaccinia-based smallpox vaccination programs is attested to by the global eradication of smallpox. The last reported naturally occurring case of smallpox was from Somalia in 1977 (Centers for Disease Control, 1991a) and the world was certified as free of naturally occurring smallpox by the World Health Assembly in 1980 (World Health Organization, 1980).

The World Health Organization has called for destruction of the world's remaining stores of smallpox virus (held under heavy guard in Atlanta and Moscow) by the end of 1993. The plan has sparked a heated debate among scientists (Altman, 1993).

With the eradication of smallpox, further inoculation of the general populace with vaccinia became both unnecessary and contraindicated.[1] The reasons for this lie in the infrequent, but severe complications sometimes observed in vaccinees. Complications of smallpox vaccination have included both abnormal skin eruptions and diseases of the central nervous system. In many instances, fatality was associated with both cutaneous and neural complications.

Many researchers have expressed the view that a vaccinia-based vaccine could be used to immunize against a wide variety of human and animal diseases. Recombinant vaccinia-based vaccines have been engineered to express the immunizing antigens of a number of pathogenic viruses, including herpesvirus, hepatitis B, influenza, human immunodeficiency virus (HIV), and, of course, rabies.

In considering the use of vaccinia virus, the wisdom of reintroducing the virus into the world has been carefully evaluated. Release of genetically engineered organisms into the environment is of global concern. In this regard, concerns have focused on the potential pathogenic side effects that vaccinia might pose, as well as the pos-

[1]Until recently, military troops of several countries, including Canada, Israel, Russia, and the United States were among the last segment of the human population to be immunized. At present, only Israel continues to vaccinate its military against smallpox (Altman, 1993).

Table 21-2

Requirements of a Live Attenuated Rabies Vaccine to be Used for the Immunization of Free-Ranging Wildlife

- Should be highly immunogenic in the target species by oral application.
- Should not be pathogenic for the target or non-target species.
- Should be incorporated into a baiting system that is readily accepted by and reaches a high proportion of the target species.
- Should not be excreted.
- Should not easily revert to higher pathogenicity.
- Should be free from pathogenic contamination.
- Should be readily storable.
- Should remain stable under a variety of environmental conditions and for variable periods of time.
- Should be easy and inexpensive to produce.
- Should bear at least one genetic marker.

From Wandeler, A. I., Capt, S., Kappeler, A., and R. Hauser. Oral immunization of wildlife against rabies: Concept and first field experiments. *Rev. Infect. Dis.* 10(Suppl. 4): S649, 1988.

sibility that the engineered virus might behave in an unpredictable fashion. These risks, however unlikely, have been carefully weighed against the potential benefits (Wokatsch, 1972; Arita and Fenner, 1985; Dietzschold et al, 1985; Dumbell, 1985; Karzon, 1985; Neff, 1985; Paoletti et al, 1985; Yilma et al, 1985; Murphy, 1985; Quinnan, Jr., 1985; Sussman et al, 1988; Ferguson, 1991).

Using established recombinant technology, certain genes from the rabies virus have been inserted into the genetic material of the vaccinia virus (Panicali et al, 1983; Paoletti et al, 1984). This has led to production of a recombinant vaccinia virus (V-RG) which expresses the set of rabies genes incorporated into it. In particular, the genes coding for the rabies G glycoprotein have been encoded into the vaccinia genome and this glycoprotein is, therefore, produced by the genetically altered vaccinia virus (Kieny et al, 1984).

Although a variety of mechanisms are important in protection against rabies, the glycoprotein moiety, which exists on the surface of the rabies virus, is very important in eliciting a protective immune response against the rabies virus (Cox et al, 1977). In fact, the glycoprotein complex is the most important component of the virus to induce formation of and react with rabies-neutralizing antibodies (Sikes et al, 1971). It also acts as a target for virus-immune T helper cells and cytotoxic T cells.

The recombinant vaccinia virus will elaborate a glycoprotein qualitatively indistinguishable from that produced by the ERA strain (see Table 23-7) of rabies virus. This will induce an immune response in inoculated animals. It cannot cause rabies and it shows great promise as a means of oral immunization of wildlife.

The nucleoprotein is also a major antigen and induces activity in T helper cells. Recombinant glycoprotein vaccines complemented with genes expressing the nucleoprotein antigen may have an enhanced effectiveness (Fu et al, 1991; Sumner et al, 1991; World Health Organization, 1992; Lodmell et al, 1991, 1993).

Experimental trials have shown the recombinant vaccinia vaccine to be both safe and effective in various target, as well as nontarget, species (including various birds that have been shown to consume baits or that might prey on small mammals consuming baits). No abortifacient, teratogenic, or oncogenic side effects have been observed (Wiktor et al, 1984; Dietzschold et al, 1985; Blancou et al, 1986; Rupprecht et al, 1986, 1987, 1992b; Tolson et al, 1988; Pastoret et al, 1988; Brochier et al, 1988, 1991; Bachmann et al, 1990; Desmettre et al, 1990; Anderson, 1991; Artois et al, 1990, 1992; Pastoret and Brochier, 1992; World Health Organization, 1992).

Other recombinant vaccine products have been evaluated. A live raccoon poxvirus vaccine has been shown to be effective in inducing rabies-neutralizing antibody in raccoons and in conferring protection against lethal challenge with raccoon street virus (Esposito et al, 1988). Similar results were obtained in mice (Lodmell et al, 1991). Efficacy studies of raccoon poxvirus recombinant vaccines in protecting skunks against rabies infection is ongoing (Fedaku et al, 1991). Favorable results have been obtained using a recombinant human adenovirus vaccine to immunize skunks and foxes against rabies (Charlton et al, 1992; Kalicharran et al, 1992). Baculovirus recombinants expressing both G and N proteins have also been engineered (World Health Organization, 1992; Fu et al, 1993; Tordo et al, 1993). Avipox viruses, such as canarypox, may be of value in formulation of human recombinant vaccines and are under investigation (Cadoz et al, 1992; World Health Organization, 1992).

Field Trials of Recombinant Vaccine Products

Limited testing of a vaccinia-derived vaccine was conducted in Argentina in 1986, but testing was stopped because of apparent failure of the Pan American Health Organization to obtain proper official sanction from Argentine health authorities (Cordes, 1988; Crawford, 1987, 1988; Editorial, 1988).

The Wistar Institute submitted a proposal for testing the efficacy of a recombinant vaccinia rabies vaccine for immunizing raccoons in the United States. Proposed test sites included isolated islands off the coast of South Carolina (Cedar and Murphy Islands) and Virginia (Parramore Island). The value of these locales for initial testing was that the water provided a barrier to migration of test raccoons into or out of the area, and the islands were free of rabid raccoons or endangered species. The islands were rarely used for recreation and were accessible only by boat (Sun, 1989a).

The Virginia Department of Health granted approval for testing. Final approval, however, was required from the Nature Conservancy, a private group which owns Parramore Island, Virginia (Cheston, 1989; Sun, 1989b). Despite an assessment by the United States Department of Agriculture (USDA), Animal and Plant Health Inspection Service (APHIS) concluding that these tests would have no "significant impact on the quality of the human environment," approval of testing was held up by state officials in South Carolina (Fox, 1989; Sun, 1989a). The Health Commissioner of South Carolina did not believe that the health of South Carolina's environment or citizens could be assured if these vaccine trials were carried out (Cheston, 1989). In July, 1989, final approval was granted for testing on Parramore Island and the first field tests in the United States began in August, 1990 (Gershon, 1990; Rupprecht et al, 1992b).

The major objective of this initial field trial was to evaluate the relative safety of the V-RG vaccine in a relatively controlled island setting, with a limited, but readily live-trapped, free-ranging animal population (Rupprecht et al, 1992b). In this trial, a majority of raccoons in the area (80%) consumed the vaccine-laden baits. Over 800 live-trapped raccoons and nearly 600 live-trapped small mammals were evaluated for evidence of vaccine-induced pathology. None was found. A large percentage of live-trapped raccoons developed serum neutralizing antibodies against the rabies virus. More than a dozen immunized raccoons were captured and subjected to lethal challenge with rabies virus seven months later. All survived the challenge (Rupprecht, 1992; Hanlon et al, 1993).

A mainland site in Sullivan County, Pennsylvania was selected for a second field trial. This site was seleced so as to mimic the complex ecosystem in which the V-RG vaccine would be expected to operate. The objective of this study was to evaluate consumption and safety of the V-RG vaccine in nontarget species (Rupprecht et al, 1992b). No lesions suggestive of vaccine-induced disease were evident in any of the subjects which consumed the vaccine.

Possible strategies that may be employed in the application of oral vaccines will depend on the particular reason for the program (Centers for Disease Control, 1991b). These might include the elimination of rabies, prevention of its introduction into a particular region, or reduction of the number of rabid animals already present in an enzootic area. The latest field trial has recently begun in the Cape May Peninsula of New Jersey. This study will be the first attempt to prevent a raccoon epizootic from moving into an uninfected area (Rupprecht, 1992).

Still in its infancy, the fate of widespread oral

immunization of wildlife in the United States remains uncertain. Rupprecht et al (1992b) stated,

> *Currently, the United States is the only major developed country with endemic terrestrial rabies, the bio-technological capacity to control the disease in wildlife, but no coordinated national control policy in place.*

Possibility of Immunizing Bats Against Rabies

Effective immunization probably requires targeting at least 70% to 80% of a wild population. Annual immunization of bats across North America is probably not particularly feasible. An effective delivery system might involve aerosol immunization of hibernating populations, if an efficacious vaccine not harmful to humans or other nontarget species can be formulated. On the other hand, if bats could be attracted to certain sounds, this might prove helpful in development of a feeding/immunization station using an orally effective insect-borne vaccine, if one could be developed for use in bats. However, the difficulties in development and implementation of such programs may be insurmountable.

There have been very few published reports of vaccine efficacy in bats. Thomas et al (1989) reported that a recombinant rabies vaccine (VVTGgRAB 26 D 3 187 XP) induced production of rabies-neutralizing antibodies in 2 of 7 specimens of *Myotis daubentoni* housed at 25° C (77° F), but not in those housed at 4° C (39° F). This preliminary work suggests that immunization of a hibernating population of bats may be difficult, although individual studies should be carried out at the hibernaculum temperature of a particular targeted population. Kwiecinski et al (1993) reported that big brown bats as well as the tropical, Jamaican fruit bat, maintained at 25° C mounted both primary and secondary immune responses to intramuscular inoculation with an inactivated PM strain of rabies virus. No challenge studies were done.

Successful immunization of bats may be possible if an efficacious nonpathogenic recombinant vector can be found, particularly if it will transmit an appropriate gene product both horizontally and vertically. This might obviate the need for annual immunizations.

The degree to which such a program should be considered depends upon several factors, some of which include:

1) The significance attributed to rabies transmission from bats to humans.
2) The significance attributed to rabies transmission from bats to animals, both wild and domestic.
3) Concern for conservation of bat populations and the perception of what such an immunization program might convey to the public.
4) The cost involved.
5) The relative risk involved.
6) The likelihood of success.
7) The potential value that might actually derive from a successful program.

At a recent World Health Organization seminar (Geneva, Switzerland) focusing on the control of rabies in wildlife, recommendations were made for development of new vaccines that could be used to immunize bats against rabies (Muller, 1990). In its latest report, the Expert Committee on Rabies also recognized a need for further studies on the feasibility of mass immunization of bats (World Health Organization, 1992) and, at a recent Canadian meeting discussing control of rabies in the Americas, it was suggested that development of oral vaccines for immunization of vampire bats be investigated (Charlton, 1992). CNEVA (1990) reported that effective immunization of wild bat populations in Europe is probably not practical without a collaborative effort by many experts.

Eradication of rabies from terrestrial wildlife has been very successful in many European countries that have implemented such control programs. Nevertheless, some researchers have expressed the view that attempts to immunize terrestrial wildlife (let alone, bats) against rabies are inappropriate. For example, Bruggemann (1992), a staff scientist for the National Audubon Society, stated,

> *It is ironic that in the United States, where*

rabies is effectively controlled and the risk of rabies is extremely low, additional rabies control is accepted as necessary. It appears that in an affluent society, fear of rabies rather than actual risk has created the necessary market for new rabies control technologies. Developing countries where the risk of rabies is high, have limited resources, many other serious health problems to address, and offer no such market.

With exception of the special case of vampire bats in Latin America, modern scientific evidence is overwhelming in its support of the belief that the public-health hazards posed by bat rabies are extremely small. Even so, the public may not readily relinquish long-held fears. By functioning in a prophylactic capacity, such an immunization program might prove useful in helping to defuse public fears. Of course, the essentially preventative nature of this type of program would have to be stressed, lest bat rabies be mistakenly emphasized to the public. Such a program is certainly preferable to decimation of bat populations, which has been suggested by some. According to the National Association of State Public Health Veterinarians (1992, 1993, 1994), control of bat rabies by areawide depopulation efforts is neither practical nor desirable.

Amelioration of public fear of insectivorous bats is one of the primary purposes that an immunization program targeting bats would serve. It is, however, difficult to determine whether the public would perceive such a program as an attempt to help safeguard valuable natural resources (i.e., bat populations) or as support of deep-rooted cultural phobias. Public-health authorities and conservation organizations would need to carefully assess the potential ramifications of a bat-immunization program. Whether, in the long run, such a program would prove beneficial to bat populations, or needlessly spend taxpayer dollars, is unknown.

Implementation of a bat-immunization program would hopefully reduce the number of rabies-positive findings in cases of bat/human interactions. In the eventuality that a bat is not recovered, or is in a condition unsuitable for testing, an assumption of positivity would still be necessary in medical decision making.

References

Altman, L. (1993). Scientists debate destroying the last strains of smallpox. *The New York Times*. August 30: A1

Anderson, R. M. (1986). Vaccination of wildlife reservoirs. *Nature*. 322: 304

Anderson, R. M. (1991). Immunization in the field. *Nature*. 354(19): 502

Arita, I. and F. Fenner (1985). Complications of Smallpox Vaccination. In G. V. Quinnan, Jr. (ed.) *Vaccinia Viruses as Vectors for Vaccine Antigens*. Elsevior Science Publishing Co., Inc. New York.

Artois, M., Chillaud, T., Maillot, E., Rigal, P., and J. Blancou (1987). Premiere campagne de vaccination antirabique du renard par voie orale menee en France. *Ann. de Medecine Veterinaire*. 131: 457

Artois, M., Charlton, K. M., Tolson, N. D., Casey G. A., Knowles, M. K., and J. D. Campbell (1990). Vaccinia recombinant virus expressing the rabies virus glycoprotein: Safety and efficacy trials in Canadian wildlife. *Can. J. Vet. Res*. 54(4): 504

Artois, M., Guittre, C., Thomas, I., Leblois, H., Brochier, B., and J. Barrat (1992). Potential pathogenicity for rodents of vaccines intended for oral vaccination against rabies: A comparison. *Vaccine*. 10(8): 524

Bachmann, P., Bramwell, R. N., Fraser, S. J., Gilmore, D. A., Johnston, D. H., Lawson, K. F., MacInnes, C. D., Matejka, F. O., Miles, H. E., Pedde, M. A., and D. R. Voight (1990). Wild carnivore acceptance of baits for delivery of liquid rabies vaccine. *J. Wildl. Dis*. 26(4): 486

Baer, G. M. (1988). Oral rabies vaccination: An overview. *Rev. Infect. Dis*. 10(Suppl. 4): S644

Baer, G. M., Abelseth, M. K., and J. G. Debbie (1971). Oral vaccination of foxes against rabies. *Am. J. Epidemiol*. 93(6): 487

Baer, G. M., Broderson, J. R., and P. A. Yager (1975). Determination of the site of oral rabies vaccination. *Am. J. Epidemiol*. 101(2): 160

Beck, A. J. (1962). Letter to the editor. *Bat Banding News*. 3(4): 30

Blancou, J., Kieny, M. P., Lathe, R., Lecocq, J. P., Pastoret, P.-P., Soulebos, J. P., and P. Desmettre (1986). Oral vaccination of the fox against rabies using a live recombinant vaccinia virus. *Nature*. 322: 373

Bracci, L., Antoni, G., Cuis, M. G., Lozzi, L., Niccolai, N., Petreni, S., Rustici, M., Santucci, A., Soldani, P., Valensin, P. E., and P. Neri (1988). Antipeptide monoclonal antibodies inhibit the binding of rabies virus glycoprotein and alpha-bungarotoxin to the nicotinic acetylcholine receptor. *Molec. Immunol*. 25(9): 881

Brochier, B. M., Languet, B., Blancou, J., Kieny, M.

P., Lecocq, J. P., Costy, F., Desmettre, P., and P.-P. Pastoret (1988). Use of recombinant vaccinia-rabies virus for oral vaccination of fox cubs (*Vulpes vulpes*, L.) against rabies. *Vet. Microbiol.* 18: 103

Brochier, B. M., Kieny, M. P., Costy, F., Coppens, P., Bauduin, B., Lecocq, J. P., Languet, B., Chappuis, G., Desmettre, P., Aliademanyo, K., Libois, R., and P.-P. Pastoret (1991). Large-scale eradication of rabies using recombinant vaccinia-rabies vaccine. *Nature.* 354(6354): 520

Bruggemann, E. P. (1992). Rabies in the mid-Atlantic states—Should raccoons be vaccinated? *Bio-Science.* 42(9): 694

Cadoz, M., Strady, A., Meignier, B., Taylor, J., Tartaglia, J., Paoletti, E., and S. Plotkin (1992). Immunisation with canarypox virus expressing rabies glycoprotein. *The Lancet.* 339(8807): 1429

Centers for Disease Control (1991a). Recommendations of the Immunization Practices Advisory Committee (ACIP). Vaccinia (Smallpox) Vaccine. *MMWR.* 40(No. RR-14): 1

Centers for Disease Control (1991b). CDC editorial note. *J. Am. Med. Assoc.* 265(11): 1365

Charlton, K. M. (1992). Report of the meeting "Control of Rabies in the Americas." Animal Diseases Research Institute. September 11-13, 1991. *Can. Vet. J.* 33: 98

Charlton, K. M., Artois, M., Prevec, L., Campbell, J. B., Casey, G. A., Wandeler, A. I., and J. Armstrong (1992). Oral rabies vaccination of skunks and foxes with a recombinant human adenovirus vaccine. *Arch. Virol.* 123: 169

Cheston, W. (1989). Rabies vaccine trials. *Science.* 245(4919): 692

CNEVA (1990). *Les Chiropteres et La Rage en Europe.* Centre National D'Etudes Veterinaires et Alimentaires. Republique Francaise. Ministere de L'Agriculture et de La Foret.

Cordes, C. (1988). NIH urged to extend gene guidelines to tests abroad. *Chronic. Higher Educ.* February 10: A7

Cox, J. H., Dietzschold, B., and L. G. Schneider (1977). Rabies virus glycoprotein. II. Biological and serological characterization. *Infect. Immun.* 16: 754

Coyne, M. J., Smith, G., and F. E. McAllister (1989). Mathematic model for the population biology of rabies in raccoons in the mid-Atlantic states. *Am. J. Vet. Res.* 50(12): 2148

Crawford, M. (1987). NIH finds Argentine experiment did not break U. S. biotechnology rules. *Science.* 235(4786): 276

Crawford, M. (1988). Wistar proposes U. S. test of rabies vaccine. *Science.* 240(4854): 877

Debbie, J. G., Abelseth, M. K., and G. M. Baer (1972). The use of commercially available vaccines for the oral vaccination of foxes against rabies. *Am. J. Epidemiol.* 96(3): 231

Desmettre, P., Languet, B., Chappuis, G., Brochier, B., Thomas, I., Lecocq, J.-P., Kieny, M.-P., Blancou, J., Aubert, M., Artois, M., and P.-P. Pastoret (1990). Use of vaccinia rabies recombinant for oral vaccination of wildlife. *Vet. Microbiol.* 23: 227

Dietzschold, B., Wiktor, T. J., and H. Koprowski (1985). Induction of Virus Neutralizing Antibodies and Protection Against Rabies Using a Vaccinia Rabies Glycoprotein Recombinant. In G. V. Quinnan, Jr. (ed.) *Vaccinia Viruses as Vectors for Vaccine Antigens.* Elsevior Science Publishing Co., Inc. New York.

Dumbell, K. R. (1985). Aspects of the Biology of the Orthopoxviruses Relevant to the Use of Recombinant Vaccinias as Field Vaccines. In G. V. Quinnan, Jr. (ed.) *Vaccinia Viruses as Vectors for Vaccine Antigens.* Elsevior Science Publishing Co., Inc. New York.

Editorial (1988). Argentina reported upset by vaccine test. *New York Times.* February 4: B13

Esposito, J. J., Knight, J. C., Shaddock, J. H., Novembre, F. J., and G. M. Baer (1988). Successful oral vaccination of raccoons with raccoon poxvirus recombinants expressing rabies virus glycoprotein. *Virology.* 165: 313

Fedaku, M., Shaddock, J. H., Sumner, J. W., Sanderlin, D. W., Knight, J. C., Esposito, J., and G. M. Baer (1991). Oral vaccination of skunks with raccoon poxvirus recombinants expressing the rabies glycoprotein or the nucleoprotein. *J. Wildl. Dis.* 27(4): 681

Ferguson, M. (1991). Progress towards rabies control. *Trends in Biotech.* 9: 7

Flamand, A., Coulon, P., Lafay, F., Kappeler, A., Artois, M., Aubert, M., Blancou, J., and A. I. Wandeler (1992). Eradication of rabies in Europe. *Nature.* 360(6400): 115

Fox, J. L. (1989). Wistar frustrated over rabies test plans. *Biotechnology.* 7(6): 541

Frisch, R., Wolff, F., and A. Krier (1988). Oral Vaccination of Foxes in the Grand-Duchy of Luxembourg. In P.-P. Pastoret, B. Brochier, I. Thomas, and J. Blancou (eds.) *Vaccination to Control Rabies in Foxes.* Commission of the European Communities EUR 11 439. Office for Official Publications of the European Communities. Luxembourg.

Fu, Z. F., Dietzschold, B., Schumacher, C. L., Wunner, W. H., Ertl, H. C. J., and H. Koprowski (1991). Rabies virus nucleoprotein expressed in and purified from insect cells is efficacious as a vaccine. *Proc. Natl. Acad. Sci.* USA. 88(5): 2001

Fu, Z. F., Rupprecht, C. E., Dietzschold, B., Saikumar, P., Niu, H. S., Babka, I., Wunner, W. H., and H. Koprowski (1993). Oral vaccination of raccoons (*Procyon lotor*) with baculovirus-expressed rabies virus glycoprotein. *Vaccine*. 11(9): 925

Gershon, D. (1990). Better late than never for start of tests. *Nature*. 346: 785

Greenhall, A. M. (1985). Effects of Vampire Bats and Paralytic Rabies on Livestock Production. In S. M. Gaafar, W. E. Howard, and R. E. Marsh (eds.) World Animal Science B2-Disciplinary Approach. *Parasites, Pests, and Predators*. Elsevior Science Publishing Co., Inc. New York.

Hadidian, J., Jenkins, S. R., Johnston, D. H., Savarie, P. J., Nettles, V. F., Manski, D., and G. M. Baer (1989). Acceptance of simulated oral rabies vaccine baits by urban raccoons. *J. Wildl. Dis.* 25(1): 1

Hanlon, C. A., Buchanan, J. R., Nelson, E., Niu, H. S., Diehl, D., and C. E. Rupprecht (1993). A vaccinia-vectored rabies vaccine field trial: Ante- and post-mortem biomarkers. *Rev. Sci. Tech. Off. Int. Epiz.* 12(1): 99

Johnston, D. H. and D. R. Voight (1982). A baiting system for the oral rabies vaccination of wild foxes and skunks. *Comp. Immunol. Microbiol. Infect. Dis.* 5(1-3): 185

Kalicharran, K. K., Springthorpe, V. S., and S. A. Sattar (1992). Studies on the stability of a human adenovirus-rabies recombinant vaccine. *Can. J. Vet. Res.* 56(1): 28

Kappeler, A., Wandeler, A., and S. Capt (1988). Ten Years of Rabies Control by Oral Vaccination of Foxes in Switzerland. In P.-P. Pastoret, B. Brochier, I. Thomas, and J. Blancou (eds.) *Vaccination to Control Rabies in Foxes*. Commission of the European Communities EUR 11 439. Office for Official Publications of the European Communities. Luxembourg.

Karzon, D. T. (1985). Considerations of Safety, Efficacy and Potential Applications of Vaccinia Vectors for Immunoprophylaxis: An Alternative Approach for Control of Human Diseases for Which Vaccines are Available. In G. V. Quinnan, Jr. (ed.) *Vaccinia Viruses as Vectors for Vaccine Antigens*. Elsevior Science Publishing Co., Inc. New York.

Kieny, M. P., Lathe, R., Drillien, R., Spehner, D., Skory, S., Schmitt, D., Wiktor, T., Koprowski, H., and J. P. Lecocq (1984). Expression of rabies virus glycoprotein from a recombinant vaccinia virus. *Nature*. 312: 1363

Kwiecinski, G. G., Murphy, D. J., and C. E. Rupprecht (1993). An enzyme linked immunosorbant assay for detection of rabies specific IgG in bats. *23rd Annual North American Symposium on Bat Research.* Gainesville, Florida. October, 1993

le Blois, H., Tuffereau, C., Blancou, J., Artois, M., Aubert, A., and A. Flammand (1990). Oral immunization of foxes with avirulent rabies virus mutants. *Vet. Microbiol.* 23: 259

Linhart, S. B. (1993). Some factors affecting the oral rabies vaccination of free-ranging carnivores. *Rev. Sci. Tech. Off. Int. Epiz.* 12(1): 109

Linhart, S. B., Blom, F. S., Dasch, G. J., Roberts, J. D., Engerman, R. M., Esposito, J. J., Shaddock, J. H., and G. M. Baer (1991). Formulation and evaluation of baits for oral rabies vaccination of raccoons (*Procyon lotor*). *J. Wildl. Dis.* 27(1): 21

Lodmell, D. L., Sumner, J. W., Esposito, J. J., Bellini, W. J., and L. C. Ewalt (1991). Raccoon poxvirus recombinants expressing the rabies virus nucleoprotein protect mice against lethal rabies virus infection. *J. Virol.* 65(6): 3400

Lodmell, D. L., Esposito, J. J., and L. C. Ewalt (1993). Rabies virus antinucleoprotein antibody protects against rabies virus challenge in vivo and inhibits rabies replication in vitro. *J. Virol.* 67(10): 6080

MacInnes, C. D., Tinline, D. R., Voight, D. R., Broekhoven, L. H., and R. C. Rosatte (1988). Planning for rabies control in Ontario. *Rev. Infect. Dis.* 10(Suppl. 4): S665

Muller, W. W. (1990). Report on seminar of wildlife rabies control, July 2-5, 1990. Geneva, Switzerland. *Rabies Bulletin Europe*. Information Surveillance Research. World Health Organization Collaborating Centre for Rabies Surveillance and Research. Tubingen, Federal Republic of Germany. 3/90: 11

Muller, W. W. and J. Blancou (1992). Rabies in Europe: Now possible to confine and eliminate. *Br. Med. J.* 305: 725

Murphy, F. A. (1985). Considerations of Safety, Efficacy and Potential of Vaccinia Vectored Vaccines for Immunoprophylaxis Against Animal Diseases. In G. V. Quinnan, Jr. (ed.) *Vaccinia Viruses as Vectors for Vaccine Antigens*. Elsevior Science Publishing Co., Inc. New York.

National Association of State Public Health Veterinarians (1992). Compendium of Animal Rabies Control. *J. Am. Vet. Med. Assoc.* 200(2): 145

National Association of State Public Health Veterinarians (1993). Compendium of Animal Rabies Control. *J. Am. Vet. Med. Assoc.* 202(2): 199

National Association of State Public Health Veterinarians (1994). Compendium of Animal Rabies Control. *J. Am. Vet. Med. Assoc.* 204(2): 173

Neff, J. M. (1985). Vaccinia Virus Vaccines: Virulence and Attenuation of Vaccinia Strain Variation. In G. V. Quinnan, Jr. (ed.) *Vaccinia Viruses as Vectors for Vaccine Antigens*. Elsevior Science Publishing Co., Inc. New York.

Panicali, D., Davis, S. W., Weinberg, R. L., and E. Paoletti (1983). Construction of live vaccines using genetically engineered poxviruses: Biological activity of recombinant vaccinia virus expressing influenza virus hemagglutinin. *Proc. Natl. Acad. Sci.*, USA. 80: 5364

Paoletti, E., Lipinskas, B. R., Samsonoff, C., Mercer,

S., and D. Panicali (1984). Construction of live vaccines using genetically engineered poxviruses: Biological activity of vaccinia virus recombinants expressing the hepatitis B virus surface antigen and the herpes simplex virus glycoprotein. *Proc. Natl. Acad. Sci.*, USA. 81: 193

Paoletti, E., Perkus, M. E., Piccini, A., Wos, S., and B. R. Lipinskas (1985). Vaccinia Vectored Vaccines. In G. V. Quinnan, Jr. (ed.) *Vaccinia Viruses as Vectors for Vaccine Antigens.* Elsevior Science Publishing Co., Inc. New York.

Pastoret, P.-P. and B. Brochier (1992). Development of a recombinant vaccinia-rabies vaccine for oral vaccination of foxes against rabies. *Dev. Biol. Stand.* 79: 105

Pastoret, P.-P., Frisch, R., Blancou, J., Wolff, F., Brochier, B., and L. G. Schneider (1987). Campaigne internationale de vaccination antirabique du renard par voie orale menee au grandduche de Luxembourg, en Belgique et en France. *Ann. de Medicine Veterinaire.* 131: 441

Pastoret, P.-P., Brochier, B., Languet, B., Thomas, I., Paquot, A., Bauduin, B., Kieny, M. P., Lecocq, J. P., De Bruyn, J., Costy, F., Antoine, H., and Ph. Desmettre (1988). First field trial of fox vaccination against rabies using a vaccinia-rabies recombinant virus. *Vet. Rec.* 123: 481

Petkevicius, S. (1993). Oral vaccination of wild animals against rabies as practiced in Lithuania. *Rabies Bulletin Europe.* Information Surveillance Research. WHO Collaborating Centre for Rabies Surveillance and Research. Tubingen, Federal Republic of Germany. 1/93: 10

Quinnan, Jr., G. V. (1985). Special Safety Concerns. In G. V. Quinnan, Jr. (ed.) *Vaccinia Viruses as Vectors for Vaccine Antigens.* Elsevior Science Publishing Co., Inc. New York.

Rosatte, R. C. (1987). Advances in rabies research and control: Applications for the wildlife professional. *Wildl. Soc. Bull.* 15: 504

Rosatte, R. C., Howard, D. R., Campbell, J. B., and C. D. MacInnes (1990). Intramuscular vaccination of skunks and raccoons against rabies. *J. Wildl. Dis.* 26(2): 225

Rosatte, R. C., Power, M. J., MacInnes, C. D., and J. B. Campbell (1992). Trap-vaccinate-release and oral vaccination for rabies control in urban skunks, raccoons and foxes. *J. Wildl. Dis.* 28(4): 562

Rossate, R. C., MacInnes, C. D., Power, M. J., Johnston, D. H., Bachmann, P., Nunan, C. P., Wannop, C., Pedde, M., and L. Calder (1993). Tactics for the control of wildlife rabies in Ontario (Canada). *Rev. Sci. Tech. Off. Int. Epiz.* 12(1): 95

Rupprecht, C. E. (1992). Associate Professor. Department of Microbiology and Immunology, Center for Neurovirology, Thomas Jefferson University, Jefferson Medical College. Philadelphia, Pennsylvania. Personal communication.

Rupprecht, C. E., Wiktor, T. J., Johnston, D. H., Hamir, A. N., Dietzschold, B., Wunner, W. H., Glickman, L. T., and H. Koprowski (1986). Oral immunization and protection of raccoons (*Procyon lotor*) with a vaccinia-rabies glycoprotein recombinant virus vaccine. *Proc. Natl. Acad. Sci.* 83: 7947

Rupprecht, C. E., Dietzschold, B., Koprowski, H., and D. H. Johnston (1987). Development of an oral wildlife rabies vaccine: Immunization of raccoons by a vaccinia-rabies glycoprotein recombinant virus and preliminary field baiting trials. *Vaccines 87.* Cold Spring Harbor Laboratory: 389

Rupprecht, C. E., Charlton, K. M., Artois, M., Casey, G. A., Webster, W. A., Campbell, J. B., Lawson, K. F., and L. G. Schneider (1990). Ineffectiveness and comparative pathogenicity of attenuated rabies virus vaccines for the striped skunk (*Mephitis mephitis*). *J. Wildl. Dis.* 26(1): 99

Rupprecht, C. E., Dietzschold, B., Campbell, J. B., Charlton, K. M., and H. Koprowski (1992a). Consideration of inactivated rabies vaccines as oral immunogens of wild carnivores. *J. Wildl. Dis.* 28(4): 629

Rupprecht, C. E., Hanlon, C. A., Koprowski, H., and A. N. Hamir (1992b). Oral wildlife rabies vaccination: Development of a recombinant virus vaccine. *Trans. 57th N. A. Wildl. and Nat. Res. Conf:* 439

Schneider, L. and J. Cox (1988). Eradication of Rabies Through Oral Vaccination. The German Field Trial. In P.-P. Pastoret, B. Brochier, I. Thomas, and J. Blancou (eds.) *Vaccination to Control Rabies in Foxes.* Commission of the European Communities EUR 11 439. Office for Official Publications of the European Communities. Luxembourg.

Sikes, R. K., Cleary, W. F., Koprowski, H., Wiktor, T. J., and M. M. Kaplan (1971). Effective protection of monkeys against death from street virus by post-exposure administration of tissue culture rabies vaccine. *Bull. Wld. Hlth. Org.* 45: 1

Steck, F., Wandeler, A., Bichsel, P., Capt, S., and L. Schneider (1982). Oral immunisation of foxes against rabies: A field study. *Zentralblatt fur Veterinarmedizin B.* 29: 372

Sumner, J. W., Fedaku, M., Shaddock, J. H., Esposito, J. J., and W. J. Bellini (1991). Protection of mice with vaccinia virus recombinants that express the rabies nucleoprotein. *Virology.* 183(2): 703

Sun, M. (1989a). South Carolina blocks test of rabies vaccine. *Science.* 244(4912): 1535

Sun, M. (1989b). Virginia OKs rabies vaccine test. *Science.* 245(4914): 126

Sussman, M., Collins, C. H., Skinner, F. A., and D. E. Stewart-Tull (1988). *Proceedings of the First International Conference on the Release of Geneti-*

cally Engineered Microorganisms. Academic Press. New York.

Thomas, I., Brouchier, B., Bauduin, B., Costy, F., Gilson, R., Fairon, J., and P.-P. Pastoret (1989). La rage des chauves-souris en Europe. *Ann. Med. Vet.* 133: 437

Tolson, N. D., Charlton, K. M., Casey, G. A., Knowles, M. K., Rupprecht, C. E., Lawson, K. F., and J. B. Campbell (1988). Immunization of foxes against rabies with a vaccinia recombinant virus expressing the rabies glycoprotein. *Arch. Virol.* 102: 297

Tordo, N., Bourhy, H., Sather, S., and R. Ollo (1993). Structure and expression in baculovirus of the Mokola virus glycoprotein: An efficient recombinant vaccine. *Virology.* 194: 59

Uhaa, I. J., Dato, V. M., Sorhage, F. E., Beckley, J. W., Roscoe, D. E., Gorsky, R. D., and D. B. Fishbein (1992). Benefits and costs of using an orally absorbed vaccine to control rabies in raccoons. *J. Am. Vet. Med. Assoc.* 201(12): 1873

Wandeler, A. I. and G. A. Casey (1993). Rabies diagnoses in eastern Canada, January 1, 1992 - June 30, 1992. Cross-Canada Disease Report. *Can. Vet. J.* 34: 123

Wandeler, A. I., Capt, S., Kappeler, A., and R. Hauser (1988). Oral immunization of wildlife against rabies: Concept and first field experiments. *Rev. Infect. Dis.* 10(Suppl. 4): S649

Wiktor, T. J., Macfarlan, R. I., Reagan, K. J., Dietzschold, B., Curtis, P. J., Wunner, W. H., Kieny, M. P., Lathe, R., Lecocq, J. P., Mackett, M., Moss, B., and H. Koprowski (1984). Protection from rabies by a vaccinia virus recombinant containing the rabies virus glycoprotein gene. *Proc. Natl. Acad. Sci.* 81: 7194

Wilhelm, U. and L. G. Schneider (1990). Oral immunization against rabies: Practical experiences of a field trial in the Federal Republic of Germany. *Bull. Wld. Hlth. Org.* 68(1): 87

Winkler, W. G. and K. Bogel (1992). Control of rabies in wildlife. *Sci. Am.* 266(6): 86

Wokatsch, R. (1972). Vaccinia Virus. In M. Majer and S. A. Plotkin (eds.) *Strains of Human Viruses.* S. Karger. New York.

World Health Organization (1980). Declaration of global eradication of smallpox. *Wkly. Epidemiol. Rec.* 55: 145

World Health Organization (1992). *Expert Committee on Rabies. Eighth Report.* WHO Tech. Rpt. No. 824. Geneva.

Yilma, T., Mackett, M., Rose, J. K., and B. Moss (1985). Vaccinia Virus Recombinants Expressing Vesicular Stomatitis Genes Immunize Mice and Cattle. In G. V. Quinnan, Jr. (ed.) *Vaccinia Viruses as Vectors for Vaccine Antigens.* Elsevior Science Publishing Co., Inc. New York.

SECTION IV

Rabies Infection in Old World Bats

Chapter 22:
RABIES AND THE RABIES-RELATED VIRUSES OF AFRICA

The Lyssavirus Genus

The family Rhabdoviridae contains two major genera, *Vesiculovirus* and *Lyssavirus*. The genus *Lyssavirus* comprises the various field strains of rabies virus (serotype 1) and a number of serologically related viruses (serotypes 2 through 5) that may produce neurological disease in humans or animals and which have no specific vaccines available against them. Classical rabies virus, Lagos bat virus, Mokola virus, Duvenhage virus, and the European bat lyssaviruses constitute the rabies subgroup of the genus *Lyssavirus*. Prior to the identification of the European bat lyssaviruses, rabies-related viruses were believed to be restricted in their distribution to sub-Saharan Africa.

Lagos bat, Duvenhage, and Mokola viruses are widely recognized as the rabies-related viruses of sub-Saharan Africa. They share certain antigenic characteristics with classical rabies virus, but can be distinguished from rabies virus, from European bat lyssavirus, and from each other, by serologic or genetic analyses.

Lagos bat and Duvenhage viruses have been isolated from various bats and may be enzootic in certain African bat populations. However, because of the very limited number of rabies-related isolates from Africa, it is not possible, at this time, to confidently ascribe a particular reactivity pattern to a given host species of bat, as can be done for nonterrestrial isolates of rabies virus elsewhere.

The rabies-related viruses of Africa are widely distributed (Table 22-1). Their public-health significance, however, is not fully known. In view of their widespread distribution throughout Africa, cases of human and animal infection with these viruses may be more frequent than reported (Mebatsion et al, 1992). These authors stressed that the rabies-related viruses may represent a potentially significant public-health concern in sub-Saharan Africa, worsened by the difficulty in diagnosis and the possible lack of efficacious vaccines. Their public-health significance, however, is minor compared to that posed by classical rabies viruses of serotype 1.

Importation of rabies-related viruses from the African continent is considered a potential, albeit small, hazard (World Health Organization, 1984, 1992). Pets of people vacationing in Africa might conceivably become infected with a rabies-related virus via interaction with local wildlife. African wildlife destined for zoos or research facilities may also harbor one of these viruses and can potentially carry it to another country, or even continent.

In view of the discovery of multiple rabies-related viruses in Africa, Shope and Tignor (1971) suggested that the ancestral viral strain of the *Lyssavirus* genus originated there. In evolving into a neuropathic form, the rabies virus (serotype 1) induced an infected individual to propagate transmission via bite. This helped to insure its subsequent dispersal worldwide. The remaining viruses (Lagos bat, Mokola, and Duvenhage) are believed to have largely remained in Africa, representing "nontransported evolution of the ancestral virus." Of the various members of the genus *Lyssavirus*, only classical rabies virus of serotype 1 has attained a global distribution.

The source and extent of rabies-related viruses in Africa is not known. Bats may be reservoirs of Duvenhage and Lagos bat viruses and shrews or rodents may be reservoirs of Mokola virus (Schneider et al, 1985a, 1985b), but verification awaits further investigation.

Major outbreaks of rabies, such as the epizo-

Table 22-1

Isolation of Rabies-Related Viruses From Africa, by Location, Year, and Species

Location	Year	Species	Virus	Reference
Lagos Island, Nigeria	1956	Bat (*Eidolon helvum*)[a]	Lagos Bat	Boulger and Porterfield, 1958
Ibadan, Nigeria	1968-69	*Crocidura* sp.[b]	Mokola	Shope et al, 1970
Ibadan, Nigeria	1968	Human	Mokola[c]	Familusi and Moore, 1972
Transvaal, South Africa	1970	Human	Duvenhage	Meredith et al, 1971
Natal Province, South Africa	1970	Cat	Lagos Bat[d]	Schneider et al, 1983
Ibadan, Nigeria	1971	Human	Mokola	Familusi et al, 1972
Yaunde, Cameroon	1974	*Crocidura* sp.	Mokola	Le Gonidec et al, 1978
Bozo, Central African Republic	1974	Bat (*Micropteropus pusillus*[e])	Lagos Bat	Sureau et al, 1977
Natal Province, South Africa	1980	2 bats (species?)[f]	Lagos Bat[d]	Schneider et al, 1985a
Pinetown (Natal Province), South Africa	1980	8 Bats (*Epomophorus wahlbergi*)[g]	Lagos Bat[d]	Meredith and Standing, 1981
Transvaal, South Africa	1981	Bat (species?)	Duvenhage	Schneider et al, 1985a
Bulawayo, Zimbabwe	1981	Dog	Mokola	Foggin, 1983
Bulawayo, Zimbabwe	1981-82	5 Cats	Mokola	Foggin, 1983
Bangui, Central African Republic	1981	*Lophuromys sikapusi*[h]	Mokola	Saluzzo et al, 1984
Dakar, Senegal	1985	Bat (*Eidolon helvum*)	Lagos Bat	WHO, 1989
Kindia, Guinea	1985	Bat (*Nycteris gambiensis*)	Lagos Bat	Bussereau et al, 1988
Zimbabwe	1986	Cat	Lagos Bat	WHO, 1989
Zimbabwe	1986	Bat (*Nycteris thebaica*)[i]	Duvenhage	King and Crick, 1988
Durban (Natal Province), South Africa	1990	Bat (*Epomophorus wahlbergi*)	Lagos Bat	King and Turner, 1993
Addis Ababa, Ethiopia	1992	Cat	Mokola	Mebatsion et al, 1992
Addis Ababa, Ethiopia	1992	Dog	Lagos Bat	Mebatsion et al, 1992

[a]Straw-colored fruit bats; [b]White-toothed shrews; [c]Possible laboratory contaminant; [d]Formerly reported as Mokola virus; [e]Dwarf epauletted fruit bat; [f]Probably specimens of *Epomophorus wahlbergi* ; [g]Wahlberg's common epauletted fruit bat; [h]Harsh-furred mouse; [i]Hollow (slit)-faced bat.

otic among kudu antelope in Namibia,[1] of dogs in Gabon (West Africa), and in wildlife in northwest Zimbabwe, are not related to rabies-related viruses, but are caused by classical rabies viruses of serotype 1 (Bourhy et al, 1988; Kennedy, 1988). Fourteen isolates of rabies virus (group E isolates) from dogs in Nigeria were found to react with two anti-G monoclonal antibodies in a fashion previously observed only from isolates of North American bats or humans infected by bats (Koprowski et al, 1985; Rupprecht et al, 1991). According to Rupprecht et al (1991), "Although bats are ubiquitous in Nigeria, the rabies serotype has never been isolated from them. The possibility cannot be entirely excluded that certain viruses in group E came from an 'original' bat strain now adapted and circulating in dogs."

The various rabies and rabies-related viruses comprise five distinct antigenic groups (serotypes 1 through 5) within the genus *Lyssavirus*. Subclassification of some of these variants (particularly the European bat lyssaviruses) is currently in a state of flux. Relevant aspects of the various serotypes are as follows:

Serotype 1. The prototype strain of serotype 1 is the Challenge Virus Standard (CVS-24, originally derived from Pasteur's virus). This group includes the majority of terrestrial field viruses and laboratory strains from different parts of the world. Also included in serotype 1 are the isolates from insectivorous bats in North America and those from insectivorous, fruit-eating, and hematophagous bats in Latin America.

Serotype 2. The prototype strain of serotype 2 is the Lagos bat virus, first isolated in 1956 from pooled brains of straw-colored fruit bats (*Eidolon helvum*) from Lagos Island, Nigeria (Boulger and Porterfield, 1958). It was also isolated from an unidentified bat found ill in a garden in Pinetown, in the Natal Province of South Africa and subsequently from five common epauletted fruit bats (*Epomophorus wahlbergi*) in the same area (Meredith and Standing, 1981; Crick et al, 1982). Isolates from the epauletted fruit bats had been previously identified as Mokola virus (Schneider et al, 1985a; World Health Organization, 1989). The range of the straw-colored and epauletted fruit bats overlap, although the epizootiological significance of this is unknown.

Lagos bat virus has also been isolated from a straw-colored fruit bat in Dakar, Senegal (Lafon, unpublished data [cited by World Health Organization, 1989]); from dwarf epauletted fruit bats (*Micropteropus pusillus*) in Bozo, Central African Republic (Sureau et al, 1977, 1980 [cited by Foggin and Swanepoel, 1985]); and from the bat, *Nycteris gambiensis*, in Kindia, Guinea (Digoutte [cited by Bussereau et al, 1988]).

In 1986, Lagos bat virus was isolated from a cat in Zimbabwe and a virus isolated from a cat in Natal, South Africa in 1970, which was previously identified as Mokola virus, has since been reclassified as Lagos bat virus (Schneider et al, 1983 [cited by Foggin and Swanepoel, 1985]; World Health Organization, 1989). In East Africa, Lagos bat virus was recently isolated from a rabid dog in Addis Ababa, Ethiopia (Mebatsion et al, 1992). These findings may reflect sporadic spillover of a nonterrestrial rabies variant to terrestrial animals. Although transmission of serotype 1 rabies virus from nonhematophagous bats to dogs has only rarely been documented (see page 196), similar transmission to cats in the United States has been repeatedly demonstrated

[1]Early in 1977, an epizootic of rabies began among the kudu antelope (*Tragelaphus strepsiceros*) of Namibia (southwest Africa). Disease spread rapidly, expanding as much as 40 to 60 km per year. Clinical manifestations in affected animals included loss of fear of humans, profuse and continuous salivation, paralysis, occasional aggression, abnormal sounds, continuous tail-wagging, increased sexual activity, and licking or nibbling of both each other and other species. Infected kudu often died within 48 hours of onset of clinical signs. The kudu are very susceptible to oral transmission and virus is believed to have spread from animal to animal by transmucosal transmission. By nibbling and licking each other (and possibly by browsing on the same foliage), highly infectious saliva was transmitted to oral mucous membranes of susceptible animals. High population densities, especially during times of drought, and characteristic social behavior of the animals increased the likelihood of transmission. By 1985, more than 50,000 kudu had died of rabies. Viral isolates proved to be antigenically identical to the local canine variant and it is believed that jackals were responsible for initiating the outbreak (Hassel, 1982; Schneider, 1985; Hubschle, 1986). The outbreak appears to have stopped and the kudu population is growing again.

(see Table 16-2).

The Lagos bat virus causes a fatal rabies-like disease in fruit bats (Meredith and Standing, 1981) and numerous deaths were reported among the epauletted fruit bats during the Natal outbreak. It is also pathogenic for mice, dogs, and monkeys (Boulger and Porterfield, 1958; Tomori and David-West, 1985). Two monkeys inoculated intracerebrally with Lagos bat virus developed clinical signs within 1 to 2 weeks. Behavioral abnormalities in experimentally infected monkeys included initial aggression, progressing to unresponsiveness. These were accompanied by a progressive paralysis until death 22 days post-inoculation (Tignor et al, 1973). Clinical signs developed in only 1 of 6 monkeys inoculated intramuscularly. This monkey developed an ipsilateral non-progressive hemiparesis by the 22nd day post-inoculation. It was euthanatized 86 days after the onset of clinical signs (Tignor et al, 1973). Lagos bat virus is not known to cause disease in humans, but Percy et al (1973) suggested that it be considered a potential human pathogen.

In the only reported possible human exposure during the Natal outbreak, Meredith and Standing (1981) reported an incident involving a motorcyclist in Natal, South Africa, who was allegedly pursued and attacked by an unidentified bat. The bat was not captured. The man sustained bite wounds about one of his eyes. Post-exposure rabies prophylaxis was administered and the individual has remained well. Whether or not this was a manifestation of a furious form of rabies in an infected bat is not known. It is a common belief among the natives inhabiting Nigeria that bites by bats will result in madness and death (Aghomo et al, 1990).

Fruit bats (various species of which are widely distributed throughout Africa) may be reservoirs of Lagos bat virus; however, this remains speculative. Three subtypes of Lagos bat virus have been recognized by the Expert Committee on Rabies (World Health Organization, 1992): Lagos-bat 1 (from bats in Nigeria), Lagos-bat 2 (from bats in the Central African Republic), and Lagos-bat 3 (from a bat in Guinea and a cat in Zimbabwe). Antigenic differences among the isolates of Lagos bat virus (Figure 22-1 and Table 22-2) can be detected by monoclonal antibody analysis (King et al, 1990; King, 1991).

Serotype 3. The prototype strain of serotype 3 is the Mokola virus (Ibadan shrew virus, Ib An 27377), first isolated in 1968 from pooled viscera of white-toothed shrews of the genus *Crocidura*[2] in the district of Mokola, in Ibadan, Nigeria (Shope et al, 1970). Infected shrews developed a paralytic condition (Familusi et al, 1972). The virus has subsequently been isolated from rabid shrews in Yaunde, Cameroon (Le Gonidec et al, 1978 [cited by Foggin and Swanepoel, 1985]) and from a harsh-furred mouse (*Lophuromys sikapusi*) in Bangui, Central African Republic (Saluzzo et al, 1984; Foggin and Swanepoel, 1985; Sureau et al, 1985). The virus is also known to have caused a fatal, rabies-like disease in five cats and one dog in the Bulawayo area of Zimbabwe (Foggin 1982, 1983) and, more recently, in a cat from Addis Ababa, Ethiopia (Mebatsion et al, 1992).

Between 1950 and 1982, 79 cases of rabies were confirmed in domestic cats in Zimbabwe (Foggin, 1985). The five cases in which Mokola virus was isolated all occurred at a time when the country was in the midst of a rabies epizootic, due to breakdown of rabies control programs following the seven-year-war between government forces and nationalists (Lawrence et al, 1980). Clinical signs in the infected cats were those of dumb rabies, but some aggression had been observed, particularly when the animals had been handled. Histopathological examination of the brains of infected cats revealed an extensive viral-type meningoencephalitis. No Negri bodies were seen and no virus was isolated from the one salivary gland tested.

Mokola virus has produced fatal disease in experimentally infected dogs and monkeys (Tignor et al, 1973). Experimental infection of domestic cats with Mokola virus (via intramuscular and subcutaneous inoculation) has not been suc-

[2]The genus of shrews *Crocidura* of the family Soricidae occurs extensively throughout southern Europe, Asia, and Africa. In southern Africa, it ranges from the eastern escarpment of Zimbabwe to southwest Namibia and the Kalahari desert. The Namib desert is the only region of southwest Africa from which it has not been reported (Meester, 1963).

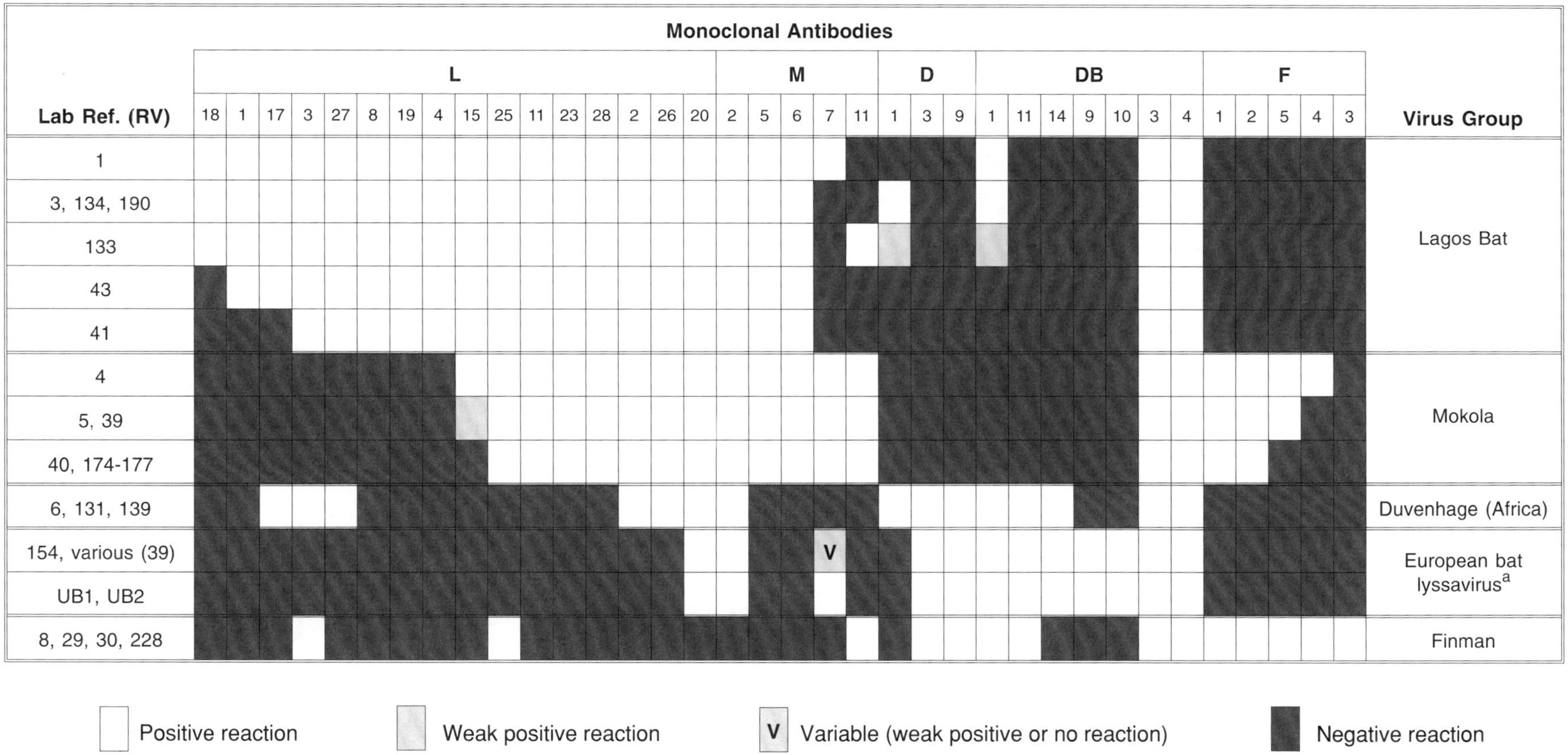

[a]Duvenhage-like (Europe)

Figure 22-1. Antigenic characterization of the rabies-related viruses. (From King, A. A. *Studies of the Antigenic Relationships of Rabies and Rabies-Related Viruses Using Anti-Nucleoprotein Monoclonal Antibodies*. Ph.D. Thesis. School of Biological Sciences, University of Surrey. Guildford, United Kingdom, 1991. Redrawn with permission.)

Table 22-2

Origin of Viral Isolates Used in Serological Studies Reported in Figure 22-1

Laboratory Reference	Geographical Location	Year of Isolation	Species Obtained From	Number Tested
		Serotype 1: Classical Rabies Viruses		
44-50	United States	-	Bats	7
108-116	Chile	-	Bats	9
156-162	Brazil	-	Bovine/Vampire	8
179	Lab. Strain	-	ERA Vaccine	1
		Serotype 2: Lagos Bat Viruses		
1	Nigeria	1956	*E. helvum*	1
3	South Africa	1983	Bat	1
134	South Africa	1982	Cat	1
190	South Africa	1980	*E. wahlbergi*	1
133	Zimbabwe	1986	Cat	1
43	Central Afr. Rep.	1974	*M. pusilus*	1
41	Senegal	1985	*E. helvum*	1
		Serotype 3: Mokola Viruses		
4	Nigeria	1968	*Crocidura sp.*	1
5	South Africa	1970	Cat	1
39	Cameroon	1971	*Crocidura sp.*	1
40	Central Afr. Rep.	1981	*L. sikapusi*	1
174-177	Zimbabwe	1981	Cats	4
		Serotype 4: Duvenhage Viruses		
6	South Africa	1970	Human	1
131	Zimbabwe	1986	Bat	1
139	South Africa	1981	Bat	1
		Serotype 5: European Bat Lyssaviruses		
8	Finland	1985	Human (Finman)	1
154	U.S.S.R.	1985	Human (Yuli)	1
29	Holland	1987	*M. dasycneme*	1
30	Holland	1987	*M. dasycneme*	1
228	Holland	1989	*M. dasycneme*	1
Various	Europe	1968-1989	Bats[a]	41

[a] Most of these bats were *Eptesicus serotinus* (serotine) bats from Denmark, France, Germany, Holland, Poland, and Spain, but three bats were of unidentified species from Germany and two (UB1 and UB2) were *Vespertilio murinus* (particolored) and *Nyctalus noctula* (noctule) bats from the Ukraine.

From King, A. A. *Studies of the Antigenic Relationships of Rabies and Rabies-Related Viruses Using Anti-Nucleoprotein Monoclonal Antibodies*. Ph.D. Thesis. School of Biological Sciences, University of Surrey. Guildford, United Kingdom, 1991. Reproduced with permission.

cessful, although one jackal and one mongoose were successfully infected. Foggin (1985) suggested that cats are relatively resistant to the virus. Regarding the five naturally occurring cases, it was postulated that they might have been exposed to high doses of virus in captured prey. However, although the cats in Zimbabwe frequently capture and play with the abundant *Crocidura* shrews, they reportedly seldom devour them. To date, the finding of Mokola-infected shrews has been reported only from Nigeria and Cameroon.

From 1950 to 1985, rabies was confirmed in 104 vaccinated dogs in Zimbabwe. Eighteen of these cases were diagnosed since 1979, when reliable tissue-culture vaccines were introduced. Foggin (1985) suggested that some of these cases may have been due to infection with a rabies-related virus. In only one of the canine cases has a confirmation of infection with Mokola virus been made. Vaccination of all dogs is required in Zimbabwe. Cat vaccination is not mandatory, but is frequently done in areas of enzootic rabies. Most countries will not allow importation of cats from Zimbabwe without evidence of prior vaccination (Foggin, 1983).

Mokola virus has been isolated from two children in Nigeria. One was a three-and-a-half-year-old girl admitted to the hospital with fever, pharyngitis, and convulsions. Diagnosed as suffering from febrile aseptic meningitis, she recovered with no apparent sequelae. Mokola virus was isolated from the child's cerebrospinal fluid (Familusi and Moore, 1972), although the possibility of laboratory contamination in this case has been raised. The second child, a six-year-old girl, presented with signs of drowsiness, fever, and paraplegia. Meningitis or encephalitis was suspected. She died 13 days after admission and Mokola virus was isolated from her brain. Postmortem examination of her brain revealed changes consistent with an encephalitis of viral origin (Familusi et al, 1972).

Mokola virus has also been isolated from the salivary glands of Nigerian shrews (*Crocidura*) and it has been suggested that the virus can be transmitted by bite (perhaps to cats which may be bitten frequently). While there was no known history of shrew bite in either of the two human cases, Kemp et al (1972) reported that Nigerian children often slept on the floor, where they might have been bitten unknowingly (especially if the incubation period was long) by one of the small night-hunting shrews. Shrews were reportedly plentiful around the homes of the two children (Familusi et al, 1972).

Dietzschold et al (1988) observed that Mokola virus may represent a potentially serious threat to human and animal health in southeast Africa. Aghomo et al (1990) reported that many Nigerian natives believe that bites from shrews will result in madness and death.

Four subtypes of Mokola virus have been recognized by the Expert Committee on Rabies (World Health Organization, 1992): Mokola 1 (from shrews and a human in Nigeria), Mokola 2 (from shrews in Cameroon), Mokola 3 (from shrews in the Central African Republic), and Mokola 5 (from dogs in Zimbabwe). Mokola virus has not been isolated from bats. Antigenic differences among the isolates of Mokola virus (Figure 22-1 and Table 22-2) can be detected by monoclonal antibody analysis (King, 1991).

Because of the limited number of Mokola isolates identified, it has been difficult to define a reservoir species for this virus in nature. To date, it has been isolated from white-toothed shrews (*Crocidura sp.*), a harsh-furred mouse, a dog, six cats, and two (one questionable) children.

Despite the fact that Mokola virus has never been isolated from any species of bat, King (1991, 1993) speculated that bats should not be ruled out as a potential reservoir species. Monoclonal antibodies (MAbs F1 through F5) prepared against a human rabies-related viral isolate ("Finman") of bat origin from a case in Finland (see page 239) recognized epitopes on viral isolates from the bat, *Myotis dasycneme*. MAbs F1, F2, F4, and F5 also recognized epitopes on isolates of the prototype variant of Mokola virus (King, 1991). In fact, these monoclonal antibodies could be used to classify isolates of Mokola virus into three distinct reactivity patterns (Figure 22-1 and Table 22-2). These antibodies have never been shown to react with serotype 1 virus of terrestrial origin. Because of the observed antigenic relationships between Mokola isolates, the human nonterrestrial isolate from Finland, and isolates from *Myotis dasycneme*, King (1991) speculated that a species of bat might yet be implicated as a reservoir of virus. If ultimately verified, King's hypothesis could account for the very limited number of isolations of this virus, reflecting the rarity with which nonterrestrial viruses are known to be transmitted to terrestrial species.

Serotype 4. The prototype strain of serotype 4 is the Duvenhage virus, first isolated in 1970 from the brain of a 31-year-old man (after whom the virus is named) who died with rabies-like signs in Transvaal, South Africa (see page 238 for additional medical details). While asleep, he had been bitten on the lip by a bat (believed to have been the insectivorous Natal clinging bat, *Miniopterus schreibersi natalensis*) one month prior to the onset of clinical signs (Meredith et al, 1971; Tignor et al, 1977). The farm where the bite occurred was situated on the main migration route for this species and located 38 km from the Sandspruit Cave, a maternity site for this bat. The farm was well within the normal foraging range of the bats (van der Merwe, 1982). This is the only reported human death from bat-induced rabies in Africa.

The bat was not tested and its role as a viral vector has remained an assumption. Experimental studies with the virus isolated from this patient have shown it to produce encephalitic disease in dogs after intracerebral, but not intramuscular or intravenous, inoculation (Fedaku et al, 1988). The virus has also been shown to be lethal for mice following intracerebral, footpad, or oral inoculation (Fedaku et al, 1988).

In 1981, Duvenhage virus was isolated from an unidentified bat (fitting the description of an insectivorous species) from Louis Trichardt town in the northern Transvaal province of South Africa (about 250 km north of the farm), lending credence to the belief that a bat exposure was responsible for the index case (Foggin and Swanepoel, 1985; Schneider et al, 1985a). The bat had been captured by a domestic cat. In trying to rescue the bat, a child was bitten or scratched by either the cat or the bat. Thus, the bat was submitted for testing. The viral isolate obtained from this bat caused a rabies-like disease, with salivary excretion of virus, in experimentally infected dogs. A third isolate of Duvenhage virus was made from a hollow-faced bat (*Nycteris thebaica*) near Bulawayo, Zimbabwe by Foggin in 1986 (King and Crick, 1988; Smith, 1991).

Three subtypes of Duvenhage virus have been recognized by the Expert Committee on Rabies (World Health Organization, 1992): Duvenhage 1 (from a human in South Africa), Duvenhage 2 (from bats in South Africa), and Duvenhage 3 (from a bat in Zimbabwe).[3] These isolates of Duvenhage virus are antigenically distinguishable from other rabies-related viruses (Figure 22-1 and Table 22-2), but not from each other (King et al, 1990; King, 1991).

Serotype 5. In recent years, Duvenhage-like viruses, collectively referred to as the European bat lyssaviruses (EBL 1 and EBL 2), have been isolated from European bat species (discussed more fully in Chapter 23). It has recently been proposed that a fifth serotype of *Lyssavirus* be established (King et al, 1990; Montano Hirose et al, 1990; World Health Organization, 1990; Bourhy et al, 1992; Caffrey, 1992). Included in serotype 5 would be isolates of European bat lyssavirus from the serotine bat (*Eptesicus serotinus*) and various other European bat species, as well as a human isolate related to bat exposure in Finland, and two from the former Soviet Union.[4] Recent studies (see Tables 23-4 and 23-5) have led to a molecular classification of the *Lyssavirus* genus.

References

Aghomo, H. O., Ako-Nai, A. K., Oduye, O. O., Tomori, O., and C. E. Rupprecht (1990). Detection of ra-

[3]Both Lagos bat (serotype 2) and Duvenhage (serotype 4) viruses have been isolated from bats in southern Africa; however, little information is available regarding the significance of bats as viral vectors in this region. In a recent survey of wild-caught bats in southern Africa, no evidence of infection with either rabies or rabies-related viruses was found in 547 bats of 13 species. Although this does not preclude the possibility of low-level enzootic disease, it does suggest that bats are not significant agents in the spread of these viruses in this region (Oelofsen and Smith, 1993).

[4]Both serotype 1 and serotype 5 viruses have been reported from bats in the former Soviet Union. Additional nonterrestrial isolates from this region should be carefully investigated.

bies virus antibodies in fruit bats (*Eidolon helvum*) from Nigeria. *J. Wildl. Dis.* 26(2): 258

Boulger, L. R. and J. S. Porterfield (1958). Isolation of a virus from Nigerian fruit bats. *Trans. Roy. Soc. Trop. Med. Hyg.* 52(5): 421

Bourhy, H., Lafon, M., Berthonneau, M. C., Renner, Y., Rollin, P. E., and P. Sureau (1988). Rabies in vaccinated dogs in Gabon. *Vet. Rec.* 122 (15): 361

Bourhy, H., Kissi, B., Lafon, M., Sacramento, D., and N. Tordo (1992). Antigenic and molecular characterization of bat rabies virus in Europe. *J. Clin. Microbiol.* 30(9): 2419

Bourhy, H., Kissi, B., and N. Tordo (1993). Molecular diversity of the *Lyssavirus* genus. *Virology.* 194(1): 70

Brown, F., Bishop, D. H. L., Crick, J., Francki, R. I. B., Holland, J. J., Hull, R., Johnson, R., Martell, G., Murphy, F. A., Obijeski, J. F., Peters, D., Pringle, C. R., Reichmann, C. R., Schneider, M. E., Shope, R. E., Simpson, D. I. H., Summers, D. F., and R. R. Wagner (1979). Rhabdoviridae. *Intervirology.* 12: 1

Bussereau, F., Vincent, J., Coudrier, D., and P. Sureau (1988). Monoclonal antibodies to Mokola virus for identification of rabies and rabies-related viruses. *J. Clin. Microbiol.* 26(12): 2489

Caffrey, J. P. (1992). Definition of the Status "Rabies Free Countries." *Report of the Meeting of the OIE Ad Hoc Group on Rabies Control.* Paris, France, April 22-23, 1992

Crick, J., Tignor, G. H., and K. Moreno (1982). A new isolate of Lagos bat virus from the Republic of South Africa. *Trans. Roy. Soc. Trop. Med. Hyg.* 76(2): 211

Dietzschold, B., Rupprecht, C. E., Tollis, M., Lafon, M., Mattei, J., Wiktor, T. J., and H. Koprowski (1988). Antigenic diversity of the glycoprotein and nucleocapsid proteins of rabies and rabies-related viruses: Implications for epidemiology and control of rabies. *Rev. Infect. Dis.* 10(Suppl. 4): S785

Familusi, J. B. and D. L. Moore (1972). Isolation of a rabies-related virus from the cerebrospinal fluid of a child with aseptic meningitis. *Afr. J. Med. Sci.* 3: 93

Familusi, J. B., Osunkoya, B. O., Moore, D. L., Kemp, G. E., and A. Fabiyi (1972). A fatal human infection with Mokola virus. *Am. J. Trop. Med.* 21(6): 959

Fedaku, M., Shaddock, J. H., Chandler, F. W., and D. W. Sanderlin (1988). Pathogenesis of rabies virus from a Danish bat (*Eptesicus serotinus*): Neuronal changes suggestive of spongiosis. *Arch. Virol.* 99: 187

Foggin, C. M. (1982). Atypical rabies virus in cats and a dog in Zimbabwe. *Vet. Rec.* 110: 338

Foggin, C. M. (1983). Mokola virus infection in cats and a dog in Zimbabwe. *Vet. Rec.* 113: 115

Foggin, C. M. (1985). Mokola Virus Infection in Domestic Cats in Zimbabwe. In E. Kuwert, C. Merieux, H. Koprowski, and K. Bogel (eds.) *Rabies in the Tropics.* Springer-Verlag. New York.

Foggin, C. M. and R. Swanepoel (1985). Rabies in Africa with Emphasis on Rabies-Related Viruses. In H. Koprowski and S. A. Plotkin (eds.) *World's Debt to Pasteur.* The Wistar Symposium Series. Vol. 3. Alan R. Liss, Inc. New York.

Frazier, C. L. and R. E. Shope (1979). Serologic Relationships of Animal Rhabdoviruses. In D. H. L. Bishop (ed.) *Rhabdoviruses.* Vol. I. CRC Press, Inc. Boca Raton, Florida.

Hassel, R. H. (1982). Incidence of rabies in Kudu in South West Africa/Namibia. *S. Afr. J. Sci.* 78: 418

Howell, P. G. (1982). Rabies and rabies-like viruses. *S. Afr. J. Sci.* 78: 409

Hubschle, O. (1986). Rabies in Kudus. *Rabies Control Symposium.* Washington, D. C. November 3-5, 1986

Kantorovich, R. A. (1957). The etiology of "madness" in polar animals. *Acta Virol.* 1: 220

Kemp, G. E., Ottis, R. C., Moore, D. L., Odelola, A., and A. Fabiyi (1972). Mokola virus: Further studies on Ib An 27377, a new rabies-related etiologic agent of zoonoses in Nigeria. *Am. J. Trop. Med. Hyg.* 21: 356

Kennedy, D. J. (1988). An outbreak of rabies in northwestern Zimbabwe 1980 to 1983. *Vet. Rec.* 122: 129

King, A. A. (1991). *Studies of the Antigenic Relationships of Rabies and Rabies-Related Viruses Using Anti-Nucleoprotein Monoclonal Antibodies.* Ph.D. Thesis. School of Biological Sciences, University of Surrey. Guildford, United Kingdom. Courtesy of Dr. Arthur A. King.

King, A. A. (1993). Rabies Reseach Leader. Central Veterinary Laboratory. New Haw, Addelstone, Surrey. United Kingdom. Personal communication.

King, A. and J. Crick (1988). Rabies-Related Viruses. In J. B. Campbell and K. M. Charlton (eds.) *Rabies.* Kluwer Academic Publications. Boston.

King, A. A. and G. S. Turner (1993). Rabies: A review. *J. Comp. Path.* 108(1): 1

King, A., Davies, P., and A. Lawrie (1990). The rabies viruses of bats. *Vet. Microbiol.* 23: 165

Koprowski, H., Wiktor, T. J., and M. K. Abelseth (1985). Cross-Reactivity and Cross-Protection: Rabies Variants and Rabies-Related Viruses. In E. Kuwert, C. Merieux, H. Koprowski, and K. Bogel (eds.) *Rabies in the Tropics.* Springer-Verlag. New York.

Lafon, M. (unpublished data). Rabies Unit. World Health Organization Collaborating Center for Rabies, Pasteur Institute. Paris, France.

Lawrence, J. A., Foggin, C. M., and R. A. I. Norval (1980). The effect of war on the control of diseases of livestock in Rhodesia (Zimbabwe). *Vet. Rec.* 107: 82

Le Gonidec, G., Rickenbach, A., Robin, Y., and G. Heme (1978). Isolement d'une souche de virus Mokola au Cameroun. *Ann. Microbiol. (Inst. Pasteur).* 129A: 245

Mebatsion, T., Cox, J. H., and J. W. Frost (1992). Isolation and characterization of 115 street rabies virus isolates from Ethiopia by using monoclonal antibodies: Identification of two isolates as Mokola and Lagos bat viruses. *J. Infect. Dis.* 166(5): 972

Meester, J. (1963). *A Systematic Revision of the Shrew Genus Crocidura in Southern Africa.* Transvaal Museum Memoir No. 13. Transvaal Museum. Pretoria.

Meredith, C. D. and E. Standing (1981). Lagos bat virus in South Africa. *The Lancet.* I(8224): 832

Meredith, C. D., Rossouw, A. P., and H. Van Praag Koch (1971). An unusual case of human rabies thought to be of chiropteran origin. *S. Afr. Med. J.* 45: 767

Montano Hirose, J. A., Bourhy H., and M. Lafon (1990). A reduced panel of anti-nucleocapsid monoclonal antibodies for bat rabies virus identification in Europe. *Res. Virol.* 141: 571

Oelofsen, M. J. and M. S. Smith (1993). Rabies and bats in a rabies-endemic area of southern Africa: Application of two commercial test kits for antigen and antibody detection. *Onderstepoort J. of Vet. Res.* 60(3): 257

Percy, D. H., Bhatt, P. N., Tignor, G. H., and R. E. Shope (1973). Experimental infection of dogs and monkeys with two rabies serogroup viruses, Lagos bat and Mokola (IbAn 27377). Gross pathologic and histopathologic changes. *Vet. Path.* 10: 534

Porterfield, J. S., Hill, D. H., and A. D. Morris (1958). Isolation of a virus from the brain of a horse with "staggers" in Nigeria. *Br. Vet. J.* 114: 425

Rupprecht, C. E., Dietzschold, B., Wunner, W. H., and H. Koprowski (1991). Antigenic Relationships of Lyssaviruses. In G. M. Baer (ed.) *The Natural History of Rabies.* 2nd Edition. CRC Press, Inc. Boca Raton, Florida.

Sacramento, D., Badrane, H., Bourhy, H., and N. Tordo (1992). Molecular epidemiology of rabies virus in France: Comparison with vaccine strains. *J. Gen. Virol.* 73: 1149

Saluzzo, J. F., Rollin, P. E., Dauguet, C., Digoutte, J. P., Georges, A. J., and P. Sureau (1984). Premier isolement du virus Mokola a partir d'un rongeur (*Lophuromys sikapusi*). *Ann. Virol.* 135E: 57

Schneider, H. P. (1985). Rabies in South West Africa/Namibia. In E. Kuwert, C. Merieux, H. Koprowski, and K. Bogel (eds.) *Rabies in the Tropics.* Springer-Verlag. New York.

Schneider, L. G., Barnard, B. J. H., and H. P. Schneider (1983). Application of Monoclonal Antibodies for Epidemiological Investigations and Oral Vaccination Studies. I. African Viruses. *Proceedings of the International Conference on Rabies in the Tropics,* Tunis. October 3-6, 1983

Schneider, L. G., Barnard, B. J. H., and H. P. Schneider (1985a). Application of Monoclonal Antibodies for Epidemiological Investigations and Oral Vaccination Studies. I. African Viruses. In E. Kuwert, C. Merieux, H. Koprowski, and K. Bogel (eds.) *Rabies in the Tropics.* Springer-Verlag. New York.

Schneider, L. G., Cox, J. H., Wandeler, A. I., Blancou, J., and S. Meyer (1985b). Application of Monoclonal Antibodies for Epidemiological Investigations and Oral Vaccination Studies. III. Oral Rabies Vaccine. In E. Kuwert, C. Merieux, H. Koprowski, and K. Bogel (eds.) *Rabies in the Tropics.* Springer-Verlag. New York.

Shope, R. E. and G. H. Tignor (1971). Rabies and Serologically-Related Viruses from Africa. In Y. Nagano and F. M. Davenport (eds.) *Rabies.* University Park Press. Baltimore.

Shope, R. E., Murphy, F. A., Harrison, A. K., Causey, O. R., Kemp, G. E., Simpson, D. I. H., and D. L. Moore (1970). Two African viruses serologically and morphologically related to rabies virus. *J. Virol.* 6: 690

Smith, J. S. (1991/1993). Research Microbiologist. Rabies Laboratory, Centers for Disease Control. Atlanta, Georgia. Personal communication.

Sureau, P., Germain, M., Herve, J.-P., Geoffroy, B., Cornet, J.-P., Heme, G., and Y. Robin (1977). Isolement du virus Lagos-bat en Empire Centrafricain. *Bull. Soc. Pathol. Exotique.* 70: 467

Sureau, P., Tignor, G. H., and A. L. Smith (1980). Antigenic characterization of the Bangui strain (ANCB-672d) of Lagos bat virus. *Ann. Virol. (Inst. Pasteur).* 131E: 25

Sureau, P., Rollin, P. E., Lafon, M., and G. Libeau (1985). Caracteristiques de Souches de Virus de Rage et de Virus Apparentes a la Rage, Isolees en Europe, Afrique, et Asie. In E. Kuwert, C. Merieux, H. Koprowski, and K. Bogel (eds.) *Rabies in the Tropics.* Springer-Verlag. New York.

Tesh, R. B., Travassos Da Rosa, A. P. A., and J. S. Travassos Da Rosa (1983). Antigenic relationships among Rhabdoviruses infecting terrestrial vertebrates. *J. Gen. Virol.* 64: 169

Thiery, G. (1959). Particularities de la rage dans l'ouest Africain. *Bull. Epiz. Dis. Africa.* 7: 265

Tignor, G. H., Shope, R. E., Bhatt, P. N., and D. H. Percy (1973). Experimental infection of dogs and monkeys with two rabies serogroup viruses, Lagos bat and Mokola (IbAn 27377): Clinical, serologic, virologic, and fluorescent-antibody studies. *J. Infect. Dis.* 128(4): 471

Tignor, G. H., Murphy, F. A., Clark, H. F., Shope, R.

E., Madore, P., Bauer, S. P., Buckley, S. M., and C. D. Meredith (1977). Duvenhage virus: Morphological, biochemical, histopathological and antigenic relationships to the rabies serogroup. *J. Gen. Virol.* 37: 595

Tomori, O. and K. B. David-West (1985). Epidemiology of Rabies in Nigeria. In E. Kuwert, C. Merieux, H. Koprowski, and K. Bogel (eds.) *Rabies in the Tropics.* Springer-Verlag. New York.

van der Merwe, M. (1982). Bats as vectors of rabies. *S. Afr. J. Sci.* 78: 421

World Health Organization (1984). Hazard of importing rabies-like viruses from Africa. *Information Circular* #15. WHO Mediterranean Zoonoses Control Centre.

World Health Organization/Veterinary Public Health (1989). *Report of the Fifth WHO Consultation on Monoclonal Antibodies in Rabies Diagnosis and Research.* Geneva. March 3, 1989. WHO/Rab. Res./ 89.33. Unpublished document (reviewed with permission).

World Health Organization/Veterinary Public Health (1990). *Report of the Sixth WHO Consultation on Monoclonal Antibodies in Rabies Diagnosis and Research.* The Wistar Institute. Philadelphia, Pennsylvania, USA. April 2-3, 1990. WHO/Rab. Res./ 90.34. Unpublished document (reviewed with permission).

World Health Organization (1992). *Expert Committee on Rabies. Eighth Report.* WHO Tech. Rpt. No. 824. Geneva.

Chapter 23: RABIES-RELATED VIRUSES FROM BATS IN EUROPE AND ASIA

Reports of Bat Rabies in Europe

Rabies in bats was first reported from Europe in 1954, when an unidentified rabid specimen was found in Hamburg, West Germany. The bat was tested because it bit the finger of a boy who picked it up. The bat died the following day. Although Negri bodies could not be identified in the bat's brain, they were plentiful in brains of mice experimentally infected with virus isolated from the bat (second passage). No viral isolates from this original specimen are currently available for serologic or genetic analysis. In 1968 and 1970, two isolates of a Duvenhage-like virus were recovered from unidentified sick bats at different locations (Stade and Hamburg), less than 90 km apart along the north shore of western Germany. This was the first apparent identification of a rabies-related virus outside of the African continent.

In the past few decades, infection of bats with a rabies-related virus has only rarely been reported from Europe (Stirbu et al, 1973; World Health Organization, 1987a). In recent years, however, reports have occurred with increasing frequency (Table 23-1). Thus, 14 positive cases were reported in Europe between 1954 and 1984, and 278 cases were reported between 1985 and 1987. As many as 4,700 bats had been examined across Europe by 1989. Between 1977 and 1992, 446 infected bats were identified throughout Europe (Muller, 1992). From 1988 to 1990, the number of reported cases ranged from 37 to 53 annually (Bourhy et al, 1992; Caffrey, 1992; Muller and Blancou, 1992). Less than two dozen cases were reported in 1991. These findings suggest that the apparent epizootic among insectivorous bats that developed (or was merely recognized) between 1985 and 1987 has declined and that the disease is now enzootic among certain European bat populations. However, they may also reflect a reduction in the number of bats investigated after 1987 (Bourhy et al, 1992; King, 1993), perhaps related to the time required for repopulation of dwindling numbers (King, 1991). Although disease was probably present in European bats for an untold period of time prior to its discovery, its seeming "increased prevalence" in recent years may, in part, be a reflection of intensified searching on the part of public-health authorities.

Rabid bats have been reported frequently from several European countries, notably Norway, Denmark, the Netherlands, the former Federal Republic of Germany (West Germany), and the former Soviet Union (Schneider, 1983; Bitsch et al, 1986; Mollgaard, 1985, 1986; Grauballe et al, 1987; Seidler et al, 1987; Veterinary Chief Inspectorate of Public Health, Netherlands, 1987, 1989, 1991; Zoffman et al, 1987; Krogsrud and Odegaard, 1988; Nieuwenhuis, 1988; Stougaard, 1986, 1989; Haagsma, 1989; Remmert et al, 1989; Schneider et al, 1989; Muller, 1990a, 1990b, 1990c; Khozinski et al, 1990; Nieuwenhuijs, 1989, 1990a, 1990b, 1990c, 1992, Nieuwenhuijs et al, 1992). Sporadic cases have been reported from Spain, France, the former German Democratic Republic (East Germany), Poland, Turkey, the former Socialist Federal Republic of Yugoslavia, and Czechoslovakia (Nikolic and Jelesic, 1956; Anonymous, 1958; Schindler and Dennig, 1958; Schneider, 1982, 1983; Twardowski and Barancewicz, 1986; Barrat et al, 1989 [cited by Montano Hirose et al, 1990]; de Felipe Gardon, 1989; Gardner, 1989; Schneider et al, 1989; Sureau et al, 1989 [cited by Bourhy et al, 1990]; Bourhy et al, 1992). In September of 1992, the first rabid bat was reported from Switzerland (Kappeler, 1992).

Table 23-1

Isolation of European Bat Lyssavirus, by Location, Year, and Species[a]

Location	Year	Number	Species
Federal Republic of Germany[b]			
Hamburg	1954	1	undetermined
Hamburg	1968	1	*Eptesicus serotinus*
Stade	1970	1	undetermined
Berlin	1973	1	*Myotis myotis*
Bremerhaven	1982	1	undetermined
Aurich	1983	1	*Eptesicus serotinus*
Rodenberg	1983	1	*Eptesicus serotinus*
Rodenberg	1985	1	*Eptesicus serotinus*
Bremerhaven	1985	1	*Eptesicus serotinus*
Nienburg	1985	1	*Eptesicus serotinus*
North Germany	1986	9	*Eptesicus serotinus*
Luneberg	1986	1	*Myotis daubentoni*
Hagen-Bremen	1986	1	*Pipistrellus nathusii*
Tubingen	1986	1	*Eptesicus fuscus*[d]
Ottweiler	1986	1	undetermined
Peine	1986	1	*Eptesicus serotinus*
Nienburg	1986	2	*Eptesicus serotinus*
Luneberg	1986	1	undetermined
Dorum	1986	1	undetermined
Steinau	1986	1	undetermined
Luneberg	1986	1	*Myotis sp.*
Offenwarden	1986	1	*Myotis sp.*
Loxsteldt-Neuenlande	1986	1	*Eptesicus serotinus*
unreported	1987	2	*Pipistrellus pipistrellus*
unreported	1989	4	undetermined
unreported	1990	1	undetermined
Niedersachsen	1990	9	undetermined
Schleswig-Holstein	1990	5	undetermined
Nordhein-Westfalen	1990	1	undetermined
Berlin	1990	1	undetermined
Federal Republic of Germany[c]			
Berlin	1991	2	undetermined
Berlin	1992	1	undetermined
Schleswig-Holstein	1992	1	undetermined
Niedersachsen	1992	3	undetermined
Democratic Republic of Germany[e]			
Jena	1963	1	*Eptesicus serotinus*
unreported	1985	1	undetermined
Bezirk Neubrandenburg	1986	1	undetermined
unreported	1985-1989	1	*Eptesicus serotinus*

[a]The majority of rabid bat specimens in Europe have been of the species *Eptesicus serotinus*; [b]Former Federal Republic of Germany (West Germany); [c]Federal Republic of Germany (unified); [d]*Eptesicus fuscus* (imported from Canada - serotype 1 variant); [e]Former German Democratic Republic (East Germany); [f]Former Socialist Federal Republic of Yugoslavia; [g]Unique subtype.

Table 23-1 (Cont'd)

Isolation of European Bat Lyssavirus, by Location, Year, and Species

Location	Year	Number	Species
Denmark			
Jutland	1985	10	*Eptesicus serotinus*
Jutland	1986	103	*Eptesicus serotinus*
Jutland	1986	1	*Myotis daubentoni*
Jutland	1986	1	*Myotis dasycneme*
Jutland	1987	47	*Eptesicus serotinus*
Jutland	1987	1	*Myotis daubentoni*
unreported	1989	1	undetermined
Yugoslavia[f]			
unreported	1954	3	*Nyctalus noctula*
unreported	1956	1	*Nyctalus noctula*
unreported	1957	1	*Nyctalus noctula*
Turkey			
unreported	1956	1	*Rhinolophus ferrumequinum*
unreported	1963	1	*Rhinolophus ferrumequinum*
Poland			
Krakau	1972	1	undetermined
Gdansk	1985	1	*Eptesicus serotinus*
Danzig	1985	1	*Eptesicus serotinus*
Gdansk	1986	1	*Eptesicus serotinus*
The Netherlands			
unreported	1987	3	*Myotis dasycneme*
unreported	1987	83	*Eptesicus serotinus*
unreported	1988	43	*Eptesicus serotinus*
unreported	1989	22	*Eptesicus serotinus*
unreported	1989	1	*Myotis dasycneme*
unreported	1990	22	*Eptesicus serotinus*
unreported	1991	12	*Eptesicus serotinus*
unreported	1992	5	*Eptesicus serotinus*
unreported	1992	10	undetermined
unreported	1993	1	undetermined
Finland			
Helsinki	1985	1	Human[g]
Norway			
unreported	1987	48	undetermined
Spain			
Valencia	1987	1	undetermined
Granada	1987	1	undetermined
unreported	1985-1989	5	*Eptesicus serotinus*
Czechoslovakia			
unreported	1989	1	undetermined
France			
Briey	1989	1	*Eptesicus serotinus*
Bainville	1989	1	*Eptesicus serotinus*
Switzerland			
Fribourg	1992	1	*Myotis daubentoni*

Information derived principally from reports of the World Health Organization. *Rabies Bulletin Europe.* Information Surveillance Research. WHO Collaborating Centre for Rabies Surveillance and Research. Tübingen, Federal Republic of Germany. Numbers are approximate in some cases due to discrepancies in reporting.

Table 23-2

Species of British Bats Examined for the Presence of Rabies Antigen

Species Tested	Common Name	Number Tested
Barbastellus barbastellus	Barbastelle	1
Eptesicus serotinus	Serotine	29
Myotis bechsteini	Bechstein's	1
Myotis brandti	Brandt's	2
Myotis daubentoni	Daubenton's	17
Myotis mystacinus	Whiskered	29
Myotis nattereri	Natterer's	31
Nyctalus leisleri	Leisler's	2
Nyctalus noctula	Noctule	21
Pipistrellus nathusii [a]	Nathusii's Pipistrelle	8
Pipistrellus pipistrellus	Pipistrelle	673
Plecotus auritus	Brown Long-eared	172
Plecotus austriacus	Grey Long-eared	3
Rhinolophus ferrumequinum	Greater Horseshoe	2
Rhinolophus hipposideros	Lesser Horseshoe	1
Unidentified	-	67

[a] Mainland species found on offshore oil rigs.

From King, A. A. *Studies of the Antigenic Relationships of Rabies and Rabies-Related Viruses Using Anti-Nucleoprotein Monoclonal Antibodies*. Ph.D. Thesis. School of Biological Sciences, University of Surrey. Guildford, United Kingdom, 1991. Reproduced with permission.

There is no evidence that the United Kingdom's rabies-free status has been affected by the changing status of bat rabies on the European mainland. King (1991) examined the brains of 1,051 British bats that were found ill or dead and eight specimens of the mainland species, *Pipistrellus nathusii* (the latter collected from offshore oil rigs, where they had been grounded). He found no evidence of infection with rabies or rabies-related viruses in any of these samples (Table 23-2). However, in view of the widespread distribution of rabies-related infection in specimens of *Eptesicus serotinus* throughout mainland Europe, the limited number (29) of serotine bats surveyed in King's study may have been too small a sample size to reliably conclude that the serotine populations of Britain remain free of infection.

Infection in European bats is most commonly reported between July and September (Figure 23-1), corresponding to the increased breeding or migratory activity in many bat populations (Haagsma, 1989; Muller, 1992; World Health Organization, 1990a, 1992a; Nieuwenhuijs et al, 1992). As is the case in North America, the number of rabid bats identified does, to a large extent, mirror efforts made to find them, which are also known to be seasonably related.

The species of bat most commonly reported to be infected in Europe is *Eptesicus serotinus* (Figure 23-2), variously referred to as the common serotine, wide-winged bat, large dark brown bat, or European house bat (Mollgaard, 1985, 1986; Stougaard, 1986; World Health Organization, 1986a, 1986b, 1986c, 1987a, 1992b; Haag-

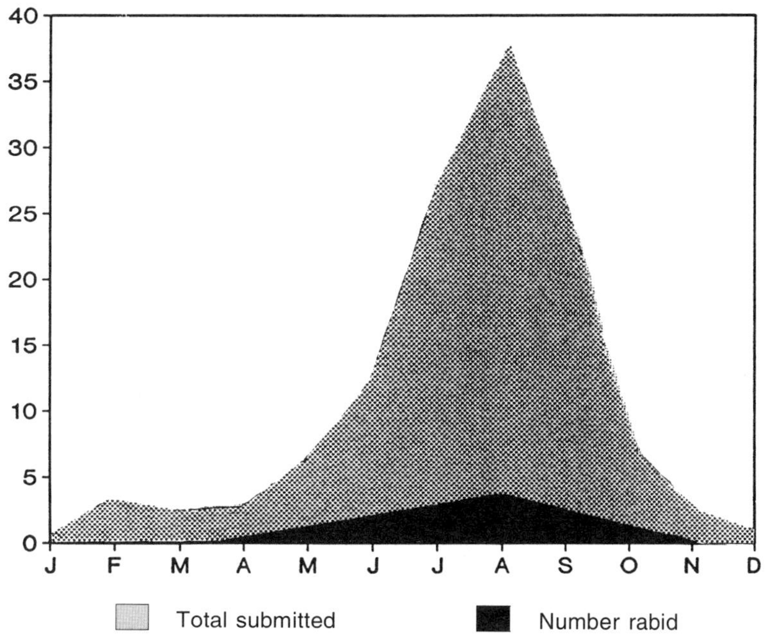

Figure 23-1. Number of bats submitted and those found rabid in the Netherlands, by month, 1987-1991 (From Nieuwenhuijs, J., Haagsma, J., and P. Lina. Epidemiology and control of rabies in bats in the Netherlands. *Rev. Sci. Tech. Off. Int. Epiz.* 11(4): 1155, 1992 Redrawn with permission.)

sma, 1989; Bourhy et al, 1992; Muller, 1992). As shown in Figure 23-3A, this species is widely distributed throughout Europe (Stebbings and Griffith, 1986; Stebbings, 1988). Apparent prevalence of infection in this species may be related, in part, to their colonial habits and roosting behavior (see page 142), which increase their chance of contact with humans (Bourhy et al, 1992). Nonserotine bats in which infection has been reported include *Myotis daubentoni*, *Myotis dasycneme*, *Myotis myotis*, *Myotis blythi*, *Pipistrellus pipistrellus*, *Pipistrellus nathusii*, *Rhinolophus ferrumequinum*, *Nyctalus noctula*, *Vespertilio nilssonii*, and *Vespertilio murinus*.

A steady decline in numbers of bats, as a consequence of habitat destruction and pollution (e.g., use of pesticides to reduce numbers of insects), has caused concern over dwindling populations of endangered species (Table 23-3). European researchers and public-health authorities have, therefore, been urged to educate the public towards a better understanding of bats and bat rabies, rather than create needless hysteria over the potential spread of bat-borne disease (World Health Organization, 1987a; Judes, 1988; Stebbings, 1988; CNEVA, 1990; Kappeler, 1989, 1992; Nieuwenhuijs et al, 1992).

Because of the endangered status accorded insectivorous bats in Europe, large-scale survey studies, as have been carried out in the United States, have not been undertaken. Information regarding prevalence of infection in European bat populations is, therefore, limited (Muller, 1990a). Furthermore, bats are protected by law in Europe and any activity which threatens their survival is illegal. This includes eviction of bats from roost sites, which may lead to reduced rearing of young (Brigham and Fenton, 1987; Ward, 1994). In Great Britain, the *Wildlife and Countryside Act* of 1981 mandates that permission must be obtained from the Nature Conservancy Council before bats may be eliminated from any dwelling (Fenton, 1992). Important international wildlife legislation related to bats includes the "Bern" and "Bonn" Conventions, which are designed to help conserve bats and their natural habitats, to protect migratory species throughout their range, and to promote international cooperation in bat conser-

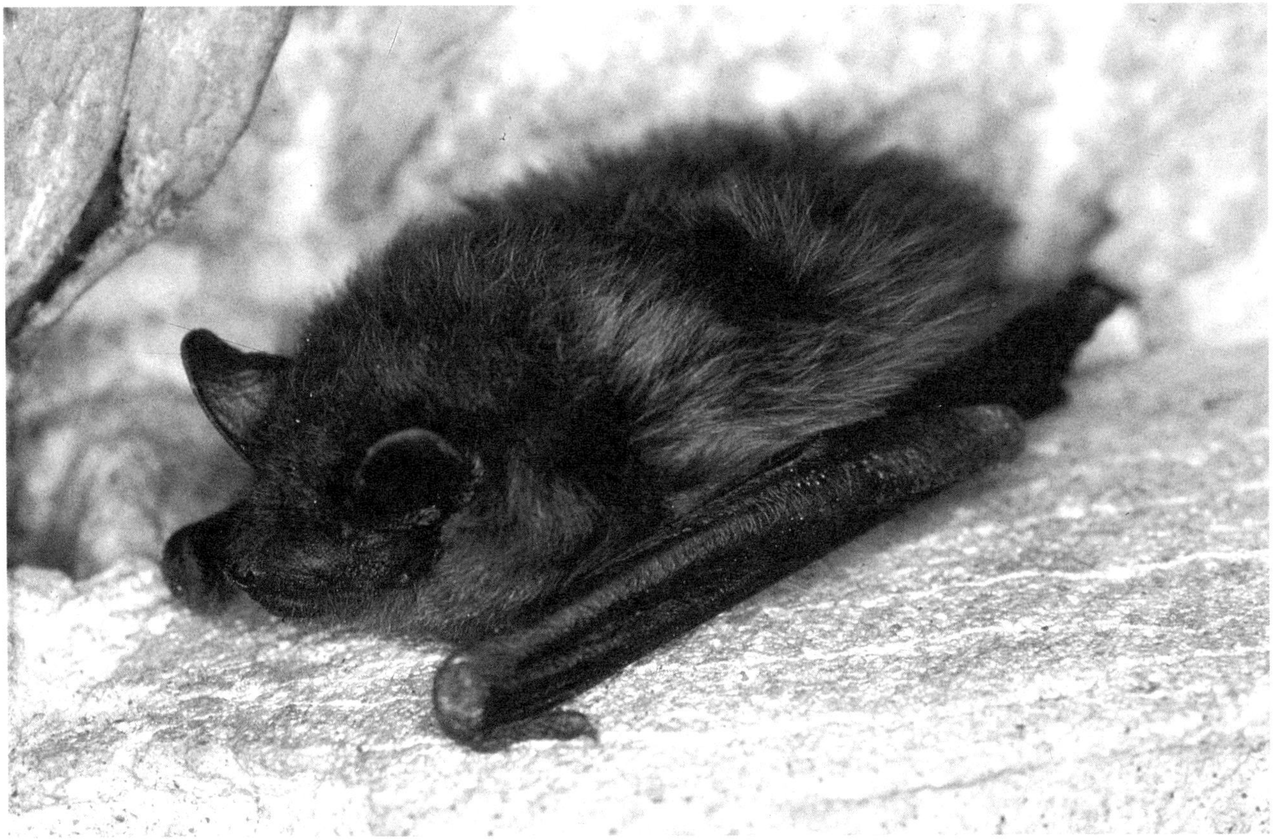

Figure 23-2. *Eptesicus serotinus* is the species of bat most commonly reported rabid (EBL 1) in Europe. Photo courtesy of Mr. F. Schwaab - Groupe D'Etude des Mammifères de Lorraine - Association Lorraine des Cinéastes et Photographes de la Nature (France).

vation (Stebbings, 1988). Laws protecting bats have been enacted in almost all European countries (Stebbings, 1988).

Antigenic Characterization of Rabies Isolates from European Bats

Collectively, the rabies-related isolates from European bats comprise a group referred to as the European bat lyssaviruses. Many of the viruses isolated from bats in Europe have been characterized by monoclonal antibody panels as being antigenically related to serotype 4 isolates (Duvenhage virus) of African origin (see Figure 22-1 and Table 22-2). Although there are antigenic similarities to the Duvenhage viruses, significant differences exist which clearly distinguish bat viruses of African and European origin.

Distinct antigenic variants of European bat lyssaviruses have been identified (Montano Hirose et al, 1990; Schneider, 1982; Dietzschold et al, 1988; World Health Organization, 1989; King et al, 1990; King, 1991). In particular, isolates from rabid specimens of *Myotis dasycneme* in Holland can be antigenically distinguished from those of serotine bats (see Figure 22-1 and Table 22-2).

Preliminary studies recently completed at the Pasteur Institute in Paris (Bourhy et al, 1992, 1993) and at the Centers for Disease Control in the United States (Smith, 1993) have documented the fact that marked genetic differences also exist between rabies isolates obtained from European species of *Myotis* and those from specimens of *Eptesicus serotinus*. These results confirm the existence of a second viral variant, so far known only from specimens of *Myotis dasycneme*. Studies of isolates from Swiss specimens of *Myotis daubentoni* are yet to be published. Because multiple variants of virus may exist among populations of nonserotine bats in Europe, continued

Table 23-3

Status of European Bats: A Summary

Species	Status[a]	Species	Status
Family Rhinolophidae		Family Vespertilionidae (Cont'd)	
Rhinolophus ferrumequinum	E	*Pipistrellus pipistrellus*	V
Rhinolophus hipposideros	E	*Pipistrellus nathusii*	V
Rhinolophus blasii	E	*Pipistrellus kuhli*	V
Rhinolophus euryale	V	*Pipistrellus savii*	V
Rhinolophus mehelyi	R (?E)	*Eptesicus serotinus*	Nt
Family Vespertilionidae		*Eptesicus nilssonii*	Nt
Myotis mystacinus	V	*Vespertilio murinus*	R
Myotis brandtii	V	*Nyctalus noctula*	V
Myotis emarginatus	E	*Nyctalus leisleri*	V
Myotis capaccinii	V (?E)	*Nyctalus lasiopterus*	R
Myotis daubentonii	?Nt	*Miniopterus schreibersii*	E
Myotis dasycneme	E	*Plecotus auritus*	V
Myotis nattereri	V	*Plecotus austriacus*	V
Myotis bechsteinii	R(?E)	*Barbastella barbastellus*	V(?E)
Myotis myotis	E	Family Molossidae	
Myotis blythi	E	*Tadarida teniotis*	V

a The status recorded here is for European bats as a whole, but individual countries may have different categories. Even bats labeled here as endangered are common in some areas.

(E) = Endangered. Species in danger of extinction and whose survival is unlikely if the causal factors continue to operate. Included are species whose numbers have been reduced to a critical level or whose habitats have been so drastically reduced that they are in immediate danger of extinction. (V) = Vulnerable. Species believed likely to move into the endangered category in the near future if causal factors continue to operate. (R) = Rare. Species with small known populations which are not at present endangered or vulnerable, but are at risk. These species are usually localized within specific geographical areas or habitats, or are thinly scattered over a more extensive range. (Nt) = Not threatened. Species which are neither rare nor threatened.

From Stebbings, R. E. *The Conservation of European Bats*. Christopher Helm, Ltd. London, 1988. Reproduced with permission.

study of viral isolates is important to further our understanding of this complex multi-species epizootiology.

With a limited availability of appropriate monoclonal antibodies and only a fledgling understanding of the relationships between European bat viruses and those of the African continent, it had been difficult for researchers to definitively classify the early isolates of rabies-related virus from European bats.

Based upon initial monoclonal antibody studies, they were originally referred to as Duvenhage-like viruses. However, they have since been classified as a distinct group, the European bat

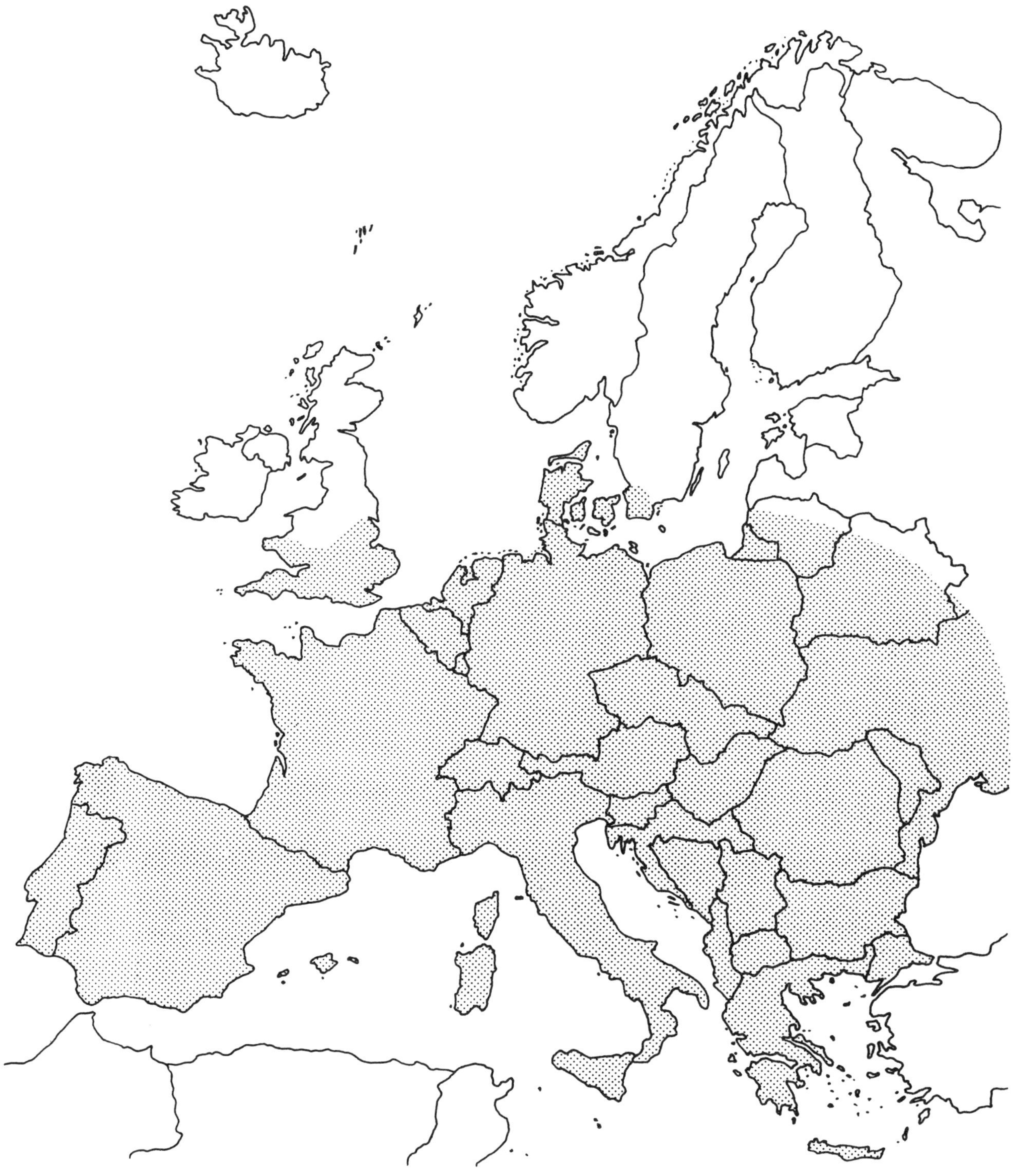

Figure 23-3A. Distribution of *Eptesicus serotinus* in Western Europe. This species is colonial and nonmigratory in habit, and common over large areas of its range. It is often found roosting in buildings and it tends to feed in sheltered urban areas, increasing the likelihood of interaction with humans. It is the species of bat most commonly reported rabid in Europe. (From Stebbings, R. E. and F. Griffith. *Distribution and Status of Bats in Europe.* Natural Environmental Research Council Institute of Terrestrial Ecology. Huntingdon, Great Britain, 1986. Redrawn with permission.)

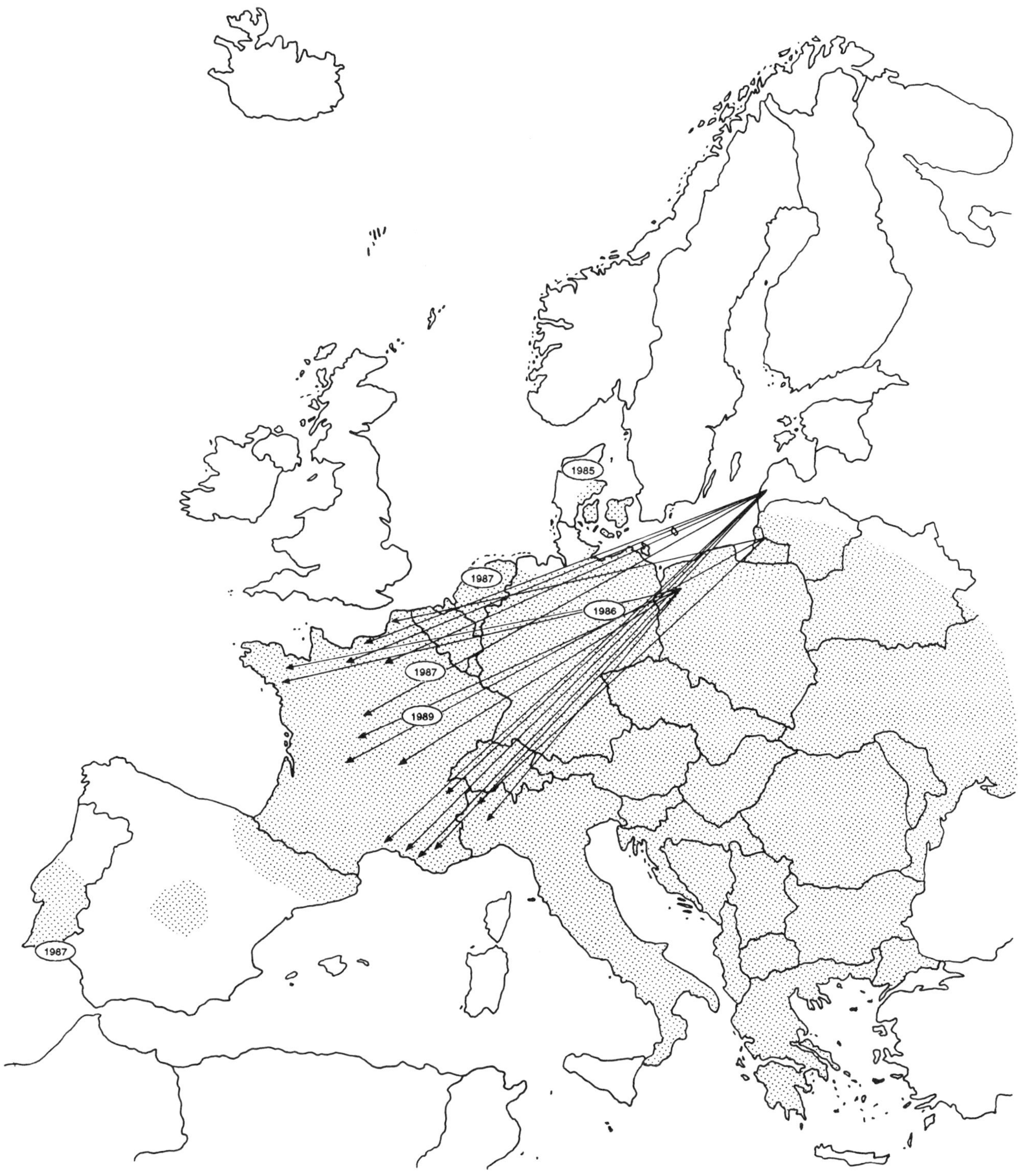

Figure 23-3B. Distribution and recorded migrations of *Pipistrellus nathusii* in Western Europe. Dates represent the geographical progression of reported cases of rabies infection in European bats, 1985-1989. (From Brosset, A. Les migrations de la pipistrelle de Nathusius, *Pipistrellus nathusii*, en France. Ses incidences possibles sur la propagation de la rage. *Mammalia*. 54(2): 207, 1990. Redrawn with permission. Distribution information from Stebbings, R. E. *The Conservation of European Bats*. Christopher Helm, Ltd. London, 1988. Redrawn with permission.)

Table 23-4

Similarity Matrix of the N Coding Region of Representative *Lyssavirus* Isolates of Genotypes 1, 2, 3, 4, 5, and 6[a]

Virus	Number	Mokola	Lagos Bat 8619NGA	Duvenhage DUV1AS	EBL1 8615POL	EBL1 8918FRA	EBL2 9007FIN	EBL2 9018HOL	Fox 9004FRA	PV
Mokola			87.1	82.1	81.3	81.6	78	77.8	79.6	79.8
Lagos Bat	8619NGA	76.2		85.8	83.1	83.8	79.1	79.1	82	81.6
Duvenhage	DUV1AS	72.7	73.3		92.7	93.3	86.2	85.8	87.1	87.6
EBL1	8615POL	71.4	74.4	79.3		98.7	87.3	86.4	87.6	88
EBL1	8918FRA	71	74.4	79.8	95.7		88	87.6	87.8	88.2
EBL2	9007FIN	71.1	72.4	76	77.2	78.1		97.8	86.9	86.9
EBL2	9018HOL	69.9	73.5	75.8	76.1	76.9	96		86.4	86.4
Fox	9004FRA	71	73.6	74.9	75.6	75.5	74.4	74.5		97.1
PV		72.1	73.2	74.5	75.4	75.3	74.4	74.6	92.8	

[a] Source of viral isolates used in this study were as follows: Mokola - cat, Zimbabwe, 1986; Lagos bat virus (8619NGA) - *Eidolon helvum*, Lagos Island, Nigeria, 1958; Duvenhage (1AS) - human, Republic of South Africa, 1971; EBL 1 (8615POL) - *Eptesicus serotinus*, Poland, 1985; EBl 1 (8918FRA) - *Eptesicus serotinus*, Briey, France, 1989; EBL 2 (9007FIN) - human, Finland, 1986; EBL 2 (9018HOL) - *Myotis sp.*, the Netherlands, 1986; Fox (9004FRA) - *Vulpes vulpes*, France, 1986; PV - vaccinal strain.

Note: The percentages of amino acid (top) and nucleotide (bottom) similarity are given.

From Bourhy, H., Kissi, B., and N. Tordo. Molecular diversity of the *Lyssavirus* genus. *Virology.* 194(1): 70, 1993. Reproduced with permission.

lyssaviruses. Based upon monoclonal antibody analyses, recommendations were made that the European bat lyssaviruses assume the status of a fifth serotype within the rabies subgroup of the *Lyssavirus* genus and that they be subdivided into two biotypes (EBL type 1 and EBL type 2), collectively forming the serotype 5 group (Montano Hirose et al, 1990; World Health Organization, 1990b; Bourhy et al, 1992).

EBL 1 is the principal variant found in *Eptesicus serotinus* throughout Europe and includes those isolates formerly identified as Duvenhage 3 to 5 (from the former Federal Republic of Germany [West Germany]), Duvenhage 6 (from Poland), and Duvenhage 7 (from Denmark). A human isolate (Yuli virus) and isolates from several nonserotine species from the former Soviet Union have also been classified as EBL 1. EBL 2 is currently known only from species of *Myotis* and from a single human isolate from Finland. Further analyses will be required to define the number and characteristics of rabies variants found in nonserotine bats in Europe. At this time, the classifications remain provisional.

Genetic Analysis of Rabies-Related Lyssaviruses

Antigenic analyses do not fully describe the relationship of the rabies-related viruses to each other and to classical (serotype 1) rabies virus. However, genetic typing studies are proving to be of value in further defining relationships among these viruses (Bourhy et al, 1992, 1993; Mebatsion et al, 1992; Sacramento et al, 1992; World Health Organization, 1992b; Smith, 1993).

Bourhy et al (1993) reported the first complete analysis of the genetic diversity of the lys-

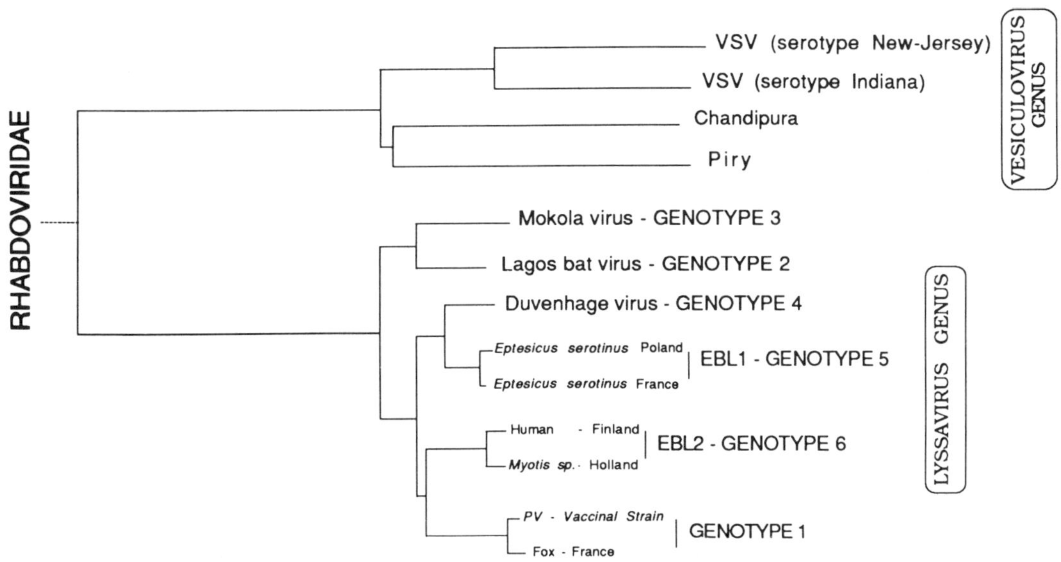

Figure 23-4. Phylogenetic tree of the genera *Lyssavirus* and *Vesiculovirus* based on alignment of the deduced amino acid sequence of 13 N proteins. Horizontal branch lengths are indicative of the evolutionary distances. Vertical lines are included for clarity. (From Bourhy, H., Kissi, B., and N. Tordo. Molecular diversity of the *Lyssavirus* genus. *Virology*. 194(1): 70, 1993. Reproduced with permission.)

saviruses, constructing a phylogenetic tree based on alignment of amino acid sequences of the N (nucleoprotein) gene (Figure 23-4). The N gene tends to be highly conserved over time and is, therefore, of value in studying evolutionary relationships among the *Lyssavirus* genus.

Based upon their genetic data, a genotypic grouping of the genus *Lyssavirus* was proposed. Six genotypes were defined on the basis of their percentage amino acid similarity (Tables 23-4 and 23-5). The lowest percentage of amino acid similarity between two isolates of the same genotype was 97.1% and the highest percentage of similarity between isolates of different genotypes was 93.3% (Table 23-4).

Genotypes 1, 2, 3, and 4 are concordant with respective serotype groupings (classical rabies, Lagos bat, Mokola, and Duvenhage viruses, respectively). The European bat lyssaviruses were divided into two independent genotypes. Genotype 5 includes isolates of the biotype identified as EBL 1 and genotype 6 includes isolates of the biotype identified as EBL 2.

The genetic analysis supported results of antigenic studies demonstrating that Mokola virus is the most divergent of the rabies-related viruses. Based on this study, genotypes 2 (Lagos bat virus) and 3 (Mokola virus) are the most distantly related to vaccinal and classical rabies viruses of genotype 1. Genotypes 4 (Duvenhage virus) and 5 (EBL 1) are closely related to each other.

Migratory Behavior of Bats and the European Bat Lyssaviruses

Although the development of a wildlife rabies epizootic following accidental importation of an infected animal is extremely unlikely, it remains an ongoing concern of public-health authorities in rabies-free countries. Bat "stowaways" have been found aboard both ships and planes (see review by Wiles and Hill, 1986). With respect to the origin of rabies-related viruses in European bats, some workers suggested that infected bats may have originally reached Europe via ship from sub-Saharan Africa, speculating that this accounted for the initial reports of viral isolation from bats in maritime regions of northern Germany (Schneider, 1982; World Health Organization, 1984a; Matouch, 1986; King, 1987; Caffrey, 1992). During the course of such ocean passage, however, stowaway bats would probably have become severely dehydrated and others believe it to

Table 23-5

Antigenic and Molecular Classifications of the Genus *Lyssavirus*

Antigenic Classification		Molecular Classification[a]	
Serotype 1	Classical rabies virus	Genotype 1	Classical rabies virus
Serotype 2	Lagos bat virus	Genotype 2	Lagos bat virus
Serotype 3	Mokola virus	Genotype 3	Mokola virus
Serotype 4	Duvenhage virus (Africa)	Genotype 4	Duvenhage virus (Africa)
Serotype 5	European bat lyssavirus EBL 1 EBL 2	Genotype 5	European bat lyssavirus EBL 1
		Genotype 6	European bat lyssavirus EBL 2

[a] Based on the work of Bourhy, H., Kissi, B., and N. Tordo (1993). Molecular diversity of the *Lyssavirus* genus. *Virology*. 194(1): 70

be unlikely that a stowaway could have survived such a journey. Because of the widespread distribution of infection in European bat populations as well as the marked differences in environmental conditions between Europe and Africa, several researchers have suggested that African importation may have been an unlikely source of virus (Lafon et al, 1988; King, 1991; Rupprecht et al, 1991).

Smith (1993) has recently shown that two genetically distinct variants of virus obtained from naturally infected European bats are also quite different in genetic makeup from African isolates of Duvenhage virus. These findings support the belief that the European bat lyssaviruses do not represent a transported form of African Duvenhage virus.

In view of the extensive migrations of *Pipistrellus nathusii* (Figure 23-3B), Brosset (1990) suggested that this species may play an important role as a migrating vector of the European bat lyssavirus over long distances throughout Europe. During the course of its migration, the pipistrelle may share roosts with *Eptesicus serotinus*, a relatively sedentary, nonmigratory species. Brosset (1990) considered it likely that this resulted in the gradual transmission of virus from infected pipistrelles to populations of serotine bats across much of Europe. Accordingly, Brosset hypothesized that both the historic and geographic spread of disease in bats across Europe coincides with the migration patterns of *Pipistrellus nathusii* (Figure 23-3B). At present, there is no significant evidence to support an important role for this species in the epidemiology and epizootiology of bat rabies in Europe and the hypothesis remains purely speculative.

In view of the report by Speakman et al (1991), suggesting that *Pipistrellus nathusii* may be a more frequent visitor to Britain than commonly believed, one might speculate that the pipistrelle's migration may ultimately affect the rabies status of British bats. Continued monoclonal and genetic analyses of viral isolates from European bats will provide additional information regarding the possibility of viral transmission from pipistrelle to serotine bats. To date, no antigenic or genetic analyses of isolates from *Pipistrellus nathusii* have been reported (Lafon, 1993) and the species is rarely implicated as a significant agent of disease in Europe.

Certain other aspects of the complex epizootiology of rabies in migratory bats have recently come under scrutiny by public-health officials in Europe. The Office International des Épizooties (the world animal health organization), is an inter-governmental organization which facilitates international cooperation among veterinary authorities. The primary functions of the OIE are to:

1) Inform governments on the course of animal diseases and control methods.

2) Promote and coordinate research activities of national veterinary services on animal diseases.

3) Standardize rules and procedures for the international trade of animals and animal products.

The OIE also determines the guidelines for defining whether a country is free of rabies or not. OIE recommendations are subsequently incorporated into the International Animal Health Code. A country has generally been considered to be free of rabies if, in the presence of adequate surveillance and an effective importation policy, no case of indigenously acquired rabies has occurred in humans or any animal species for the preceeding two years. The rabies-free status of a country is unaffected by the detection of cases in quarantine stations or in humans who were infected elsewhere.

Making recommendations to the OIE, Caffrey (1992) addressed both the public-health significance of rabies in insectivorous bats, and the relationship between migratory behavior of potentially rabid bats and the rabies status of a particular European country. In the face of widespread geographic dispersal of infected bats throughout much of Europe, the adequacy of previous guidelines for defining a country's rabies status has recently been questioned. What status, for example, should be accorded a rabies-free country that sporadically reports cases of rabies in migratory bat species?

At a recent meeting in Paris, the OIE Ad Hoc Group on Rabies Control considered the recommendation that the status of an otherwise rabies-free country not be affected by the sporadic isolation of European bat lyssavirus (Caffrey, 1992). At the most recent meeting of its General Session in Paris (May, 1993), this recommendation was adopted by the OIE International Committee (Chillaud, 1993). Currently, the criteria defining a rabies-free status, as per the International Animal Health Code (Office International des Épizooties, 1993), are as follows:

1) The disease is compulsorily notifiable.

2) An effective disease surveillance system is in effect.

3) All regulatory measures for the prevention and control of rabies, including effective importation procedures, have been implemented.

4) No imported cases of rabies in a carnivore have been confirmed outside of a quarantine facility within six months.

5) No case of indigenously acquired rabies has been confirmed in humans or any animal species during the preceding two years.

6) The rabies-free status of a country is not affected by the isolation of European bat lyssavirus (EBL 1 or EBL 2).

King (1991) emphasized the importance to a rabies-free country not only of being able to identify the rabies and rabies-related viruses, should their presence be suspected, but of being able to characterize them as well. The response of public-health officials, following identification of a rabies or rabies-related isolate, would, in large measure, be determined by the nature of the virus. Accordingly, King wrote,

> *...if the virus was shown to be of bat origin, the contingency plans for wildlife destruction [in England] may be restricted or not brought into play at all since, although bat viruses can spill over into terrestrial animals, there is no evidence to suggest that a cycle of infection within these animals can become established.*

Pathogenicity of European Bat Lyssaviruses

Danish isolates obtained from specimens of *Eptesicus serotinus* have produced lethal disease in adult and suckling mice following intracerebral, footpad, and oral inoculation. Intracerebral inoculation was lethal in dogs and cats. Lesions in the central nervous system of dogs, cats, and mice infected with the Danish isolate were more severe than those observed following infection with other street viruses and were characterized by spongiosis.

In dogs and cats that were infected by the intracerebral route, virus was confined to the CNS. In mice and cats infected by peripheral routes, however, virus was found in various tissues, including the salivary glands. Cats so exposed could, therefore, transmit disease either to other animals or to humans (Fedaku et al, 1988a). Although isolates of EBL 1 have been transmitted experimentally to sheep and foxes by intramuscular administration, the virulence of virus in these animals was considered to be low (Soria Baltazar et al, 1988).

Pathogenicity of European bat lyssaviruses in the reservoir hosts themselves has been poorly studied, principally because these bats are considered to be endangered species in Europe and are, therefore, protected (Bourhy et al, 1992). In limited studies, however, Botvinkin et al (1992) reported that two species of *Myotis* (*M. daubentoni* and *M. brandtii*) had a reduced susceptibility to intramuscular administration of EBL 1 virus (Stade and Yuli isolates).

Transmission of Nonterrestrial Virus to Terrestrial Species in Europe

With the increase in number of reported EBL-positive findings in European bats in recent years comes a concern regarding the potential for viral transmission to other animals, both wild and domestic, as well as to humans. In this respect, rabies (or rabies-related) infection in terrestrial animals had been unknown in Denmark for three years prior to identification of the first rabid bat (Mollgaard, 1985) and is reportedly minimal in those areas of the former Federal Republic of Germany (West Germany) where EBL-infected bats have been prevalent. Brains of more than 10,000 terrestrial species throughout Europe have been examined for evidence of infection with European bat lyssaviruses. None have been found to be infected.

Virus isolated from a sheep in the former Socialist Federal Republic of Yugoslavia and from a fox in France were tested with a reduced panel of monoclonal antibodies. Results were consistent with EBL 2 variants of virus. However, when these isolates were tested with a larger panel of monoclonal antibodies, they were shown to be terrestrial variants of serotype 1 virus (Montano Hirose et al, 1990; Lafon, 1993). The authors considered it probable that some isolates of serotype 1 may share a common nucleocapsid epitope (in this case, one which reacts with MAb IP7) with isolates of EBL 2, leading to the possibility of an error in differentiation when reduced panels are used.

To date, no variant of European bat lyssavirus has been isolated from a naturally infected terrestrial species. The probability of transmission to other species is very low (Grauballe et al, 1987; Soria Baltazar et al, 1988; Thomas et al, 1989; CNEVA, 1990; World Health Organization, 1990b; Bourhy et al, 1992; Caffrey, 1992; Nieuwenhuijs et al, 1992). In areas where enzootic fox rabies has been brought under control by oral vaccination, evidence is consistent with the premise that ongoing infection of foxes following interaction with bats will not occur. As is the case for bat rabies in North America, epidemiologic investigations support the conclusion that rabies-related infections in European bat populations have no significant impact on terrestrial animals.

Human Exposure to European Bat Lyssavirus

Many human contacts with bats have been reported in Europe, primarily from handling sick or injured animals. In fact, in each European country in which European bat lyssavirus has been reported, the initial finding was made after a person was allegedly bitten by a bat. In 1990 and 1991, 239 people across Europe (159 and 80, respectively) received post-exposure rabies prophylaxis following contact with a bat (World Health Organization, 1993a, 1993b). Between 1987 and 1991, 174 people (43, 17, 24, 69, and 21, respectively) in the Netherlands alone received post-exposure rabies prophylaxis following direct contact with an infected bat (Nieuwenhuijs et al, 1992). A definite, albeit very small, risk of viral transmission to humans now exists in Europe (Lafon et al, 1986; Haagsma, 1989; Remmert et al, 1989; Thomas et al, 1989). One human fatality from bat-inflicted disease has been reported from Finland, and two from the former Soviet Union. Risk of exposure can be greatly minimized simply

Table 23-6

Isolation of Nonterrestrial Rabies and European Bat Lyssavirus From Regions of the Former Soviet Union, by Location and Year

Location	Year	Species	Virus	Reference
Kiev (Ukraine)	1964	*Eptesicus serotinus*	not tested	Selimov et al, 1986
Voroschilovgrad (Ukraine)	1977	Human case of bat origin	not tested	Selimov et al, 1986
Novosibirsk (RSFSR)	1981	*Myotis daubentoni*	Serotype I	Selimov et al, 1986
Omsk (RSFSR)	1984	*Vespertilio murinus*	Serotype I	Selimov et al, 1986
Belgorod (RSFSR)	1985	Human case of bat origin (Yuli isolate)	European bat lyssavirus	Selimov et al, 1986
Volin (Ukraine)	1987	*Vespertilio murinus*	European bat lyssavirus	Khozinski et al, 1990
Volin (Ukraine)	1987	*Nyctalus noctula*	European bat lyssavirus	Khozinski et al, 1990
Yakutia (Taiga)	1987	*Vespertilio nilssonii*	Serotype I	Khozinski et al, 1990
Volynsky Region (Ukraine)	1990	*Nyctalus noctula*	European bat lyssavirus	Selimov et al, 1991
Volynsky Region (Ukraine)	1990	*Vespertilio murinus*	European bat lyssavirus	Selimov et al, 1991
Kyrgyzstan (Osh Province)	1992	*Myotis blythi* (Aravan isolate)	European bat lyssavirus	Kuzmin et al, 1992

by not disturbing or handling bats (Grauballe et al, 1987).

On October 9, 1985, a Swiss biologist in Helsinki, Finland was admitted to the emergency ward of Meilahti Hospital in Helsinki with an ascending paralysis, resembling the Guillain-Barré syndrome (additional medical details can be found on page 239). Rabies was suspected because of the clinical signs and a history of multiple bat bites. The patient was a bat biologist and he had been bitten by a bat four and a half years earlier in Malaysia, one year earlier in Switzerland, and 51 days earlier in Finland (the latter identified as *Myotis daubentoni*, but unavailable for testing). Apart from his trip to Malaysia, he had never been out of Europe, had never been in close contact with bats in other European countries, and had reportedly never sustained any other animal bites. He had also never been pre-exposure immunized against rabies. He died on October 29.

Postmortem viral analysis confirmed the causative agent as being related to Duvenhage virus (Berger, 1986; Lumio et al, 1986; Roine et al, 1988; Bussereau et al, 1989; King et al, 1990). Continued study of this isolate showed it to be related to EBL isolates from bats (*Myotis dasycneme*) in Holland (see Figure 22-1 and Table 22-2), but distinct from other European bat lyssaviruses that had so far been identified (King, 1991).

Finland has enjoyed a rabies-free status for a considerable period of time. The last reported case of human rabies occurred in 1934 and the last reported case of animal rabies was in 1959. The Veterinary Department of the Ministry of Agriculture has conducted limited survey studies of Finland's nine species of insectivorous bats for rabies infection (Berger, 1986; Lumio et al, 1986; Roine et al, 1988). No evidence of infection with rabies or rabies-related viruses has been found in bat populations of Finland. European bat lyssavirus has since been isolated from *Myotis daubentoni* in Switzerland (Kappeler, 1992) and studies comparing these viral isolates with the human variant from Finland continue. The source of exposure remains undetermined.

Bat Rabies in the Former Soviet Union

Of 11 nonterrestrial viruses isolated from regions of the former Soviet Union, six have been classified as European bat lyssaviruses. Three may be serotype 1 viruses (Table 23-6). Two isolates had never been tested (Botvinkin et al, 1988; Khozinski et al, 1990; King et al, 1990; Kuzmin et al, 1992). The identification of both serotype 1 and EBL viruses was an unusual and unexpected finding. Of these 11 reported isolations of nonterrestrial viruses, two were marked by human fatality (Selimov et al, 1986 [cited by Selimov et al, 1989]).

Rabies infection in bats of the former Soviet Union was first identified in 1964, when a 35-year-old man from Kiev (Ukrainian S.S.R.) was bitten by a bat, subsequently identified as *Eptesicus serotinus*. The man received post-exposure rabies prophylaxis and did not develop rabies. The bat was not immediately tested and it died 20 days later, with no apparent clinical symptoms. An identification of rabies virus was subsequently made (Ryaboshapka and Kroveletskaya, 1967 [cited by World Health Organization, 1987b]). The viral isolate in this instance has not been further characterized.

On August 16, 1977, a 15-year-old girl from Voroshilovgrad (Ukrainian S.S.R.) was bitten on a finger by a bat. She died about five weeks later and rabies was confirmed as the cause of death (Shcherbak, 1984 [cited by World Health Organization, 1987b]). The viral isolate in this instance has not been further characterized.

In 1985, an 11-year-old girl from Belgorod (Russian Soviet Federative Socialist Republic) died four weeks after being bitten on the lower lip by a bat. The viral isolate obtained from this child (Yuli isolate) is antigenically related to the European bat lyssaviruses, behaving essentially like Stade (EBL 1) isolates (Selimov et al, 1987, 1989, 1991; World Health Organization, 1987b, 1989). Yuli virus is presently classified as an EBL 1 virus, belonging to sero(geno)type 5. Selimov et al (1991) reported the isolation of virus antigenically identical to the Yuli isolate from the carcasses of two species of insectivorous bats (*Nyctalus noctula* and *Vespertilio murinus*) found in hollow trees along the Pripyat River (Volynsky region of the Ukrainian S.S.R.), near the Polish border.

Bat Rabies in Asia

There have been few reports of bat rabies in Asia. However, in view of the relatively low prevalence of infection in healthy-appearing insectivorous bats in the United States, negative findings in limited surveys of bats worldwide should not be taken as definitive evidence of a rabies-free bat population. On the other hand, the finding of very limited numbers of rabies-positive bats in resident species might reflect the occasional sporadic spillover of virus from infected terrestrial wildlife (such as an arboreal quadruped), leading to dead-end infection (Constantine, 1985). There have been no published reports of terrestrial rabies variants isolated from infected bats. It is important that all such isolates from bats be characterized as to their essential antigenic or genetic nature.

Limited surveys in Indonesia, the Philippines, Bangladesh, and Malaysia have not substantiated the presence of rabies in native bat populations (Ressang et al, 1963; Steele, 1966; Beran and de Mira, 1966; Tacal and Boado, Jr., 1966; Tan et al, 1969; Beran et al, 1972; Ali et al, 1983). Rabies has been reported in a greater horseshoe bat (*Rhinolophus ferrumequinum*) from Turkey (Tuncman, 1958 [cited by King and Crick, 1988]) and in two (of 79) dog-faced fruit bats (*Cynopterus brachyotis*) from Thailand (Smith et al, 1967), although the validity of the latter determination has been questioned (Constantine, 1988). Meesomboon (cited by King, 1991) reported finding one rabid bat in Khonken Province, Thailand in 1986 and in its World Survey of Rabies for the year 1991, the World Health Organization (1993b) reported the finding of a rabid bat in Thailand.

In India, rabies has been identified in a fruit bat, the flying fox (*Pteropus poliocephalus*). This bat had been found dead in front of a home during a winter storm on March 11, 1978 (Pal et al, 1980). There is one report from India of a human death due to rabies following the bite of an unidentified bat. This occurred in 1954 in Srikakulam District, Andhra State. A railway pointsman was bitten near his wrist by an injured bat that he had picked up. Clinical signs began three months later and he died within four days (Veeraraghavan, 1954). The bat was not examined.

Public-Health Recommendations

Despite limited data regarding the prevalence of infection in European bat populations, the World Health Organization (1988) maintains that no active surveillance studies should be carried out. Rather, in keeping with ongoing conservation measures, it has been recommended that information gathering should be confined to passive surveillance studies alone. Furthermore, the Expert Committee on Rabies maintains that specific population control measures directed at reducing disease prevalence in bats are not justified and has reemphasized the importance of leaving bat colonies unmolested (World Health Organization, 1992b). Continued surveillance will be necessary to define the changing epidemiologic significance of bat rabies in Europe. In this respect, recommendations of European public-health officials have included the following (Muller, 1990a):

1) Conduction of public-awareness campaigns to provide essential information about bat rabies.

2) Fundamental research into bats and bat rabies in cooperation with biologists, virologists, epidemiologists, and those making decisions in animal and human health fields.

3) Establishment of uniform guidelines for dealing with bats presented for examination. These must include provision for species identification. Detailed information must be obtained for cases in which species other than *Eptesicus serotinus* are involved.

4) Development of new vaccines that may be used to immunize bats.

5) Need for ongoing research to answer the following questions:

   a) how does infection spread?

   b) how many virus strains are involved?

   c) does infection between different bat species occur?

Vaccination Against European Bat Lyssaviruses

In view of the demonstrated antigenic and genotypic differences between rabies (sero[geno] type 1) and the rabies-related viruses (sero[geno] types 2 through 6), concern has been voiced regarding the efficacy of today's human and animal vaccines (which are formulated against sero [geno]type 1 viruses) to protect against exposure to the rabies-related lyssaviruses. This has become a more significant concern since the discovery that rabies-related isolates are no longer restricted in their distribution to sporadic findings on the African continent. Despite the fact that there is currently no evidence to suggest that rabies-related viruses will cause alarming epizootics among terrestrial animals or significant human fatality, ongoing discussion addresses the possible need for development of vaccines specifically tailored against these particular viral variants. The existence of multiple rabies-related variants has encouraged a careful reexamination of currently recommended strategies of pre- and post-exposure rabies prophylaxis.

Studies seeking to establish vaccine efficacy have taken advantage of viral-neutralization studies (will vaccine induce appropriate antibody production?) and protection experiments (will vaccine protect against challenge with a lethal dose of virus?). The capacity of a vaccine to confer protection against a particular rabies or rabies-related isolate has been shown to vary with the strain of virus used to manufacture the vaccine (Table 23-7), the nature of the infecting virus, and the species involved (Koprowski et al, 1985; Dietzschold et al, 1987; Lafon et al, 1988). Animal responses can be expected to vary with dosage and route of inoculation (Charlton et al, 1982).

Schneider (1982) and Lafon et al (1988) immunized mice with rabies vaccines derived from the Pitman-Moore (PM) strain of virus and then challenged them with isolates of EBL 1 (Stade or Hamburg) obtained from bats in the former Federal Republic of Germany (West Germany). The PM strain of virus serves as the basis for the widely used human diploid cell vaccine produced by the Merieux Institute. The PM-derived vaccines failed to protect mice against the German bat isolates.

A vaccine derived from the Flury LEP strain also failed to protect mice against EBL 1 (Hamburg strain) challenge (Lafon et al, 1988). However, immunization of mice with a vaccine derived from the PV4 virus strain did confer protection (Lafon et al, 1988). An ERA-derived vaccine protected mice against lethal challenge with an isolate of EBL 1 from Poland (Dietzschold et al, 1987).

Dietzschold et al (1987) examined the capacity of various vaccine strains, including those derived from PM, ERA, and EBL 1 (Polish isolate) viruses, to induce protective neutralizing antibody and anamnestic responses (immunologic memory). Primary immunization of mice with an ERA- or EBL 1-derived vaccine induced significant neutralizing antibody against an EBL 1 virus (Polish isolate). Mice immunized with a PM-derived vaccine developed serum neutralizing antibody against serotype 1 virus only.

EBL 1-derived booster vaccines induced anamnestic responses (as measured by higher titers of viral-neutralizing antibody) against EBL 1 virus (Polish isolate) in mice primed with an ERA- or EBL 1-, but not PM-derived, vaccine. In the PM-primed mice, antibody titers following EBL 1 boosters were not significantly different from those of mice immunized with an EBL 1-derived vaccine alone. Mice primed with a PM-derived vaccine and subsequently boosted with a PM strain of virus, mounted an anamnestic response to serotype 1 virus only (Dietzschold et al, 1987).

High titers of neutralizing antibody against serotype 1 virus were found in the sera of mice immunized with vaccines derived from PM, Flury LEP, or PV4 strains of virus. Mice immunized with PV4 also developed serum neutralizing antibody against EBL 1 (Hamburg strain). Despite the fact that PM, PV4, and CVS strains of virus have a common origin from the virus originally isolated by Louis Pasteur in 1882, the PV4 strain may now be more closely related than the others to EBL 1 virus (Lafon et al, 1988).

Mice immunized with human diploid cell vaccine were protected against lethal challenge with several serotype 1 rabies viral variants, as well as EBL 1 (Danish isolate) and an African isolate of Duvenhage (obtained from an infected human bitten by a rabid bat in South Africa). They were not protected against Lagos bat virus (serotype 2) obtained from an infected bat in Nigeria and only partial protection was afforded against the human isolate of EBL 2 from Finland (Fedaku et al, 1988b).

Two animal vaccines (Rabisin and Rabiffa) derived from the PM strain of virus protected mice against lethal challenge with a variety of serotype 1 rabies viruses and against challenge with Lagos bat virus (Nigerian isolate). Only partial protection was afforded against the human isolate of EBL 2 from Finland (Fedaku et al, 1988b). Dogs immunized with Rabisin were protected against lethal challenge with the Danish bat isolate (Fedaku et al, 1988b).

In rabbits primed with either an ERA- or PM-derived vaccine, an EBL 1 (Polish isolate) booster induced anamnestic responses to the EBL 1 virus (Dietzschold et al, 1987).

Animal models of vaccine efficacy include both the capacity of the vaccine to stimulate production of viral-neutralizing antibody, as well as to confer protection against lethal challenge with virus. In humans, on the other hand, antibody production is the only endpoint that can be measured (Celis et al, 1988).

Lafon et al (1986) obtained serum from human volunteers immunized with various rabies vaccines (human diploid cell/PM, purified vero rabies/PM, purified duck-embryo/PM, fetal bovine kidney cell/PV, and purified chick-embryo/Flury LEP). All vaccines were found to induce high titers of neutralizing antibody against EBL 1 (Stade isolate). Herzog et al (1991) reported that 73% of human patients receiving post-exposure rabies prophylaxis (for exposure to an animal other than a bat) with a PM-derived rabies vaccine developed specific neutralizing antibody against the Stade isolate. However, rabies-

Table 23-7

Origin and Passage History of Selected Strains of Fixed Rabies Virus Used in Vaccine Production

Viral Strain	Passage History
Pasteur Virus	Originally isolated by Louis Pasteur in 1882 from the brain of a rabid cow. It was then serially passaged 90 times by intracerebral passage in rabbits and harvested from their spinal cords.
Pitman-Moore Strain (PM)	Believed to be derived from the original Pasteur virus. It has an unrecorded passage history between 1940 and 1945. In 1964, virus from one of the rabbit passages was used to prepare the human diploid cell strain (HDCS). This strain was used to develop the human diploid cell rabies vaccine (HDCV) by the Merieux Institute.
PV_4 Strain	Believed to be derived from the original Pasteur virus. Its passage history is unknown. After one passage on rabbit brain at the Pasteur Institute, it was adapted to primary bovine fetal kidney cells and then to baby hamster kidney cells.
Street Alabama Dufferin Strain (SAD)	Originally isolated from the brain of a rabid dog by the Communicable Disease Center in Montgomery, Alabama in 1953. It was maintained by serial passage in mice until adapted to primary hamster kidney cells in 1960.
Evelyn Rockitnicki Abelseth Strain (ERA)	Produced by passage of the SAD strain of virus in chicken embryos and then porcine kidney cells.
Flury Low Egg Passage Strain (LEP)	Originally isolated in 1939 from a girl, named Flury, who died of rabies in Georgia, USA. Brain tissue was inoculated into one-day-old chicks and passaged in chick- embryo brain and chick embryo. Further passage in embryonated chicken eggs resulted in development of the Flury High Egg Passage (HEP) Strain.

neutralizing antibody was undetectable in 27% of patients.

Passive transfer of preformed antibodies in human rabies immunoglobulin (HRIG) or equine rabies immunoglobulin (ERIG) is an integral component of post-exposure rabies prophylaxis. Specific neutralizing antibody activity against the Stade isolate and against an EBL 2 (Finnish isolate) virus was determined in samples of HRIG, ERIG, and hyperimmune horse serum. Antibody titers were shown to vary from batch to batch. Higher titers of neutralizing antibody against EBL 1 and EBL 2 were observed in hyperimmune horse serum or ERIG than in HRIG (Herzog et al, 1991). Lafon et al (1986) reported that four batches of HRIG, as well as one concentrated preparation of HRIG, had high neutralizing antibody activity against EBL 1 (Stade isolate), although lower than that produced against serotype 1 virus. King (1991) reported that HRIG prepared in the United Kingdom neutralized viruses of serotypes 2 through 4 much less efficiently than it neutralized serotype 1 viruses.

A World Health Organization conference was held in Marburg, Germany in May of 1986 to discuss the questions raised by the presence of European bat lyssavirus in bat populations of Europe. Representatives from Denmark, Finland, France, Germany, Poland, Switzerland, the United Kingdom, and the United States agreed that all persons working with bats in Europe should be pre-exposure immunized against rabies and all persons bitten by a bat should receive the standard post-exposure rabies prophylaxis (Centers for Disease Control, 1986).

It has generally been recommended that human post-exposure rabies prophylaxis against the European bat lyssavirus consist of rabies vaccine and human rabies immunoglobulin, as per standard recommendations of the World Health Organization Expert Committee on Rabies (Lafon et al, 1986; World Health Organization, 1986d, 1992b). Celis et al (1988) suggested that vaccines formulated against a serotype 1 rabies virus may facilitate the capacity to mount an initial immune response and, therefore, confer an additional measure of protection.

Others have recommended investigating the use of highly specific EBL-targeting immunoglobulins in post-exposure rabies prophylaxis. The use of a "cocktail" of monoclonal antibodies may also be of value in the future (Dietzschold et al, 1990; Lafon et al, 1990; Enssle et al, 1991; Herzog et al, 1991; Montano-Hirose et al, 1993).

Montano-Hirose et al (1993) reported that passive protection of mice against lethal challenge with EBL 1 (Stade isolate) could be obtained using an intraperitoneally administered murine monoclonal antibody (MAb 8-2). Complete protection was afforded against EBL 1 using 50 EU of MAb 8-2. Only 62.5% of mice were protected using 2.5 EU of MAb 8-2. HRIG or ERIG (11 IU) alone protected only 25% of mice against EBL 1 challenge. A combination of HRIG (11 IU) and MAb 8-2 (2.5 EU) conferred 75% protection against EBL 1 challenge.

The need for development of a vaccine specifically formulated against the European bat lyssaviruses has also been suggested. Tordo et al (1993) recently reported development of the first recombinant vaccine against the Mokola virus. This baculovirus-derived recombinant vaccine effectively protected mice against lethal intracerebral challenge and fulfills international standards for protection.

References

Ali, M. W., Majumder, M. J., Huq, F., Latif, M. A., Bari, I. F., and S. A. Alam (1983). Study of the presence of rabies virus in indigenous bats. *Bangladesh Med. Res. Counc. Bull.* 9(2): 33

Anonymous (1958). Rabies in bats, moles, and cattle. *Vet. Bull.* 132: 469

Barrat, J., Artois, M., and H. Bourhy (1989). Two bats diagnosed rabid in France. *Rabies Bulletin Europe.* Information Surveillance Research. WHO Collaborating Centre for Rabies Surveillance and Research. Tubingen, Federal Republic of Germany. 13/89: 10

Beran, G. W. and O. de Mira (1966). Communitywide campaign on rabies in Dumaguete City, Philippines. *Pub. Hlth. Repts.* 81(2): 169

Beran, G. W., Nocete, A. P., Elvina, O., Gregorio, S. B., Moreno, R. R., Nakao, J. C., Buchett, G. A., Canizares, H. L., and F. F. Macasaet (1972). Epidemiological and control studies on rabies in the Philippines. *Southeast J. Trop. Med. Pub. Hlth.* 3(3): 433

Berger, R. (1986). A human rabies case in Finland possibly of bat origin. *Rabies Bulletin Europe.* Information Surveillance Research. WHO Collaborating Centre for Rabies Surveillance and Research. Tubingen, Federal Republic of Germany. 4: 12

Bitsch, V., Westergaard, J., and M. Valle (1986). Bat Rabies—Europe. *MMWR.* 35(26): 430

Botvinkin, A. D., Vakhrushev, A. V., and M. A. Selimov (1988). Isolation of rabies virus from a bat in western Siberia, USSR. *Zhurnal Mikrobiologii Epidemiologii i Immunobiologii.* No. 7: 97 (English abstract) in *Vet. Bull.* (1988). 58(11): 927

Botvinkin, A. D., Kuzmin, I. V., and S. M. Chernov (1992). The experimental infection of bats with *lyssavirus* serotypes 1 and 4 (English abstract). *Vopr-Virusol.* 37(4): 215.

Bourhy, H., Sureau, P., and N. Tordo (1990). From rabies to rabies-related viruses. *Vet. Microbiol.* 23: 115

Bourhy, H., Kissi, B., Lafon, M., Sacramento, D., and N. Tordo (1992). Antigenic and molecular characterization of bat rabies virus in Europe. *J. Clin. Microbiol.* 30(9): 2419

Bourhy, H., Kissi, B., and N. Tordo (1993). Molecular diversity of the *Lyssavirus* genus. *Virology.* 194(1): 70

Brigham, M. and M. Brock Fenton (1987). The effect of roost sealing as a method to control maternity colonies of big brown bats. *Can. J. Pub. Hlth.* 78(1): 47

Brosset, A. (1990). Les migrations de la pipistrelle de Nathusius, *Pipistrellus nathusii*, en France. Ses incidences possibles sur la propagation de la rage. *Mammalia.* 54(2): 207 English translation courtesy of Mme. Michèle Fressinier.

Bussereau, F., Vincent, J., and P. Sureau (1989). Caracterisation d'une souche Finlandaise, d'origine humaine de virus rabique, par des anticorps monoclonaux: anti-virus Mokola. *Rec. Med. Vet.* 165(11): 895. English translation courtesy of Mme. Michèle Fressinier.

Caffrey, J. P. (1992). Definition of the Status "Rabies Free Countries." *Report of the Meeting of the OIE Ad Hoc Group on Rabies Control.* Paris, France. April 22-23, 1992

Celis, E., Dawei, O. U., Dietzschold, B., and H. Koprowski (1988). Recognition of rabies and rabies-related viruses by T cells derived from human vaccine recipients. *J. Virol.* 62(9): 3128

Centers for Disease Control (1986). Bat rabies—Europe. *MMWR.* 35(26): 430

Charlton, K. M., Casey, G. A., Boucher, D. W., and

T. J. Wiktor (1982). Antigenic variants of rabies virus. *Comp. Immunol. Microbiol. Infect. Dis.* 5(1-3): 113

Chillaud, T. (1993). Head, Information and International Trade Development. Office International des Épizooties. Paris, France. Personal communication.

Clark, H. F. and T. J. Wiktor (1972). Rabies Virus. In M. Majers and S. A. Plotkin (eds.) *Strains of Human Viruses*. S. Karger. New York.

CNEVA (1990). *Les Chiropteres et La Rage en Europe*. Centre National D'Etudes Veterinaires et Alimentaires, Republique Francaise. Ministere de L'Agriculture et de La Foret. English translation courtesy of Mme. Michèle Fressinier.

Constantine, D. G. (1985). Disease exchange between bats and researchers: Problems and precautions. *Austr. Mammal.* 8(3/4): 325

Constantine, D. G. (1988). Health Precautions for Bat Researchers. In T. H. Kunz (ed.) *Ecological and Behavioral Methods for the Study of Bats*. Smithsonian Institution Press. Washington, D. C.

de Felipe Gardon, J. L. (1989). Rabies in Spain. *Rabies Bulletin Europe*. Information Surveillance Research. WHO Collaborating Centre for Rabies Surveillance and Research. Tubingen, Federal Republic of Germany. 2/89: 7

Dietzschold, B., Tollis, M., Rupprecht, C. E., Celis, E., and H. Koprowski (1987). Antigenic variation in rabies and rabies-related viruses: Cross-protection independent of glycoprotein-mediated virus-neutralizing antibody. *J. Infect. Dis.* 156(5): 815

Dietzschold, B., Rupprecht, C. E., Tollis, M., Lafon, M., Mattei, J., Wiktor, T. J., and H. Koprowski (1988). Antigenic diversity of the glycoprotein and nucleocapsid proteins of rabies and rabies-related viruses: Implications for epidemiology and control of rabies. *Rev. Infect. Dis.* 10(Suppl. 4): S785

Dietzschold, B., Gore, M., Casali, P., Ueki, Y., Rupprecht, C. E., Notkins, A. L., and H. Koprowski (1990). Biological characterization of human monoclonal antibodies to rabies virus. *J. Virol.* 64(6): 3087

Enssle, K., Kohler, K. R., Muller, H., Kanzy, E. J., Hilfenhaus, J., and F. R. Seiler (1991). A rabies-specific human monoclonal antibody that protects mice against lethal rabies. *Hybridoma.* 10(5): 547

Fedaku, M., Shaddock, J. H., Chandler, F. W., and D. W. Sanderlin (1988a). Pathogenesis of rabies virus from a Danish bat (*Eptesicus serotinus*): Neuronal changes suggestive of spongiosis. *Arch. Virol.* 99: 187

Fedaku, M., Shaddock, J. H., Sanderlin, D. W., and J. S. Smith (1988b). Efficacy of rabies vaccines against Duvenhage virus isolated from European house bats (*Eptesicus serotinus*), classic rabies and rabies-related viruses. *Vaccine.* 6: 533

Fenton, M. B. (1992). *Bats*. Facts on File, Inc. New York.

Gardner, S. D. (1989). Bat rabies in Europe. *J. Infect.* 18: 205

Grauballe, P. C., Baagoe, H. J., Fedaku, M., Westergaard, J. M., and H. Zoffmann (1987). Bat rabies in Denmark. *The Lancet.* I(8529): 379

Haagsma, J. (1989). Rabies en vleermuizen; hoe te handelen? *Ned. Tijdschr. Geneeskd.* 133(11): 550. (Rabies in bats: How should it be treated?). English translation courtesy of Dr. Nathan M. Appel.

Hentschke, J. and E. Hellmann (1975). Nachweis der tollwut bei einer fledermaus in Berlin (Diagnosis of rabies in a bat in Berlin). *Berliner und Munchener tierarztliche Wochenschrift.* 88(5): 92 (English abstract) in *Vet. Bull.* (1975). 45(7): 502

Herzog, M., Fritzell, C., Lafage, M., Montano Hirose, J. A., and D. Scott-Algara (1991). T and B cell human responses to European bat lyssavirus after postexposure rabies vaccination. *Clin. Exp. Immunol.* 85: 224

Judes, U. (1988). On the problem of "rabies" in bats. *Macroderma.* 4(1): 11

Kappeler, A. (1989). Bat rabies surveillance in Europe. *Rabies Bulletin Europe.* Information Surveillance Research. WHO Collaborating Centre for Rabies Surveillance and Research. Tubingen, Federal Republic of Germany. 13(4): 12

Kappeler, A. (1992). 4.2 First case of rabies in a bat in Switzerland. *Rabies Bulletin Europe*, 3rd quarter. Information Surveillance Research. WHO Collaborating Centre for Rabies Surveillance and Research. Tubingen, Federal Republic of Germany. 3/92: 11

Khozinski, V. V., Selimov, M. A., Botvinkin, A. D., King, A., Antonova, L. A., Smekhov, A. M., Shablovskaya, E. A., Klueva, E. V., and T. A. Aksenova (1990). Summary of rabies in Europe, 1st quarter 1990. Rabies virus of bat origin in the USSR. *Rabies Bulletin Europe.* Information Surveillance Research. WHO Collaborating Centre for Rabies Surveillance and Research. Tubingen, Federal Republic of Germany. 14(1): 10

King, A. (1987). Bat rabies "established in Europe." *Vet. Rec.* 121(13): 291

King, A. A. (1991). *Studies of the Antigenic Relationships of Rabies and Rabies-Related Viruses Using Anti-Nucleoprotein Monoclonal Antibodies.* Ph.D. Thesis. School of Biological Sciences, University of Surrey. Guildford, United Kingdom. Courtesy of Dr. Arthur A. King.

King, A. A. (1993). Rabies Reseach Leader. Central Veterinary Laboratory. New Haw, Addelstone, Surrey. United Kingdom. Personal communication.

King, A. and J. Crick (1988). Rabies-Related Viruses. In J. B. Campbell and K. M. Charlton (eds.) *Rabies.*

Kluwer Academic Publications. Boston.

King, A., Davies, P., and A. Lawrie (1990). The rabies viruses of bats. *Vet. Microbiol.* 23: 165

Koprowski, H., Wiktor, T. J., and M. K. Abelseth (1985). Cross-Reactivity and Cross-Protection: Rabies Variants and Rabies-Related Viruses. In E. Kuwert, C. Merieux, H. Koprowski, and K. Bogel (eds.) *Rabies in the Tropics*. Springer-Verlag. New York.

Krogsrud, J. and O. Odegaard (1988). Rabies situation—Current position in Norway. *Vet. Bull.* (1989). 59(2): 123

Kuzmin, I. V., Botvinkin, A. D., and A. B. Baialiev (1992). A lyssavirus with an unusual antigenic structure isolated from a bat in southern Kyrgyzstan (English abstract). *Vopr-Virusol.* 37(5-6): 256

Lafon, M. (1993). Rabies Unit. World Health Organization Collaborating Center for Rabies, Pasteur Institute. Paris, France. Personal communication.

Lafon, M., Herzog, M., and P. Sureau (1986). Human rabies vaccines induce neutralising antibodies against the European bat rabies virus (Duvenhage). *The Lancet.* II(8505): 515

Lafon, M., Bourhy, H., and P. Sureau (1988). Immunity against the European bat rabies (Duvenhage) virus induced by rabies vaccines: An experimental study in mice. *Vaccine.* 6: 362

Lafon, M., Edelman, L., Bouvet, J. P., and M. Lafage (1990). Human monoclonal antibodies specific for the rabies virus glycoprotein and N protein. *J. Gen. Virol.* 71: 1689

Lumio, J., Hillbom, M., Roine, R., Ketonen, L., Haltia, M., Valle, M., Neuvonen, E., and J. Lahdevirta (1986). Human rabies of bat origin in Europe. *The Lancet.* I(8477): 378

Matouch, O. (1986). Nakazova situace vztekliny v Evrope a CSSR vobobi 1981-1985. (Rabies situation in Europe and Czechoslovakia, 1981-85.) *Veterinarstvi.* 36(12): 551 (English abstract) in *Vet. Bull.* (1987). 57(6): 470

Mollgaard, S. (1985). Bat-rabies in Denmark, 3rd quarter 1985. *Rabies Bulletin Europe.* Information Surveillance Research. WHO Collaborating Centre for Rabies Surveillance and Research. Tubingen, Federal Republic of Germany. 3: 8

Mollgaard, S. (1986). Bat-rabies in Denmark (DEN), 4th quarter 1985. *Rabies Bulletin Europe.* Information Surveillance Research. WHO Collaborating Centre for Rabies Surveillance and Research. Tubingen, Federal Republic of Germany. 4: 11

Montano-Hirose, J. A., Bourhy H., and M. Lafon (1990). A reduced panel of anti-nucleocapsid monoclonal antibodies for bat rabies virus identification in Europe. *Res. Virol.* 141: 571

Montano-Hirose, J. A., Lafage, M., Weber, P., Badrane, H., Tordo, N., and M. Lafon (1993). Protective activity of a murine monoclonal antibody against European bat lyssavirus 1 (EBL1) infection in mice. *Vaccine.* 11(12): 1259

Muller, W. W. (1990a). Report on seminar of wildlife rabies control, July 2-5, 1990. Geneva, Switzerland. *Rabies Bulletin Europe.* Information Surveillance Research. World Health Organization Collaborating Centre for Rabies Surveillance and Research. Tubingen, Federal Republic of Germany. 3/90: 11

Muller, W. W. (1990b). Summary of rabies in Europe, 1st quarter 1990. Rabies in the Federal Republic of Germany. *Rabies Bulletin Europe.* Information Surveillance Research. WHO Collaborating Centre for Rabies Surveillance and Research. Tubingen, Federal Republic of Germany. 1/90: 5

Muller, W. W. (1990c). Summary of rabies in Europe, 3rd quarter 1989. Rabies in the Federal Republic of Germany (DEU). *Rabies Bulletin Europe.* Information Surveillance Research. WHO Collaborating Centre for Rabies Surveillance and Research. Tubingen, Federal Republic of Germany. 3/90: 5

Muller, W. W. (1992). 4.3 Review of reported rabies case data in Europe to the WHO Collaborating Centre Tubingen from 1977 to 1992. 4.3.3 Bat rabies cases. *Rabies Bulletin Europe*, 4th quarter. Information Surveillance Research. WHO Collaborating Centre for Rabies Surveillance and Research. Tubingen, Federal Republic of Germany. 4/92: 18

Muller, W. W. and J. Blancou (1992). Rabies in Europe: Now possible to confine and eliminate. *Br. Med. J.* 305: 725

Muller, W. W. and T. Muller (1992). 3. Rabies in individual countries—Germany, Federal Republic. *Rabies Bulletin Europe*, 4th quarter. Information Surveillance Research. WHO Collaborating Centre for Rabies Surveillance and Research. Tubingen, Federal Republic of Germany. 2/89: 6

Nieuwenhuijs, J. H. M. (1987). Rabies bij vleermuizen (Rabies in bats). *Tijdschrift voor Diergeneeskunde.* 112(20): 1193 (English abstract) in *Vet. Bull.* (1988). 58(2): 98

Nieuwenhuijs, J. H. M. (1989). Rabies in Europe, 2nd quarter 1989. Rabies in the Netherlands (NET). *Rabies Bulletin Europe.* Information Surveillance Research. WHO Collaborating Centre for Rabies Surveillance and Research. Tubingen, Federal Republic of Germany. 2/89: 6

Nieuwenhuijs, J. H. M. (1990a). Summary of rabies in Europe, 1st quarter 1990. Rabies in the Netherlands (NET). *Rabies Bulletin Europe.* Information Surveillance Research. WHO Collaborating Centre for Rabies Surveillance and Research. Tubingen, Federal Republic of Germany. 2/90: 7

Nieuwenhuijs, J. H. M. (1990b). Summary of rabies in Europe, 2nd quarter 1990. Rabies in the Netherlands (NET). *Rabies Bulletin Europe.* Information Surveillance Research. WHO Collaborating Centre for Rabies Surveillance and Research. Tubingen, Federal Republic of Germany. 2/90: 6

Nieuwenhuijs, J. H. M. (1990c). Summary of rabies in Europe, 3rd quarter 1989. Rabies in the Netherlands (NET). *Rabies Bulletin Europe*. Information Surveillance Research. WHO Collaborating Centre for Rabies Surveillance and Research. Tubingen, Federal Republic of Germany. 3/90: 6

Nieuwenhuijs, J. H. M. (1992). Summary of rabies in Europe, 4th quarter 1992. 3. Rabies in individual countries. Netherlands (NET). *Rabies Bulletin Europe*. Information Surveillance Research. WHO Collaborating Centre for Rabies Surveillance and Research. Tubingen, Federal Republic of Germany. 4/92: 12

Nieuwenhuijs, J., Haagsma, J., and P. Lina (1992). Epidemiology and control of rabies in bats in the Netherlands. *Rev. Sci. Tech. Off. Int. Epiz.* 11(4): 1155

Nieuwenhuis, H. U. (1988). The rabies situation in The Netherlands. *Parrassitologica*. 30(1): 123

Nikolic, M. and Z. Jelesic (1956). Isolation of rabies virus from insectivorous bats in Yugoslavia. *Bull. Wld. Hlth. Org.* 14: 801

Office International des Épizooties (1993). Chapter 3.1.5. Rabies. *International Animal Health Code*. Office International des Épizooties. Paris, France.

Pal, S. R., Arora, B., Chhuttani, P. N., Broor, S., Choudhury, S., Joshi, R. M., and S. D. Ray (1980). Rabies virus infection of a flying fox bat, *Pteropus poliocephalus* in Chandigarh, Northern India. *Trop. Geogr. Med.* 32: 265

Remmert, H. P., Rumke, H. C., and T. J. F. Savelkoul (1989). Rabies en vleermuizen; hoe te handelen? *Ned. Tijdschr. Geneeskd.* 133(22): 1142. (Rabies in bats: How should it be treated?) English translation courtesy of Dr. Nathan M. Appel.

Ressang, A. A., Gwan, S. I., and S. Hardjosworo (1963). Bats, rodents and rabies in Indonesia. *Communications Veterinaire*. 7: 33

Roine, R. O., Hillbom, M., Valle, M., Haltia, M., Ketonen, L., Neuvonen, E., Lumio, J., and Lahdevirta, J. (1988). Fatal encephalitis caused by a bat-borne rabies-related virus. *Brain*. 111: 1505

Rupprecht, C. E., Dietzschold, B., Wunner, W. H., and H. Koprowski (1991). Antigenic Relationships of Lyssaviruses. In G. M. Baer (ed.) *The Natural History of Rabies*. 2nd Edition. CRC Press, Inc. Boca Raton, Florida.

Schindler, R. and H. K. Dennig (1958). The role of bat rabies in Europe. *Monatsh. f. Tierheilk.* (1958) 10: 169 cited by *J. Am. Vet. Med. Assoc.* (1959). 134: 92

Schneider, L. G. (1982). Antigenic variants of rabies virus. *Comp. Immunol. Microbiol. Infect. Dis.* 5(1-3): 101

Schneider, L. G. (1983). A new case of bat-rabies in Germany (DEU). *Rabies Bulletin Europe*. Information Surveillance Research. WHO Collaborating Centre for Rabies Surveillance and Research. Tubingen, Federal Republic of Germany. 4/82: 17

Schneider, L. G., Muller, W. W., and K. P. Hohnsbeen (1989). Rabies in Europe, 3rd quarter. *Rabies Bulletin Europe*. Information Surveillance Research. WHO Collaborating Centre for Rabies Surveillance and Research. Tubingen, Federal Republic of Germany. 4/82: 17

Seidler, M., Brehmer, H.-J., Pott, B., Cox, J. H., and H. Zinke (1987). Tollwut bei fledermausen in Niedersachsen (Rabies in bats in Lower Saxony). *Berl. Munch. Tierarztl. Wschr.* (English translation) 100: 199

Selimov, M. A., Tatarov, A. G., Antonova, L. A., Shcherbak, Y. N., Shablovskaya, E. A., Smekhov, A. M., and B. Y. Mogilevsky (1986). To the issue of chiropteric rabic infection. *Rabies Information Exchange*. June 14: 9

Selimov, M. A., Tatarov, A., Botvinkin, A., Kulikova, L., and N. Khismatullina (1987). The rabies-related Yuli virus and its identification with a panel of antinucleocapsid monoclonal antibodies (NC MCAb). *Rabies Information Exchange*. June 16: 5

Selimov, M. A., Tatarov, A. G., Botvinkin, A. D., Klueva, E. V., Kulikova, L. G., and N. A. Khismatullina (1989). Rabies-related Yuli virus: Identification with a panel of monoclonal antibodies. *Acta Virol.* 33: 542

Selimov, M. A., Smekhov, A. M., Antonova, L. A., Shablovskaya, E. A., King, A. A., and L. G. Kulikova (1991). New strains of rabies-related viruses isolated from bats in the Ukraine. *Acta Virol*. 35: 226

Shcherbak, Y. N. (1984). Virological Studies of Rabies in the Ukrainian Soviet Socialist Republic. In: *Viruses and Viral Diseases*. 12: 11, Kiev (in Russian).

Smith, J. S. (1993). Research Microbiologist. Rabies Laboratory, Centers for Disease Control. Atlanta, Georgia. Personal communication.

Smith, P. C., Lawhaswasdi, K., Vick, W. E., and J. S. Stanton (1967). Isolation of rabies virus from fruit bats in Thailand. *Nature*. 216: 385

Soria Baltazar, R. S., Blancou, J., and M. Artois (1988). Etude du virus de la rage isole d'une chauve-souris Europenne (*Eptesicus serotinus*) pouvoir pathogene pour les ovins et le renard roux. *Revue. Med. Vet.* 139(7): 615

Speakman, J. R., Racey, P. A., Hutson, A. M., Webb, P. I., and A. M. Burnett (1991). Status of Nathusius' pipistrelle (*Pipistrellus nathusii*) in Britain. *J. Zool. (Lond.)*. 225: 685

Stebbings, R. E. (1988). *The Conservation of European Bats*. With the assistance of the IUCN/SSC Chiroptera Specialist Group. Christopher Helm, Ltd. London.

Stebbings, R. E. (1993). The Robert Stebbings Consultancy Limited. Species Ecologists and Habitat Assessors. Peterborough, Cambridgeshire, England. Personal communication.

Stebbings, R. E. and F. Griffith (1986). *Distribution and Status of Bats in Europe*. Natural Environment Research Council Institute of Terrestrial Ecology. Huntingdon, Great Britain.

Steele, J. H. (1966). *Rabies Survey—Territory of Papua and New Guinea. Appendix D - Indonesia*. Communicable Disease Center. U. S. Public Health Service. Atlanta, Georgia. September 17 - October 9, 1966

Stirbu, A., Filotti, A., and E. Toacsen (1973). Epidemo-epizootia de turbare in Romania si rolul liliecilor in transmiterea acestei boli (The rabies epidemic in Roumania and the role of bats in transmission). *Studii si Cercetari de Virusologie*. 24(2): 95 (English abstract) in *Vet. Bull.* (1973). 43(10): 551

Stougaard, E. (1986). Rabies in Denmark. *Rabies Bulletin Europe*. Information Surveillance Research. WHO Collaborating Centre for Rabies Surveillance and Research. Tubingen, Federal Republic of Germany. 3/86: 3

Stougaard, E. (1989). Rabies in Europe, 2nd quarter 1989. Rabies in Denmark (DEN). *Rabies Bulletin Europe*. Information Surveillance Research. WHO Collaborating Centre for Rabies Surveillance and Research. Tubingen, Federal Republic of Germany. 2/89: 3

Sureau, P., Bourhy, H., and M. Lafon (1989). La rage des chauve-souris en France. *Bull. Epidemiol. Hebdomadaire*. 40: 167. English translation courtesy of Mme. Michèle Fressinier.

Tacal, Jr., J. V. and P. A. Boado, Jr. (1966). Examination for Negri bodies of the brains of a species of Philippine bat (*Scotophilus temminckii horsfield*). *Acta Medica Philippina*. 3(2) ser. 2: 103

Tan, D. S. K., Beck, A. J., and M. Omar (1969). The importance of Malaysian bats in the transmission of viral disease. *Med. J. Malaya*. XXIV(1): 32

Thomas, I., Brouchier, B., Bauduin, B., Costy, F., Gilson, R., Fairon, J., and P. P. Pastoret (1989). La rage des chauves-souris en Europe. *Ann. Med. Vet.* 133: 437. English translation courtesy of Mme. Michèle Fressinier.

Tordo, N., Bourhy, H., Sather, S., and R. Ollo (1993). Structure and expression in baculovirus of the Mokola virus glycoprotein: An efficient recombinant vaccine. *Virology*. 194: 59

Twardowski, H. and M. Barancewicz (1986). Przypadki wscieklizny u syczura i nietoperza (Rabies in a rat and a bat). *Medycyna Weterynaryjna*. 42(1): 15 (English abstract) in *Vet. Bull.* (1986). 56(10): 892

Veeraraghavan, N. (1954). I. Rabies. E. A case of hydrophobia following bat bite. The Pasteur Institute of Southern India, Coonoor. Section E. Scientific Report. Abstract from Burke-Gaffney, H. J. (1955). *Trop. Dis. Bull.* 52: 764

Veterinary Chief Inspectorate of Public Health, Netherlands (1987). Rabies bij vleermuizen (Rabies in bats). *Tijdschrift voor Diergeneeskunde*. 112(13): 809 (English abstract) in *Vet. Bull.* (1987). 57(11): 915

Veterinary Chief Inspectorate, Netherlands (1990). Rabies bij vleermuizen (Rabies in bats). *Tijdschrift voor Diergeneeskunde*. 115(15/16): 752 (English abstract) in *Vet. Bull.* (1991). 61(3): 249

Veterinary Public Health Directorate (1989). Rabies bij vleermuizen (Rabies in bats). *Tijdschrift voor Diergeneeskunde*. 114(17): 913 (English abstract) in *Vet. Bull.* (1990). 60(3): 256

Ward, C. (1994). Bats in church. *The Lancet*. 343(8896): 552

Wersching, S. and L. G. Schneider (1969). A second case of rabies in a bat in Hamburg. *Berl. Munch. tierarztl. Wschr.* 82: 293 (English abstract) in *Vet. Bull.* (1970). 40(4): 282

Wiles, G. J. and J. E. Hill (1986). Accidental aircraft transport of a bat to Guam. *J. Mammal.* 67(3): 600

World Health Organization (1984a). Hazard of importing rabies-like viruses from Africa. *Information Circular* #15. WHO Mediterranean Zoonoses Control Centre.

World Health Organization (1984b). *Expert Committee on Rabies. Seventh Report*. WHO Tech. Rpt. No. 709. Geneva.

World Health Organization (1986a). Occurrence of bat rabies in Europe. *Rabies Bulletin Europe*. Information Surveillance Research. WHO Collaborating Centre for Rabies Surveillance and Research. Tubingen, Federal Republic of Germany. 1: 9

World Health Organization (1986b). Bat-rabies cases in the Federal Republic of Germany (DEU). *Rabies Bulletin Europe*. Information Surveillance Research. WHO Collaborating Centre for Rabies Surveillance and Research. Tubingen, Federal Republic of Germany. 2: 8

World Health Organization (1986c). Rabies in Germany, Federal Republic (DEU). *Rabies Bulletin Europe*. Information Surveillance Research. WHO Collaborating Centre for Rabies Surveillance and Research. Tubingen, Federal Republic of Germany. 3: 4

World Health Organization (1986d). Present human rabies vaccines and neutralising antibody activity against the bat strain DUVENHAGE recently isolated in Poland (POL), Denmark (DEN), and the Federal Republic of Germany (DEU). *Rabies Bul-*

letin Europe. Information Surveillance Research. WHO Collaborating Centre for Rabies Surveillance and Research. Tubingen, Federal Republic of Germany. 2: 9

World Health Organization (1987a). Table of bat rabies cases 1954-1986. *Rabies Bulletin Europe*. Information Surveillance Research. WHO Collaborating Centre for Rabies Surveillance and Research. Tubingen, Federal Republic of Germany. 4/86: 12

World Health Organization (1987b). Bat rabies in the Union of Soviet Socialist Republics. *Rabies Bulletin Europe*. Information Surveillance Research. WHO Collaborating Centre for Rabies Surveillance and Research. Tubingen, Federal Republic of Germany. 4/86: 12

World Health Organization/Veterinary Public Health (1988). *Report of WHO Consultation on Rabies (European Bat Rabies, Postexposure Treatment and Potency Testing for Rabies Vaccine)*. Essen. FRG. July 8, 1988. WHO/Rab. Res./88.30/Rev. 1. Unpublished document (reviewed with permission).

World Health Organization/Veterinary Public Health (1989). *Report of the Fifth WHO Consultation on Monoclonal Antibodies in Rabies Diagnosis and Research*. Geneva, March 3, 1989. WHO/Rab. Res./ 89.33. Unpublished document (reviewed with permission).

World Health Organization (1990a). Summary of rabies in Europe, 3rd quarter 1989. Rabies in Poland. *Rabies Bulletin Europe*. Information Surveillance Research. WHO Collaborating Centre for Rabies Surveillance and Research. Tubingen, Federal Republic of Germany. 3/90: 6

World Health Organization/Veterinary Public Health (1990b). *Report of the Sixth WHO Consultation on Monoclonal Antibodies in Rabies Diagnosis and Research*. The Wistar Institute, Philadelphia, Pennsylvania, USA. April 2-3, 1990. WHO/Rab. Res./ 90.34. Unpublished document (reviewed with permission).

World Health Organization (1990c). Summary of rabies in Europe. *Rabies Bulletin Europe*. Information Surveillance Research. WHO Collaborating Centre for Rabies Surveillance and Research. Tubingen, Federal Republic of Germany. 14 (1): 3

World Health Organization (1991a). Summary of rabies in Europe. *Rabies Bulletin Europe*. Information Surveillance Research. WHO Collaborating Centre for Rabies Surveillance and Research. Tubingen, Federal Republic of Germany. 15 (2): 3

World Health Organization (1991b). Summary of rabies in Europe. *Rabies Bulletin Europe*. Information Surveillance Research. WHO Collaborating Centre for Rabies Surveillance and Research. Tubingen, Federal Republic of Germany. 15 (3): 14

World Health Organization (1992a). Summary of rabies in Europe, 3rd quarter 1992. *Rabies Bulletin Europe*. Information Surveillance Research. WHO Collaborating Centre for Rabies Surveillance and Research. Tubingen, Federal Republic of Germany. 3/92: 3

World Health Organization (1992b). *Expert Committee on Rabies. Eighth Report*. WHO Tech. Rpt. No. 824. Geneva.

World Health Organization (1992c). Summary of rabies in Europe, 2nd quarter 1992. *Rabies Bulletin Europe*. Information Surveillance Research. WHO Collaborating Centre for Rabies Surveillance and Research. Tubingen, Federal Republic of Germany. 16 (2): 3

World Health Organization (1993a). *World Survey of Rabies 26 (for the year 1990)*. World Health Organization, Veterinary Public Health Unit, Division of Communicable Diseases, Geneva, Switzerland. WHO/Rabies/93.208, 1993. Unpublished document (reviewed with permission).

World Health Organization (1993b). *World Survey of Rabies 27 (for the year 1991)*. World Health Organization, Veterinary Public Health Unit, Division of Communicable Diseases, Geneva, Switzerland. WHO/Rabies/93.209, 1993. Unpublished document (reviewed with permission).

World Health Organization (1993c). Summary of rabies in Europe, 1st quarter 1993. Netherlands. *Rabies Bulletin Europe*. Information Surveillance Research. WHO Collaborating Centre for Rabies Surveillance and Research. Tubingen, Federal Republic of Germany. 1/93: 7

Zoffmann, H., Baagoe, H., Fedaku, M., Grauballe, C., and J. M. Westergaard (1987). Rabies hos flagermus i Danmark. Forekomst, betydning og forholdsregler (Rabies in bats in Denmark. Occurrence, significance, and precautions). *Dansk. Veterinaertidsskrift*. 70(14): 699 (English abstract) in *Vet. Bull.* (1988). 58(3): 162

SECTION V

Public Health Concerns

Chapter 24:
BAT RABIES AND THE GENERAL PUBLIC

A cloud of confusion has existed in the rabies literature, and especially in popular accounts regarding the role of bats in the epidemiology of this disease. Numerous interpretations of early investigators are still widely cited, despite the fact that they are no longer supported by modern scientific evidence. Contradiction and ambiguity, mistakes and misinterpretations have been perpetuated over decades. The difficulty lies in ferreting out the true from the seemingly true, the false from the seemingly false. Reasoned debate has been invited by the literature, serving as the stimulus which is the lifeblood of science.

As in all considerations of human/animal relationships, complex ethical questions surround the issue of bat rabies. Concerns for both human and animal welfare have been raised. Regrettably, many of these issues have been grossly magnified and carried far out of proper perspective by irresponsible, sensation-seeking reporting, designed to prey on deep-rooted cultural phobias. Not infrequently, insectivorous bats are likened to vampire bats and the lay public is not often encouraged to recognize a difference. In fact, some people even cling to the mistaken belief that insectivorous bats, when rabid, become transformed into "blood-sucking" vampire bats. The reckless narratives that characterize tabloid journalism have continued to fuel public fear of bats, helping to forge an image of these animals not at all consistent with scientific fact.

Routes of Human Exposure

Compared to the more significant threat posed by canine rabies worldwide, the public-health hazards associated with insectivorous bats are of minor importance. They cannot, however, be completely dismissed. Education of the public about the potential dangers of handling bats remains the single most important safeguard against bat-borne disease.

Human exposure to bat rabies might occur through one of several possible routes of transmission. Primary transmission of virus may result directly from bite (and possibly scratch) wounds, or may follow from the inhalation of an infectious aerosol. Secondary transmission may occur following exposure to a terrestrial animal, itself previously infected by a bat. Secondary transmission also includes the indirect transmission of a bat variant of virus via corneal transplantation from an undiagnosed rabid donor, as well as the possibility of mechanical transmission of short-lived virus in the saliva of a cat or dog that has just had a rabid bat in its mouth.

Transmission of rabies virus via inhalation of an infectious aerosol is extremely rare. Only four human cases have been reported. This mode of infection should not be of even remote concern to the general public, since it is a phenomenon confined to the research laboratory and possibly to the exploration of certain unique underground environments.

Transmission of rabies virus following corneal transplant is also very rare, only six cases having been reported. Only one of these cases involved a nonterrestrial variant of virus. The likelihood of infection from this type of exposure is extremely remote, particularly in view of the fact that it is now a well-recognized phenomenon. The Expert Committee on Rabies currently recommends that organs from any donor with neurological disease not be used for transplantation (World Health Organization, 1992).

There have been no documented cases of human rabies following mechanical transfer of virus; however, the possibility is of occasional concern to public-health authorities in the medical management of certain cases. At present, such a mode of transmission remains only a theoretical possibility.

Primary transmission via bite is, by far, the most significant route of human exposure to rabies virus. Examination of reports of bat-inflicted bites reveals three probable patterns of exposure:

1) The overwhelming majority of bat bites have occurred when people have handled sick or moribund animals. Both the curious passerby and the Good Samaritan (and children in particular) risk exposure to bite when handling grounded animals.
2) Less common are reports of encounters with bats that have wandered into homes or even been brought in by the family pet.
3) Least common are reports of deranged behavior and seemingly unprovoked (or, at least, unknowingly provoked) aggression caused by the neuropathic condition of rabies.

Handling of Bats

In England, *The Wildlife and Countryside Act* of 1981 affords protection to wild bats, as well as roosts and hibernation sites. In fact, it is a crime for an unlicensed person in England to even touch a bat. According to section 10(3) of this statute, however, Good Samaritans are allowed to retain disabled bats for the purpose of rendering first aid and nursing care, if deemed necessary (Editorial, 1986; Routh, 1991).

In this regard, sick or injured bats are being presented to veterinary practitioners and wildlife rehabilitation centers in England with increasing frequency. The care and devotion towards injured bats displayed by well-intentioned individuals is noteworthy and remains a reflection of our collective humanity and our increasing concern for the environment and the myriad of creatures it supports. England, however, currently enjoys a rabies-free status and so the risks involved in handling sick and injured wildlife are considerably decreased. Nevertheless, the Ministry of Agriculture, Fisheries, and Food requires that any dead bat be submitted for rabies testing (Routh, 1991).

In view of the dramatic increase in the number of reported cases of bat rabies in Europe, and especially Denmark, Turner and Crick (1987) wrote,

> *In Britain, bats now receive a lot of attention in the media and are being promoted as charming and harmless animals—as indeed they normally are. Geographical isolation makes it unlikely that British bats might be involved in any way [with cases of bat rabies on the European mainland]; nor should reports from mainland Europe be cause for public alarm. Nevertheless, 102 of the 104 positive isolations [of European Bat Lyssavirus from 550 bats examined in Denmark] were from Eptesicus serotinus, a species that is not uncommon in Britain. Perhaps the enthusiasm of bat conservationists, which encourages children to touch and handle bats, should be tempered by a little prudence in view of the Danish report.*

Bats should never be handled without good reason. It is extremely important that obviously ill or moribund bats, or those behaving in what seems to be an abnormal fashion, not be handled at all. The majority of persons who have been bitten by bats have been exposed by handling sick or injured animals. In countries in which enzootic bat rabies exists (including the United States), no attempts at rehabilitating wild bats should be made by inexperienced individuals, and bat conservation groups should not encourage such attempts.

Veterinary clinicians and wildlife rehabilitators, who may be presented with ill or injured bats, should be wary of ministering to them, particularly if they are inexperienced in the proper care and management of these animals.[1] Moreover, they should carefully question all people directly involved, ascertain the probability that they may have been exposed to infectious saliva, and guide them towards visiting with a physician, if warranted.

[1]Notable exceptions might include endangered species or those individual bats which have been in residence at zoological gardens for extended periods of time. Some zoos, however, introduce wild-caught insectivorous bats into their exhibits without allowing an adequate period of time in quarantine.

Table 24-1

Dog and Cat Contacts With Bats Submitted for Rabies Testing in New York State, 1985-1991

	1985	1986	1987	1988	1989	1990	1991
Total No. Bats Submitted	1,184	953	1,312	1,177	1,271	1,782	1,663
No. (%) Submitted Bats Having Contact with a Cat	429 (36.2)	396 (41.6)	485 (37)	452 (38.4)	499 (39.3)	713 (40)	826 (50)
No. (%) Submitted Bats Having Contact with a Dog	62 (5.2)	38 (4.0)	51 (3.9)	52 (4.4)	79 (6.2)	123 (6.9)	99 (6.0)
No. (%) Rabies-Positive Submissions	43 (3.6)	46 (4.8)	48 (3.7)	38 (3.2)	54 (4.2)	84 (4.7)	79 (4.8)
No. (%) Rabies-Positive Bats Having Contact with a Cat	11 (25.6)	11 (23.9)	18 (37.5)	6 (15.8)	11 (20.4)	25 (29.8)	24 (30.4)
No. (%) Rabies-Positive Bats Having Contact with a Dog	7 (16.3)	4 (8.7)	8 (16.7)	5 (13.2)	5 (9.3)	14 (16.7)	16 (20.3)

Data from Trimarchi, C. V. *Rabies Annual Summaries, 1985-1991.* Rabies Laboratory, Wadsworth Center for Laboratories and Research, New York State Department of Health. Albany, New York.

Potential Exposure of Pets

Although rabid cats and dogs represent a small proportion of animals confirmed rabies positive each year in the United States, they do represent a high proportion of suspect submissions. In a 12-month survey of 20 states in 1981, approximately 23% and 32% of post-exposure rabies prophylaxis resulted from exposures to cats and dogs, respectively (Helmick, 1983). Between 1981 and 1987, each rabid cat identified in Maryland exposed an average of 9.7 humans (Fischman et al, 1992). In view of the vast number of people who sustain bites from cats or dogs, any encounter that a cat or dog might have with a rabid bat has potential public-health significance.

Being quite agile, cats frequently capture and play with bats (Dean et al, 1960; Scatterday et al, 1960; Trimarchi, 1983, 1990; Frantz and Trimarchi, 1984; Trimarchi et al, 1986; Delpietro et al, 1987; Nieuwenhuijs et al, 1992; Hoff et al, 1993). Dogs may also play with sick and moribund bats. Although cats interact with bats much more frequently than dogs do, they are much less likely to be immunized against rabies. Delpietro et al (1987) reported observing both cats and dogs actively hunting bats in Argentina. Pet owners should be wary of such habits (Barker, Jr. and Francis, 1972).

Although most states do not keep adequate records of animal exposure to bats, information from those that do indicates that the potential for such interaction may be significant. Between 1985 and 1991, 41% of bats submitted to the New York State Department of Health and 27% of those confirmed rabies positive had interacted with a cat. Comparable figures for interaction with dogs were 5.4% and 15%, respectively (Table 24-1). Between January, 1990 and September, 1993, 19.8% of 180 bats confirmed rabid in Arizona interacted with a dog or cat (Levy, 1993).

In England, 50% (16 of 32) of bats seen at one veterinary clinic over a two-year period had been injured by a domestic cat (Routh, 1991) and Stebbings (1988) reported that approximately 33% of 450 bats found dead in Britain over a seven-year period were captured by cats. This latter determination was based on identification of characteristic injuries found during necropsy of dead bats (Stebbings, 1993). It is unknown how many of these bats were active and actually captured in flight and how many were already ill and grounded when found by a cat. There have been only three reports of transmission of rabies virus from a bat to a dog (Whetstone et al, 1984; Neill, 1993; Smith, 1994). The validity of the first report has been questioned; however, the two most recent reports have been confirmed. There have been close to two dozen confirmed reports of such transmission to cats in the United States (see Table 16-2).

Cats may capture bats outside or interact with those that have found their way into homes. They are also known to bring captured bats home with them, often releasing them once inside. In the face of confirmed reports of rabies transmission from bats to cats, and the significant potential for bat/cat interaction, all cats should be vaccinated against rabies.

Only about 4% of the 50 million plus pet cats in the United States are immunized against rabies (Raef, 1990). Mandatory immunization of cats against rabies is urged by the American Veterinary Medical Association, the National Association of State Public Health Veterinarians, the Cornell University Feline Health Center, and numerous epidemiologists and veterinary practitioners. Immunization of cats against rabies is particularly important in areas of enzootic terrestrial or nonterrestrial rabies (Brass, 1993; Hoff et al, 1993; Spencer, 1994).

Hazard to Human Health

Sporadic spillover of virus from bat populations to wildlife does not appear to be significant in the total spectrum of rabies epidemiology. Similar spillover to human populations, however, represents a direct human health hazard.

Alarmists may assert that since the discovery of the first rabid bat in the United States in 1953, the number of rabies-positive specimens has significantly increased from year to year. Moreover, a significant percentage of human deaths from indigenously acquired rabies infection (75% between 1980 and 1990) has been due to bat-inflicted disease. Bats are, therefore, to be considered highly significant reservoirs of this disease.

Considering numbers in a vacuum, however, does not provide a complete story and will lead to erroneous interpretations. For example, although 75% of human rabies deaths between 1980 and 1990 were, in fact, related to bats, it should be noted that this represented a total of only three of four persons. In fact, since the first report of bat rabies in the United States, only 20 cases of human rabies have been attributed to virus of bat origin (see pages 220-237). Of these, one individual survived the ordeal and one patient was infected indirectly via a corneal transplant from a donor who had died of bat-origin virus. Additionally, three human deaths due to the bite of an insectivorous bat are known from Canada, two from the former Soviet Union, and one each from India, South Africa, and Finland. Based on the absolute number of human rabies cases due to virus of insectivorous-bat origin (28 cases known globally), bat rabies can hardly be said to constitute a significant cause of human mortality.[2]

Furthermore, although the total number of bats reported rabid annually has continued to rise dramatically each year, the percentage of submitted specimens that are confirmed rabid has remained essentially unchanged. Rabies in bats is not on the rise. More rabid bats are found each year because public-health facilities are more actively searching for them. Although the prevalence of disease may be relatively high (5% to 10% or more) among suspect submissions, it is generally extremely low (<1%) in randomly collected, healthy-appearing specimens that have been adequately sampled (although prevalence may be higher in migratory species during annual migrations or in certain species of nonmigratory bats). The human health hazards posed by rabid insectivorous bats are extremely low.

By equating the dangers of bat-associated rabies with death rate alone, however, we arrive at a falsely low assessment of risk. Fortunately, due to the efficacy of post-exposure rabies prophylaxis, human deaths from rabies in the United States and other industrialized nations are not common. As Table 3.1 shows, since 1980, human rabies deaths have averaged less than three cases annually in the United States. Of these, 44% (7 of 16) were exposed by contact with animals outside the United States (Centers for Dis-

[2]A number of cases of human rabies believed to have been due to interaction with nonhematophagous bats have been reported from Latin America. Unfortunately, an accurate assessment of the number of such cases or the epidemiologic circumstances surrounding them is impossible.

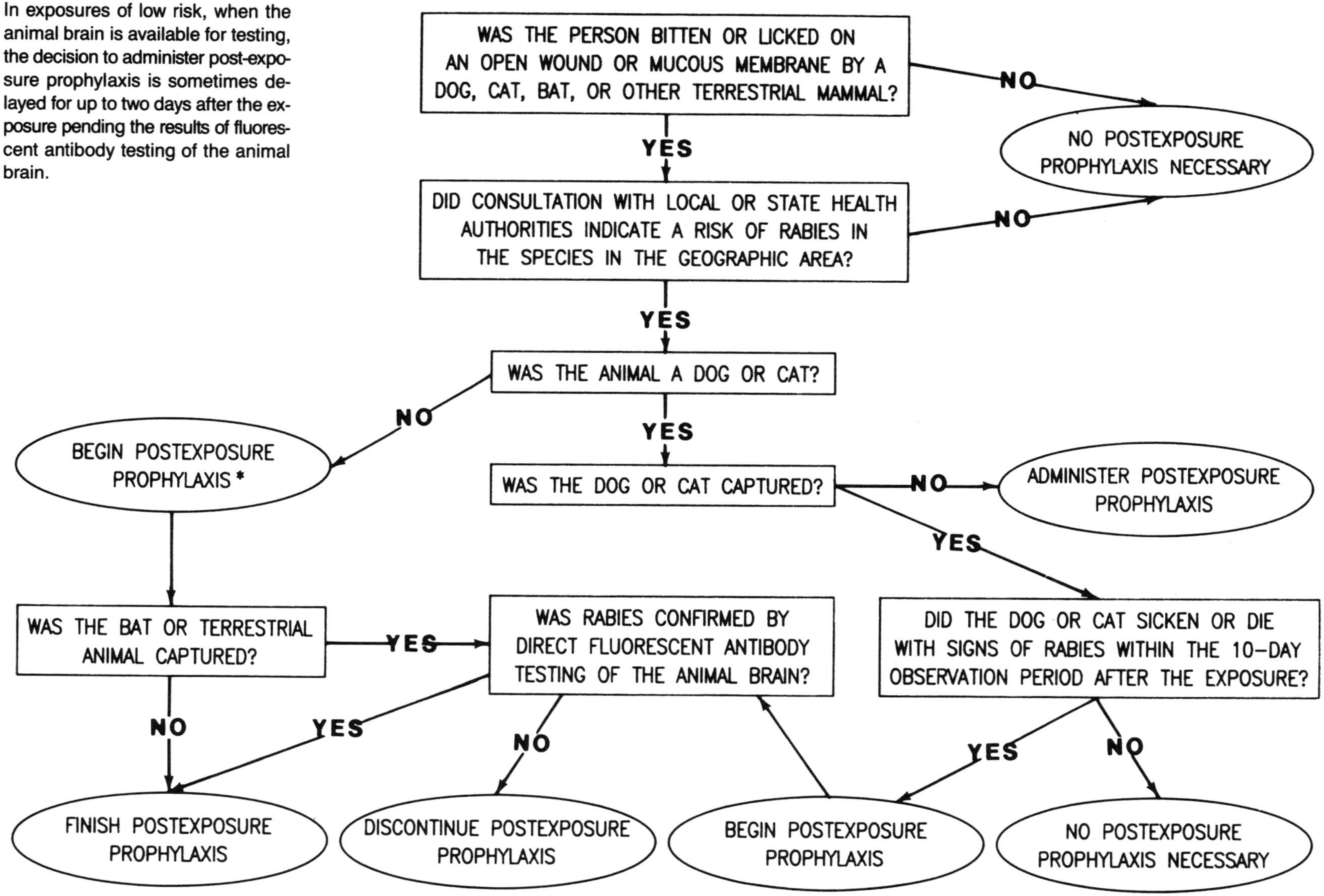

* In exposures of low risk, when the animal brain is available for testing, the decision to administer post-exposure prophylaxis is sometimes delayed for up to two days after the exposure pending the results of fluorescent antibody testing of the animal brain.

Figure 24-1. An algorithm for human post-exposure rabies prophylaxis. (From Fishbein, D. B. Pre-exposure and Postexposure Immunization Against Rabies. In D. B. Fishbein, L. A. Sawyer, and W. G. Winkler (eds.) *Rabies Concepts for Medical Professionals*. 2nd Edition, 1986. Merieux Institute. Miami, Florida. Reproduced by permission of Connaught Laboratories.)

ease Control, 1993).

A closer approximation to the real public-health significance of bat-inflicted rabies may be related to the number of humans who are bitten by rabid bats. Unfortunately, this number cannot be accurately determined. Sporadic reports from various public-health facilities provide some information; however, the availability of accurate information is extremely limited. Furthermore, it is impossible for public-health authorities to validate many reports of alleged human encounters with insectivorous bats (see page 217).

All persons who have sustained a bite or scratch from a bat, or a nonbite exposure involving contamination of open lesions or mucous membranes with saliva or other potentially infectious materials, must be considered at high risk of exposure to rabies until such time as the bat is proven to be free of rabies by a qualified laboratory. As such, the presence of bats in homes may lead to anxiety due to concern over potential exposures of family members and pets. If disturbed by the presence of bats roosting in a home, effective and economical means exist for building them out by batproofing the premises.

First Aid For Bat Bite

If bitten or scratched by a bat, reasonable attempts should be made to capture the animal, if possible, taking adequate precautions not to sustain another bite. As little damage as possible should be done to the animal's head, since examination of the brain is the method used to determine whether or not the animal is rabid. The bat should be brought to a public-health laboratory as soon as possible. Local physicians and veterinarians can advise on the nearest location of a laboratory capable of performing the fluorescent antibody test required for identification of the rabies virus.

The wound should be washed with soap and water as quickly as possible, followed by application of alcohol or tincture or aqueous solution of iodine. The victim should seek medical attention immediately. If possible, wounds should not be sutured. Figure 24-1 illustrates a flow chart of possible scenarios following human exposure to a potentially rabid animal. Post-exposure rabies prophylaxis is not routinely recommended for "animal encounters." The need for more aggressive treatment must be carefully evaluated on an individual basis by medical professionals. Administration of antibiotics or tetanus prophylaxis, if indicated, should follow local wound treatment.

Role of Pre-Exposure Rabies Prophylaxis

It is imperative that pre-exposure immunized persons understand the nature of the immunity established. Guaranteed protection against the threat of rabies following the bite of a rabid animal is not the goal of pre-exposure rabies prophylaxis. Rather, it is aimed at providing a measure of immediately available protection that will function until such time as medical attention is obtained, or hopefully provide adequate protection in the case of an unknown exposure. This, in and of itself, may be lifesaving. However, if bitten by what is believed to be a potentially rabid animal, all pre-exposure immunized persons should receive post-exposure rabies prophylaxis. However, in this instance, an abbreviated treatment regimen is used, which may save the victim hundreds of dollars in the cost of medicinals. Attending medical personnel must be informed of the immune status of the victim prior to initiation of post-exposure rabies prophylaxis.

References

Barker, Jr., W. H. and B. J. Francis (1972). Rabies in the Northwest. Epidemiology 1930-1969. *Northwest Med.* 71(3): 179

Beran, G. W. (1988). Professor of Veterinary Epidemiology and Public Health. Department of Veterinary Microbiology and Preventive Medicine, College of Veterinary Medicine, Iowa State University. Ames, Iowa. Personal communication.

Brass, D. A. (1993). Insectivorous bats as reservoirs of rabies. *Compen. Cont. Educ. Pract. Vet.* 15(12): 33

Campbell, A. G. M. (1993). Is a change in rabies vaccine schedule necessary for travellers? *The Lancet.* 341(8843): 500

Centers for Disease Control (1993). Editorial Note. *MMWR.* 42(41): 805

Dean, W. D., Maddy, K. T., Cockrum, E. L., and H. G. Crecelius (1960). Rabies in insectivorous bats of Arizona. *Arizona Med.* 17(2): 69

Delpietro, H., Fabregas, F., and M. Diaz (1987). Riesgo de transmision rabica en la predacion de quiropteros por carnivoros domesticos. (Risk of rabies transmission to cats and dogs by predation on bats.) *Vet. Arg.* IV(32): 119 (English abstract) in *Vet. Bull.* (1987) 57(9): 734

Editorial (1986). Oh for the life of a bat!! *NSS (Natl. Speleol. Soc.) News.* 44(7): 275

Fischman, H. R., Grigor, J. K., Horman, J. T., and E. Israel (1992). Epizootic of rabies in raccoons in Maryland from 1981-1987. *J. Am. Vet. Med. Assoc.* 201(12): 1883

Frantz, S. C. and C. V. Trimarchi (1984). Bats in human dwellings: Health concerns and management. In D. J. Decker (ed.) *Proceedings of the First Eastern Wildlife Damage Control Conference.* pp. 299-308. Cornell University. Ithaca, New York. September 27-30, 1983.

Helmick, C. G. (1983). The epidemiology of human rabies postexposure prophylaxis, 1980-1981. *J. Am. Med. Assoc.* 250(15): 1990

Hoff, G. L., Mellon, G. F., Thomas, M. C., and D. H. Giedinghagen (1993). Bats, cats, and rabies in an urban community. *South. Med. J.* 88(10): 1115

Levy, C. (1993). Epidemiology Specialist. Division of Disease Prevention, Vector-Borne and Zoonotic Diseases, Arizona Department of Health Services. Phoenix, Arizona. Personal communication.

Neill, S. U. (1993). Supervisor, Medical Virology. Texas Department of Health. Austin, Texas. Personal communication.

Nieuwenhuijs, J., Haagsma, J., and P. Lina (1992). Epidemiology and control of rabies in bats in the Netherlands. *Rev. Sci. Tech. Off. Int. Epiz.* 11(4): 1155

Prins, B. and K. Loewen (1988). Bat rabies in British Columbia 1971-1985. *Can. Vet. J.* 29: 41

Raef, T. A. (1990). AVMA encourages mandatory rabies vaccinations for cats. *J. Am. Vet. Med. Assoc.* 196(4): 528

Routh, A. (1991). Bats in the surgery: A practitioner's guide. *Vet. Rec.* 128(14): 316

Scatterday, J. E., Schneider, N. J., Jennings, W. L., and A. L. Lewis (1960). Sporadic animal rabies in Florida. *Pub. Hlth. Repts.* 75(10): 945

Smith, J. S. (1994). Research Microbiologist. Rabies Laboratory, Centers for Disease Control. Atlanta, Georgia. Personal communication.

Spencer, L. M. (1994). Taking a bite out of rabies. *J. Am. Vet. Med. Assoc.* 204(4): 479

Stebbings, R. E. (1988). *The Conservation of European Bats.* With the assistance of the IUCN/SSC Chiroptera Specialist Group. Christopher Helm, Ltd. London.

Stebbings, R. E. (1993). The Robert Stebbings Consultancy Limited. Species Ecologists and Habitat Assessors. Peterborough, Cambridgeshire, England. Personal communication.

Trimarchi, C. V. (1983). The Epidemiology and Control of Bat Rabies in New York State. *Proceedings of the North American Symposium on Wildlife Rabies.* Johns Hopkins University. Baltimore. November 7-8, 1983.

Trimarchi, C. V. *Rabies Annual Summaries, 1985-1991.* Rabies Laboratory, Wadsworth Center for Laboratories and Research, New York State Department of Health. Albany, New York.

Trimarchi, C. V., Rudd, R. J., and M. K. Abelseth (1986). Experimentally induced rabies in four cats inoculated with a rabies virus isolated from a bat. *Am. J. Vet. Res.* 47(4): 777

Turner, G. S. and J. Crick (1987). Bat rabies and the UK. *The Lancet.* I(8535): 744

Whetstone, C. A., Bunn, T. O., Emmons, R. W., and T. J. Wiktor (1984). Use of monoclonal antibodies to confirm vaccine-induced rabies in ten dogs, two cats, and one fox. *J. Am. Vet. Med. Assoc.* 185(3): 285

World Health Organization (1992). *Expert Committee on Rabies. Eighth Report.* WHO Tech. Rpt. No. 824. Geneva.

Chapter 25:
CONCERNS IN CAVE EXPLORATION

Encounters with Bats in Restricted Passageway

Avid spelunkers (cavers) may spend hundreds of hours underground annually. Depending on the location and nature of their excursions, cavers may come into close proximity to enormous numbers of bats during the course of a year's activity. With respect to the potential for exposure to bat-transmitted rabies virus, it is justified that the responsibility and safety of such activity be explored.

In negotiating restricted passage (crawlways, narrow stoopways, etc.), it is not uncommon for cavers to pass close to, or sometimes even lightly brush against, an unseen bat (Figure 25-1). Most conscientious cavers try to avoid disturbing bats as much as possible, but such encounters are usually inevitable in cave exploration. The degree to which human encounters may distress these bats is highly variable, as is a bat's individual reaction to the disturbance. Bats so disturbed may respond in a variety of ways. They may remain essentially motionless (seemingly unaffected, although metabolically possibly not), they may "look about" in seemingly alert fashion, they may vocalize, or they may simply up and fly away. Regarding individual reactions to such human intrusion, there are usually no overt signs by which cavers might predict a bat's response (Barker, Jr. and Francis, 1972). Students of bat ethology might be more keenly observant of predictive signs, but for the caving community in general, bat response must be regarded as unpredictable. Certainly, time of year, time of day, nature of the disturbance, as well as individual and species-specific characteristics play a role. So, too, does the health of the animal. Lack of predictability of bat behavior may be magnified by rabies infection.

It is not unusual for bats to lightly brush cavers, or even have momentary collisions with them, while in flight through restricted cave passages. Cavers should note that this is not reflective of a rabies-induced disorientation. The echolocative skills of bats enable them to build a neural/sonic representation of their complex three-dimensional underground world.[1] Once learned, they may fly passageways by memory, without resorting to echolocation. Thus, they may not be echolocating when they unexpectedly brush against a caver in the middle of their intended flight path. Pregnant bats may also occasionally collide with cavers. Constantine et al (1968) reported that they may lack the necessary maneuverability to navigate around unexpected obstacles in their flight path.

Risk to Cave Explorers

Regarding a face-to-face encounter with a bat disturbed by human passage, cavers are justified in seeking answers to certain questions. Could this bat be rabid? Would I recognize a rabid bat if I saw one? Am I subjecting myself to a potential exposure to virus? In the unlikely eventuality that this bat is rabid, will it manifest signs of spontaneous aggression? Am I unknowingly provoking it? Will it be strong enough to hang onto the wall if I bump into it? Might it fall down onto my shoulder? Will it bite me?

[1]Echolocation refers to the mechanism by which bats direct their flight, avoid obstacles in their path, and locate and track prey. They do this by emitting a high-frequency sound and assessing the quality of the reflected echo. Auditory processing of emitted frequencies and returning echoes (usually held at an over-represented frequency) allows them to gather information about the size, shape, speed, and direction of intended prey, as well as to construct an acoustic image of their surrounding environment.

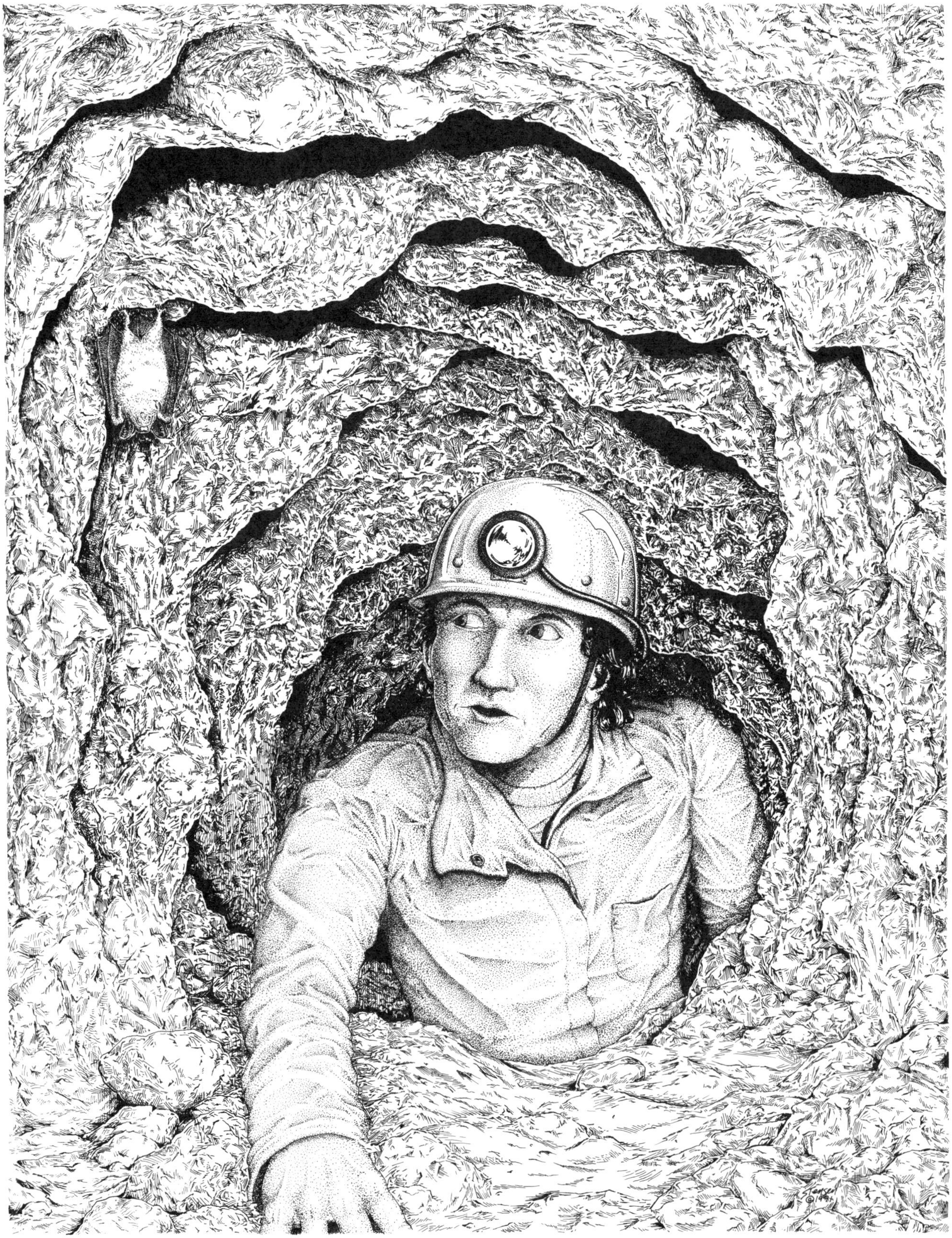

Figure 25-1. Cavers frequently encounter bats in narrow passageway. Care should be taken to avoid disturbing them.

Although these are questions with no definitive answers, make no mistake about it, the likelihood of a caver encountering an individual rabid bat in restricted passageway is exceedingly small. Similarly, the risk of contracting rabies while traveling underground is remote in the extreme. Despite the hundreds of thousands of man hours spent underground annually by members of the National Speleological Society,[2] there has been no report of bat-inflicted rabies in a caver secondary to a bite sustained while underground. However, while this fact certainly attests to the rarity of the phenomenon, it does not mean that it cannot occur.[3]

Consider, for example, that 1 in 500 (0.2%) bats in a given population is rabid. Between the number of bats disturbed by close passage and those passed beneath at some distance, active cavers may have relative encounters with 500 bats in a short span of time. In a statistical sense, one may consider this span of time as representing one potential encounter with a rabid individual, the behavior of which must be regarded as only marginally predictable.

The likelihood of this potential exposure being a tragic one is unbelievably small. As in other considerations of caver safety, however, it is important that a presumably safe track record not lead to a state of complacency. Many instances are known of people sustaining bites by handling debilitated bats, and grounded (ill or injured) bats are sometimes observed by cavers. It is extremely important that cavers encountering such bats not unwittingly expose themselves to bites by handling them.

Finally, it is not impossible (however rare) for a caver to sustain an unprovoked (or even unknowingly provoked) attack by a rabid bat. At least one such incident is known to have occurred. In his survey of American Caving Accidents, Knutson (1981) reported the following account:

In late August [1977], a 19-year-old Oklahoma City woman went with friends to Henson's Cave in McDonald County, Missouri. Past the entrance crawl, the woman was standing in some water when she was bitten by a bat. A companion struck the bat with a coat. In Oklahoma City, the bat was determined to be rabid by health officials. The woman was treated for rabies. The cave was later closed by the Missouri Department of Highways.

It is not known how many cavers may have experienced bites by bats (rabid or nonrabid), provoked or unprovoked in nature. There has been only this one report of such an exposure in cave accident-analysis files. However, others may have gone unreported. Survey studies aimed at evaluating population densities of bats are not uncommon. They may involve the handling of individual specimens by persons relatively inexperienced in doing so. The author has witnessed survey participants handling bats barehanded during the course of identification and Halliday (1958) reported cavers frequently handling bats (although responsible cavers rarely handle bats today). It is unknown if any unreported bites may have been sustained by those involved.

By increasing his time underground, a caver may be increasing his probability of exposure to a rabid bat. The fact that no caver, to date, is known to have contracted bat rabies is a reflection of the low prevalence of natural infection in wild bats, the general lack of aggression in rabid cave-dwelling Chiropteran species, and the willingness of the overwhelming majority of cavers to leave cave-dwelling creatures unmolested. In this regard, most cavers adhere to the time-honored motto of the National Speleological Society, a maxim that should serve as an umbrella for wilderness travelers everywhere:

Take nothing but pictures,
Leave nothing but footprints,
Kill nothing but time.

[2]The National Speleological Society (NSS) is an American-based organization that has grown to international proportion. With a membership of over 10,000 individuals, the Society is devoted to the exploration, conservation, and scientific study of caves.

[3]It should be noted that two persons are believed to have contracted bat rabies in Frio Cave or a similar Mexican free-tailed bat nursery. Their respective sojourns, however, were so far removed from the mainstream of American caving activity that they might arguably be excluded from a consideration of general caver exposure.

Can Probabilities of Exposure Be Defined?

The overwhelming number of instances of caver encounters with bats at close range (and these are frequent) will present as little more than momentary diversions from other caving activities. Invariably, the bat will suffer more than the caver. Indeed, at the wrong time of the year, forcing a bat to arouse out of its torpid state may needlessly kill it (Brady, 1983). In this regard, spelunkers and speleologists have both inadvertently been responsible for major declines in many bat populations (Mohr, 1972).[4]

The fact that underground interactions between bats and humans frequently result in adverse effects on bat populations should not be construed as a guarantee of absolute safety. Wilderness travel underground should always be approached in a conservative fashion and cavers should address relevant safety issues. Is an anchor safe? Yes, but it should be backed up anyway. Is a rope likely to break? No, but responsible cavers are very cognizant of where their ropes are set down, how they are handled, and how any given technical excursion relates to a rope's previous history. Is available lighting adequate for the planned trip? Yes, but not carrying spare light sources is one of the cardinal sins of underground travel. Is a caver likely to encounter a rabid bat? No, but in this respect, there is no single train of thought universally shared by students of either bat biology or bat rabies. Experts remain sharply divided in their assessment of exposure risk. It is, therefore, incumbent upon each caver to arrive at his own conclusions regarding the relative risks involved. In assessing the potential risk of bat-inflicted rabies from stray encounters with bats underground, some thoughts that merit consideration by cavers include the following:

1) **What is the probability of a caver being bitten by a bat?** Very rare. According to Dr. Merlin Tuttle (1986), an internationally recognized expert on bats and founder of Bat Conservation International, "The odds of ever being attacked by a bat, rabid or otherwise, are extremely remote, as attested by the fact that neither I nor any of my colleagues have witnessed such an event over the last 25 years and, to my knowledge, none occurred before that." It should be noted, however, that nationwide, many bites by insectivorous bats have been reported above ground by public-health authorities, although cave-dwelling species are generally not involved in these instances.

Unprovoked attacks most often involve solitary species or colonial big brown bats. Some health-department officials have expressed the view that authentic recorded attacks by bats are extremely rare, and Tuttle and Kern's (1981) concerns regarding the validity of such reports have merit. However, while it is likely that many alleged reports may have no real basis in actual fact, it is quite clear that many of them do. At least one well-documented report exists of a caver sustaining an unprovoked attack by a rabid bat while underground (Knutson, 1981).

2) **If bitten by a bat, what is the probability that the bite will pierce the skin?** Unknown. This depends on various circumstances, such as site of bite, presence and type of clothing, fury of the attack, species of bat, etc. Many bats, for example, are not able to exert sufficient biting force to effectively penetrate the skin (Griffin, 1958). Of commonly infected species, the little brown bat's bite rarely breaks the skin, being more of a pinch. Solitary bats can produce small lacerations, but these bats are not likely to be encountered by cavers. The big brown bat has nee-

[4]When a bat enters into a state of winter hibernation, its body is laden with fat deposits to insure survival through its long tenure in a dormant state. With metabolism geared down to a bare minimum, stored fat depots provide an acceptable energy reserve. Unnatural disturbances, such as human intrusion, frequently arouse bats out of torpor. With arousal comes a dramatic increase in metabolism and a consequent drain on available energy reserves. Even small depletions of energy stores may result in the death of aroused animals. Death does not ensue immediately, but is a gradual process as depleted reserves are gradually utilized, with no hope of replenishment. At the present time, a more conservation-minded generation of cavers avoids exploration in various caves at those times of the year when bat populations are most sensitive to the detrimental effects of human intrusion. Seasonal closure of many caves to human intrusion helps prevent a traffic of persons less interested in cave ecology and conservation.

dle sharp teeth and powerful jaws. Its bite often causes lacerations and bleeding (Daniels et al, 1960). This is another species not usually found in caves unless in a state of hibernation (although the majority probably hibernate in buildings [Whitaker, Jr. and Gummer, 1992]). Bites from Mexican free-tailed bats may break the skin if their canine teeth are sharp. Baer (1992) believes that bites by bats with small teeth may still pierce the skin. This is particularly true if bitten in an area where the skin is very thin, or on an especially delicate area such as the lip.

3) **If bitten, what is the probability that the bat is rabid?** Not very great. Nationwide, the prevalence of rabies among healthy-appearing wild colonial species is believed to be less than 1% (approximating 0.1% to 0.5%). Healthy bats, however, do not randomly target humans as bite victims and the likelihood of a healthy bat inflicting an unprovoked bite is considerably less than that of a rabid individual (although the probability of either remains very low). Any bat, healthy or not, abused by human interaction may bite in self-defense. From a medical perspective, any bat bite must be considered as an exposure to a potentially rabid animal until proven otherwise.

4) **If bitten by a rabid bat, what is the probability of viral transmission?** Unknown. It has been suggested that virus may be present intermittently in the saliva of some rabid animals. At any given moment, viral levels in the saliva may vary greatly. Probability of disease among untreated persons bitten by confirmed rabid dogs varies between 15% to 60%, depending on numerous factors. Certainly, severity of the bite wound (did it break the skin?) is significant.

5) **If infected, what is the probable outcome?** If treated promptly and appropriately, the risk of contracting rabies is almost nonexistent.[5] If untreated, agonizing death is a virtual certainty once clinical signs appear.

Exposure to Viral Aerosols

The development of human rabies following exposure to aerosolized virus has been reported in only four instances. The two alleged human cases of natural infection are known only from the unique environment of heavily populated nursery colonies in the Southwest. In fact, although widely accepted, the evidence that inhalation of aerosolized virus was involved in these two human deaths remains questionable. The inhalant risks for humans entering this type of ecosystem remain poorly defined. It is prudent, however, to consider that unprotected humans entering Mexican free-tail maternity colonies may be at increased risk of exposure.

The dangers associated with such locales can be eliminated completely by simply avoiding them altogether. There is, in fact, no reason for any lay person to enter the environment of one of these nursery colonies while a maternity roost is in residence. No one other than a properly immunized scientist with valid reasons has any business whatsoever in a free-tailed bat nursery. It is not a place for sport cavers; it is not a place for boy-scout trips; it is not a place for school or family outings; it is not a place for adventurous or mischievous little boys. Proper education and entry control may both preserve these sites as valuable natural nurseries and diminish their status as attractive hazards. In considering these sites as aerosol infection centers for local wildlife, it must be emphasized that there is no evidence to indicate that this actually occurs.

The densely populated maternity caves of the southwestern United States are hardly typical of most caves in the country and the likelihood of an airborne rabies hazard in caves elsewhere is remote (Constantine, 1986a). Mahan (1973) tested air samples from caves in Tennessee and Alabama with summer populations of several thousand bats in residence. Winkler and Adams (unpublished data cited by Winkler, 1975) tested air samples from several caves in Oklahoma, Alabama, and Tennessee. Tennessee and Alabama are major karst zones and are heavily trafficked by cavers. With 4,500 and 2,713 known caves, respectively, these two states account for 18.3% of known caves in the United States (Thorne,

[5]Discussion of rare instances of vaccine failure can be found in reports by Centers for Disease Control (1987), Lumbiganon et al (1987), Shill et al (1987), Editorial (1988), Fishbein et al (1988), and Fescharek et al (1994).

1987). All caves studied were well ventilated. Neither group found evidence of airborne virus. Winkler (1975) reported that the prevalence of rabies among the resident bat populations had remained constant at approximately 0.5% for several years.

Conditions in north temperate-zone caves are probably not conducive to airborne transmission of virus (Trimarchi, 1978; Constantine, 1986a). The risk to cavers exploring in caves other than the Mexican free-tailed bat nurseries of the southwestern United States is virtually nonexistent.

It must be emphasized that the presence of such incredible numbers of bats in southwest maternity caves creates a unique environment, markedly different from those systems frequented by cavers (or tourists visiting commercial caves). It is plainly evident that the labyrinths of Frio Cave and similar locales do not constitute environments wherein the typical caver would find himself engaged in exploration. The likelihood of a caver inadvertently finding his way into such a place is remote. It is, therefore, not possible to unwittingly stumble into a Frio Cave-like ecosystem and unknowingly expose oneself to aerosolized virus. Like the gaudy monarch butterfly, dressed in its orange-red warning coloration, the caves signal their potential danger to all who care to heed their warning. In this regard, at least, exposure to aerosolized rabies virus of bat origin cannot be regarded as a realistic hazard to even the most intrepid of hard-core cavers. Statements such as the following, which appeared in *Medical World News* (1965), are misleading and should not be accepted at face value,

> *...and it has even been shown that men can contract rabies merely by walking into a cave inhabited by infected bats.*

Unfortunately, such misleading statements are still made today. The vast majority of caves in the United States do not support large enough populations of bats to make aerosol transmission of virus even a remote concern. Even in areas where infected bats may be present, it is highly unlikely that viral dissemination can result in an infectious aerosol. This points to the insignificance of such a route of infection in the epidemiology of human rabies and cavers should not be unduly concerned about the threat of such an exposure.

Maximizing Safety Underground

In the course of an average year, an active dry caver or sump diver may spend innumerable hours underground. Even though the probability is very small that bats in any given cluster are rabid, there is little doubt but that most active cavers have passed, unknowingly, beneath many rabid bats in the course of their stygian adventures.

Should cavers, in fear of bat rabies, stop caving? Hardly. Should they advance underground harboring fear and trepidation with every footstep? Most certainly not. They should, however, recognize that, as a group, the caving community constitutes a population that might be at greater potential risk of exposure to bats than almost any other. Caving is a sport that is not without risk. It enjoys a reputation (deserved or not) in a class with mountaineering, technical rock climbing, hang gliding, skydiving, scuba diving, base jumping, and others. As such, it demands a responsibility of action for safe participation, part of which must necessarily include a consideration of unique biological hazards, including exposure to rabies of bat origin.

Safety underground can be increased in many ways, not the least of which are such obvious precautions as adequate lighting, adequate clothing, careful rigging when required, safety belays when necessary, proper route finding, and the acquisition of skill and experience in discrete increments. Protection against singular, potential health hazards must also be included in any consideration of safety and responsibility in wilderness travel.

Should Cavers Seek Pre-Exposure Rabies Prophylaxis?

With regard to bat rabies, the caver's best possible protection derives from common-sense caution in handling bats and from prompt wound care and post-exposure rabies prophylaxis in the unlikely eventuality that a bite from a rabid bat (or from one unavailable or unsuitable for testing) is sustained. The need for pre-exposure rabies immunization remains controversial.

Varying opinions have been expressed regarding the need for pre-exposure immunization of the caving community. The diverse convictions of bat biologists, conservationists, physicians, veterinarians, public-health officials, and experts in rabies notwithstanding, the hazards to cavers posed by rabies in bat populations are extraordinarily remote.

Tuttle, for example, claims that only cavers who have legitimate reasons for handling or being in close contact with bats should be pre-exposure immunized (Tuttle, 1986). It is certainly prudent for all persons who handle bats to be pre-exposure immunized. It is equally prudent for all others to leave bats strictly alone. In view of the rarity of reported instances of apparently unprovoked bat attacks upon cavers (only one documented case), pre-exposure rabies immunization of the general caving community may not be warranted (Brass, 1993).

However, the fact that cavers do not routinely pass through maternity passage harboring tens of millions of bats (with consequent potential exposure to aerosolized virus) is not sufficient justification, in itself, to recommend against immunization.[6] That one caver has suffered an apparently unprovoked attack by a rabid bat while underground is sufficient enough justification to think that another can. In this regard, Dr. George Baer (1992), former Chief, Rabies Laboratory, Centers for Disease Control and advisor to the World Health Organization Expert Committee on Rabies; Dr. George Beran (1992), a consultant to the World Health Organization Expert Committee on Rabies and Professor of Veterinary Epidemiology and Public Health, Iowa State University; and Dr. Denny Constantine (1986a), Public Health Veterinarian, California Department of Health Services, a leading expert on bats and renowned authority on the relationship between bats and public health—all advise that anyone exploring caves be pre-exposure immunized. This latter view is shared by the Immunization Practices Advisory Committee (Centers for Disease Control, 1991).

Even though the risk of bat-inflicted rabies palls to near insignificance in comparison with more familiar underground hazards, consideration of pre-exposure rabies immunization is merited. Suffice it to say, each person must assess for himself the risks associated with bat rabies, and weigh them against the risks, benefits, and costs of pre- versus post-exposure rabies prophylaxis.

Cavers who decline to seek pre-exposure immunization are certainly not in imminent danger of bat-inflicted rabies. Likelihood of bat bite, let alone infection from a rabid individual, remains extremely remote.

A special case may exist among those cavers who routinely mount expeditions into Latin America. In recent years, this area (particularly Mexico) has become something of a new frontier of exploration, to which cavers worldwide have been attracted in increasing numbers. As home range of the vampire bat, this region should be one of particular concern to cavers. Possibly within caves, but particularly in the rustic setting of primitive campsites, cavers may be exposed to vampire bats and thus may invite attack.

The habits of these bats in seeking blood meals is of significance. Attacks on humans by vampire bats are not uncommon and several hundred people have died of vampire-transmitted rabies. The caver who exposes himself to potential encounters with these bats places himself at possible risk. Members of such expeditions should take special precautions, and it is this author's belief that pre-exposure immunization should be mandatory safety protocol for any caver embarking on an extended expedition to this part of the world.

Of additional concern to cavers traveling from the United States to Mexico (or deeper into Latin America) is the significant presence of en-

[6]Although it is true that conservation-minded cavers should not engage in exploration of areas where large numbers of bats are present, the unfortunate truth of the matter is that not all persons traveling underground are particularly concerned about bat conservation. Ethical concerns in wilderness usage notwithstanding, to many cavers, bats represent little more than a nuisance to exploration. They regard them as creatures whose hibernation or reproductive cycles often force periodic, if not permanent, closure of favored caving sites. It is an attitude that cannot be condoned by more ecologically responsible segments of the caving community.

zootic rabies in the canine population. Rabies in dogs is common from Mexico to Argentina and has been responsible for many human fatalities. From 1988 to 1990, dogs accounted for 93.5% (35,678 of 38,149) of the cases of animal rabies diagnosed in Mexico. Of 208 human deaths due to rabies in Mexico during this time period, 184 (88.5%) were due to exposure to rabid dogs (Centers for Disease Control, 1989; Reid-Sanden et al, 1990; Uhaa et al, 1992). Although studies are currently underway in attempts to develop oral vaccination programs for free-roaming rabid dogs in Mexico (Fishbein et al, 1992; Frontini et al, 1992), tourists traveling to Latin America remain at increased risk.

Regardless of a caver's immunization status, safety guidelines include common-sense caution in handling bats and appropriate post-exposure rabies prophylaxis, if warranted. In this respect, it is extremely important to realize that pre-exposure immunization does not guarantee protection if bitten by a rabid animal. Although it may afford considerable protection (particularly in cases of unrecognized exposure or those involving delayed medical attention), an abbreviated post-exposure regimen is still necessary to insure safety following exposure to rabies virus.

Specific Recommendations for the Caving Community

1) Only properly immunized individuals, with a demonstrated adequate serum antibody titer, should explore maternity caves harboring enormous numbers of Mexican free-tailed bats (such as those of the southwestern United States)—and then, only with good reason. Responsible sport cavers have no business being in such locales. Heedless exploration of these caves needlessly endangers both bats and cavers and cannot be condoned.

2) Fortunately, rescue call-outs for accidents in southwestern maternity caves are uncommon. In the event of an emergency, only pre-exposure-immunized persons should be involved in rescue operations (National Cave Rescue Commission, 1981). The NCRC should maintain an updated national roster of pre-exposure-immunized rescue personnel.[7] Should the need for a call-out arise, resources should be selectively drawn from this list. Additionally, it would be well advised for the NCRC to maintain a local cache of specialized rescue gear to help minimize exposure of underground personnel to the potential threat of aerosolized virus or noxious gas. The necessity for post-exposure rabies prophylaxis of rescue personnel following an extended period in a Frio Cave-like environment is questionable. Consideration must focus on duration of stay, density of bat population, proximity of bats to caving activity, patterns of air flow, etc. Beran (1992) observed that these factors must be carefully evaluated on an individual basis. Public-health authorities should be consulted prior to engaging in rescue operations.

3) All caves harboring large bat populations should be avoided during times of mass movement. Cavers caught in a "bat storm" may be jeopardizing their safety to an unknown degree. Unfortunately, the number of bats that constitute a "large enough" population cannot be adequately defined. Furthermore, cavers should not disturb either maternity colonies or hibernating populations of bats, since irrevocable damage to the population may be sustained.

4) Constantine (1988) reiterated a number of points of potential importance to cavers, particularly those studying bats in the field. Cavers should recognize that the presence of large populations of cave-dwelling bats does not necessarily imply the existence of an atmosphere safe for humans to breathe. High concentrations of noxious and toxic gases have been found in southwestern maternity bat caves and individuals may succumb to their debilitating effects if not adequately protected (Knutson, 1984). If poisonous gases have recently been used to control vampire bats in Latin America, residues may persist in caves and present a health hazard to cavers. Similarly, in-

[7]Formed in 1977, the National Cave Rescue Commission (NCRC) was developed to coordinate cave rescue resources throughout the United States. It is a national communication network serving to locate and mobilize the specialized manpower and equipment required for cave rescue operations across the country.

discriminate smearing of anticoagulants along cave walls, in attempts to kill vampire bats, may present a danger to cavers who inadvertently contact the material. Fortunately, these methods of control are rarely used. Cavers should, nonetheless, be attentive to signs suggestive of vampire habitation and avoid exploration in systems known to or suspected of harboring vampire bats.

5) Cavers should avoid caves where large-scale die-offs of bats have recently occurred. Although major die-offs of bats due to rabies outbreaks have not been documented, such losses may be indicative of other potential public-health hazards, such as noxious gases. Public-health authorities should be notified immediately of any observed increase in numbers of dead bats. It is difficult to say when one could safely venture back into such a cave. Public-health officials, concerned with human safety, may be overly cautious in this regard. But, their recommendations should be given every consideration by the caving community.

6) Although cavers should generally avoid handling bats, there are times when bat handling is justified. In particular, bat surveys and bat-banding studies conducted by properly trained conservation personnel are important yardsticks for assessing population dynamics of various species. This information is essential to conservation programs. No person, however, should ever handle a bat without receiving proper training from experienced individuals. All persons participating in bat surveys, bat-banding programs, or otherwise handling bats, should be pre-exposure immunized against rabies. Experts have repeatedly emphasized that bats should not be handled without gloves (Orr, 1958; Davis, 1960; Martin, 1961; Schnurrenberger et al, 1964; Greenhall, 1972; Constantine, 1985, 1986b; Carpenter, 1986; Raisweiler, IV, 1977, 1986; Wimsatt, 1986; Haagsma, 1989; Schmidly, 1991; Fenton, 1992). Conservation personnel should, in addition, maintain a national roster of pre-exposure-immunized cavers to call upon for survey assistance. Requests of the general caving community for aid in population surveys should never be made if handling of bats will be involved. Cavers asked to participate in such surveys should, in their own best interest, decline if they have not been pre-exposure immunized against rabies.

7) Cavers should give serious consideration to pre-exposure rabies prophylaxis. This should include a post-vaccination blood sample, followed by one at least every two years to assess serum antibody titers. Should antibody titers fall below an adequate level, a booster injection is required to maintain an acceptable level of immunity. This echoes recommendations made by others (Centers for Disease Control, 1966 [cited by Davis, 1966]; Sikes [see Constantine, 1967]; Smith, 1971; Koprowski, 1979; McClurg, 1980; Halliday, 1982; Corey, 1983; McChesney et al, 1983; Immunization Practices Advisory Committee - Centers for Disease Control, 1984, 1991; Elliot et al, 1985; Constantine, 1986a; Webster et al, 1987; Vodopija and Clark, 1991; Baer, 1992; Beran, 1992).

Compared to the individual expense, cost of pre-exposure immunization is tremendously reduced if a group is involved. For cavers who are members of university-sponsored outdoor or caving clubs, expense may be reduced even further by utilizing the assistance of university health services for administration of the vaccine (Brown, 1971; Lewis, 1990).

Cavers should, however, recognize that others do not consider there to be a pressing need for generalized pre-exposure immunization of the caving community. Based upon the rarity of reported bat attacks on cavers, there may be no need for widespread caver immunization (Tuttle, 1986; Brass, 1993). It remains for cavers themselves to judge the relative risks involved.

8) Cavers planning expeditions in Mexico, or Central or South America should be pre-exposure immunized against rabies well in advance of departure.

9) Cavers should recognize that bats are not vicious creatures. They are neither malignant nor malevolent. To the contrary, they are generally harmless and quite beneficial to human society. In their habits, bats remain both unique and fascinating. Many species of bats are essential components of tropical and desert ecosystems and insectivorous bats devour untold quantities of insects worldwide. Bats do, indeed, play integral

roles in the complex web of life and, all aspects considered, the world of man is a better place because of them.

Cavers, Caves, and Caving—A Perspective

In the aftermath of wilderness tragedy, public sentiment is often particularly acute. Many of us have been witness to a typical public response—wilderness travelers must be protected from themselves. Crags have been closed to climbing; caves have been posted, gaited, or blasted shut; dive sites have been rendered inaccessible; wilderness travel banned; etc. In considering the possible ramifications that human intrusion into wilderness areas might have, responsible activity by the caving community has lasting justification. Part of this responsibility must include minimizing the risk of bat-inflicted rabies.

In placing bats, rabies, cavers, caves, and caving in perspective, some might argue that recommendations for cavers to consider pre-exposure immunization will be construed by the public as application of yet another onerous label to an already overly maligned animal. These recommendations are not meant to affix such labels. If a caver contracts rabies from an encounter with a bat, a shudder will likely pass through the local community. Moreover, outcries of "Killer Bats/ Killer Caves" may start anew, and the public might well move in the direction of closing local caves and mounting anti-bat campaigns. This is a very real response scenario. Local authorities often go to great lengths to insure the safety of wilderness travelers, even if this manifests itself as closing off the wilderness. In any event, local community reaction is not likely to be in the best interest of bats, caves, or cavers.

By further minimizing an admittedly minimal risk, we provide a measure of protection for both bats and cavers. At best, this can be achieved through mass education and pre-exposure immunization of the caving community. Realistically, however, an acceptable safety alternative would probably derive from a mass education of the caving community towards an awareness of the potential hazards in handling bats and an understanding of how to proceed in the unlikely eventuality that a bat bite is sustained.

By caving softly and wisely, and by minimizing interactions with fragile underground life, the caving community can lessen its impact on the underground environment. Furthermore, by demonstrating a united responsibility of action and a willingness to police their own safety, cavers can help forestall legislation restricting public access to wilderness terrain. This, in turn, will help to preserve the freedom of wilderness travel that we all have come to hold so dear.

References

Baer, G. M. (1992). Former Chief, Rabies Laboratory. Centers for Disease Control. Atlanta, Georgia. Personal communication.

Barker, Jr., W. H. and B. J. Francis (1972). Rabies in the Northwest. Epidemiology 1930-1969. *Northwest Med.* 71(3): 179

Beran, G. W. (1992). Professor of Veterinary Epidemiology and Public Health. Department of Veterinary Microbiology and Preventive Medicine, College of Veterinary Medicine, Iowa State University. Ames, Iowa. Personal communication.

Brady, J. T. (1983). Cave management for the endangered Indiana bat (*Myotis sodalis*) and gray bat (*Myotis grisescens*). *NSS (Natl. Speleol. Soc.) News* 41(11): 298

Brass, D. A. (1993). Rabies in bats. Proceedings of the Arizona Regional Association (NSS). *The Desert Caver.* Newsletter of the Escrabrosa Grotto, Inc. National Speleological Society. 23(1): 2

Brown, R. C. (1971). Pre-exposure rabies prophylaxis in amateur spelunkers. *J. Am. College Hosp. Assoc.* 20: 132

Carpenter, R. E. (1986). Old World Fruit Bats. In M. E. Fowler (ed.) *Zoo and Wild Animal Medicine.* 2nd Edition. W. B. Saunders Co. Philadelphia.

Centers for Disease Control (1984). Possible rabies exposure from bats—Texas. *MMWR.* 33(26): 375

Centers for Disease Control (1987). Editorial note. *MMWR.* 36(46): 759

Centers for Disease Control (1989). *Rabies Surveillance Report. Annual Summary for the Year 1988.* U. S. Department of Health and Human Services, Public Health Service. Atlanta, Georgia.

Centers for Disease Control (1991). Recommendations of the Immunization Practices Advisory Committee (ACIP). Rabies Prevention—United States, 1991. *MMWR.* 40(No. RR-3): 1

Constantine, D. G. (1967). Bat rabies in the southwestern United States. *Pub. Hlth. Repts.* 82(10): 867

Constantine, D. G. (1985). Disease exchange between

bats and researchers: Problems and precautions. *Austr. Mammal.* 8(3/4): 325

Constantine, D. G. (1986a). Public Health Veterinarian. Department of Health Services, State of California—Health and Welfare Agency, Veterinary Public Health Unit. Berkeley, California. Personal communication.

Constantine, D. G. (1986b). Insectivorous Bats. In M. E. Fowler (ed.) *Zoo and Wild Animal Medicine.* 2nd Edition. W. B. Saunders Co. Philadelphia.

Constantine, D. G. (1988). Health Precautions for Bat Researchers. In T. H. Kunz (ed.) *Ecological and Behavioral Methods for the Study of Bats.* Smithsonian Institution Press. Washington, D.C.

Constantine, D. G., Tierkel, E. S., Kleckner, M. D., and D. M. Hawkins (1968). Rabies in New Mexico cavern bats. *Pub. Hlth. Repts.* 83(4): 303

Corey, L. (1983). Rabies and Other Rhabdoviruses. In R. G. Petersdorf, R. D. Adams, E. Braunwald, K. J. Isselbacher, J. B. Martin, and J. D. Wilson (eds.) *Harrison's Principles of Internal Medicine.* W. B. Saunders Co. Philadelphia.

Daniels, J. B., Stuart, G., Wheeler, R. E., Gifford, C., Ahearn, J. P., Philbrook, F. R., Hayes, R. O., and R. A. MacCready (1960). A search for encephalitis and rabies in bats of eastern Massachusetts. *New Engl. J. Med.* 263(10): 516

Davis, W. H. (1960). Be careful. *Bat Banding News.* 1: 4

Davis, W. H. (1966). Accidental exposure of individuals to airborne rabies. *Bat Res. News.* 7(2): 18

Editorial (1988). Rabies vaccine failures. *The Lancet.* 1(8591): 917

Elliot, D. W., Tolle, S. W., Goldberg, L., and J. B. Miller (1985). Pet-associated illness. *New Engl. J. Med.* 313(16): 985

Fenton, M. B. (1992). *Bats.* Facts on File, Inc. New York.

Fescharek, R., Franke, V., and M. R. Samuel (1994). Do anesthetics and surgical stress increase the risk of postexposure rabies treatment failure. *Vaccine.* 12(1): 12

Fishbein, D. B., Sawyer, L. A., Reid-Sanden, F. L., and E. H. Weir (1988). Administration of human diploid-cell rabies vaccine in the gluteal area. *New Engl. J. Med.* 318(2): 124

Fishbein, D. B., Frontini, M. G., Dobbins, J. G., Collins, E. F., Huerta, G. Q., Rodriguez, J., Woo-Ming, B., Ramos, J. G., Belotto, A. J., Torres, J. M. B., Yenne, K. M., Linhart, S. B., and G. M. Baer (1992). Prevention of canine rabies in rural Mexico: An epidemiologic study of vaccination campaigns. *Am. J. Trop. Med. Hyg.* 47(3): 317

Frontini, M. G., Fishbein, D. B., Ramos, J. G., Collins, E. F., Torres, J. M. B., Huerta, G. Q., Rodriguez, J., Belotto, A. J., Dobbins, J. G., Linhart, S. B., and G. M. Baer (1992). A field evaluation in Mexico of four baits for oral rabies vaccination of dogs. *Am. J. Trop. Med. Hyg.* 47(3): 310

Greenhall, A. M. (1972). Identification of the vampire bat. *Wld. Anim. Rev.* 2: 44

Griffin, D. (1958). *Listening in the Dark—The Acoustic Orientation of Bats and Men.* Yale University Press. New Haven, Connecticut.

Haagsma, J. (1989). Rabies en vleermuizen; hoe te handelen? *Ned. Tijdschr. Geneeskd.* 133(11): 550. (Rabies in bats: How should it be treated?) English translation courtesy of Dr. Nathan M. Appel.

Halliday, W. R. (1958). Medical hazards to cave explorers. *Gen. Pract.* XVIII(1): 80

Halliday, W. R. (1982). *American Caves and Caving—Techniques, Pleasures, and Safeguards of Modern Cave Exploration.* Barnes and Noble Books. New York.

Knutson, S. (1981). American Caving Accidents, 1976 through 1979. *NSS (Natl. Speleol. Soc.) News* (part 2). 39(5): A31

Knutson, S. (1984). American Caving Accidents, 1983. *NSS (Natl. Speleol. Soc.) News.* 42(11): 353

Koprowski, H. (1979). Rabies. In P. B. Beeson, W. McDermott, and J. B. Wyngaarden (eds.) *Cecil's Textbook of Medicine.* W. B. Saunders Co. Philadelphia.

Lewis, W. C. (1990). Airborne rabies in bat maternity caves. *NSS (Natl. Speleol. Soc.) News.* 48(11): 282

Lumbiganon, P., Bunyahotra, V., and C. Pairojkul (1987). Human rabies despite treatment with rabies immune globulin and human diploid cell rabies vaccine—Thailand. *MMWR.* 36(46): 759

Mahan, W. E. (1973). *An Evaluation of the Relationship Between Cave-Dwelling Bats and Fox Rabies in Appalachia.* M.S. Thesis. University of Georgia. Athens, Georgia.

Martin, R. L. (1961). Current aspects of U. S. bat rabies problem. *Bat Banding News.* 2(3): 23

McChesney, T. C., Spatz, H., and M. Edelman (1983). Bat rabies in Arkansas. *J. Arkansas Med. Soc.* 80(4): 181

McClurg, D. (1980). *Exploring Caves—A Guide to the Underground Wilderness.* Stackpole Books. Harrisburg, Pennsylvania.

Medical World News (1965). Growing menace of rabies. August 27, 1965. p. 58

Mohr, C. E. (1972). The status of threatened species of cave-dwelling bats. *Bull. Natl. Speleol. Soc.* 34(2): 33

National Cave Rescue Commission (1981). Hazardous Atmospheres. In T. L. Williams (ed.) *Manual of U. S. Cave Rescue Techniques.* National Cave Rescue Commission, National Speleological Society. Huntsville, Alabama.

Orr, R. T. (1958). Keeping bats in captivity. *J. Mam-*

mal. 39(3): 339

Rasweiler, IV, J. J. (1977). Bats as Laboratory Animals. In W. A. Wimsatt (ed.) *Biology of Bats.* Vol. III. Academic Press. New York.

Rasweiler, IV, J. J. (1986). American Leaf-Nosed Bats. In M. E. Fowler (ed.) *Zoo and Wild Animal Medicine.* W. B. Saunders Co. Philadelphia.

Reid-Sanden, F. L., Dobbins, J. G., Smith, J. S., and D. B. Fishbein (1990). Rabies surveillance in the United States during 1989. *J. Am. Vet. Med. Assoc.* 197(12): 1571

Schmidly, D. J. (1991). *The Bats of Texas.* Texas A and M University Press. College Station, Texas.

Schnurrenberger, P. S., Beck, J. R., and F. Burson (1964). Bat rabies: A discussion of problems existing in Ohio. *Ohio State Med. J.* 60: 361

Shill, M., Baynes, R. D., and S. D. Miller (1987). Fatal rabies despite appropriate post-exposure prophylaxis. *New Engl. J. Med.* 316(20): 1257

Smith, C. W. (1971). Rabies and the caver: A review of the pertinent literature. *NSS (Natl. Speleol. Soc.) News.* 29: 60

Thorne, J. (1987). How many caves are there? *NSS (Natl. Speleol. Soc.) News.* 45(8): 298

Trimarchi, C. V. (1978). Rabies in insectivorous temperate-zone bats. *Bat Res. News.* 19(1): 7

Tuttle, M. D. (1986). President, Bat Conservation International. Austin, Texas. Personal communication.

Tuttle, M. D. and S. J. Kern (1981). Bats and Public Health. *Contributions in Biology and Geology.* No. 48. Milwaukee Public Museum.

Uhaa, I. J., Mandel, E. J., Whiteway, R., and D. B. Fishbein (1992). Rabies surveillance in the United States during 1990. *J. Am. Vet. Med. Assoc.* 200(7): 920

Vodopija, I. and H. F. Clark (1991). Human Vaccination Against Rabies. In G. M. Baer (ed.). *The Natural History of Rabies.* 2nd Edition. CRC Press, Inc. Boca Raton, Florida.

Webster, W. A., Casey, G. A., Charlton, K. M., Sayson, R. C., McLaughlin, B., and M. A. Noble (1987). A case of human rabies in western Canada. *Can. J. Pub. Hlth.* 78: 412

Whitaker, Jr., J. O. and S. L. Gummer (1992). Hibernation of the big brown bat, *Eptesicus fuscus*, in buildings. *J. Mammal.* 73(2): 312

Wimsatt, W. A. (1986). Vampire Bats. In M. E. Fowler (ed.) *Zoo and Wild Animal Medicine.* W. B. Saunders Co. Philadelphia.

Winkler, W. G. (1975). Airborne Rabies. In G. M. Baer (ed.) *The Natural History of Rabies.* Vol. II. Academic Press. New York.

INDEX

A

Addis Ababa, rabies-related viruses and, 266
Adenovirus, use in recombinant rabies vaccine, 254
Aerosol transmission of rabies, 6, 35, 169-174, 236-237, 315-316
Africa, rabies-related viruses of, 263-270
Aggression in rabid bats
- insectivorous bats, 152-153
- interspecific, 163, 166
- intraspecific, 166
- vampire bats, 46, 51, 93-94

Agrarian activity, human depredation by vampires and, 108
Alaska, bat rabies in, 137
Alberta
- bat rabies in, 212-213
- human rabies of bat origin in, 237-238

Amino acid sequencing, 203
Amplification, of virus, 8
Amputation, of bitten limb, 8
Antibody, see Rabies-neutralizing antibody
Anticoagulants
- vampire-bat control and, 86, 88, 116-122
- in vampire-bat saliva, 73-75

Antigenic reactivity, see Monoclonal antibodies
Antigenic stability, of rabies virus, 189, 191
Antigenicity, of rabies glycoprotein, 253
Antirabies therapy, see Post-exposure rabies prophylaxis
Anti-vampire antibodies, 113
Aravan isolate, 289
Argentina
- bovine paralytic rabies in, 86-87, 89
- human deaths due to vampire-bat rabies in, 105-106
- population studies of vampire bats in, 41
- vampire epizootics in, 95

Aristotle, historical account of rabies, 3
Arsenic, use in vampire-bat control, 116
Artibeus sp., 51-53, 159, 255
Artificial insemination, imported rabies and, 7
Asia, bat rabies in, 290
Associations, causal, 181-183
Asymptomatic carrier state, see Salivary carrier state
Attack rates, 172-173
Audition, in vampire bats, 66-67
Aujesky's disease, see Pseudorabies
Australia
- imported human rabies in, 139
- long incubation periods in, 29, 34, 139
- quarantine program of, 7
- survey for bat rabies in, 139

Auto-vampirism, 58
Availability of animal hosts, human depredation by vampires and, 105, 107, 112
Avipox virus, use in recombinant rabies vaccine, 254
Axonal transport, of rabies virus, 8

B

B-1 to B-4 groups of bat virus, 209, 211-212
Baculovirus, use in recombinant rabies vaccine, 294
Baiting
- aid in vampire-bat control, 65, 118
- distribution of wildlife vaccines and, see Baits

Baits, as vehicles for oral vaccines, 251-252, 254-255
Bangladesh, survey for bat rabies in, 290
Bangui-M7 bat virus, 154
BAT, see Brown adipose tissue
Bat bite
- distribution of vampire bites, 67-70
- Good Samaritan and, 219, 304
- provoked versus unprovoked, 152-153, 313
- real or imagined, 217
- recognition of, 101, 108
- severity of, 314-315
- solitary versus colonial species, 132-133, 166, 217

Bat colonies
- in buildings, 243-244, 279
- control of, see Batproofing
- maternity, 169-170, 243
- of vampire bats, 88, 97

Bat infestation, 243-247
Bat-PA, see Plasminogen activators
Bat poisoning, public-health hazards of, 245-246
Batproofing
- animal enclosures, 105, 111
- homes, 101, 111, 247-249

Bat salivary gland virus, see Rio Bravo virus
Behavioral abnormalities, 8-9, 13, 17-18, 20, 22, 51, 143, 151
Belgorod, bat rabies in, 290
Bern Convention, 279-280
Big brown bat
- antigenic characterization of isolates, 191, 198-199, 212
- attacks on humans by, 234
- geographic associations of, 147, 207
- habits of, 146, 207
- home infestations and, 243-244
- immune response in, 158-159, 255
- prevalence of rabies in, 142-146, 207, 209

Biological warfare, as a means of vampire control, 115
Birdnetting checkvalves, use in batproofing, 247-248
Bite wounds
- experimental viral transmission by, 83, 177-180
- incidence of, human, 3, 6, 21
- insectivorous bats and, 133, 136, 217, 275, 289, 308, 314-315
- post-exposure rabies prophylaxis and, 307-308
- provoked versus unprovoked, 152-153, 313
- survival following, 132
- vampire bats and, 67-71, 93, 101-103, 107

Blood craving, among humans, 58

Blood lapping, by vampire bats, 72-73
Blood loss, following vampire attack, 41, 72-74, 85
Bolivia, human deaths due to vampire-bat rabies in, 105-106
Bonn Convention, 279
Bovine anti-vampire antibodies, 113
Bovine paralytic rabies
- in Brazil, 43-44, 86-87, 89
- cattle at risk from, 85
- changing incidence of in Latin America, 122
- clinical signs of, 44
- control of, 105, 111-124
- distribution of vampire-bat bites and, 67-70
- early misdiagnosis of, 43-47
- economic importance of, 41-42, 47, 85-87, 89
- estrous cycle and, 65-66
- immunization of cattle against, 112-113
- incubation period of, 113
- meat consumption and, 107
- in Mexico, 86-87, 89
- official reports of, 86
- propagation of migrating epizootic, 47, 94-95, 113
- protection against, 111-124
- seasonal influences on, 47, 97
- slaughter of livestock and, 107
- in Trinidad, 44-47, 86-87, 89
- vampire bats and, 85-88, 94-97

Brain, rabies and, 8, 155
Brazil
- bovine paralytic rabies in, 43-44, 86-87, 89
- human deaths due to vampire-bat rabies in, 103-108
- Santa Catarina, 43

Brazilian free-tailed bat, 165
British Columbia, bat rabies in, 212-213
British Guiana, see Guyana
Brown adipose tissue
- role in hibernation, 155-156
- viral deposition in, 155

Brujas, in Mexican folklore, 57
Bukalosa bat virus, 154

C

Calendar guidelines for batproofing homes, 248
California myotis, 180
Cameroon, rabies-related viruses and, 266, 268
Canada
- antigenic characterization of bat rabies in, 191, 209, 211-212
- human exposure to bats in, 213-214
- human rabies of bat origin in, 199, 214-215, 237-238
- migration of bats and, 207, 210-211
- nonterrestrial reservoirs in, 207-208
- prevalence of bat rabies in, 207, 209, 212-213, 306
- terrestrial rabies of bat origin in, 199-200, 208
- terrestrial reservoirs in, 131, 207

Canine rabies
- antigenic characterization of isolates, 104
- of bat origin, 196-197, 199, 305-306
- general aspects of, 19-21

Carrier state, see Salivary carrier state
Categories of injury, 28, 32
Cats, interactions with bats, 195, 199, 219, 221-225, 245, 303-306
Cattle rabies, see Bovine paralytic rabies
Cave exploration
- post-exposure rabies prophylaxis and, 318
- pre-exposure rabies prophylaxis and, 27, 316-320
- risk of bat rabies and, 311-316
- specific recommendations for, 318-320

Cedar Island, wildlife vaccine testing and, 254
Central African Republic, rabies-related viruses and, 265-266, 268
Centrifugal migration, of rabies virus, 8-9
Centripetal migration, of rabies virus, 8
Chacachacare, presence of vampire bats on, 94
Channel Tunnel, 7
Children
- incidence of rabies in, 25-26, 29
- insectivorous bats and, 213, 219-225, 229, 244, 275
- post-exposure rabies prophylaxis and, 25, 28
- vampire attacks and, 102

Chlorophacinone, use in vampire control, 118
Coadaptation of virus and host, 9-10
Coagulation cascades, 75
Cochliomyia hominivorax, see Myiasis
Colombia, human deaths due to vampire-bat rabies in, 105-106
Colonial bats
- aggressive behavior and, 166
- colony structure of, 166
- prevalence of rabies in, 139-147

Colony, rabies in captive bat, 4, 83
Color, vampire feeding and, 69
Commensal pests, see Bat infestation
Common circumstances of human exposure to bats, 219, 304
Common vampire bat, see Vampire bat
Compartmentalization of virus, 131-132, 189-191
Competence, as rabies vector, 85, 132, 180
Conservation of bats, 279, 288, 291
Continuity of viral transmission, 9-10
Control of rabies
- in domestic animals, 105
- in humans, 26-29, 31, 108-109, 111, 248-249, 293, 307-308, 316-320
- in insectivorous bats, 240, 255-256, 291-294, 318, 320
- recombinant vaccines and, 252-255
- in vampire bats, 109, 111-124
- in wildlife (terrestrial), 251-255

Corneal transplantation, rabies transmission and, 7, 230, 233-234
Coyote rabies
- aerosol transmission of virus to, 170-171
- of bat origin, 213

Craving for blood, by humans, 58
Crocidura shrew, see White-toothed shrew
Cultured fetal bat cells, 167
Cynopterus brachyotis, see Dog-faced fruit bat
Cytoplasmic inclusion bodies, see Negri bodies
Czechoslovakia, bat rabies in, 275, 277

D

Daily torpor, rabies pathogenesis and, 157
Dam construction, human depredation by vampires and, 107
Dangerous Dogs Act, 177
Daytime activity, of rabid animals, 13
Daytime flying
  bat rabies and, 51, 143, 151-152
  in nonrabid bats, 152
DDT, 246
Dead-end hosts, 34, 234
Deforestation, human depredation by vampires and, 107
Democritus, historical account of rabies and, 3
Denmark, bat rabies in, 275
Dental formula, of vampire bats, 71
Dentition, of vampire bats, 71, 74
Derriengue, see Bovine paralytic rabies
Descending lateral trigeminal tract, see Thermal sense
Desmodus rotundus, see Vampire bat
Desmokinase, 73-75
Diaemus youngi, see White-winged vampire bat
Diagnosis of rabies
  fluorescent antibody test and, 53, 155, 308
  mouse inoculation test and, 155
  Negri bodies and, 52
  polymerase chain reaction and, 155
Diagnostic laboratories
  availability of human exposure data from, 218
  Colorado State Department of Health, 218
  identification of specimens by, 140
  New York State Department of Health, 134-135, 218
  testing of suspect submissions by, 139-140, 146, 208-209, 212-213, 304
Die-offs, of bats, 158, 319
Diphacinone, use in vampire control, 117
Diphenadione, use in vampire control, 113, 116-118, 121
Diphylla ecaudata, see Hairy-legged vampire bat
Disorientation, bat rabies and, 151-152
Dissecting bats, possible health hazard associated with, 94, 222
Diuresis, in vampire bats, 66, 76
Dog-faced fruit bat, 290
Dogs
  human bites from, 3, 6, 153, 317-318
  interaction with bats, 195-196, 199, 305-306
Dracula, 60
Drug-withdrawal time, vampire control and, 120
Dumb rabies, see Paralytic rabies
Duvenhage virus, 270
Duvenhage-like virus, see European bat lyssavirus
Dwarf epauletted fruit bat, Lagos bat virus and, 264-265
Dynamiting, as a means of vampire control, 114, 123

E

East Germany, bat rabies in, 275-276
EBL type 1, 284
EBL type 2, 284
Echolocation, 311
Eclipse phase, 8
Ecotypes, of rabies virus, 189
Education, regarding rabies exposure
  of the caving community, 318, 320
  of the general public, 109, 240, 291
  of health-care workers, 109
Eidolon helvum, see Straw-colored fruit bat
El Niño, 97
El Salvador, human deaths due to vampire-bat rabies in, 105-106
Electrocution, as a means of vampire control, 114
Enamel, of vampire teeth, 71
Encephalitis, 3, 266, 269
Encephalomyelitis, 3, 8, 34
Entebbe bat salivary gland virus, 154
Epauletted fruit bat, Lagos bat virus and, 264-265
Epidemiology, 4
  of rabies in insectivorous bats, 217-240
  of rabies in vampire bats, 101-109
Epizootiology, 4
  of rabies in insectivorous bats, 177-204
  of rabies in vampire bats, 85-97
Epomophorus wahlbergi, see Epauletted fruit bat
Eptesicus fuscus, see Big brown bat
Eptesicus serotinus, see Serotine bat
Equine rabies, of bat origin, 195, 199
Equine rabies immunoglobulin
  use in post-exposure rabies prophylaxis, 29, 293
  and protection against European bat lyssavirus, 293-294
ERA strain of virus, 293
Escape variants, 29
Eschnunna, Laws of, 3
Estrous cycle (bovine), host selection by vampire bats and, 65-66
Ethiopia, rabies-related viruses and, 266, 268
Europe
  bat conservation in, 279, 291
  control of sylvatic rabies in, 185, 251
  human rabies of bat origin in, 239, 288
  post-exposure rabies prophylaxis in, 293-294
  terrestrial rabies of bat origin in, 288
European bat lyssavirus
  antigenic characterization of isolates, 280-284
  bat-to-bat transmission of, 286-287
  countries reported from, 275-277
  EBL type 1, 284
  EBL type 2, 284
  Eptesicus serotinus and, 275-290
  genetic analysis of, 284-286
  genotype 5 virus, 285-286
  genotype 6 virus, 285-286
  historical distribution of, 275, 282-283, 286
  human deaths due to, 239-240, 289-291
  International Animal Health Code and, 287
  isolation from western Europe, 275-277
  Myotis dasycneme and, 269
  nonserotine bats and, 279, 291
  pathogenicity of, 287-288
  Pipistrellus nathusii and, 278-279, 283, 286-287
  post-exposure rabies prophylaxis and, 292-294
  prevalence of, 275, 279

rabies-free status and, 286-287
relation to Duvenhage virus, 281, 284-286
seasonal reports of, 278-279
serotype 5 virus, 270, 286
in the former Soviet Union, 289-290
transmission to terrestrial species, 288
transport from Africa, 284-285
Yuli virus, 270, 284, 290
Evelyn Rockitnicki Abelseth, see ERA strain
Exposure to rabies virus
abroad, 33, 308
of bat origin, 101-109, 213-215, 217-240, 266, 270, 289-291
first-aid for, 308
hospital personnel and, 234
recognition of source, 101, 108, 229
validity of reports, 217-218
versus infection, 7
Extermination of bats, health concerns and, 245

F

Facial pit organs, see Thermal sense
FAT, see Fluorescent antibody test
Federal Republic of Germany, see West Germany
Feline rabies
of bat origin, 22, 195, 199, 305
general aspects of, 21-22
Fetal bat cells, 167
Fibrinolysis, vampire-bat saliva and, 73-75
Filoviridae, 4
Finland
antigenic characterization of human isolate, 284
human rabies of bat origin in, 239, 284, 289
Mokola virus and, 269
Myotis dasycneme and, 269
survey for bat rabies in, 289
First-aid, for bat bite, 308
Fixed virus, 5, 35, 165
Florida, bats and raccoon rabies in, 183, 198-199
Florida yellow bat, 133, 147, 191
Flying fox, 152, 290
Fluorescent antibody test, 53, 155
Flury low egg passage strain, see LEP strain
Formication, 34
Fossil record, of vampire bats, 62-63
Fox rabies
aerosol transmission of virus to, 170-173
of bat origin, 181-185, 197-198
control of in Europe, 185, 251
general aspects of, 17-19
France, bat rabies in, 275, 277
Freeze-dried blood, as food for vampire bats, 64
Frio Cave
aerosol transmission of rabies in, 6, 158, 169-174, 236-237, 315-316
bat inhabitants of, 169-170
human deaths in, 169, 173-174
predators of bats and, 177
Frugivorous bats, rabies in, 51-52, 159, 255, 264-266
Furious rabies
in cats, 21
in dogs, 20, 153
in humans, 34
in insectivorous bats, 152
in vampire bats, 46, 51
viral distribution in brain and, 8

G

G protein, see Glycoprotein
Ganglionic lesions, 8
Gassing, in control of vampire bats, 114, 123
Genetic characterization
of bat-rabies isolates, 163, 166, 191
epidemiologic associations and, 5, 203-204
phylogenetic relationships based on, 284-286
of rabies-related viruses, 284-286
of terrestrial isolates, 204
Genotypes of lyssaviruses, 284-286
Georgia, caves and fox rabies in, 183
German Democratic Republic, see East Germany
Gliosis, 8
Glycoprotein
antigenic stability of, 189
immune response to, 253
Good Samaritan, at risk, 219, 304
Gray foxes, bat rabies in New York State and, 197-198
Great Britain
Channel Tunnel, 7
Dangerous Dogs Act, 177
interaction of cats and bats in, 305
pressures from EC, 7
quarantine program of, 7
survey for bat rabies in, 278
Wildlife and Countryside Act, 279, 304
Greater horseshoe bat, 290
Grooming, see Social grooming
Guano mining, 169, 171
Guerilla activity, human depredation by vampires and, 107
Guillain-Barré syndrome, 233
Guinea, rabies-related viruses and, 265-266
Gulf of Paria, migration of vampires across, 94
Guyana, human deaths due to vampire-bat rabies in, 103, 105-106

H

Hairy-legged vampire bat
dental formula of, 71
dietary preferences of, 62
distribution of, 61
as reservoir of rabies, 58
Handling bats, 119, 152-153, 213-215, 304, 319
Handling infected cattle, 107
Hanging jaw, 21
Hank's Bat Excluder, 247
Harsh-furred mouse, Mokola virus and, 264, 269
Hawaii
imported bat rabies in, 137, 139

quarantine program of, 7
HDCV, see Human diploid cell vaccine
Hematophagous bats, see Vampire bat
Hibernation
and immunization of bat colonies, 255
role in rabies pathogenesis, 155-157
susceptibility of bats to intrusion during, 314
Hip disease of cattle, see Bovine paralytic rabies
Histoplasmosis, 171
Hoary bat
antigenic characterization of isolates, 191, 194
attacks on humans by, 133, 219
behavior when grounded, 219
geographic associations of, 147
home infestations and, 243
migration of, 210
prevalence of rabies in, 143
Holoendemic, 4
Hollow-faced bat, Duvenhage virus and, 270
Home infestation, with bats, 243-249, 279
Horizontal transmission, 166, 255
Host/parasite relationships, 9-10
Host selection, by vampire bats, 62, 64-65
Howl, rabies, 20
HRIG, see Human rabies immunoglobulin
Human diploid cell vaccine
post-exposure rabies prophylaxis and, 29, 31
pre-exposure rabies prophylaxis and, 28
protection against rabies-related viruses and, 293
Human exposure, to bat rabies, 213-215, 217-240
Human rabies
acute neurologic phase, 33-35
aerosol transmission of virus, 6, 35, 169-174, 236-237, 303, 315-316
animal bite, incidence of, 25
cat bites and, 21-22
clinical signs of, 33-35, 45, 101-102
coma, 34-35
complications of disease, 35
corneal transplant and, 7, 229, 233-234, 303
diagnosis of, 35
dog bites and, 3, 6, 19-21, 25, 317-318
domestic animals and, 6, 26
exposure abroad, 33, 308
exposure to rabid bats and, 133, 136-137, 213-240, 289
furious, 34
global incidence of, 3
hospital personnel, risk to, 234
human-to-human transmission of, 34-35, 234
hydrophobia and, 34
hyperesthesia and, 34
impending doom, feeling of, 34, 239
imported, 139
incubation period of, 29, 34, 139
insectivorous bats and, 35, 133, 136-137, 199, 214-215, 229-240, 270, 289-291
intensive care and, 35
jungle communities and, 103-104, 107-109
long incubation period of, 29, 34, 139
misdiagnosis of, 35, 45, 103
nonbite routes of exposure, 6-7, 35, 169-174, 180-181
paralytic, 35
paresthesia and, 34
populations at increased risk of disease, 107-109
populations at increased risk of exposure, 26-28, 107-109, 248-249
post-exposure rabies prophylaxis, 25-26, 28-29, 292-294, 307-308
pre-exposure rabies prophylaxis, 26-28, 31, 108-109, 111, 248-249, 293, 308
prevalence of, 25
prodromal phase, 34
recognition of source, 101, 108, 229
recovery from, 35, 172
relationship to age, 25-26, 28
risk factors of, 109
in rural settings, 25, 27
seasonal occurrence of, 25-26
in urban settings, 25, 27, 131
vampire bats and, 45, 101-109
wildlife and, 6, 26
Human rabies immunoglobulin, post-exposure rabies prophylaxis and, 29, 31-32, 293
Hunting, in vampire bats, 62
Hunting clubs
fox rabies and, 18-19
raccoon rabies and, 16
Hydrophobia, 21, 34
Hyperendemic, 4
Hyperesthesia, 20, 34
Hypoendemic, 4

I

IgG-class antibody, 158-159
IgM-class antibody, 158-159
Immunization, against rabies
of cats, 22, 306
of cattle, 112-113
compliance with local ordinances, 22
of dogs, 19, 21
of free-ranging wildlife, 251-256
of humans, 26-28, 31, 108-109, 111, 248-249, 293, 308
of insectivorous bats, 255-256
oral vaccination of foxes in Europe, 185, 251
recombinant vaccines for, 252-255
of vampire bats, 123
Immunization Practices Advisory Committee, 27, 31, 33, 108
Immunodeficiency, rabies in bats and, 159
Impending doom, feeling of, 34
Importation, of bats, 4, 94, 137, 139
Imported rabies
in Africa, 263
in Australia, 139
bat rabies in Canada and, 207
bat rabies in Europe and, 94, 276, 285-287
bat rabies in the U. S. and, 137, 139
establishment of disease and, 3
International Animal Health Code and, 286-287
quarantine requirements and, 4, 7

rabies-free countries and, 137, 139, 286-287
vampire bats and, 94, 163-166
Inclusion bodies, see Negri bodies
Incubation period, of rabies
age of victim and, 34
in cats, 21
in cattle, 113
in cold-adapted bats, 155-157
density of peripheral nerves and, 34
in dogs, 19
dose of virus and, 34
of fixed virus, 5, 165
in foxes, 18
in humans, 29, 34, 139
immunologic status and, 34
in insectivorous bats, 151
intramuscular harborage of virus and, 8
long, 34, 139
quarantine programs and, 7, 304
in skunks, 13
in vampire bats, 83
viral variant and, 34
in warm-adapted bats, 155-157
wound location and, 34
India, bat rabies in, 290-291
Indonesia, survey for bat rabies in, 290
Infection, versus exposure, 7
Ingestion, rabies transmission by, 107, 180-181
Inhalation exposure, see Aerosol transmission
Insectivorous bats, see Rabies in insectivorous bats
International Animal Health Code, 3, 286-287
Interspecific aggression, 166
Intramuscular
administration of anticoagulants, 115, 117, 119-120
harborage of virus, 8
Intranuclear inclusion bodies, see Negri bodies
Intraruminal administration of anticoagulants, 113-114, 116-117, 119-120
Intraspecific aggression
among insectivorous bats, 166
among vampire bats, 46, 51, 93-94
In utero, rabies infection, 167
Ireland, quarantine program of, 7

J

Jumbie, in Trinidad folklore, 57
Jungle communities, at risk of rabies, 103-109

K

Keen's myotis, 193, 211
Kiev, bat rabies in, 289-290
Kudu antelope, rabies epizootic in, 265
Kyrgyzstan, bat rabies in, 289

L

L protein, see Large viral polymerase
Lagos bat virus, 265-266
Large viral polymerase, 189
Lasionycteris noctivagans, see Silver-haired bat
Lasiurus borealis, see Red bat
Lasiurus cinereus, see Hoary bat
Lasiurus intermedius, see Florida yellow bat
Lasiurus seminola, see Seminole bat
Latent state, see Salivary carrier state
Latin America
bovine paralytic rabies in, 43-44, 85-89
canine rabies in, 43-44, 47, 51, 103-104, 318
human rabies in, 101-109, 229
insectivorous-bat rabies in, 94, 229
vampire-bat rabies in, see Rabies in hematophagous bats
LEP strain of virus, 293
Lethal cycle of infection in bats, 151
Limbic system, 8
Limping illness, see Bovine paralytic rabies
Little brown bat, 156, 193, 207, 211, 243
Livestock, vampire bats and
breathing sounds of, as vampire attractant, 66-67
distribution of vampire bats and, 41, 60, 64, 105, 108, 114
estrous cycle of, and vampire depredation, 65-66
hyperactivity of, and vampire depredation, 65
milk production of, 41, 120-121
population at risk, 85
rabies in, see Bovine paralytic rabies
reproductive capacity of, 41
stress of foraging in vampire bats and, 41
weight gain of, 41, 120-121
Long-eared myotis, 193, 207
Longevity, of vampire bats, 59
Lophuromys sikapusi, see Harsh-furred mouse
Lymphoplasmacytic infiltration, 8
Lyssavirus
genotypes of, 285
serotypes of, 265-270

M

M_1 and M_2 proteins, see Matrix proteins
MAb 8-2, use in post-exposure rabies prophylaxis, 294
Malaise, 34
Malarial prophylaxis, pre-exposure rabies prophylaxis and, 28
Malaysia, survey for bat rabies in, 290
Mal de caderas de bovinos, see Bovine paralytic rabies
Management
of home infestations of bats, 243-249, 279
of rabies in insectivorous bats, 109, 240, 255-256, 291, 293, 318, 320
of rabies in vampire bats, 111-124
of rabies in wildlife, 251-256
Maternity colonies, 169-170, 243
Matrix proteins, 189
Mechanical transmission of virus, 174, 221-222, 303
Mesoendemic, 4
Methyl bromide, 246
Metivier, H. V., contributions to rabies epidemiology, 47

Mexican free-tailed bat
- aerosol transmission of virus and, 169-174, 236-237, 315-316
- antigenic characterization of isolates, 165, 191-192, 197, 203
- cohabitation with vampire bats, 163, 165
- colony structure of, 166, 170, 243
- fed on by vampire bats, 163
- geographic associations of, 147
- hibernation and rabies pathogenesis in, 155-157
- home infestations and, 243
- intraspecific transmission of virus in, 159, 166, 193
- migration of, 143, 163-164, 170
- prevalence of rabies in, 142-143, 146
- Project X-Ray and, 115
- rabies-neutralizing antibody in, 151, 157-158
- Rio Bravo virus and, 154

Mexico
- bovine paralytic rabies in, 47-48, 86-87, 89
- human deaths due to vampire-bat rabies in, 48, 105-106
- public-health concerns at U. S. border, 48

Micropteropus pusillus, see Dwarf epauletted fruit bat
Mid-Atlantic raccoon epizootic, 15-17
Migration of bats
- bat rabies in Canada and, 207, 210-211
- bat rabies in Europe and, 283, 285-287
- bat rabies in the U. S. and, 133, 143, 163, 170, 184
- Chacachacare, 94
- home infestations and, 243, 248
- International Animal Health Code and, 286-287
- potential role as migrating vectors, 132-133, 283, 285-287
- public-health programs and, 133
- rabies-free status and, 286-287
- vampire bats and, 94, 163

Migration of virus
- centrifugal, 8-9
- centripetal, 8

Migratory epizootic, of vampire rabies
- in Mexico, 47
- predictability of, 45, 51, 121-122
- related to season, 47, 97

Military activity
- exposure to rabies and, 27
- human depredation by vampires and, 107

Mining activity, human depredation by vampires and, 103-108
Miniopterus shreibersi natalensis, see Natal clinging bat
Misdiagnosis, of bovine paralytic rabies, 43-47
MIT, see Mouse inoculation test
Mokola virus, 266-270, 284, 294
Monoclonal antibodies
- abbreviated panels, 196
- antigenic characterization of isolates, 14, 94, 104, 163, 165, 189-203, 209, 211-213, 267-268
- anti-glycoprotein MAbs, 189, 265
- anti-nucleocapsid MAbs, 189
- epidemiologic associations and, 5, 94, 107, 189-203, 265
- European bat lyssavirus and, 280-281, 284
- limitations of, 196, 203
- post-exposure rabies prophylaxis and, 29, 294
- production of, 191

Mononegavirales, 4
Montana Myotis leukoencephalitis (MML) virus, 154
Moonlight, feeding of vampire bats in relation to, 62, 111
Mount Elgon bat virus, 154
Mouse inoculation test
- as backup test, 155
- salivary carrier state and, 155

Mucous membranes, as site of infection, 6
Murphy Island, wildlife vaccine testing and, 254
Muscle, rabies virus and, 8
Myiasis, vampire wounds and, 41-42
Myotis blythi, 279, 289
Myotis brandtii, 288
Myotis californicus, see California myotis
Myotis dasycneme, 279-280, 289
Myotis daubentoni, 255, 279-280, 288-289
Myotis evotis, see Long-eared myotis
Myotis lucifugus, see Little brown bat
Myotis sp.
- antigenic profile of isolates from, 192-193, 211-212
- interspecific transmission of virus and, 147, 192
- prevalence of rabies in, 207, 212-213

N

N protein, see Nucleocapsid protein
Naphthalene, 246
Nasal mucosa, rabies virus in, 170
Natal clinging bat, 238, 270
National Cave Rescue Commission (NCRC), 318
National Pest Control Association, 247, 249
National Speleological Society (NSS), 313
Negri bodies, 5, 8, 46, 52-53
Netherlands
- bat rabies in, 275, 277
- quarantine program of, 7

Neurotropism, of rabies virus, 8
Neutralizing antibody, see Rabies-neutralizing antibody
New Guinea, survey for bat rabies in, 139
New Jersey, wildlife vaccine testing and, 254
New York
- bat rabies in, 144-145, 305
- big brown bats in, 196
- dog and cat exposure to bats in, 196, 305-306
- gray-fox rabies in, 197-198
- public-health program of, 133-135

New Zealand, quarantine program of, 7
Newcastle disease virus, use in vampire-bat control, 115
Nigeria, rabies-related viruses and, 264-266, 268
Nigerian natives
- fear of bats, 266
- fear of shrews, 269

Nonbite routes of exposure
- aerosol, 6, 35, 169-174, 236-237, 315-316
- corneal transplant, 7, 229, 234
- ingestion, 107, 180-181
- licks, 226
- mucous membranes, 6

scratch, 308
transmammary, 93
transplacental, 93, 167
Nonlethal cycle of infection in bats, 151
Nonserotine bats
infected with EBL, 279
isolates from, 280, 284-286
migration of, 285-287
Nonterrestrial reservoirs of rabies, 147, 190-193, 207-208
Norway, bat rabies in, 275, 277
Nosferatu, 60
Nova Scotia, human rabies of bat origin in, 238
Novosibirsk, bat rabies in, 289
Nucleocapsid protein
antigenic stability of, 189
immune response and, 253
Nucleotide sequencing, 203-204
Nyctalus noctula, 289-290
Nycteris gambiensis, Lagos bat virus and, 264-265
Nycteris thebaica, see Hollow-faced bat

O

Office International des Épizooties (OIE), 286-287
Old World bats, rabies infection in, 261-294
Olfaction
host detection by vampire bats and, 65-66
urine of vampire bat and, 76
Olfactory epithelium, see Nasal mucosa
Omsk, bat rabies in, 289
Opossum, aerosol exposure to rabies, 170, 173
Oral immunization against rabies, 185, 251-255
Osh Province, bat rabies in, 289
Outbreaks of rabies in bats, 139, 207

P

Pallid bat, 156
Pan American Zoonoses Center, surveillance program of, 86, 89, 109
Pandemic, 4
Paralytic rabies
distribution of virus in brain and, 8
in dogs, 20-21
in humans, 35
in insectivorous bats, 151-152
in livestock, see Bovine paralytic rabies
in vampire bats, 83
The Paralytic Rabies Regulations, 111
Paramyxoviridae, 4
Parasites (viral), coadaptations with reservoir host, 9-10
Paresthesia, at inoculation site, 34
Parramore Island, wildlife vaccine testing and, 254
Pasteur virus, 293
Pathology, of rabies infection, 8
Pawan, J. L., contributions to rabies epidemiology, 47
PCR, see Polymerase chain reaction
Pennsylvania, wildlife vaccine testing and, 254
Perinatal transmission, of rabies, 167
Perivascular cuffing, 8
Peru, human deaths due to vampire-bat rabies in, 103-108
Philippines, survey for bat rabies in, 290
Photophobia, 20
Pica, 20
Pima Indians, fear of bats, 137
Pipistrellus nathusii
distribution of, 283
possible role as migrating vector, 283, 286-287
Pitman Moore strain of virus, 293
Plasminogen activators
in saliva of vampire bats, 73-75
therapeutic potential of, 73-75
Pleistocene deposits, of vampire bats, 62
PM strain, see Pitman Moore strain
Pneumonia, 171
Poison gas, as a means of vampire control, 114
Poisoned bats, 245-246
Poland, bat rabies in, 275, 277
Polymerase chain reaction
diagnosis of rabies and, 155, 203
genetic analysis of viral isolates and, 203
Population reduction
and control of bovine paralytic rabies, 113-123
as means of rabies control, 251, 256
nonselective, 114-115, 123-124
selective, 115-120
Port-of-Spain, Trinidad, bovine paralytic rabies in, 44
Post-exposure management, of pets, 21-22
Post-exposure rabies prophylaxis
age of victim and, 25, 28
algorithm for, 307
bat exposure and, 213-215, 217-228, 308
bat scratch and, 308
categories of exposure and, 28, 32
cost of, 25, 29, 308
decision making and, 28, 153
enzootic dog rabies and, 28
European bat lyssavirus and, 292-294
extent of in the United States, 25
failure of, 315
monoclonal antibodies and, 29, 294
population density and, 25, 27, 32
pregnancy and, 29, 223
rabies-related viruses and, 291-294
season and, 25-26
sex of victim and, 28
Poxvirus, use in recombinant rabies vaccine, 253-254
Predators, of bats, 177
Pre-exposure rabies prophylaxis
of cattle in Latin America, 112-113
of cavers (spelunkers), 27, 316-320
of domestic animals, 19, 22, 306
of high-risk jungle populations, 108-109
of human populations at increased risk, 26-28, 31, 108-109, 248-249, 293, 308
of insectivorous bats, 255-256
intradermal administration, 28
intramuscular administration, 28
malarial prophylaxis and, 28
rabies-related viruses and, 293
recombinant viral vaccines and, 252-255

of terrestrial wildlife, 251-255
of vampire bats, 123
Prenatal transmission, of rabies, 167
Prevalence of rabies, in insectivorous bats
in apparently healthy bats, 142-143, 146, 306
artifacts of reporting, 139-140, 142-143, 146
biased reporting and, 139-140, 147
in colonial species, 142-143
in European bat populations, 275, 279
limitations of surveillance data, 139-141, 147
in solitary species, 142-143
in suspect submissions, 140, 146, 209, 212-213
Prevalence of rabies, in vampire bats
relation to migrating epizootic, 95-96
seasonal influences on, 47, 97
Primary screw-worm, see Myiasis
Prodromal period
in cats, 21
in dogs, 19
in foxes, 18
in humans, 34
in skunks, 14
Project X-ray, 115
Propagation, of the vampire epizootic, 47, 94-95, 113
Prophylaxis, see Pre- or post-exposure rabies prophylaxis
Provoked attacks by bats, 152-153
Pruritus, 34
Pseudorabies, 43, 53
Pteropus poliocephalus, see Flying fox
Public perceptions, of bats, 147, 217, 244, 256, 303, 320
PV_4 strain of virus, 293

Q

Quarantine programs, 4, 7, 47, 304
Queen's Park Savannah, Trinidad, 44-45

R

Rabia paralitica, see Bovine paralytic rabies
Rabia paresiante, see Bovine paralytic rabies
Rabies
behavioral abnormalities in, 8-9, 13-22, 51, 143, 151
clinical progression of, 13
CNS lesions in, 8
compartmentalization of virus and, 131-132, 189-190
control programs for, 105, 111-124, 251-256
countries free of, 3-5, 286-287
in developing nations, 4, 131, 318
diagnosis of, 20, 35, 155
in domestic animals, 19-22
Eschnunna Code and, 3
fear, loss of, 13-14, 17
in frugivorous bats, see Rabies in frugivorous bats
furious form of, see Furious rabies
global distribution of, 3-4
histopathology and, 8
in humans, see Human rabies
imported, 138-139, 263
incubation period of, 5, 7, 13, 18-19, 21, 29, 34, 83, 139, 151
in industrialized nations, 4, 131
in insectivorous bats, see Rabies in insectivorous bats
nonterrestrial reservoirs of, 13, 147, 190-193, 207-208
paralytic form of, see Paralytic rabies
pathogenesis of infection, 6-9
prodromal period, 14, 18-19, 21, 34
recovery from, 35, 172, 235-236
routes of transmission, 6-7, 93, 107, 166-174, 180-181, 303
single-species involvement, 131
species susceptibility to, 13, 131, 170
spillover from reservoir species, 131, 147, 192-202, 212, 265, 305-306
surveillance studies and, 86, 109, 139-141, 147, 218-219
sylvatic rabies cycles, see Sylvatic rabies
terrestrial reservoirs of, 13, 131-132
testing, see Diagnostic laboratories, FAT, MIT
translocation of animals and, 16, 18-19
urban rabies cycles, see Urban rabies
in vampire bats, see Rabies in hematophagous bats
in terrestrial wildlife, 13-19
Rabies dendrogram, phylogenetic relationships and, 204
Rabies-free countries, 3-5, 286-287
Rabies in frugivorous bats, 51-53, 158-159, 255, 264-266
Rabies in hematophagous (vampire) bats
antigenic characterization of isolates, 104, 165-166
in Brazil, 43-44, 51
in captive specimens, 4
cave exploration and, 317
clinical signs in, 51, 83-84
control of, 105, 111-124
cyclic nature of, 54, 94-95
discovery of, 51
early history of, 43-48
economic importance of, 47, 85-87
epidemiology of, 101-109
epizootiology of, 85-97
experimental studies and, 46, 51-54, 83, 93
genetic characterization of isolates, 204
human deaths due to, 45, 101-109
immunization of bats, 123
incubation period of, 83
livestock and, see Bovine paralytic rabies
in Mexico, 47-48, 86-87, 89, 105-106
migrating epizootics of, 45, 47, 94-97, 121-122
nonselective control of, 115, 123-124
prevalence of, 53-54
selective control of, 115-120, 255
social grooming and, 88
surveillance studies and, 86, 109
in Trinidad, 44-47, 51
Rabies Importation of Dogs and Cats or Other Mammals Order, 7
Rabies in insectivorous bats
aerosol transmission and, 169-174, 236-237, 303, 315-316
in Africa, 270
antigenic characterization of isolates, 165, 189-203, 209, 211-212, 280-284

in Asia, 291
in Canada, 199, 207-215
in Chile, 165
clinical signs in, 151-153, 214
in colonial species, 139-143, 146, 166
correlated with cave locations, 184
discovery of, 133
distribution of in the U. S., 136-137, 139
in Europe, 275-294
experimental transmission studies and, 170-172, 179-181
flight abnormalities and, 51, 143, 151-153
furious versus paralytic disease, 151-153
genetic analysis of isolates, 166, 191, 284-286
in Hawaii, 137, 139
hibernation and, 155-157
historical accounts of, 133, 136-137
human deaths due to, 133, 136-137, 214-215, 229-240, 289-290
human exposure to, 213-240, 289
incubation period of, 151, 155-157
interspecific transmission and, 192-193, 197-198
intraspecific transmission and, 159, 193
in Latin America, 53, 165
lethal cycle in, 151
migration of bats and, 132-133, 143, 163, 170, 207, 210-211, 283, 285-287
in New York State, 133-135, 144-145, 195-198, 218, 305
nonlethal cycle in, 151
outbreaks of disease, 139, 207
pets, exposed to, 219, 221-224, 303-306
prevalence of, 139-141, 144-146, 306
provoked versus unprovoked attacks and, 152-153, 219, 313
public-health programs and, 133-135
raccoons and, 16, 183, 198-199
recovery from infection, 154-155, 179
risks in cave exploration, 311-320
salivary carrier state, see Salivary carrier state
seasonal nature of, 142-143, 146, 158, 170, 278
in solitary species, 139-143, 146, 166
source of virus in, 163-166
species-associated distribution of, 147
species found positive, 137-138, 276-279, 290
states reporting, 136-137, 144-145
in suckling bats, 167
surveillance studies and, 143
transmission to bats, 147, 159, 166
transmission to cats, 195, 199, 305-306
transmission to dogs, 196-197, 199, 305
transmission to foxes, 181-185, 195, 197-198
transmission to humans, 217-240, 270, 289-291, 303
transmission to terrestrial wildlife, 132-133, 177-185, 193-202, 208, 288-289
vampire bats and, 163-166
virus in saliva and, 151, 179

Rabies-neutralizing antibody
development of immunity and, 29, 31, 158, 291-294
experimental, 157-158
in frugivorous bats, 158-159, 255
ingestion of virus and, 158
in insectivorous bats, 157-159, 255
maternally derived, 158
naturally occurring, 157-158
pre-exposure immunization and, 255
protection of newborn bats and, 158-159
in terrestrial carnivores, 157-158
in vampire bats, 95-96, 158

Rabies-related viruses, 4, 263-270

Rabies in vampire bats, see Rabies in hematophagous bats

Rabies virus
antigenic characterization of isolates, 5-6, 16, 94, 104, 107, 163-166, 189-203, 209, 211-212, 267, 280-281, 284
antigenic diversity of, 5-6
antigenic stability of, 189, 191
centrifugal migration of, 8-9
centripetal migration of, 8
coadaptation with reservoir host, 9-10
compartmentalization of, 131-132, 189-190
dimensions of, 5
disinfection and, 5
distribution in tissue, 8-9, 155
eclipse period of, 8
fixed virus, 5, 35, 165
genetic diversity of, 166, 284-286
genotypes of, 284-286
glycoprotein of, 5, 189, 253
intramuscular harborage, 8
morphology of, 4-6
neurotropism of, 8
nonterrestrial variants of, 163-166, 189-203, 209, 211-212, 280-284
nucleocapsid of, 189, 253
olfactory mucosa and, 170
pathogenesis of infection, 6-9
prophylaxis against, see Pre-exposure rabies prophylaxis
protein components of, 189
replication of, 8-9
resistance to environmental factors, 5
retrograde transport of, 8
routes of transmission, 6-7, 93, 107, 166-167, 169-174, 180-181, 303
serotypes of, 265-270
species susceptibility to, 13, 131, 170
spillover from reservoir species, 131, 147, 192-202, 212, 265, 305-306
virions, 4

Raccoon poxvirus, use in recombinant vaccine, 253-254

Raccoon rabies
aerosol transmission of virus to, 172
general aspects of, 14-17
insectivorous bats and, 16, 183, 198-199

Range, of vampire bats, 60-63

rDSPα_1, 74-75

Reciprocal altruism, in vampire bats, 91

Reciprocal food sharing, in vampire bats, 90-92

Reciprocity theory, 92

Recombinant rabies vaccine, field trials, 254-255

Recombinant rabies vaccines, 252-255

Recovery, in human rabies, 35, 172, 235-236
Red bat
    antigenic characterization of isolates, 191, 194
    geographic associations of, 147
    home infestations and, 243
    prevalence of rabies in, 143
Rehabilitation, of ill or injured bats, 304
Reservoirs, of rabies
    nonterrestrial, 13, 147, 190-193, 207-208
    terrestrial, 13, 131-132
Reservoirs, of rabies-related viruses
    African, 266, 269-270
    European, 278
Respiratory system, inhalation of virus and, 170
Retrograde transport, of rabies virus, 8
Retrospective analyses
    associations on a local level, 181-183
    associations on a national level, 183-184
Rhabdoviridae, 4, 263-270
Rhinolophus ferrumequinum, see Greater horseshoe bat
Rio Bravo virus, 84, 154-155
Road construction, human depredation by vampires and, 107
Rockefeller Foundation, 47
Rodent rabies
    of bat origin, 208
    Mokola virus and, 266-270
Roosts, of vampire bats, 76, 97, 111
Rozol Tracking Powder, 245
Russian Soviet Federative Socialist Republic, human rabies of bat origin in, 239, 290

S

SAD strain of virus, 293
Saliva
    anticoagulants in, 73-75
    exchange among vampire bats, 88, 92
    presence of rabies virus in, 9, 52, 84, 88, 131-132, 151, 179, 226
    salivary cycle of viral secretion, 179
    salivary gland viruses in, 84, 154-155
    of vampire bats, 73-75
Salivary carrier state
    in dogs, 154
    in insectivorous bats, 154-155, 179
    in vampire bats, 83-84
Salivary glands, 9
Santa Catarina, Brazil, 43
Saskatchewan, human rabies of bat origin in, 238
Screw-worm, see Myiasis
Season
    identification of rabies-positive bats and, 142-143, 146, 170, 209, 278-279
    influence on bovine paralytic rabies, 47, 97
    submission of suspect bats and, 142-143, 146, 209, 278-279
Selection pressure, G antigen and, 189
Seminole bat, 133
Senegal, rabies-related viruses and, 265, 268
Serial murders, blood craving and, 58
Serotine bat, 275-290
Serotypes, of lyssavirus, 265-270
Sheep rabies, of bat origin, 196, 288
Silver-haired bat
    antigenic characterization of isolates, 191
    attacks on humans by, 133
    geographic associations of, 147, 207
    home infestations and, 243
    prevalence of rabies in, 143, 213
    relation to human deaths, 229-231
Single-species involvement, 131
Siparia, Trinidad, 94
Skunk rabies
    attenuated vaccines and, 252
    of bat origin, 200
    general aspects of, 13-14
Smoke and fire, as a means of vampire control, 114
Social grooming, in vampire bats
    exploited for vampire-bat control, 88, 118-119, 121
    identification of group members and, 91
    maintenance of rabies enzootic and, 88
    reciprocal food sharing and, 90-92
    time spent in activity, 88
Socioeconomic class, human depredation by vampires and, 69, 101
Solitary bats
    prevalence of rabies in, 142-143, 146
    sampling studies of, 139-141
    unprovoked attacks by, 133, 152-153
Soucouyant, in Trinidad folklore, 57
Sound, hyperesthesia to, 226
South Africa, rabies-related viruses and, 266, 268
Soviet Union
    antigenic characterization of bat rabies in, 288, 290
    bat rabies in, 270, 275
    human rabies of bat origin in, 239-240, 288, 290-291
Spain, bat rabies in, 275, 277
Spelunkers, see Cave exploration
Squirrel rabies, of bat origin, 208
St. Ann's Savannah, Trinidad, 44
Steroid hormones, feeding of vampire bats and, 65
Straw-colored fruit bat
    Lagos bat virus and, 264-265
    rabies-neutralizing antibody in, 158
Street Alabama Dufferin, see SAD strain
Street virus, 5
Strychnine, use in vampire-bat control, 115-116
Supernatural, see Jumbie, Soucouyant
Suriname, human deaths due to vampire-bat rabies in, 105-106
Surveillance studies
    of bovine paralytic rabies, 86
    diagnostic laboratories and, 140, 146, 208-209, 212-213, 217-218, 304
    of human rabies, 109
    International Animal Health Code and, 3, 286-287
    limitations of, 105, 143, 217-218
    of post-exposure rabies prophylaxis, 218-219
Switzerland, bat rabies in, 275, 277, 289
Sylvatic rabies, 131
Synanthropic pests, see Bat infestation

T

Tacaribe virus, 84, 154
Tadarida brasiliensis, see Mexican free-tailed bat
Taiga, bat rabies in, 289
Tamana bat virus, 84, 154
Teeth of vampire bats, see Dentition
Tennessee, caves and fox rabies in, 181-183
Terrestrial rabies, of bat origin, 132-133, 181-185, 193-203
Thailand, bat rabies in, 290
Thegosis, 71
Thermal sense, of vampire bats, 67, 69
Thermoregulation, of vampire bats, 61
Timbering activity, human depredation by vampires and, 108
Tobago, 44-45
Topical treatment
  of bite wounds, 29, 32, 308
  of cattle with anticoagulants, 118-121
  of vampire bats with anticoagulants, 118-121
Torpor, rabies pathogenesis and, 157
Torres Strait, survey for bat rabies in, 139
Toxicants, use in bat infestations, 245-247
T-PA, 75
Translocation of rabid animals, 16, 18-19
Transmammary transmission, 7, 93
Transmission of virus
  bite wounds, 6, 303, 314-315
  continuity of, 9-10
  human-to-human, 234
  mechanical, 303
  nonbite modes of, 6-7, 93, 169-174, 180-181, 303
Transplacental transmission, 7, 93, 167
Trap-vaccinate-release programs, 251
Trinidad
  bovine paralytic rabies in, 44-47, 86-87, 89
  canine rabies and, 47
  human deaths due to vampire-bat rabies in, 45, 101-102, 105-106
  quarantine program of, 47
Tumbi baba, see Bovine paralytic rabies
Turkey, bat rabies in, 275, 277, 290

U

Ukraine
  bat rabies in, 289
  human rabies of bat origin in, 240, 289-290
United Kingdom, bat rabies in, 278, 285, 304
United States
  animal bites, incidence of, 3, 21
  bat rabies in, 131-147
  compartmentalization of rabies and, 147, 189-190
  epidemiologic surveillance in, 139-146, 218-219
  human deaths due to bat rabies in, 229-240
  prevalence of bat rabies in, 139-147, 306
  sylvatic rabies in, 131
  urban rabies in, 14, 16, 19, 131
Unprovoked attacks
  by insectivorous bats, 133, 152-153, 303
  by vampire bats, 51
Urban rabies
  in developing nations, 131
  in industrialized nations, 14, 16, 19, 131
Urination, see Diuresis
Urine, as olfactory attractant for vampires, 66, 76
U.S.S.R., see Soviet Union

V

Vaccination, see Immunization
Vaccination failure, 315
Vaccine baits, efficacy in target species, 254-255
Vaccine delivery systems, 252
Vaccine strains of virus, 293
Vaccines
  attenuated (modified live), 112, 185, 251-252
  genetically engineered, 123, 252-255
  killed, 112, 251
  use of, see Post-exposure rabies prophlyaxis
Vaccinia virus, 252-254
Vampir, 57
Vampire bat
  agility of, 59-60
  anatomic characteristics of, 59
  anticoagulants in control of, 86, 116-123
  anticoagulants in saliva of, 73-75
  appetite of, 41, 72, 75
  as asymptomatic carriers of rabies, 83-84
  audition of, 66-67
  bite wounds from, 71, 101
  blood lapping by, 72-73
  cohabitation with insectivorous bats, 163-166
  colony structure of, 88, 90, 97
  dental formula of, 71
  detection of hosts by, 65-67
  dietary preferences of, 59, 62, 64, 66-67
  duration of feeding, 72
  economic importance of, 47, 85-87, 89
  energetics of, 60-61
  failure to feed, 62, 92
  feces of, 59-60
  feeding habits of, 61, 64, 66-67, 93-94, 97
  flight of, 75
  food sharing in, 90-92
  foraging flights of, 76
  fossil remains of, 62-63
  gestation period of, 113
  group associations of, 88, 90, 97
  hairy-legged, 58, 60-62, 66-67, 77
  host selection by, 62-65
  human deaths due to, 45, 101-109
  human depredation by, 101-109
  human vampires, 58
  hunting characteristics of, 62
  immunization against rabies, 123, 255
  importation of, 163
  interspecific aggression and, 163
  intraspecific aggression and, 93-94
  jungle rabies cycles and, 103-109

juvenile development of, 90
livestock and, see Bovine paralytic rabies
livestock losses due to, 85-87, 89
locomotion of, 59-60
longevity of, 59
moonlight, in relation to feeding of, 62
olfaction in, 65-66, 76
outbreaks of rabies in, 94-97
plasminogen activators of, 74-75
pleistocene deposits of, 62-63
population control of, 113-124
population density of, 41
prevalence of rabies infection in, 54, 95-97
protection of humans against, 101, 108-109, 111
protection of livestock against, 105, 111-124
quarantine programs and, 4, 7
rabies in, see Rabies in hematophagous bats
rabies-neutralizing antibody in, 95-96, 158
range of, 60-61, 63
reciprocal altruism in, 90-92
regurgitation of blood by, 90-92
reproduction of, 113
as reservoirs of rabies, see Rabies in hematophagous bats
roosts of, 41, 59, 76, 97, 111
sequential feeding from a wound by, 93-94
size of, 59
social grooming in, 88
social organization of, 62, 90, 97
taxonomy of, 58
temperature requirements of, 59-61
territorial aggression in, 62, 93-94
thermoperception in, 67, 69
thermoregulation in, 61
thumbs of, 59
in the United States, 48
urination of, 66, 76
vampire pool, 59-60
as vectors of rabies, 47-48, 85
walking of, 59-60
water consumption of, 76-77
weight of, 59
white-winged, 58-62, 66-67, 74, 94
wingspan of, 59
Vampire-bat bite
blood loss following, 41, 72-74, 85
color of host and, 69
depth of, 71
distribution on animal hosts, 67-70
of humans, 64, 69, 101-107
impairment of function by, 68
reaction of hosts to, 69, 72, 101
reopening of old wounds and, 71, 93, 97, 119
types of, 71
Vampire-bat rabies, see Rabies in hematophagous bats
Vampire ghosts, 57
Vampire pool, 59-60
Vampirism, 58
Variants, of rabies virus
antigenic characterization of isolates, 5-6, 16, 94, 104, 107, 163-166, 189-203, 209, 211-212, 267, 280-284
genetic analysis of, 284-286
nonterrestrial, 190-193, 209, 211-212
terrestrial, 190
Vector competence, 85, 132, 180, 314-315
Venezuela
bovine paralytic rabies in, 91
human deaths due to vampire-bat rabies in, 105-106
Vertical transmission, 167, 255
Vesiculovirus, 263
Vespertillio murinus, 279, 289-290
Vespertillio nilssonii, 279, 289
Viral transmission studies
forced bite, 179-180
ingestion, 158, 180-181
inoculation, 179
Virus fixé, see Fixed virus
Virus rué, see Street virus
Volin, bat rabies in, 289
Voroshilovgrad, human rabies of bat origin in, 240, 289-290
V-RG, see Vaccinia virus

W

Warfarin, use in vampire control, 117-119
Water consumption, of vampire bats, 76
West Germany, bat rabies in, 275-276
White-toothed shrew, Mokola virus and, 264, 266
White-winged vampire bat
dental formula of, 71
dietary preferences of, 62, 66-67
distribution of, 61
as reservoir of rabies, 58
Wildlife
as pets, 226
rabies in, 13-19
Wildlife and Countryside Act, 279, 304
Wildlife rabies
management by population control, 251, 256, 291
oral immunization and, 185, 251-255
sampling biases and, 139-140, 142
as source of infection for domestic animals, 19, 22
trap-vaccinate-release programs, 251
Wound treatment
of cattle exposed to vampire bats, 118-120
of humans exposed to rabies, 29, 32, 308

X, Y, Z

Yakutia, bat rabies in, 289
Yugoslavia, bat rabies in, 275, 277
Yuli virus, 270, 284, 289-290
Yuma bat, 207
Zimbabwe, rabies-related viruses and, 266, 268-270

Jacket Photo Credits:
Fishing Bat (front): Stephen Dalton, © Photo Researchers.
Vampire Bat (back): Bruce Dale, © National Geographic Society.